ELECTRODIAGNOSIS IN CLINICAL NEUROLOGY

Michael J. Aminoff, B.Sc., M.D., M.R.C.P. (Lond.)

Associate Professor of Neurology
School of Medicine
University of California, San Francisco
San Francisco, California

With 21 Contributors

Churchill Livingstone

New York, Edinburgh and London   1980

Distributed in the United Kingdom by Churchill Livingstone,
Robert Stevenson House. 1-3 Baxter's Place. Leith Walk,
Edinburgh EH1 3AF and by associated companies, branches
and representatives throughout the world.

First published 1980
Printed in U.S.A.

ISBN 0-443-08021-6

7   6   5   4   3   2   1

Library of Congress Cataloging in Publication Data
Main entry under title:

Electrodiagnosis in clinical neurology.

    Bibliography: p.
    Includes index.
    1.   Electrodiagnosis.   2.   Nervous system—
Diseases—Diagnosis.   I.   Aminoff, Michael Jeffrey.
[DNLM: 1. Electrodiagnosis. 2. Nervous system
diseases—Diagnosis.   WL141.3 A517e]
RC349.E53E43   616.8'04'754   79-23579
ISBN 0-443-08021-6

Contributors

Michael J. Aminoff, B.Sc., M.D., M.R.C.P. (Lond.)
Associate Professor of Neurology
School of Medicine
University of California, San Francisco
San Francisco, California

John C. Armington, Ph.D.
Professor of Psychology
Northeastern University
Boston, Massachusetts

Mary A. B. Brazier, B.Sc., Ph.D. (Lond.)
Professor of Anatomy
School of Medicine
University of California, Los Angeles
Los Angeles, California

Gian Emilio Chatrian, M.D.
Professor and Head
Division of EEG and Clinical Neurophysiology
University Hospital
University of Washington School of Medicine
Seattle, Washington

Jasper R. Daube, M.D.
Associate Professor of Neurology
Mayo Medical School
Consultant in Neurology and Electromyography
The Mayo Clinic
Rochester, Minnesota

Alan S. Gevins
Director, EEG Systems Laboratory
Langley Porter Institute
School of Medicine
University of California, San Francisco
San Francisco, California

Denis R. Giblin, M.D.
Associate Professor of Neurology
Albert Einstein College of Medicine
Bronx, New York

J. A. R. Lenman, M.B., Ch.B., F.R.C.P. (Ed.)
Reader in Neurology
University of Dundee
Dundee
Scotland

C. Ajmone Marsan, M.D.
Director
EEG Laboratory
Jackson Memorial Hospital
University of Miami School of Medicine
Miami, Florida

W. B. Matthews, D.M., F.R.C.P.
Professor of Clinical Neurology
University of Oxford
Oxford, England

Peter A. McGregor
Chief Technologist
Sleep-Wake Disorders Center
Montefiore Hospital and Medical Center
New York, New York

Charles P. Pollak, M.D.
Assistant Professor of Neurology
Co-Director, Sleep-Wake Disorders Center
Montefiore Hospital and Medical Center
New York, New York
Assistant Professor of Neurology
Albert Einstein College of Medicine
Bronx, New York

Robert A. Schindler, M.D.
Assistant Professor of Otolaryngology
Director of Vestibular Testing Unit
School of Medicine
University of California, San Francisco
San Francisco, California

Bhagwan T. Shahani, M.D., D.Phil.
Assistant Professor of Neurology
Harvard Medical School
Assistant Neurologist and Director
of the Electromyography and
Movement Disorders Laboratory
Massachusetts General Hospital
Boston, Massachusetts

Frank W. Sharbrough, M.D.
Associate Professor of Neurology
Mayo Medical School
Consultant in Neurology and Electroencephalography
The Mayo Clinic
Rochester, Minnesota

Samuel Sokol, M.D.
Associate Professor of Ophthalmology
Tufts University School of Medicine
Boston, Massachusetts

James J. Stockard, M.D.
Department of Neurology
Section of Electroencephalography
The Mayo Clinic
Rochester, Minnesota

Janet E. Stockard, B.A.
Section of Electroencephalography
The Mayo Clinic
Rochester, Minnesota

Bary R. Tharp, M.D.
Associate Professor of Neurology
Stanford University
School of Medicine
Stanford, California

Vivian Weigel, B.S.
Vestibular Testing Unit
Medical Center
University of California, San Francisco
San Francisco, California

Elliot Weitzman, M.D.
Professor and Chairman
Department of Neurology
Director, Sleep-Wake Disorders
Center
Montefiore Hospital and Medical
Center
New York, New York

Robert R. Young, M.D.
Associate Professor of Neurology
Harvard Medical School
Associate Neurologist and Director
of the Clinical Neurophysiology
Laboratory and Movement Disorders Clinic
Massachusetts General Hospital
Boston, Massachusetts

Preface

Fifty years have passed since Hans Berger's first paper on the human electroencephalogram. Over this time, electroencephalography has evolved into an investigative technique of undoubted practical value, and technologic advances have permitted the development of a number of new electrophysiologic approaches to neurologic diagnosis. These developments have led to certain difficulties for clinicians and neurophysiologists alike. On the one hand, the present-day physician is tempted to avail himself of investigative procedures that he does not entirely understand and that provide him with information which he is often unable to interpret. On the other hand, the neurophysiologist is commonly faced with clinical problems that he fails to appreciate or to which there is no ready solution by the means at his disposal. There is therefore a need for a conveniently sized monograph that provides a general introduction to the role of electrodiagnosis in neurology and is directed at the clinical relevance of the investigative procedures that are now within the province of the electrophysiologist. In preparing the present volume, it has therefore been my aim, and that of the other contributors, to provide in simple terms a comprehensive but concise account of the clinical application of various electrophysiologic methods of investigating the function of the central and peripheral nervous systems. Some of these methods, such as electroencephalography and electromyography, are admirably covered in encyclopedic detail in certain textbooks aimed at specialists or trainees in these fields. The chapters covering these topics in the present volume are in no way intended to take the place of such works; rather, they are directed at those who need to know the principles, uses and limitations of the methods, and who have to relate the information derived from such studies to the clinical context of individual cases. Certain quantitative aspects of these subjects have also been considered, however, because of their potential clinical utility. A number of the other electrophysiologic methods that are covered in this book—such as the various evoked potential techniques—have been developed comparatively recently, and their clinical applications are as yet incompletely defined. In view of the obvious interest, shown by increasing numbers of clinicians and neurophysiologists, in setting-up facilities to undertake such studies for clinical purposes, the technical aspects of some of these subjects have been reviewed in somewhat greater detail, although the emphasis has remained on the practical relevance of the methods. Electrophysiologic techniques that are of more limited clinical utility at the present time, such as recording of the contingent negative variation, have deliberately not been considered.

I am greatly indebted to the various contributors to this book, all of whom have taken much time and trouble to survey developments in their own particular fields of interest. I am grateful also to those authors, editors and publishers who have allowed us to reproduce illustrations previously published elsewhere, and whose permission is acknowledged in the text. The advice and understanding that I received from Ms. Carole Baker and Mr. Bill Schmitt of Churchill Livingstone, the publishers, are greatly appreciated. Finally, it is a pleasure to acknowledge the help, encouragement and support that my wife, Jan, gave me during all stages of the preparation of this book.

M. J. Aminoff

Contents

1

The Emergence of Electrophysiology as an Aid to Neurology

MARY A. B. BRAZIER

INTRODUCTION

From the time of the ancients to well into the eighteenth century, electricity was regarded as a strange invisible power. It was differentiated from magnetism in 1600 by Gilbert, but its nature remained a mystery. Gradually the role of electricity in relation to the nervous system was to emerge, first from observation of the effect of applying it to the body, and eventually from the discovery that both muscle and nerve could themselves be sources of this power. The first of these—observation of its application—had had to wait for the technical development of instruments to deliver electricity; the second, for the more delicate instrumentation necessary for detection of the fine currents of nerve. The first became the ancestor of electrotherapy, the second of electrical diagnosis.

ELECTROTHERAPY

The experimenters of the eighteenth century inherited from Robert Boyle (1673, 1675) a description of electric attraction as "a Material Effluvium, issuing from and returning to, the Electrical Body." This concept, when applied to the nervous system, retained a flavor of Galenism's nervous fluids and the vis nervosa of Haller (1757–65), and permeates nearly all the writings of the experimenters in this field until vitalism finally gave way to materialism.

Working at first only with frictional machines as a source of electricity, experimenters in the early eighteenth century played with many demonstrations of its strange action at a distance. This was a period when interest in electricity was so keen that it was invoked to explain many natural phenomena, not only of animals but also of plants. According to Fée (1832), Elizabeth, the daughter of the great Linnaeus, noticed that at twilight in her father's garden near Uppsala some of the orange-colored flowers, such as marigolds and firelilies, appeared to give off flashes of light. (It was Goethe, 1810, who showed this to be a retinal contrast effect and not an electrical flash.) But those who speculated about animals and man felt they were on surer ground. Did not the cat's fur crackle when you rubbed it, and had not Theodoric, the Visigoth, thrown off sparks as he marched?

In the early part of the century it had been discovered empirically that the human body could be charged electrostatically, provided it were insulated. At first it was thought that a layer of air had to be present between the subject and the ground, for the characteristics of conductors and nonconductors were only beginning to be understood. Stephen Gray (who died in 1736) had discovered (1731) that the distribution of electric charges varied with the insulating or conducting properties of the material employed, and he had reported these findings in a series of letters to the Royal Society. These terms were not used at the time, nor was induction understood (which he had demonstrated and called "Electrical Attraction at a Distance"). He wrote of "Electrick Virtue" and said that his experiments showed that animals "receive Electrick Effluvia." His teacher, Desaguliers (1742), demonstrator for Newton, clarified the distinction between conductors and nonconductors, showing them to be essentially the "non-electrics" of Gilbert (1600) that conveyed electricity away, and the "electrics" that could be charged.

In many countries the phenomenon by which the human body could carry a charge was exploited for entertainment. Outstanding examples were the Abbé Nollet (1746) at the Court of Louis XVth, Winkler (1744), Hausen (1743) at Leipzig, Du Fay (1735) in Paris, and Kratzenstein in Halle (Fig. 1.1). Many delightful illustrations survive.

The next step was the discovery that application of electricity to muscles, even those of the dead, could evoke a contraction. Inevitably this led to the exploitation of this effect as a therapy in spite of a complete lack of understanding of its modus operandi. Some attempts were deliberate hoaxes, but the physicians at the center at Montpellier, for example, were true believers.

Also among believers was a young physician named Kratzenstein, who was raised in the unlikely atmosphere of the Stahlian school in Halle, but was greatly influenced by his teacher Gottlob Krüger (1745). Krüger, beginning to draw away from the influence of Georg Ernst Stahl (who taught that the soul was the vital force that caused muscles to contract) had experimented widely with the electrification of animals and encouraged his pupil to engage in electrotherapeutic studies. These were first printed in 1744 in the form of letters entitled "Abhandlung von dem Rutzen der Electricität in der Arznenurssenschaft."

Still using frictional electricity and noting from experiments on himself that electrification of his body caused him to sweat (the "effluvium" of Boyle?), Kratzenstein advanced the hypothesis that this loss of salt-containing fluid could have beneficial medicinal effects. No doubt this proposal stemmed from the age-old concept that bloodletting had therapeutic value.

The cures he claimed consisted of two cases in which there was restoration of movement in contracted fingers. He also noted the induction of sound sleep, forerunner of that observed in electrosleep. As the news spread around

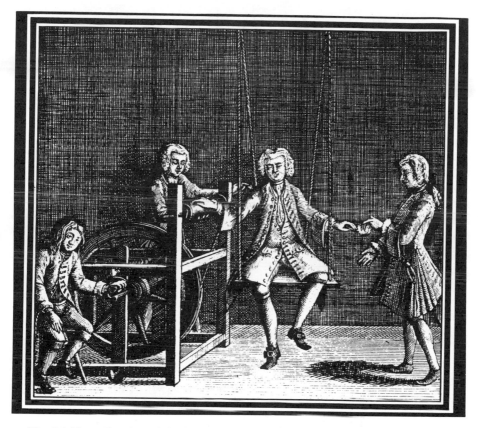

Fig. 1.1 *Electrification of the human body by frictional electricity (from Krüger, J. C. 1745. Zuschrift, 2nd edition. Hemmerde, Halle).*

Europe, attempts at cures were made in many centers. These were at first mostly in cases of paralysis. The fact that contraction of a muscle could be obtained at the moment of direct stimulation yet could not be maintained as a cure, failed of its correct interpretation, for the role of innervation was not yet understood.

The rare cases of success anteceded the understanding of hysterical paralysis and encouraged the establishment of many centers for the treatment of paralytic conditions, among the most famous being the school of Montpellier under the leadership of Boissier de la Croix de Sauvages. One of de Sauvage's pupils, Deshais, published a thesis (1749) boldly entitled "De Hemiplegia per Electricitatem Curanda" which showed his thinking to be creeping towards the recognition of the role of the nerve supply, though this was still versed in Galenist terms. Deshais wrote. "paralysis is caused by the arrest of nervous fluid destined to circulate in the brain because it meets an insuperable resistance in the nerve fibres. Thus we must increase the pressure of the nervous fluid when hemiplegia resists ordinary remedies." He added that hemiplegia could be cured or, at any rate, improved by electrification. (Fig. 1.2).

At this time electricity and its effects on the human body were a favorite

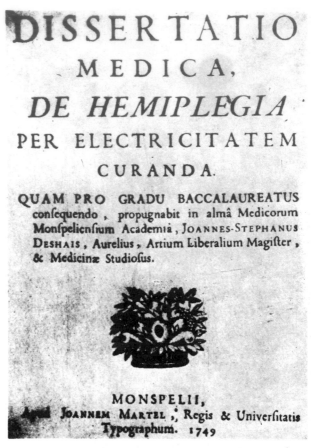

Fig. 1.2. *Title page of the doctoral thesis of J. C. Deshais on the cure of hemiplegia by electricity (by courtesy of the University of Montpellier).*

subject for theses. In the collection of unpublished manuscripts (1750–1760) by Jacques de Romas that is preserved in the City Archives of Bordeaux, there is one on electricity that includes observations on electrification of two paralytic patients. Another example is found in the thesis collection at the University of Montpellier, written in 1750 by Jean Thecla Dufay, who restricts himself to the electrical nature of the nervous fluid and does not discuss therapy. His thesis does, however, give a useful review of the experiments and knowledge of his time. He concludes his account boldly: "Ergo Fluidum nerveum est Fluidum electricum." Montpellier was at that time a center of great interest in electricity, and it was here that Boissier de Sauvages endowed a convent hospital solely for electrical therapy (1740–1760). In 1748 de Sauvages had himself received a prize from the Académie Royale des Sciences at Toulouse for a dissertation on hydrophobia and this was published in 1758. In this, in what he termed a "Digression sur l'électricité," he championed the existence of animal electricity and evolved a bizarre hypothesis about nerve and muscle activity in hydrophobia. This went as follows: given that muscular movement is proportional to the force of the nervous fluid, the venom of rabies, on mixing with it, doubles the velocity and also doubles the density of the nervous fluid—hence the nerve force and the resultant muscular movement are eight times stronger than normal. By this tortuous piece of arithmetic de Sauvages explained the violent muscular spasms in hydrophobia.

Academies were generous with prizes on medical uses of electricity, which no doubt accounts in part for the plethora of such theses at this time. Another winner was Jean Paul Marat (1784) who was to meet such a violent death in the French Revolution. His essay won the prize of the Paris Academy but drew the rebuke that his criticisms of other workers were too forcefully expressed. Many absurd claims for electrotherapy were made by physicians, and at their doors must be laid the blame for much subsequent quackery. A contemporary critic ridiculed these claims but published only anonymously. However, his gay and witty touch betrayed his identity to Nollet (1749) as that of another gentleman of the Church, the Abbé Mangin (1752). Nollet, who had himself gathered acclaim through his use of electrotherapy (though he had also done his bit to expose the quacks) scolded Mangin "d'avoir confondu les temps, les lieux, les personnes et les choses."

A more efficient source of electricity was to come to the aid of electrotherapists, though a natural one had, in fact, been used for some years, namely, the shock delivered by the marine torpedo. On being applied to the soles of the feet, this was said to relieve the pain of gout. The rationale for the treatment, however, received no elucidation from the great surgeon, John Hunter (1773) whose exquisite dissections revealed the anatomy of these electric fish, for he thought that "the will of the animal does absolutely controul the electric powers of its body." The reflex nature of the discharge was not established until the serial experiments of Matteucci and Pavi (1843–1844).

By the middle of the eighteenth century eager electrotherapists were no longer dependent on the frictional machines for producing electricity, for in 1745 van Musschenbroek, Professor of Physics at Leyden, almost by chance invented a device to store electricity and discharge it as a shock. This, the ancestor of the condenser, was the Leyden jar.

Van Musschenbroek (1746), striving to conserve electricity in a conductor and to delay the loss of its charge in air, attempted to use charged water as the conductor, insulating it from air in a nonconducting glass jar. However, when he charged the water through a wire leading from a frictional electrical machine, he found the electricity dissipated as quickly as ever. An assistant who was present while holding the jar containing charged water, accidently touched the inserted wire with his other hand and got a frightening shock. With one hand he had formed one "plate," the charged water being the other "plate," and the glass jar the intervening dielectric. A condenser was born. Experimental electricity had, in fact, reached the stage when such a development was due, for a similar discovery was made by the Dean of the Cathedral of Kamin in Pomerania whose followers gave the jar his name "Kleiste Flasche."

One of the many to espouse this new electrifying technique was the Abbé

Bertholon (1780) who travelled widely in Europe bringing back reports of strange cures of diseases that others could not replicate. He was not alone in the variety of claims he made, for this form of "therapy" had spread widely through Europe. So diverse were the diseases for which cures were being claimed that Academies in several countries offered prizes, including the Académie at Lyon which offered in 1777 a prize for the answer to the questions, "Quelles sont les maladies qui dépendent de la plus ou moins de grande quantité de fluide électrique dans le corps humain, et quels sont les moyens de remédier aux unes et aux autres?" This was a spur to many, including Bertholon (1780) who, in his two volumes on the electricity of the human body in health and disease, claimed to examine his cases as to whether electrification was the only ameliorator of the patient's condition or an additive to other therapies. A great believer in a "latent electricity" within the body, he held that it was manipulation of this inherent electricity that formed the basis of the cures he claimed. This concept was a rewording of "animal spirits" and in no way did he foresee the intrinsic electricity of nerve and muscle found (but little understood) by Galvani (1791).

We owe the next step in the invention of sources of electricity to the controversy that developed with Volta (1800) over the explanation of Galvani's results; the voltaic pile which soon replaced the Leyden jar in the hands of those espousing electrotherapy was the ancestor of the batteries of today. By the turn of the century, books were beginning to appear on the history of medical electricity—for example, by Vivenzio in 1784 and Sue in 1802.

The early ventures in applying electricity to patients with various diseases were gradually to be sorted out and achieve a rational basis thanks to the development of knowledge of basic neurophysiology with its elucidation of the relationship of nerve to muscle, of spinal cord to nerve, and of brain to all.

One method, however, for which great claims were made as a treatment has not, even today, reached the first stage of scientific rationale. This is electroconvulsive shock.

Many early experimenters, Fontana (1760) and Caldani (1784) for example, had noted the convulsions of their frogs when electricity was applied to their brains, though Galvani (1791) attempted this without success. ("Si enim conductores non dissectae spinale medullae, aut nervis, ut consuevimus, sed vel cerebro—contractiones vel nullae, vel admodum exiguae sunt.") In the first decade of the nineteenth century, his nephew Aldini was to experiment with electroshock in man (1804). Impressed by the muscular contractions he obtained on stimulating animals and cadavers, he stood close to the guillotine to receive heads of criminals in as fresh condition as possible and found that passing the current, either through ear and mouth or through exposed brain and mouth, evoked facial grimaces. The fresher the head the more remarkable the grimace. He then proceeded to apply electrical stimulation from a voltaic pile to the living. His concept was that the contractions were excited by "le developpement d'un fluide dans la machine animale" and this he held to be conveyed by the nerves to the muscles. We recognize here the explanation popularized by Bertholon (1780).

One set of these early experiments on man reaches into the twentieth century, for Aldini applied his galvanism to the mentally ill (Fig. 1.3). Having experimented on himself with electrodes in both ears or in one ear and his mouth, or on forehead and nose, he experienced a strong reaction (''une forte action''), followed by prolonged insomnia lasting several days. He found the experience very disagreeable but thought the changes it produced in the brain might be salutary in the psychoses (''la folie''). Passing the current between the ears produced violent convulsions and pain, but he claimed good results in patients suffering from melancholia.

Aldini had no instrument to tell him the amount of current passed (he recorded only the number of copper and zinc discs in the voltaic pile). In the twentieth-century adaptation of this technique (although it is current and not voltage that stimulates) we are also not told by the originator what current flowed between electrodes placed bilaterally on the frontoparietal regions, only the voltage. ''I decided to start cautiously with a low-intensity current of 80 volts for 1.5 seconds . . . The electrodes were applied again and a 110-volt discharge was applied for 1.5 seconds'' (Cerletti, 1954). We are not surprised to be told of the resultant convulsion, apnoea and cyanosis.

This report related the results of the first experiments made by Cerletti in 1932 but even now, 47 years later, no rationale has been found for the salutary effects claimed by the users, and one is reminded again of Aldini's concept of a

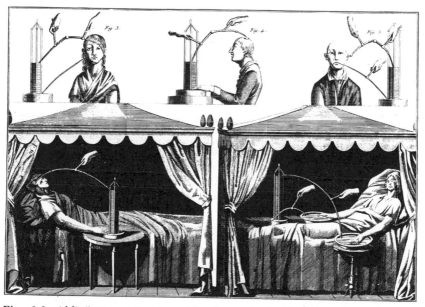

Fig. 1.3. *Aldini's experiments with electroshock 'therapy' in man. Above: mental patients with the electrodes in various positions connecting to voltaic piles for stimulation. Below: two recently dead patients connected directly, or by saline baths to voltaic piles (from Aldini, G. 1804. Essai Theorique et Expérimental sur le Galvanisme. Fournier, Paris).*

rearrangement of functions in the brain such as take place from a hit on the head—"Une chute, un coup violent porté sur la tête, ont souvent produit des altérations très sensibles dans les facultés intellectuelles."

In the years following Aldini's application of electricity to man, a revival of electrotherapy resulted from the work of Duchenne (1855, 1867) who stimulated paralyzed muscles, at first through punctures of the skin but later percutaneously. Although considerable controversy arose from his work he had, in fact, a greater understanding of electric currents than his predecessors, and by careful exploration he found the motor points for the muscles he was stimulating. From his work grew some understanding of the anatomy underlying the induced contractions of muscles, and in 1868 he published a small book on muscular paralysis in which he illustrated the muscle-fiber abnormalities he found by light microscopy. It may be said that it was Duchenne who built the bridge between electrotherapy and electrodiagnosis, leaving his name to Duchenne dystrophy.

A less controversial ancestor of modern electrical techniques (the cardiac stimulator) is found in a report given to the Accademia di Torino in 1803 in which the hearts of three decapitated felons were found to retain excitability long after the voluntary muscles ceased to respond to galvanic stimulation. The reporters were Vassalli, Giulio, and Rossi (1803).

Before the turn of the century, stimulation of the heart by alternating currents was being used in France for resuscitation by Prévost and Batelli (1899) and developed into a standard procedure in the century following this review.

ELECTRODIAGNOSIS

The several forms of electrodiagnosis used in neurology have much shorter histories than electrotherapy for they have their basis in fundamental neurophysiology rather than quasi-quackery. They include electroencephalography (EEG), electromyography (EMG), cerebral and spinal potentials evoked by sensory stimulation (EPs), the recording of the action potentials of nerve, the electroretinogram, and the contingent negative variation (CNV). Of these, the electroretinogram has had little exploration in clinical work and the CNV up to this time has proved of more interest to the psychologist than the neurologist.

In the period under review, only the EEG, the EMG, the action potential of nerve, and the evoked cortical potential have a history, a history which, however, they largely share and all stemming essentially from the discoveries of Galvani.

The epoch-making researches of Galvani have been described so many times that they are well-known to all who work in electrophysiology. Best known is his Commentarius (1791) in which he first made public his claims for intrinsic animal electricity, but this was only the culmination of years of experimentation about which he has left copious notes, now in the Archives of the University of Bologna.

These laboratory notes, written in the vernacular and plentifully illustrated by his own sketches, often including himself, begin in 1780 (Fig. 1.4). Retaining still the analogy of an electric fluid, Galvani declared his goal in the title of his notes: "Dell'azione del fluido elettrico applicato a' nervi in varie maniere."

The three chief observations that stand out from the many experiments which Galvani included in 1791 in his published Commentarius were (a) that a frog's nerve preparation, although at a distance from a sparking electrostatic machine, would twitch when touched by an observer; (b) that the atmospheric electricity of a thunderstorm could be used to stimulate frogs' legs if a long wire were stretched across the roof (the principle of the lightning conductor); and (c) that frogs' legs twitched when hung by hooks from the railing of his house even in the absence of a thunderstorm. Galvani interpreted this as evidence that the muscle contraction was caused by electricity originating in the animal tissues themselves.

It was this last experiment (Fig. 1.5) that raised the most controversy and was eventually attacked by Volta (1800) and explained as merely the current that flows between dissimilar metals. In fact, in spite of the title of Volta's famous letter (1800), two dissimilar metals are not enough to cause a current to flow. They need to be separated by an electrolyte. In Galvani's case the metals were the brass of the hooks and the iron of the railings with the frog providing the electrolyte. Volta's insistence on the metallic origin of all of the electricity

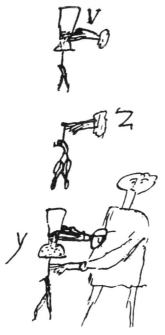

Fig. 1.4. Galvani's sketch of himself experimenting on a frog nerve-muscle preparation which he likened to a Leiden jar (from notes made December 10, 1781, preserved in the Archives of the University of Bologna).

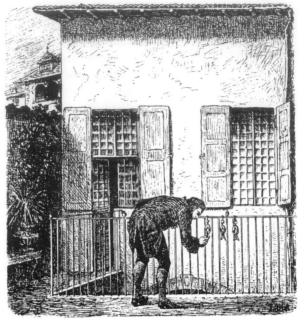

Casa Galvani Settembre 1786.

Fig. 1.5. *Drawing that Du Bois-Reymond had made by an artist from his own original sketch. This shows Galvani hanging up frogs' legs on the railings of his house in the Strada San Felice in Bologna (from Reden von Emil Du Bois-Reymond. 1887. vol. 2, Leipzig).*

in all Galvani's experiments on frogs caused him, and more especially his eager but less prudent nephew Aldini (1794), to press on to experiments omitting the dissimilar metals. Finally, an experiment was evolved and published anonymously in 1794 (but quite certainly the work of Galvani) in which no external source of electricity was present. A twitch was demonstrated in a frog's nerve-muscle preparation when the cut end of another nerve was placed on the muscle. In this case the source of the electricity was what we now recognize as the current of injury from the cut nerve, or demarcation potential as it came to be called (Fig. 1.6).

It seems strange in the light of history that this challenge based on bimetallic electricity was the one to throw the greatest doubt on Galvani's claim of intrinsic animal electricity, for he had himself, in 1786, made intensive tests of touching the frog (on a metal hook) with a second metal—gold, silver, tin, and lead—and his notes recorded on September 20 of that year make it clear that he was fully familiar with this metallic source. In fact, he described experiments with dissimilar metals in his Commentarius but failed to interpret them correctly.

Von Humboldt (1797) is the first great name in support of Galvani for he recognized that both protagonists had made discoveries of real phenomena and that Volta's brilliant development of the current flow between dissimilar metals

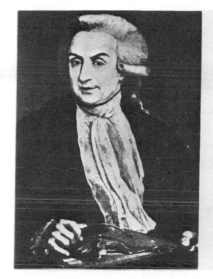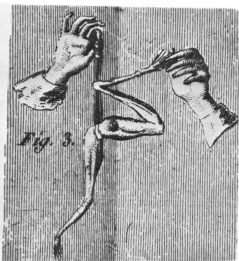

Fig. 1.6. Portrait of Galvani from the oil-painting in the library of the University of Bologna (courtesy of the late Dr. Giulio Pupilli) and his experiment on muscle contraction in the absence of all metals (from Aldini, G. 1804. Essai sur le Galvanisme. 2 vols. Paris).

did not preclude the existence of animal electricity. Not only did Humboldt expose the erroneous parts of Galvani's and Volta's interpretations but also those of the writers who had rushed in so precipitously to take up arms for one or the other protagonist—Pfaff (1798), Fowler (1793), Valli (1793), Schmück (1792)—each received his rebuke.

The next step, once the skeptics had been persuaded that nerve-muscle preparations could emit electricity, was to establish that this phenomenon was not dependent on injury. The clear proof of demarcation currents we owe to Matteucci, Professor of Physics in Pisa, who established in 1842 (publishing his findings in 1843 and 1844) that a current flowed from an injured point in a muscle to its uncut surface. By this time, thanks to the invention by Oersted (1820) in Copenhagen, galvanometers had come to the aid of the electrophysiologist and Matteucci could determine not only the presence of a current but also its direction. Matteucci became convinced (but did not prove) that in an uninjured limb a current normally flowed from the tendon to the belly and this he called the "muscle current," but he doubted the electricity of nerve.

The main center of research on this problem moved from Italy to Berlin where Hermann (1884) and Du Bois-Reymond (1848 and 1849), with their superior instrumentation, were able to differentiate currents of injury from normal electrical potentials recorded from the surface of a muscle on contraction. With Du Bois-Reymond's demonstration of this in man, electromyography was born (Fig. 1.7).

But the kind of electricity that Galvani was searching for was the "fluido elettrico," what we now call transmission—namely, the transmission of the

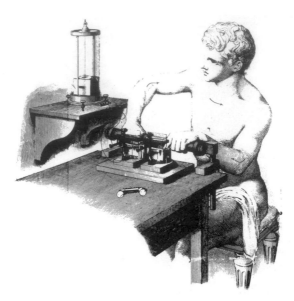

Fig. 1.7. Du Bois-Reymond's experiment on muscle currents in man. The two fingers of the subject were plunged into cups of saline. On contraction of the right arm muscles a difference of potential developed which, through wires to the solenoid, produced a deflection of the needle (from Du Bois-Reymond, E. 1849. Untersuchungen über thierische Electricität. Reimer, Berlin. Vol. 1, 1848; vol. 2, 1849).

nerve impulse that exerts control of muscle movement by the nervous system. In this concept Galvani was unquestionably correct though it was another 50 years before the electrical nature of the nerve impulse was indubitably demonstrated by Du Bois-Reymond (1848, 1849). Improving on Oersted's invention of passing a current through a single coil of wire to deflect the needle, Du Bois-Reymond increased the number of coils to 2,500 and, thereby, provided himself with an induction coil sufficiently sensitive to detect the change in potential when an impulse passed down a nerve trunk. This he detected as a "negative variation" in the demarcation potential that his predecessors had described. It was what we now know as the action potential of nerve and is the basis of electroneuronography. When in 1850 Helmholtz designed an instrument for measuring the conduction velocity of nerve, he opened the way for the modern neurologists' detection of demyelinating diseases.

Du Bois-Reymond did not underestimate the importance of his discovery. He wrote:

> If I do not greatly deceive myself, I have succeeded in realizing in full actuality (albeit under a slightly different aspect) the hundred years' dream of physicists and physiologists to wit, the identification of the nervous principle with electricity.

His discovery did indeed have importance, an importance that led even beyond his dreams of biologic electricity. Within 25 years of the publication of his massive book (Untersungen über thierische Electricität, 1848–9) the idea occurred to a young lecturer at Liverpool, in the north of England, that as nerve impulses flowed in and out of the brain their passage might be detectable. In 1874 he obtained a grant from the British Medical Association and within a year reported his findings to a meeting of the BMA on August 25, 1875. His name was Richard Caton (Fig. 1.8).

Caton had already experimented (and published, 1875) on the peripheral nerve muscle currents, but began to search for their cerebral counterparts; he not only detected them but noticed that when both of his electrodes lay on the cortical surface there was a continuous waxing and waning of potential. This oscillation of the baseline was present in the unstimulated animal and Caton proved it to be unrelated to respiratory or cardiac rhythms. He also proved these fluctuations to be biologic in origin by showing them to be vulnerable to

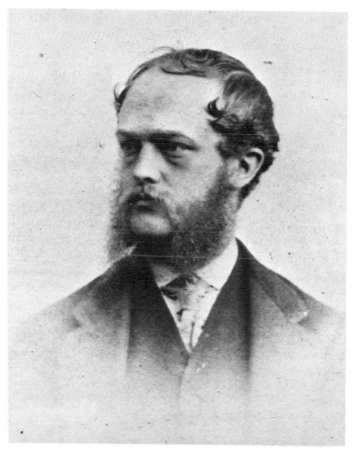

Fig. 1.8. *Richard Caton, the first to discover the EEG and to detect the evoked potential change on visual stimulation and realize its application to cortical localization (from a photograph taken in his thirties when he was working in electrophysiology. The generous gift to the writer from his daughter).*

anoxia and to anesthesia and to be abolished by the death of the animal. Caton had discovered the electroencephalogram.

The report of Caton's demonstration (1875) that the British Medical Association published contained (in part) these statements.

> Feeble currents of varying direction pass through the multiplier when the electrodes are placed on two points of the external surface, or one electrode on the grey matter, and one on the surface of the skull. . . . When any part of the grey matter is in a state of functional activity, its electric current usually exhibits negative variation. . . . Impressions through the senses were found to influence the currents of certain areas; . . .

Caton had found not only the electroencephalogram but also the cerebral potential change evoked by sensory stimulation. In these potential swings superimposed on the baseline oscillations, Caton immediately recognized a meaning for studies of cortical localization, a discovery basic to the use of evoked potentials in today's clinical neurology.

Caton's great contribution, in addition to discovering the EEG, was in providing experimentalists for the first time with a method for mapping the localization of sensory areas in the cortex, supplanting the crude ablation techniques which had until then been the only approach (other than Gall's claims for bumps on the skull, 1810–19). This was an era of intense interest in cortical localization owing to the prominence of David Ferrier's mapping of the motor cortex (1873–4), and in his subsequent work it was this aspect of his discoveries that Caton pursued.

In 1875 electronic amplifiers were unthought of and cameras had not yet come into the laboratory. To gain acceptance of his discovery Caton had to demonstrate the "brain waves" of his animals by optical magnification of the movements of the meniscus in his Thompson's galvanometer.

He went on to expand his experiments, reporting them more fully in 1877 in a Supplement to the British Medical Journal and again at the Ninth International Medical Congress in Washington, D.C., in 1887. At this meeting he reported experiments on 45 animals—cats, rabbits, and monkeys—and described his operating technique, electrodes and instrumentation.

Among these many experiments is one of special interest to electroencephalographers: he found the flicker response of the EEG, a phenomenon found again in man by Adrian in 1934. Caton wrote:

> I tried the effect of intervals of light and darkness on seven rabbits and four monkeys, placing electrodes on the region (13) stimulation of which causes movement of the eyes . . .
> In those five experiments in which I was successful the relation between the intervals of light and darkness and the movements of the galvanometer needle was quite beyond question . . .

Strangely enough, in spite of the prominent groups before whom Caton gave his demonstrations and the popular medical journal in which he reported them, his work received no attention among English-speaking physiologists.

In Poland, as it happened, a young assistant in the physiology department of the University of Jagiellonski in Crakow, Adolf Beck, not knowing of Caton's work 15 years earlier, was searching initially for the same phenomenon, namely for electrical signs in the brain of impulses reaching it from the sense organs (Fig. 1.9). Like Caton before him he succeeded, and he also found the brain wave. His animals were dogs and rabbits, and because he lacked a camera, he published the protocols of all his experiments in the Polish language for a doctoral thesis (1890). In order to reach a greater audience he sent a short account to the most widely read journal in Germany, the Centralblatt für Physiologie (1890). A spate of claims for priority for finding sensorily evoked potentials followed the German publication of Beck's findings—the first came in 1890 from Fleischl von Marxow, Professor of Physiology (and teacher of Freud) in Vienna; his claim was based on a letter he had sealed in 1883. Other claims came from Gotch and Horsley (1891), and Danilevsky (1891).

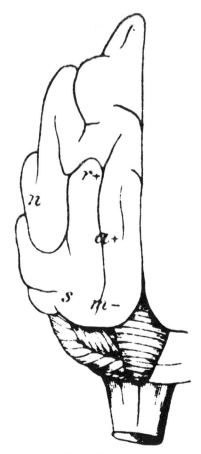

Fig. 1.9. Beck's diagram of the dog's brain in which he marked the positions of electrodes that gave him a response to light (m+, a+) and a faint response to sound (n, s) (from the Doctoral Thesis of Adolf Beck. 1891. Polska Akademija Umiejetnosci. Series 2, 187).

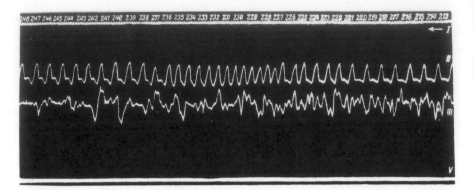

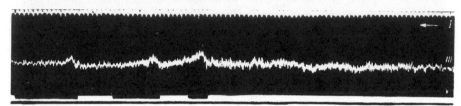

Fig. 1.10. *The first photograph to be published of electroencephalograms and of an evoked potential. The upper record shows (in trace III) the brain potentials of a curarized dog with the pulsations of an artery in the brain recorded above them.*

In the lower record the sciatic nerve is being stimulated from time to time and the decrease in activity noted by Neminsky (and by Beck before him) can be seen. The record reads from right to left, line 1 being a time-marker in fifths of a second, line III the EEG and line V the signal for stimulation at each break (from Pravdich-Neminsky, V. V. 1913. Zentralbl. Physiol., 27, 951).

It is noticeable that it was the electrical response of the brain to sensory stimulation that drew the most interest, for this was a finding that lay directly in the mainstream of current thinking about cortical localization of function.*

The completely novel idea of a continuously fluctuating electrical potential intrinsic to the ''resting'' brain, although confirmed by every worker, was of interest at that time only to its two independent discoverers, Caton and Beck.

By the end of the century the electrical activity of the brain had reached the textbooks (Schäfer, 1898) and cameras were beginning to reach the laboratory scientist. In 1913 and 1914 came the first photographs of EEGs from Pravdich-Neminsky in Russia and from Beck's old professor, Cybulski, in Poland. It was Neminsky who gave us the first photograph of an evoked potential recorded at the cortex of a dog on stimulation of the sciatic nerve (Fig. 1.10). He also demonstrated that the EEG could be recorded from the intact skull. From Cybulski (1914) came the first photograph of experimentally in-

---

*For a fuller account of this early work on the EEG and the use of the evoked cortical potential see: Brazier, M. A. B. (1961). A History of the Electrical Activity of the Brain, Pitman, London.

duced epilepsy (Fig. 1.11), although such a result had been reported previously by Kaufmann (1912) in Russia who lacked a camera. Kaufmann had read the works of Caton and Beck and the other claimants and, in fact, had written a review of them (1912). From this study he argued that an epileptic attack must surely be accompanied by abnormal discharges and, on provoking one in his animals, he found both the tonic and clonic phases.

Although successful with light as the stimulus, Caton had been disappointed by his failure to record cortical potential swings evoked by sounds, for he was searching for the auditory cortex. "Search was made," he wrote (1877), "to discover an area related to perceptions of sound. The electrodes were placed on various parts of the brain, and loud sounds were made close to the rabbit's ears by means of a bell, etc. No results were obtained." Beck, independently, had searched for a cortical area that responded electrically to sound but was rarely successful. He did, however, discover the desynchronization of the ongoing oscillatory activity on sensory stimulation, which is what we now call "alpha blocking of the EEG."

At the turn of the century this question of the localization of the auditory cortex was taken up by a student of the famous Bechterev in St. Petersburg.

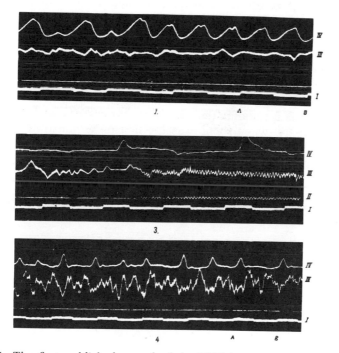

Fig. 1.11. The first published record of the EEG in experimental epilepsy in-duced by cortical stimulation in a dog. The record reads from right to left, the uppermost trace IV being the heart, III the cortex, II the stimulus (which leaks onto the EEG), and I the time-line. The lower strip is continuous with the upper one. A–B = 1 second (from Cybulski, N. and Jeleńska-Macieszyna. 1914. Bull. Sci. Krakov. Ser. B, 776).

Larionov by name, he started to attempt localization by extirpation experiments but, on learning of Caton's success with visual stimuli, he changed to a search for the evoked potential. He was fortunate in having far more sensitive instrumentation than his predecessors (a Wiedermann-D'Arsonval galvanometer) and with this he was able to map out, in cats, the topographic centers on the temporal cortex of response to the pitch of different tuning forks (1899) (Fig. 1.12).

In America and in western Europe there was no sign of interest in these many revelations of the electrical activity of the brain in spite of their obvious meaning for cortical localization. In Germany, however, there was a psychiatrist who had read all the publications and who hoped to find in the electrical activity of the brain the source of "psychic energy." This was Hans Berger at the University of Jena. He worked in secrecy and did not publish until 1929, but he kept copious notebooks and diaries from which we know that he began experiments in 1902, rapidly confirmed Caton's discovery of the EEG in animals, but failed to find the potential changes evoked by sensory stimulation. He made further attempts in 1907 and again in 1910, by which time he had a more sensitive galvanometer, but again he failed. This was a great disappointment to him for he eagerly wanted to relate such to psychic functions. Berger's failure to find these changes in his animal experiments lacks an explanation, for Caton's findings had by that time been confirmed by many workers in four different countries, all of whose works were read by Berger (Beck, 1890; Verigo, 1889; Fleischl von Marxow, 1890; Danilevsky, 1891; Larionov, 1899; Kaufmann, 1912; Pravdich-Neminsky, 1913; Cybulski, 1914). In none of Berger's publications, which began in 1929 (Fig. 1.13) and continued with rapidity to 1938, do we find him claiming the discovery of the EEG for himself; the claim he made, and justly, was that he was the first to demonstrate that, in having electrical activity in his brain, man was no different from other vertebrates, and it was he who named the spontaneous ongoing activity "Das Elektrenkephalogram."

Being of an abnormally reclusive nature, he kept his first success (the recording from a patient with a skull defect) a secret for five years, though he

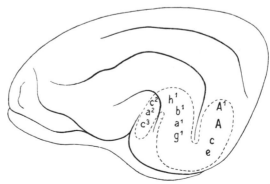

Fig. 1.12. *Schema for localizations of tones in the dog's cortex (from Larionov, V. E. 1899. Pflüg. Arch. ges. Physiol., 76, 608).*

Über das Elektrenkephalogramm des Menschen.

Von

Professor Dr. **Hans Berger**, Jena.

(Mit 17 Textabbildungen.)

(Eingegangen am 22. April 1929.)

Wie *Garten* [1], wohl einer der besten Kenner der Elektrophysiologie, mit Recht hervorgehoben hat, wird man kaum fehlgehen, wenn man jeder lebenden Zelle tierischer und pflanzlicher Natur die Fähigkeit zuschreibt, elektrische Ströme hervorzubringen. Man bezeichnet solche Ströme als bioelektrische Ströme, weil sie die normalen Lebenserscheinungen der Zelle begleiten. Sie sind wohl zu unterscheiden von den durch Verletzungen künstlich hervorgerufenen Strömen, die man als Demarkations-, Alterations- oder Längsquerschnittsströme bezeichnet hat. Es war von vornherein zu erwarten, daß auch im Zentralnervensystem, das doch eine gewaltige Zellanhäufung darstellt, bioelektrische Erscheinungen nachweisbar seien, und in der Tat ist dieser Nachweis schon verhältnismäßig früh erbracht worden.

Caton [2] hat bereits 1874 Versuche an Kaninchen- und Affenhirnen veröffentlicht, bei denen unpolarisierbare Elektroden entweder an der Oberfläche beider Hemisphären oder die eine Elektrode an der Hirnrinde, die andere an der Schädeloberfläche angelegt worden waren. Die Ströme wurden zu einem empfindlichen Galvanometer abgeleitet. Es fanden sich deutliche Stromschwankungen, die namentlich beim Erwachen aus dem Schlaf und beim Eintritt des Todes sich verstärkten, nach dem Tode schwächer wurden und dann vollständig schwanden. Schon *Caton* konnte nachweisen, daß starke Stromschwankungen bei Belichtung des Auges sich an der Hirnrinde einstellten, und er sprach bereits die Vermutung aus, daß unter Umständen diese Rindenströme zur Lokalisation innerhalb der Hirnrinde verwendet werden könnten.

Fleischl von Marxow [3] hat im Jahre 1883 zuerst beobachtet, daß bei verschiedenen Tieren bei Ableitung von zwei symmetrisch gelegenen

[1] *Garten:* Die Produktion von Elektrizität. *Winterstein* Handbuch der vergleichenden Physiologie 3. Bd., 2. Hälfte, S. 105.
[2] *Caton:* Brit. med. J. **2**, 278 (1875). Ref. Zbl. Physiol. 4, Nr 25 (1890). Nach *Bechterew:* Die Energie des lebenden Organismus. S. 102. Wiesbaden 1902.
[3] *Fleischl von Marxow:* Gesammelte Abhandlungen S. 410. Leipzig: J. A. Barth 1893 und Zbl. Physiol. 4 (1890).

Archiv für Psychiatrie. Bd. 87.   35

Fig. 1.13. *The opening page of the first publication reporting the electroencephalogram of man. Note the acknowledgement to Caton (from Berger, H. 1929. Arch. Psychiatr. Nervenkr. 87, 527).*

jotted down in his notebook that this gave him the opportunity to apply Caton's observations to man and the hope that "we may learn the physical basis of consciousness."

Disappointed as he was in his search for a physiologic basis for psychic phenomena, on which he had published a monograph in 1921 and one on telepathy in 1940, he had, as the world knows, launched the electroencephalogram as a clinical neurologic test—a test now employed in every neurologic institution in the world.

REFERENCES

Adrian, E. D. and Matthews, B. H. C. 1934. The Berger rhythm: potential changes from the occipital lobes in man. Brain, *57:* 355.

Aldini, Giovanni (1762–1834) 1794. De Animali Electricitate Dissertationes Duae. Bologna.

Aldini, Giovanni 1804. Essai Théorique et Expérimental sur le Galvanisme. 2 vols. Fournier, Paris.

Beck, Adolf (1863–1942) Presented October 1890. The determination of localization in the brain and spinal cord by means of electrical phenomena (in Polish). Rozprawy Wydzialu Matematycvno-przyrodniczych Polska Akademia, Series II, *1:* 186.

Beck, Adolf 1890. Die Ströme der Nervencentren. Centralbl. f. Physiòl., *4:* 572.
Beck, Adolf and Cybulski, Napoleon 1891. Further research on the electrical phenomena of the cerebral cortex in monkeys and dogs (in Polish). Rozprawy Wydzialu Matematycvno-przyrodniczych Polska Akademia, *32:* 369.
Berger, Hans, (1873–1941) 1921. Psychophysiologie in 12 Vorlesungen. Fischer, Jena.
Berger, Hans 1929. Über das Elektrenkephalogram des Menschen. Arch. Psychiatr. Nervenkr., *87:* 527.
Berger, Hans 1938. Das Elektrenkephalogram des Menschen. Acta Nova Leopoldina, *6:* 173.
Berger, Hans 1940. Psyche. Fischer, Jena.
Bertholon, Nicole (1742–1800) 1780. De l'Electricité du Corps Humain dans l'État de Santé et de Maladie. 2 vols. Croulbois, Paris.
Bertholon, Nicole 1783. De l'Électricité des Végétaux. Didot, Paris.
Boissier de la Croix de Sauvages, François (1706–1767) 1758. Dissertation sur la nature et cause de la rage. In: Pièces qui ont Remporté le Prix de l'Académie Royale des Sciences; Inscriptions, et Belles Lettres de Toulouse depuis l'Année 1747 jusqu'au 1750. Forest, Toulouse.
Boyle, Robert (1627–1691) 1673. Essays of the Strange Subtilty Determinate Nature, Great Efficacy of Effluviums, to which are Annext New Experiments to Make Fire and Flame Ponderable Together with a Discovery of the Perviousness of Glass. Pitt, London.
Boyle, Robert 1675. Experiments and Notes about the Mechanical Origins or Production of Electricity. London.
Caldani, Leopoldo (1725–1813) 1784. Institutiones Physiologicae et Pathologicae. Luchtmans, Leyden.
Caton, Richard (1842–1926) 1875. On the electric relations of muscle and nerve. Liverpool Medical and Chirurgical Journal.
Caton, Richard 1875. The electric currents of the brain. Br. Med. J. *2:* 278.
Caton, Richard 1877. Interim report on investigation of the electric currents of the brain. Br. Med. J., Supp. *1:* 62.
Caton, Richard 1887. Researches on electrical phenomena of cerebral grey matter. Ninth International Medical Congress *3:* 246.
Caton, Richard 1891. Die Ströme des Centralnervensystems. Centralbl. f. Physiol., *4:* 785.
Cerletti, Ugo (1877–   ) 1954. Electroshock therapy. J. Clin. Exp. Psychopathol., *15:* 191.
Comitato di Torino 1803. Classe di Scienza esatta dell'Accademia di Torino. Thermidor Année, *10:* 27.
Cybulski, Napoleon (1854–1919) and Jeleńska-Macieszyna 1914. Action currents of the cerebral cortex (in Polish). Bulletin Internationale de l'Académie des Sciences de Cracovie, Series B, 776.
Danilevsky, Vasili Yakovlevich (1852–1939) 1891. Zu Frage über die elektromotorische Vorgänge im Gehirn als Ausdruck seines Tätigkeitzustandes. Centralbl. f. Physiol., *5:* 1.
De Romas, Jacques (1713–1776). Observations sur l'Électrisation de Deux Paralytiques. Oeuvres inédites de Romas 1750–1760. Archives de la Ville de Bordeaux.
Desaguliers, Jean Théophile (1683–1744) 1742. A Dissertation Concerning Electricity. Innýs and Longman, London.
Deshais, Jean-Etienne 1749. De Hemiplegia per Electricitatem Curanda. Martel, Montpellier.
Du Bois-Reymond, Emil (1818–1896) (Vol. I 1848, Vol II 1849). Untersuchungen über thierische Electricität. Reimer, Berlin.
Du Bois-Reymond, Emil 1877. Gesammelte Abhandlungen zur allgemeinen Muskel- und Nerve-physik. Veit, Leipzig.

Duchenne, Guillaume Benjamin Amand (1806–1875) 1855. De l'Électrisation Localisée, et de son Application à la Pathologie et à la Thérapeutique. Ballière, Paris.

Duchenne, G. B. A. 1867. Physiologie des Mouvements Démontrée à l'Aide de l'Expérimentation Électrique et de l'Observation Clinique et Applicable a l'Étude des Paralysies et des Déformations. Ballière, Paris.

Duchenne, G. B. A. 1868. De la Paralysie Musculaire, Pseudo-hypertrophique ou Paralysie Myo-sclérosique. Asselin, Paris.

Du Fay, Charles de Cisternai (1698–1739) 1735. Quatrième mémoire sur l'électricité. In: Mémoires de l'Académie Royale des Sciences, p. 457, Paris.

Dufay, Jean Thecla Felicitas 1750. An Fluidum Nerveum sit Fluidam Electricum? Martel, Montpellier.

Fée, A. 1832. Vie de Linné. Mémoires de la Societé Royale des Sciences de Lille.

Ferrier, David (1843–1928) 1873–74. The localisation of function in the brain. Proc. Roy. Soc., 22: 229.

Fleischl von Marxow, Ernst (1846–1892) 1890. Mittheilung betreffend die Physiologie der Hirnrinde. Centralbl. f. Physiol., 4: 538.

Fontana, Felice Gaspar Ferdinand (1730–1805) 1760. Letter to Urbain Tosetti. In: Mémoires sur les Parties Sensibles et Irritables du Corps Animal. von Haller, A., Ed. 3: 159.

Fowler, Richard 1793. Experiments and Observations Relative to the Influence Lately Discovered by M. Galvani, and Commonly Called Animal Electricity. Duncan, Edinburgh.

Gall, Franz Joseph (1758–1828) and Spurzheim, Johann Christophe (1776–1832) 1810–1819. Anatomie et Physiologie du Système Nerveux et Général et du Cerveau en Particulier, avec des Observations Intellectuelles et Morales de l'Homme et des Animaux, par Configuration de leur Têtes. Schoell, Paris.

Galvani, Luigi (1737–1798) 1791. De viribus electricitatis in motu musculare commentarius. De Bononiensi Scientiarum et Artium Instituto atque Academia Commentarii, 7: 363.

(Galvani, Luigi) Anon. 1794. Dell'Uso e dell'Attivita dell'Arco Conduttore nelle Contrazioni dei Muscoli. Bologna.

Galvani, Luigi 1937. Memorie ed Esperimenti Inediti di Luigi Galvani. Capelli, Bologna.

Gilbert, William (1540–1603) 1600. De Magnete, Magneticisque Corporibus et de Magno Magnete Tellure. Peter Short, London.

Goethe, Johann Wolfgang (1740–1832) 1810. Farbenlehre.

Gotch, Francis (1853–1913) and Horsley, Victor Alexander Haden (1857–1916) 1891. Über den Gebrauch der Elektricität für die Lokalisierung der Erregungsscheinungen im Centralnervensystem. Centralbl. f. Physiol., 4: 649.

Gray, Stephen (died 1736) 1731. A letter to Cromwell Mortimer, M.D., Secretary of the Royal Society containing several experiments concerning electricity. Phil. Trans., 37–38: 18 and 405.

Hausen, Christian August (1693–1743) 1743. Novi Profectus in Historia Electricitatis. Schwann, Leipzig.

Hermann, Ludimar (1838–1914) 1884. Über sogennanten secondär-electromotorische Erschneinungen an Muskeln und Nerve. Pflüger's Arch. f. d. ges. Physiol., 33: 103.

Hunter, John (1728–1793) 1773. Anatomical observations on the torpedo. Phil. Trans., 63: 481.

Kaufmann, Pavel Yrevich (1877–1951) 1912. Electrical phenomena in cerebral cortex (in Russian). Obzory Psikhiatrii Nevrologii i Eksperimental'noi Psikhologii, 7–8: 403.

Kratzenstein, Johann Heinrich (1726–1790) 1744. Abhandlung von dem Rutzen der Electricität in Arznenwissenschaft. Hemmerde, Halle.

Krüger, Johann Gottlob (1715–1759) 1745. Zuschrift an seine Zuhörer worinnen er ihren seine Gedancken von der Electricität mittheilet. Hemmerde, Halle.

Larionov, Vladimir Efimovich 1899. Galvanometric determination of cortical currents in the area of the tonal centres under stimulation of peripheral acoustic organs (in Russian). Nevrologicheskii Vestnik 7: 44.

Larionov, Vladimir Efimovich 1899. Über die musikalischen Centren des Gehirns. Pflüger's Arch. f. d. ges. Physiol., 76: 608.

Mangin, l'Abbé de (died 1772) 1752. Histoire Générale et Particulière de l'Électricité ou ce qu'en Dit de Curieux et d'Amusant Quelques Physiciens de l'Europe. 3 vols. Rollin, Paris.

Marat, Jean-Paul (1744–1793) 1784. Mémoire sur l'Électricité Médicale. Méguignon, Paris.

Matteucci, Carlo (1811–1868) 1843. Mémoire sur l'existence du courant électrique musculaire dans les animaux vivants ou récemment tués. Annal. de Chimie, 7: 425.

Matteucci, Carlo 1844. Traité des Phénomènes Électro-physiologiques des Animaux Suivi d'Études Anatomiques sur le Système Nerveux et sur l'Organe Électrique de la Torpille par Paul Savi. Fortin et Masson, Paris.

Nollet, Jean-Antoine (1700–1770) 1749. Recherches sur les Causes Particulières des Phenomènes Électriques. Guerin, Paris.

Oersted, Christian (1777–1851) 1820. Experimenta circa Effectum Conflictis Electrici in Acum Magneticum. Copenhagen.

Pfaff, Christophe-Henri (1773–1858) 1798. Abhandlung über die sognnante thierische Electrizität. Gren's Journal der Physik, 8: (2) 196.

Pravdich-Neminsky, Vladimir Vladimirovich (1879–1952) 1913. Ein Versuch der Registrierung der elektrischen Gehirnerscheinungen. Zentralbl. Physiol., 27: 951.

Prévost, J. L. and Batelli, F. 1899. La mort par les courants électriques alternatifs à bas voltage. Journal de Physiologie et de Pathologie générale, 1: 399.

Schäfer, Edward Albert (1850–1935) 1898. Textbook of Physiology, Pentland, London.

Schmück, Edmund Joseph 1792. Beiträge zur neuern Kenntniss der thierische Elektricität. Mannheim.

Stahl, Georg Ernst (1600–1734) 1708. Theoria Medica Vera. Halle.

Sue, Pierre (1739–1816) 1802–1805. Histoire du Galvanisme. 4 vols. Bernard, Paris.

Valli, Eusèbe (1755–1816) 1793. Experiments in Animal Electricity. Johnson, London.

Van Musschenbroek, Petrus (1692–1761) 1746. Quoted in J-A Nollet. Mémoires de l'Académie des Sciences, Paris.

Verigo, B. F. 1889. Action currents of the brain and medulla (in Russian). Vestnik Klinicheskoi i sudebnoi Psikhiatrii i Nevropathologii 7.

Verigo, B. F. 1889. Action currents of the frog's brain. Report of the 3rd Congress of Russian physiologists and biologists, St. Petersburg (in Russian), Vrach, 10: 45.

Vivenzio, G. 1784. Istoria dell'Elettricitá Medica. Naples

Volta, Allessandro Giuseppe Antonio (1745–1827) 1800. Letter to Sir Joseph Banks, March 20, 1800 on electricity excited by the mere contact of conducting substances of different kinds. Phil. Trans., 90: 403.

Von Haller, Albrecht (1708–1777) 1757 and 1765. Elementa Physiologiae Corporis Humani. 8 vols. Bousquet, Lausanne.

Von Helmholtz, Hermann (1821–1894) 1850. Messungen über den zeitlichen Verlauf der Zuchung animalischer Muskeln und die Fortpflanzungsgeschwindigkeit der Reizung in den Nerven. Archiv für Anatomie und Physiologie, 277.

Von Humboldt, Frederick Alexander (1769–1859) 1797. Versuche über die gereizte Muskel und Nervenfaser. 2 vols. Decker, Posen und Rottman, Berlin.

Van Kleist, Ewald Jurgen. Quoted in Winkler, J. H. 1745. Eigenschaften der electrischen Materie und des electrischen Feuers. Breitkopf, Leipzig.

Winkler, Johann Heinrich (1703–1770) 1744. Gedanken von den Eigenschafen Wirkungen und Ursachen der Electricität. Breitkopf, Leipzig.

2

Electroencephalography

M. J. AMINOFF

The electroencephalogram (EEG) is a record of the electrical activity of the brain, and is obtained by means of electrodes placed on the scalp. Many clinical neurologists and neurosurgeons do not fully appreciate the potential value or limitations of electroencephalography and this is reflected in the manner that they use it in clinical practice. On the one hand, patients are often referred indiscriminately for study and little, if any, information is provided about their clinical background. On the other hand, patients in whom electroencephalography might be expected to provide clinically useful information are not investigated by this means at all.

Electroencephalography is most useful in the investigation and management of patients with epilepsy. The presence of "epileptiform" activity (p. 41) in the EEG of a patient with suspected epilepsy does not establish the diagnosis beyond doubt, since similar activity may be found in occasional patients who have never had a seizure. It is, however, one more factor that must be taken into account when the patient is evaluated clinically. In patients with an established seizure disorder, the EEG findings may help to classify the disorder, to identify a focal or lateralized epileptogenic source, to indicate the most appropriate medication that should be prescribed, to provide a guide to prognosis, and to follow the course of the disorder.

Electroencephalography is also an important, noninvasive means of localizing structural abnormalities such as brain tumors. Localization is generally by indirect means, however, depending on the production of abnormalities by viable brain in the neighborhood of the lesion. Moreover, it is sometimes disappointingly inaccurate, and the findings themselves provide no reliable indication of the type of underlying pathology. In this context, it is hardly surprising that recent advances in the radiologic detection of structural abnormalities in the brain—in particular by the development of computerized axial tomography—have led to a reduction in this use of electroencephalography as a screening procedure. Nevertheless, it still has an important role in examining the function of the brain, and it is, therefore, complementary to, rather than an inconsequential alternative of, these newer procedures.

The third major use of electroencephalography is in the investigation of patients with other neurologic disorders. Certain of these disorders produce characteristic EEG abnormalities which, though nonspecific, help to suggest, establish, or support the diagnosis. This is well exemplified by the repetitive slow wave complexes sometimes seen in herpes simplex encephalitis, and which should suggest this diagnosis if found in patients with an acute cerebral illness. The electrical findings are best regarded as one more physical sign, however, and as such should be evaluated in conjunction with the other clinical and laboratory data. A further use of electroencephalography—and one which is increasing in importance with the development of quantitative techniques for assessing the data that it provides—is in the screening or monitoring of patients with metabolic disorders, for it provides an objective measure of improvement or deterioration that may precede any change in the clinical state of the patient. Electroencephalography is also used as a means of evaluating patients with altered levels of consciousness. Finally, it is used in studying natural sleep and its disorders, and as a help in the determination of brain death. Further comment on these aspects is deferred to Chapters 16 and 17, while the clinical utility of the EEG in the investigation of infants and children is considered separately in Chapter 3.

PRACTICAL CONSIDERATIONS

The EEG is recorded from metal electrodes placed on the scalp. The electrodes are coated with a conductive paste, applied to the scalp, and held in place by adhesives, suction, or pressure from caps or headbands; alternatively, needle electrodes can be inserted directly into the scalp. Until recently, there was no general agreement about the most suitable placements for recording electrodes, but most laboratories are now using the International 10-20 system proposed by Jasper (1958) in which electrode placements are based on measurements from four standard positions on the head, namely the nasion, inion, and right and left pre-auricular points, as illustrated in Figure 2.1. The potential differences between electrodes are amplified and recorded on continuously moving paper by a number of pen-writers. The electrodes are connected with amplifiers in predetermined patterns or montages to permit the electrical activ-

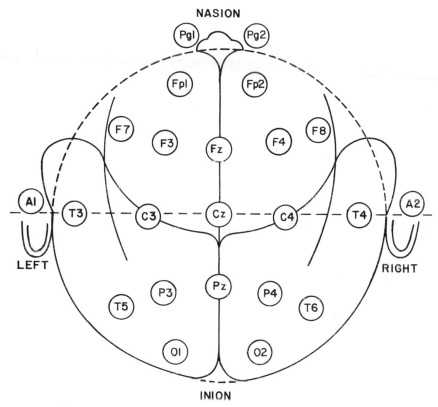

NASION

LEFT

RIGHT

INION

Fig. 2.1. The International 10-20 system of electrode placement. A, earlobe; C, Central; F, Frontal; Fp, Frontal Polar; P, Parietal; Pg, Nasopharyngeal; T, Temporal; O, Occipital; right sided placements are indicated by even numbers, left sided placements by odd numbers, and midline placements by Z.

ity of various areas to be recorded in sequence. The recording arrangements can be varied so that the potential difference is measured either between pairs of scalp electrodes (bipolar derivation), or between individual electrodes and a common reference point. In the latter circumstance, the reference point can either be at a relatively inactive site on the scalp or elsewhere, or it can be a point connected to all the electrodes in use so that it reflects the average of the potentials at those electrodes. Each technique has its own advantages and drawbacks, but for routine purposes at least two of these methods for deriving the EEG should be used. Montages are generally selected so that recordings are made from rows of equidistant electrodes running from front to back of the head, or transversely across it. In most laboratories, traces from the right side of the head are displayed above those from the left, and those from anterior regions are above those from more posterior areas.

The more detailed technical and practical aspects of EEG recording are beyond the scope of this chapter, and the interested reader is referred to the review by Cooper, Osselton, and Shaw (1974). There is, however, one general point that must be made clear. As already indicated, the potential difference between pairs of electrodes—or between an electrode and its reference point—is amplified before being displayed on moving paper. The input leads of the individual amplifiers are designated as black (input terminal 1) and white (input terminal 2). They are so arranged that when the electrode connected with the black lead is relatively more negative than that connected to the white one, the recording pen makes an upward deflection. With bipolar derivations, the conventional recording arrangement is for the most anterior electrode of each pair to be connected with the black lead when recording from front to back of the head, and for the right hand electrode of any pair to be connected with the black lead when recording across the head. With the reference derivations, the active scalp electrodes are each connected to the black lead of an amplifier, while all the white leads are connected with the common reference point.

Both the bipolar derivation and the use of a common reference permit abnormalities to be localized, but the former method is less satisfactory for localizing widespread changes or for demonstrating areas in which activity is suppressed. With bipolar derivations, the source of localized EEG abnormalities is determined by locating the electrode at which the activity shows a reversal of its phase or polarity, when recordings are made simultaneously from at least two rows of electrodes at right angles to each other, i.e. from rows of electrodes in the anteroposterior and transverse axes of the head. With common reference derivations, localization of abnormalities is primarily on the basis of amplitude.

Various special electrodes have been devised for recording the activity of inaccessible regions of the brain, since such activity may not be detected by electrodes placed on the scalp. A nasopharyngeal electrode, consisting of a flexible, insulated rod or wire with a small silver electrode at its tip, can be inserted into the nostril and advanced until the terminal electrode is in contact with the mucosa of the posterior nasopharynx. This permits recording of electrical activity from the anteromedial surface of the temporal lobe. Activity from the anteroinferior portion of the temporal lobe can be recorded by sphenoidal electrodes. These are less likely to lead to artifacts than are nasopharyngeal electrodes, but their application is more difficult. The electrode consists of a sterile needle or fine wire which is insulated except at its tip, and it is inserted percutaneously under local anesthesia by a physician so that it lies adjacent to the sphenoid bone, a little in front of the foramen ovale.

The EEG examination is usually undertaken in quiet, relaxed circumstances, with the patient seated or lying comfortably with eyes closed. Recordings are initially made for up to about 5 minutes from each of several different standard montages, for a total of about 30 minutes. Depending on the findings, the examination can then be continued by recording with less conventional montages. During the recording of activity from each montage, the patient may be asked to lie with his eyes open for about 20 seconds before closing them again, so that the responsiveness of the background activity can be assessed.

When this routine part of the examination has been completed, recording continues while activation procedures are undertaken in an attempt to provoke abnormalities.

Hyperventilation for 3 to 4 minutes is a harmless method of provoking EEG abnormalities. The patient is asked to take deep breaths at his normal respiratory rate until instructed to stop. The resultant fall in arterial pCO_2 leads to a cerebral vasoconstriction which may activate EEG abnormalities. Certain quantitative techniques have been suggested in an endeavor to establish a more uniform procedure, but these are not in routine use. The EEG is recorded during the period of hyperventilation and for the following 2 minutes, using a montage that encompasses the area where it is suspected that abnormalities may be found on clinical or other grounds, or—in the absence of any localizing clues—that covers as much of the scalp as possible. Hyperventilation usually causes more prominent EEG changes in children than in adults, but there is considerable variation in the response of individual subjects.

Recording during sleep or after a 24-hour period of sleep deprivation may also provoke EEG abnormalities that might otherwise be missed, and is similarly harmless. It has been used most widely in the investigation of patients with suspected epilepsy.

An electronic stroboscope is used to cause rhythmic photic stimulation while the EEG is recorded using a bipolar recording arrangement that covers, particularly, the occipital and parietal regions of the scalp. At any given flash rate the EEG is recorded with the patient's eyes open for about 5 seconds and then while his eyes are closed for a further 5 seconds. Flash rates of up to 30 per second are generally used, but an even wider range of frequencies is employed in some laboratories.

A number of different pharmacologic activating procedures have been described, but since these are not in general use and may carry some risk to the patient they will not be discussed. Brief reference is, however, made in a later section to the technique of injecting amobarbital or pentylenetetrazol intraarterially.

THE ACTIVITY RECORDED IN THE EEG

There is now considerable evidence from studies in experimental animals to suggest that the rhythmic activity normally recorded from the scalp has a cortical origin, being derived from the postsynaptic potentials of cortical neurons. In particular, it is the pyramidal neurons—cells that are vertically oriented with regard to the cortex and have a large apical dendrite extending toward the surface—that are important in this respect, while potentials arising from neuronal activity in subcortical structures or from horizontally oriented cortical cells contribute little, if anything, to the normal, scalp-recorded EEG.

The cortical activity has a regular rhythmicity which seems to depend on the functional integrity of subcortical mechanisms. In the cat, for example, rhythmic cortical activity persists after the brainstem has been sectioned between, or just above, the colliculi (Bremer, 1935), but is much reduced when the cortex is isolated by cutting its connections to other parts of the brain (Bremer, 1938). The results of other lesion experiments (Kristiansen and Courtois, 1949; Jasper, 1949; Andersen, Andersson, and Lømo, 1967) suggest that it is the thalamus which serves as pacemaker of certain of the cortical rhythms that are recorded at electroencephalography. Following their series of stimulation experiments, Dempsey and Morison (1942) suggested that the midline nuclei of the thalamus were important in this respect, and this concept was subsequently modified by Jasper (1949) who emphasized that the activity from these nuclei relayed in various other intrathalamic nuclei before being projected to the cortex (Fig. 2.2). More recent work has indicated, however, that the medial nuclei are not essential for the generation of rhythmic cortical activity, the primary sensory relay nuclei themselves being capable of rhythmic activity and of influencing cortical activity. This has led to the so-called facultative

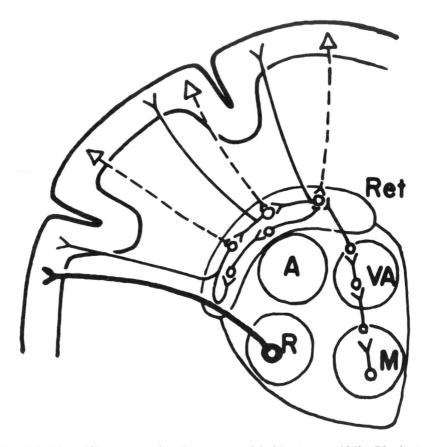

Fig. 2.2. *The midline pacemaker theory as modified by Jasper (1949). Rhythmic activity is imposed upon widespread cortical areas via a multineuronal system, including the intralaminar nuclei, the anterior thalamic nucleus (VA), and the thalamic reticular nucleus (Ret). (A) Association, (M) medial thalamic nuclei. The cortical projection from the relay nuclei (R) is separate from the rhythm-inducing system (from Andersen, P. and Andersson, S. A. 1968. Physiological Basis of the Alpha Rhythm, Appleton-Century-Crofts, New York, with permission of Plenum).*

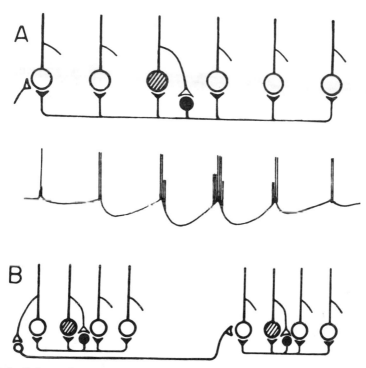

Fig. 2.3. *Schematic representation of the proposed inherent mechanism giving rhythmic discharges of thalamic neurons. (A) a discharge of the cell (hatched) causes recurrent inhibition via an interneuron (black) that hyperpolarizes many neighboring projection cells. During the postinhibitory rebound, many of these cells discharge action potentials and an increasing number of cells participate during the successive cycles (A, lower part). Alternatively, intrathalamic connections via distributor neurons (B) spread the rhythmic activity from one group to other parts of the thalamus (from-left-to-right group) (from Andersen, P. and Andersson, S. A. 1968. Physiological Basis of the Alpha Rhythm, Appleton-Century-Crofts, New York, with permission of Plenum).*

pacemaker theory (Andersen and Sears, 1964; Andersen and Andersson, 1968) in which thalamic rhythmicity is related to a recurrent inhibitory process, as shown in Fig. 2.3. Postsynaptic inhibitory potentials have a synchronizing effect on the activity of thalamic cells, thereby leading to the generation of a series of excitatory waves and governing the interval between successive waves (Andersen and Sears, 1964). Rhythmic activity can arise in any or all of the thalamic nuclei, can spread from one nucleus to another, and is imposed on the cortex via the thalamocortical projections (Fig. 2.4.). Further details are given by Andersen and Andersson (1968, 1974) in their recent reviews.

The physiologic basis of the abnormal rhythms that are encountered at electroencephalography, and the mechanisms responsible for the hypersynchronization that underlies seizure activity, remain less clearly defined and will not be discussed.

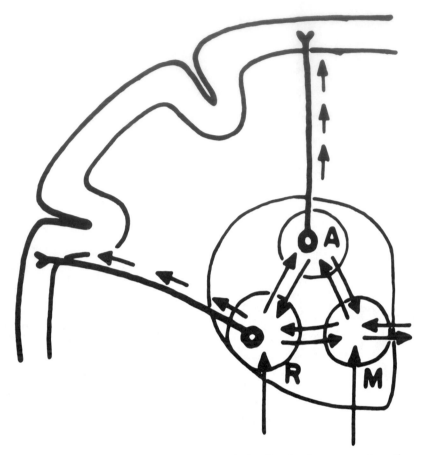

Fig. 2.4. *Diagrammatic representation of the facultative pacemaker theory. Rhythmic activity is assumed to be an inherent property of groups of cells in all thalamic nuclei. The rhythm (series of arrows) is imposed upon the cortex in a topographic pattern determined by the specific thalamocortical fibers from the relay and association nuclei. The arrows between the thalamic nuclei indicate mutual connections between various thalamic parts. These connections determine the degree of synchrony of the rhythmic activity in the thalamus and cortex (from Andersen, P. and Andersson, S. A. 1968. Physiological Basis of the Alpha Rhythm, Appleton-Century-Crofts, New York, with permission of Plenum).*

Alpha Rhythm

Alpha rhythm has a frequency of between 8 and 13 Hz, is found over the posterior portions of the head during wakefulness, and is best seen when the patient is resting with eyes closed. It is attenuated or abolished by visual attention (Fig. 2.5), and transiently by other sensory stimuli. Alpha activity is well-formed and prominent in some normal subjects, while in others it is relatively inconspicuous. Its precise frequency is usually of little diagnostic significance, unless information is available about its frequency on earlier occasions.

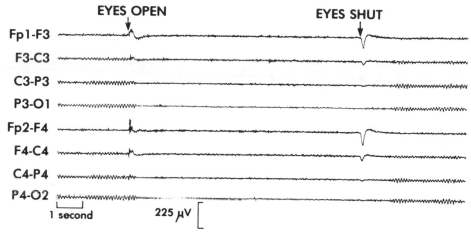

Fig. 2.5. Normal 9–10 Hz alpha rhythm recorded in the EEG of a 64-year-old man. The posterior distribution and responsiveness to eye-opening of the rhythm can be seen.

Slowing occurs with advancing age, as a consequence of certain medication such as anticonvulsant drugs, and in patients with clouding of consciousness, metabolic disorders, or virtually any type of cerebral pathology. The alpha activity may increase in frequency in children as they mature, and in older subjects who are thyrotoxic. A slight asymmetry is often present between the two hemispheres with regard to the amplitude of alpha activity and the degree to which it extends anteriorly. In particular, alpha rhythm may normally be up to 50 percent greater in amplitude over the non-dominant hemisphere (Kiloh, McComas, and Osselton, 1974). A more marked asymmetry of its amplitude may have lateralizing significance but is difficult to interpret unless other EEG abnormalities are present, because either depression or enhancement may occur on the side of a hemisphere lesion. Similarly, a persistent difference in alpha frequency of more than 1 Hz between the two hemispheres is generally regarded as abnormal, but it is usually difficult to be certain which is the abnormal side unless other abnormalities are also found.

Beta Activity

Any rhythmic activity which has a frequency greater than 13 Hz is referred to as beta activity. Activity of this sort, responsive to eye opening, is sometimes found over posterior portions of the hemispheres and is then best regarded as a fast variant of the alpha rhythm. Beta activity that fails to respond to eye opening is a common finding and usually has a generalized distribution, but in some instances it is located centrally and is attenuated by contralateral movements. It usually has an amplitude of less than about 30 μV. There is considerable variation in the amount of such activity that is found in different normal subjects. Beta activity may, however, be induced by a number of different drugs, particularly barbiturates and the benzodiazepine compounds. Focal or lateralized spontaneous beta activity, or asymmetric drug-induced fast activity, raises the possibility of localized cerebral pathology, but in such circumstances it must be borne in mind that the amplitude of beta activity may be increased either ipsi- or contralateral to a cerebral lesion (Green and Wilson, 1961). Moreover, if beta activity is increased in amplitude over the area of a skull defect, this may merely relate to the greater proximity of the recording electrodes to the surface of the brain.

Theta Activity

Activity with a frequency between 4 and 7 Hz is referred to as theta activity. Theta and slower activity is usually very conspicuous in children, but becomes less prominent as maturation proceeds. Some theta activity is often found in young adults, particularly over the temporal regions and during hyperventilation, but in older subjects theta activity with an amplitude greater than about 30 μV (Mundy-Castle, 1951) is seen less commonly except during drowsiness. Focal or lateralized theta activity may be indicative of localized cerebral pathology. More diffusely distributed theta activity is a common finding in patients with a wide variety of neurologic disorders, but may also be due to nothing more than a change in the patient's state of arousal.

Delta Activity

Activity that is slower than 4 Hz is designated delta activity. Activity of this sort is the predominant one in infants, and is a normal finding during the deep stages of sleep in older subjects. When present in the EEG of awake adults, delta activity is an abnormal finding.

Polymorphic Delta Activity. Polymorphic delta activity is continuous, irregular slow activity that varies considerably in duration and amplitude with time, persists during sleep, and shows little variation with change in the physiologic state of the patient. It has been related to deafferentation of the involved area of the cortex (Hirsch et al, 1966), or to metabolic factors. Such activity may be found postictally, and in patients with metabolic disorders. It is commonly seen, with a localized distribution, over destructive cerebral lesions involving subcortical white matter (Fig. 2.6.), but is generally not found with lesions restricted to the cerebral cortex itself (Rhee, Goldensohn, and Kim, 1975; Gloor, Ball, and Schaul, 1977). It may be found either unilaterally or bilaterally in patients with thalamic tumors, but its distribution in such circumstances is somewhat variable. Thus, although diffuse irregular slow activity may be found over one hemisphere in some cases (Gloor et al, 1977), in others it may be restricted to, or more conspicuous in, the projection area of the involved thalamic nucleus (Nakamura and Ohye, 1964). Polymorphic delta activity occurs diffusely in patients with white matter encephalopathies (Gloor, Kalabay, and Giard, 1968), and following acute or extensive lesions of the upper brainstem. Unilateral lesions of the midbrain tegmentum—unlike bilateral

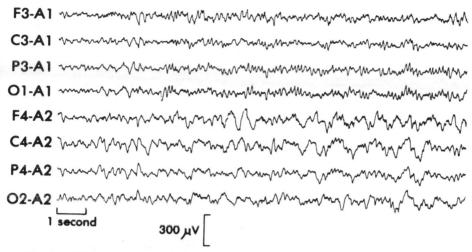

F3-A1

C3-A1

P3-A1

O1-A1

F4-A2

C4-A2

P4-A2

O2-A2

1 second

300 μV

Fig. 2.6. EEG of a 52-year-old man who had a right parietal glioma. There is a polymorphic slow wave focus in the right central region, and a diffusely slowed background.

lesions—did not, however, produce delta activity in the experimental studies performed by Gloor et al (1977) in cats.

Intermittent, Rhythmic, Delta Activity. Slow activity of this sort is paroxysmal, has a relatively constant frequency, and is usually synchronous over the two hemispheres. It is often more prominent occipitally in children (Daly, 1968) or frontally in adults (Fig. 2.7), may be enhanced by hyperventilation or drowsiness, and is usually attenuated by attention. Its origin is unclear, but it probably relates to dysfunction of subcortical centers influencing the activity of cortical neurons.

Mu Rhythm

This activity has a frequency that is usually in the alpha range, is seen over the central region of one or both hemispheres, is unaffected by eye opening, but is blocked bilaterally by movement or the thought of movement (Fig. 2.8). When present bilaterally, it is often asynchronous and there may be amplitude asymmetries between the two hemispheres. The negative portions of the waves are sharpened, while the positive portions are generally rounded. It is often associated with centrally-located beta rhythm that is also attenuated by contralateral movement. In most instances, mu rhythm has no diagnostic significance.

Lambda Waves

These are electropositive sharp waves that may occur in the occipital region in normal subjects who are looking at something in a well-illuminated field,

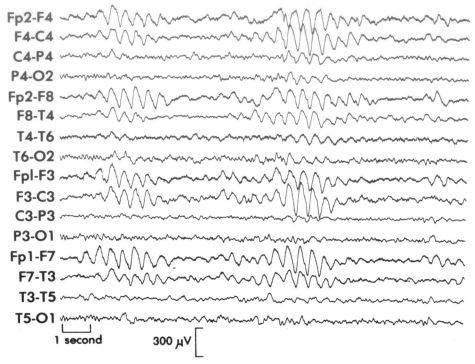

Fig. 2.7. *Frontal intermittent rhythmic delta activity recorded in the EEG of a 14-year-old boy with obstructive hydrocephalus.*

particularly if their attention and interest are aroused. Morphologically similar activity is sometimes seen during nonREM sleep. The nature of these potentials is unclear, and they have no known diagnostic significance at the present time.

Spike Discharges

As indicated earlier, one of the major uses of electroencephalography is in the investigation of patients with suspected epilepsy. In this regard, the presence in the EEG of interictal spike discharges or sharp waves is often held to be suggestive of an epileptic disturbance. A spike is arbitrarily defined as a potential having a sharp outline and a duration of 80 msec or less, while a sharp wave has a duration of between 80 and 200 msec. Since such activity may occur in nonepileptic subjects, its presence must be interpreted with caution. The distinction between epileptiform and non-epileptiform sharp transients is usually made intuitively, but Maulsby (1971) and Gloor (1975) have recently documented some of the criteria that are taken into account in such circumstances. Epileptiform transients are usually asymmetric in appearance, are frequently followed by a slow wave, have a duration that differs from that of the ongoing background activity, may be bi- or triphasic, and often occur on a background containing irregular slow elements (Fig. 2.9).

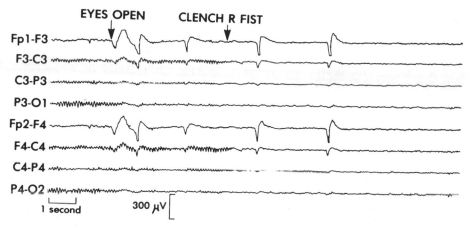

Fig. 2.8. *Bilateral mu rhythm recorded in the EEG of a 26-year-old woman with no neurologic disorder. The effect on the rhythm of clenching the right fist can be seen.*

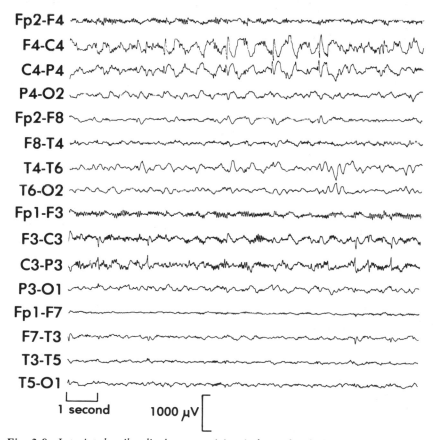

Fig. 2.9. *Interictal spike discharges arising independently in the central region of either hemisphere in the EEG of a patient with seizures since infancy.*

Paroxysmal Activity

This refers to activity which has an abrupt onset and termination, and can be clearly distinguished from the background activity. It may occur as a normal phenomenon during hyperventilation in young adults, and in response to arousal or sensory stimuli during sleep.

In pathologic circumstances, paroxysmal slow activity may result from a destructive lesion, or from pressure and concomitant distortion, affecting midline subcortical structures, and in particular the diencephalon and rostral midbrain. Intermittent rhythmic delta activity with a frontal predominance is seen. Such activity can sometimes be provoked or blocked by arousal, especially when the conscious level is depressed. Similar activity is also seen with deep frontal lesions.

In an extremely useful study, Gloor et al (1968) related EEG changes to the distribution of the pathologic process in 32 cases of diffuse encephalopathy. They found that generalized paroxysmal disturbances, consisting of either slow activity, slow wave and spike activity, or sharp transients, were seen in patients with a diffuse encephalopathic process involving predominantly the cortical and subcortical gray matter, but not when the white matter alone was involved. If both were affected, generalized paroxysmal activity occurred on a background of continuous polymorphic slow activity. Bilaterally synchronous spike and wave activity was seen in diffuse gray matter encephalopathies, and was usually more slow and irregular than is found in patients with primary epilepsy.

Paroxysmal activity of various sorts also occurs in patients without structural abnormalities. It may be found either ictally or interictally in patients with epilepsy, as is discussed in detail in a later section of this chapter, and is also encountered not infrequently in patients with metabolic disorders.

Repetitive paroxysmal slow and/or sharp wave discharges may occur with a regular periodicity in a number of conditions. Such periodic complexes are seen most conspicuously in subacute sclerosing panencephalitis, Creutzfeldt-Jakob disease, and herpes simplex encephalitis, are sometimes found in patients with liver failure (Bickford and Butt, 1955), and are also seen as a lateralized phenomena (designated "periodic lateralized epileptiform discharges" or PLEDs) in patients with hemispheric lesions due, most commonly, to cerebral infarction or tumors (Chatrian, Shaw, and Leffman, 1964; Markand and Daly, 1971). In the latter circumstances, there may be a concomitant seizure disorder, and the complexes, which usually occur every 1 to 2 seconds, generally disappear spontaneously with time. Periodic complexes that exhibit, to a greater or lesser extent, a regular rhythmicity in their occurrence may also be found in patients with cerebral lipidosis, progressive myoclonus epilepsy, anoxic encephalopathy (Pampiglione, 1962), head injury (Zappoli, 1959), subdural hematomas (Watson, Flynn, and Sullivan, 1958), occasionally after grand mal seizures (Cobb and Hill, 1950), and in rare instances in other circumstances. Their diagnostic value therefore depends upon the clinical circumstances in which they are found.

Low Voltage Records

A number of normal subjects have generally low voltage EEGs, consisting of an irregular mixture of activity with a frequency ranging between 2 and 30 Hz (Adams, 1968), and an amplitude of less than 20 μV (Adams, 1959). A little alpha activity may, however, be present at rest or during hyperventilation. Similar findings are occasionally encountered in patients with various neurologic disorders, but are of no diagnostic value.

Other EEG Patterns

Over the years, special pathologic significance has been attributed without adequate justification to a number of EEG patterns which are known to occur as a normal phenomenon in some healthy subjects, particularly during drowsiness or sleep. It seems unlikely, therefore, that such activity as 6 Hz spike and wave complexes, 14 and 6 Hz positive spikes, and so-called small sharp spikes has any useful diagnostic significance.

THE EEG RESPONSES TO SIMPLE ACTIVATING PROCEDURES

Hyperventilation

The response to hyperventilation varies considerably in different subjects, and is enhanced by hypoglycemia. Typically, there is buildup of diffuse slow activity, first in the theta and then in the delta frequency ranges, such activity settling over about 30 seconds following the conclusion of overbreathing. The response depends very much on the age of the subject, however, and in normal children or young adults it may be quite striking, with continuous or paroxysmal rhythmic, high voltage delta activity coming to dominate the EEG record. Persistence of the response for an excessive period after hyperventilation has ceased is generally regarded as abnormal, as is an asymmetric response. However, individual variability in the response to hyperventilation can make it difficult to evaluate the findings provoked by the maneuver.

In patients with cerebrovascular disease, irregular theta and delta activity appears earlier and more conspicuously on the affected side than the other, while in some instances repetitive paroxysmal discharges may be seen in a restricted distribution (Naquet et al, 1961). In patients with tumors, hyperventilation may enhance the abnormalities seen on the resting record, or provoke changes that are otherwise not apparent. Spike and wave discharges can certainly be provoked in patients with petit mal epilepsy, and also in grand mal or myoclonic epilepsy, while focal abnormalities may be enhanced in patients with partial epilepsy. Delta rhythm notched by faster activity is an occasional nonspecific finding, and should not be taken as evidence of epilepsy (Kiloh et al, 1974).

Photic Stimulation

In response to photic stimulation, it is usual to see a so-called "driving response" over the posterior regions of the head. This consists of rhythmic activity which is time-locked to the stimulus and has a frequency identical or harmonically related to that of the flickering light. A mild amplitude asymmetry is sometimes seen in normal subjects, and even when the amplitude difference between the two hemispheres is greater than 50 percent, an underlying structural lesion is unlikely if no other EEG abnormality is present. An asymmetry in the development of a driving response is more likely to be associated with focal slowing and other EEG abnormalities, and with the presence of a structural lesion, although the site of the latter may vary markedly in different subjects (Coull and Pedley, 1978).

Paroxysmal activity is sometimes found during photic stimulation, even when the EEG is otherwise normal. Polyspike discharges following each flash of light may be seen, particularly during stimulation while the eyes are closed. The discharges are muscular in origin, are most conspicuous frontally, stop when stimulation is discontinued, and may occur without clinical accompaniments although in other cases a fluttering of the eyelids is seen. Activity of this sort is generally referred to as a photomyoclonic type of response (Fig. 2.10), and is regarded as a normal response to high-intensity light stimulation, being found not uncommonly in healthy subjects (Bickford et al, 1952). It must be distinguished from the photoconvulsive response (Fig. 2.10) that occurs in some epileptic patients, particularly those with generalized seizures, and in occasional patients with diverse CNS and metabolic disorders (Klass and Fischer-Williams, 1976). This consists of bursts of slow wave and spike or polyspike activity that have a discharge frequency unrelated to that of the flashing light, and may outlast the stimulus; the activity is cerebral in origin and is usually generalized, bilaterally symmetrical, and bisynchronous, although it may have a frontocentral emphasis. It is sometimes associated with such clinical phenomena as speech arrest, transient absence, or deviation of the eyes or head, and if photic stimulation is continued a generalized seizure may result. Similar activity can occur with a more restricted distribution in the occipital region, particularly in patients with an epileptogenic lesion in that area.

Natural Sleep

The electrophysiologic changes that occur during sleep are discussed in Chapter 16, and only brief mention of them will be made here. As the patient becomes drowsy (Stage 1), the alpha rhythm becomes attenuated and the EEG is characterized mainly by theta and beta rhythms. During light sleep (Stage 2) theta activity becomes more conspicuous, and single or repetitive vertex sharp transients may occur spontaneously or in response to sensory stimuli. Bursts of high voltage biphasic slow waves may also occur either spontaneously or following sensory stimuli, and these so-called K-complexes are often associated

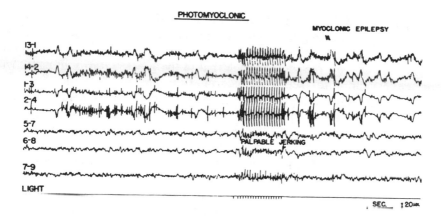

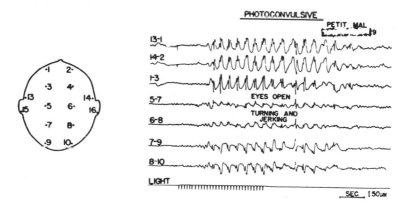

Fig. 2.10. Comparison of photomyoclonic and photoconvulsive responses to photic stimulation (from Bickford, R. G., Sem-Jacobsen, C. W., White, P. T. and Daly, D. 1952. Electroencephalogr. Clin. Neurophysiol., 4, 275).

with bursts of diffuse 12 to 14 Hz activity which are referred to as sleep spindles. The spindles are usually most prominent in the central regions and may occur independently of the K-complexes. Positive occipital sharp transients may also occur sponaneously, either singly or repetitively, during this stage of sleep. As sleep deepens, the EEG slows further until up to 50 to 60 percent (Stage 3), or more (Stage 4) of the record consists of irregular delta activity at 2 Hz or less. During REM sleep, the heart and respiratory rates become irregular, irregular eye movements occur, and the EEG comes to resemble that of Stage 1 sleep.

As already indicated, the EEG is sometimes recorded during sleep or following a period of sleep deprivation, especially when patients with suspected epilepsy are being evaluated. The incidence of epileptiform discharges is certainly increased when the EEG is recorded during sleep as well as during wakefulness, and the additional yield is greatest when patients with suspected psychomotor seizures are being investigated (Merlis, Grossman, and Henriksen, 1951). However, the yield is such that in the great majority of cases with suspected psychomotor seizures, recording during sleep is unnecessary, at least as a routine procedure (Gloor et al, 1957; Gloor, Tsai, and Haddad, 1958). Thus, in a recent study, Currie et al (1971) found that recording during sleep provided findings of diagnostic significance in only 6 percent of cases after one or more routine EEGs obtained during wakefulness were negative. Slow, atypical, spike and wave discharges are usually more conspicuous during sleep (Gastaut et al, 1966; Markand, 1977), but this is not always the case. Blume, David, and Gomez (1973), for example, found that sleep augmented slow spike and wave activity in 12 cases, had no effect in 7, and diminished it in 2. Focal spike discharges can be enhanced or precipitated during any stage of nonREM sleep, but most interictal epileptiform discharges—whether focal or generalized—are usually seen less frequently during REM sleep (Finley, 1972). Classical 3 Hz slow wave and spike activity is seen more often but is less well-organized during nonREM sleep than during wakefulness, while during REM sleep it occurs less frequently but is similar in form, rhythmicity, and regularity to its appearance in the waking record (Ross, Johnson, and Walter, 1966).

Thus, recording during sleep can be useful on occasions, although interpretation of EEGs obtained in such circumstances can be complicated by difficulty in determining whether particular findings represent normal electrical accompaniments of sleep or are of pathologic significance. Indeed, Niedermeyer (1966) has stressed that abnormal epileptiform activity may sometimes be associated with, and distributed like, K-complexes.

Sleep Deprivation

Sleep deprivation is also a harmless activating procedure and is, therefore, undertaken in many laboratories. Mattson, Pratt, and Calverley (1965) studied 89 patients with seizures of various sorts who had normal or equivocal resting interictal EEGs, reexamining them electrophysiologically after they had been deprived of sleep for 26 to 28 hours. They found that 30 patients (34 percent) showed clear activation of spike-wave, focal spike, or electrographic seizure activity, and these abnormalities could not be related to drowsiness or sleep. Pratt et al (1968) similarly investigated 114 epileptic patients with normal or equivocal interictal EEGs, performing a second recording after sleep deprivation for 24 to 26 hours. Activation occurred in 41 percent of cases, abnormalities consisting usually of focal spikes or sharp waves, or spike and wave complexes. This increased diagnostic yield was attributed to the effect of increasing the EEG sampling time by the additional record in 18 percent of these cases, to sleep or drowsiness in 28 percent, and to activation of the EEG by sleep deprivation itself in the remainder.

EEG FINDINGS IN PATIENTS WITH NEUROLOGIC DISORDERS

Epilepsy

Although the EEG is recorded from a very restricted portion of the brain and for only a limited time, it is an invaluable adjunct to the management of patients with epilepsy. The recording of electrocerebral activity during one of the patient's clinical attacks may be particularly helpful in determining whether the attacks are indeed epileptic in nature, and whether they have a focal origin. Since attacks usually occur unpredictably, however, the chances of a recording actually being in progress during an attack are not particularly good unless prolonged recordings are made or attacks are deliberately provoked. Moreover, even if an attack can be recorded, the EEG may be so obscured by muscle and movement artifact that little useful information can be gained from it.

Fortunately, the interictal EEG is also abnormal in many patients, and exhibits features that help to establish the diagnosis. In this connection, the presence of paroxysmal activity consisting of spike, polyspike, or sharp wave discharges, either alone or in association with slow waves, is of prime importance. Such epileptiform activity may be focal, multifocal, or diffuse, and may appear unilaterally or bilaterally; if bilateral it may be synchronous or asynchronous, and symmetrical or asymmetrical. When multiple foci are present, three principal types of relationship may exist between them (Lugaresi and Pazzaglia, 1975). First, one of the foci may be the primary one, generating a mirror focus in the homologous region of the contralateral hemisphere. Second, there may be a single deep focus that discharges to homologous regions of the cortex, and in such circumstances the EEG may reveal either a focus that shifts from side to side, or bilaterally synchronous discharges (Jasper, Pertuisset, and Flanigin, 1951). Finally, the epileptogenic foci may be distinct from each other, with discharges occurring from them asynchronously. In a study of patients with independent multifocal spike discharges in the EEG, Noriega-Sanchez and Markand (1976) found that most had extensive, bilateral cerebral lesions, and that clinical seizures of different types could be associated with this type of EEG appearance.

Epileptiform activity is an occasional finding in subjects who have never experienced a seizure, and its presence must not be taken as establishing in itself a diagnosis of epilepsy. Similarly, a normal interictal record does not exclude a diagnosis of epilepsy. Such a diagnosis must be based on clinical judgement, and the electrophysiologic findings can only be interpreted in a supportive way in the context of the case. In interpreting the EEG findings it must also be borne in mind that anticonvulsant medication may influence them by reducing, or in some cases—surprisingly—by enhancing, paroxysmal epileptiform activity, and by causing excessive fast and/or slow activity to appear in the background.

In discussing the EEG findings in patients with seizure disorders, an attempt has been made to follow the international classification of the epilepsies as published in *Epilepsia* (1970). Not all types of seizure will be considered, attention being confined instead to the more common varieties that are encountered in clinical practice. Furthermore, the basic mechanisms underlying the epileptic phenomena to be described will not be discussed as they are beyond the scope of this book.

Primary Generalized Epilepsy. The background activity of the interictal record is usually relatively normal, although some posterior slow (theta and delta) activity may be present in patients with petit mal epilepsy. Generalized, bilaterally symmetrical and bisynchronous paroxysmal epileptiform activity is often seen, especially during such activation procedures as hyperventilation or photic stimulation. In patients with absences of the petit mal type, this paroxysmal activity consists of well-organized 2.5 to 3 Hz slow wave and spikes (Fig. 2.11) which may be seen both interictally—especially during hyperventilation—and ictally, while in patients with myoclonic attacks bursts of spike or polyspike and wave activity are found. In those with tonic-clonic (grand mal) seizures, generalized, bilaterally synchronous spike discharges and/or bursts of slow wave and spike or polyspike activity may be seen interictally (Fig. 2.12), the latter sometimes being identical to that found in petit mal.

The earliest change during a tonic-clonic convulsion is often the appearance of low voltage fast activity. This then becomes slower, more conspicuous and more extensive in distribution and, depending upon the recording technique, may take the form of multiple spike or repetitive sharp wave discharges that have a frequency of about 10 Hz and are seen during the tonic phase of the attack. In other instances, seizure activity may be initiated by a flattening (desynchronization) of electrocerebral activity, or by paroxysmal activity such as occurs in the interictal period. In any event, as the seizure continues into the clonic phase there is a buildup of slow waves and the EEG comes to be characterized by slow activity with associated spike or polyspike discharges. Following the attack the EEG may revert to its pre-ictal state, although there is usually a transient attenuation of electrocerebral activity. Irregular polymorphic slow activity is then seen and may persist for several hours or even longer, while in a few cases the EEG is characterized by periodic complexes (Cobb and Hill, 1950).

As already indicated, generalized, bilaterally symmetrical and bisynchronous slow wave and spike activity is the expected finding in patients with primary generalized epilepsy, but it may also be found in the secondary form. Indeed, similar bilaterally synchronous activity may occasionally arise from a unilateral cortical focus, particularly on the medial surface of the hemisphere, and this is referred to as secondary bilateral synchrony (Tükel and Jasper, 1952). In such circumstances, the paroxysmal activity usually has a faster or slower frequency than that of the 2.5 to 3 Hz activity seen in primary generalized epilepsy, and the form and relationship of the spike to the wave component of the complex is less regular. Moreover, there may be an asymmetry of amplitude and wave form between the hemispheres, the activity being

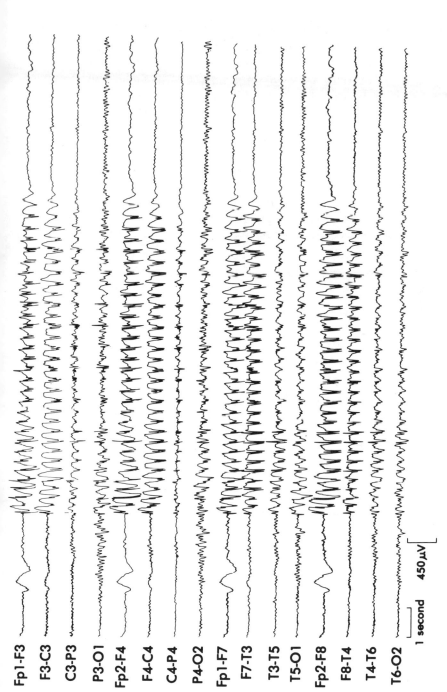

Fp1-F3
F3-C3
C3-P3
P3-O1
Fp2-F4
F4-C4
C4-P4
P4-O2
Fp1-F7
F7-T3
T3-T5
T5-O1
Fp2-F8
F8-T4
T4-T6
T6-O2

1 second 450μV

Fig. 2.11. Paroxysmal, generalized, bilaterally synchronous and symmetrical 2.5–3 Hz slow wave and spike activity recorded interictally in the EEG of a patient with generalized seizures of the petit mal type.

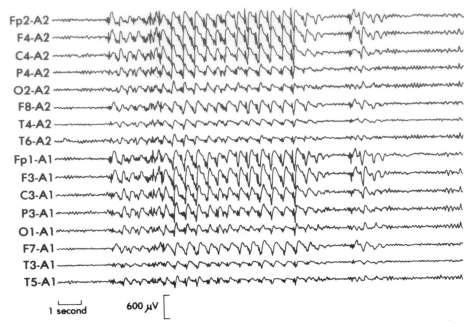

Fp2-A2
F4-A2
C4-A2
P4-A2
O2-A2
F8-A2
T4-A2
T6-A2
Fp1-A1
F3-A1
C3-A1
P3-A1
O1-A1
F7-A1
T3-A1
T5-A1

1 second   600 μV

Fig. 2.12. Paroxysmal, generalized, bilaterally synchronous, slow wave and spike or polyspike discharges seen interictally in the EEG of a 62-year-old woman with tonic-clonic seizures due to primary generalized epilepsy.

either more or less conspicuous on the affected side. Recognition of the cortical origin of such activity is facilitated when isolated focal discharges from one side precede the bursts of bilaterally synchronous activity, but can otherwise be difficult unless the paroxysmal discharges have a focal or lateralized onset. It has been suggested that when patients are being evaluated for possible surgical treatment of epilepsy, the intra-arterial injection of amobarbital or pentylenetetrazol may sometimes be useful in determining whether independent bilateral spike discharges, or generalized, bilaterally synchronous paroxysmal discharges, have a unilateral dependence. Studies of this type are potentially hazardous, however, and often fail to provide helpful information (Gloor, 1975).

Bilaterally synchronous wave and spike activity may also be seen in rare instances in patients with structural subtentorial or midline lesions (Ajmone Marsan and Lewis, 1960), in unselected nonepileptic patients (Zivin and Ajmone Marsan, 1968), and in the clinically unaffected sibs of patients with primary generalized epilepsy (Metrakos and Metrakos, 1961).

Secondary Generalized Epilepsy. In patients with secondary generalized epilepsy (such as the Lennox-Gastaut syndrome) the background activity of the interictal EEG is usually abnormal, containing an excess of diffuse theta or delta activity which is poorly responsive to eye opening and which may show a focal or lateralized emphasis. Single or independent multiple spike discharges may also be found (Markand, 1977). However, interictal paroxysmal activity characteristically consists of wave and spike or polyspike discharges that are usually slower and less well organized than in the primary generalized epilepsies, having a frequency that varies between 1 and 4 Hz but is usually about 2 Hz (Fig. 2.13). This activity exhibits a characteristic irregularity in frequency, amplitude, morphology, and distribution in different paroxysms (Markand, 1977). In some instances it is generalized and exhibits bilateral symmetry and synchrony, while in others it is markedly asymmetric, showing a clear emphasis over one hemisphere or even over a discrete portion of that hemisphere (Gastaut et al., 1966). This variability may be seen in individual subjects, often during the course of the same examination. Hyperventilation and flicker stimulation are generally much less effective as activating agents than in the primary epilepsies, but nonREM sleep can certainly increase the frequency of the paroxysmal discharges (Gastaut et al, 1966; Markand, 1977).

Such paroxysmal activity may also occur as an ictal phenomenon accompanying absence attacks. However, the most common EEG changes associated with clinical seizures are a relative or total desynchronization (flattening), with sudden disappearance of any ongoing spike-wave activity, or the development of rhythmic activity (usually at about 10 Hz, or faster) which increases in amplitude, has a focal or generalized distribution, and is followed by irregular slow waves; in some instances, an initial desynchronization of the traces is followed by this rhythmic activity. Tonic seizures are probably the most common type of attack experienced by patients with the Lennox-Gastaut syndrome, and they are accompanied by EEG changes of this sort, as is shown in Figure 2.14.

In patients with myoclonus epilepsy the background is also diffusely slowed, and bursts of spikes, polyspikes or sharp waves, or of spikes and slow waves, are seen either uni- or bilaterally. Flicker stimulation may lead to bursts of wave and spike or polyspike activity. The spike activity may or may not be time-locked to the myoclonic jerking which the patient exhibits.

Partial Epilepsy. There may be considerable variability in the interictal EEG findings at different times in patients with partial (focal) epilepsy, and especially those with complex symptomatology. The interictal record (Fig. 2.9) may

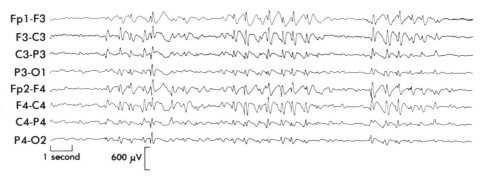

Fig. 2.13. Interictal 2 Hz spike and wave activity in the EEG of a 17-year-old boy with the Lennox-Gastaut syndrome.

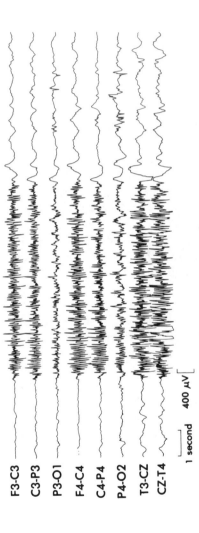

Fig. 2.14. Tonic seizure recorded in the EEG of an 11-year-old girl with the Lennox-Gastaut syndrome.

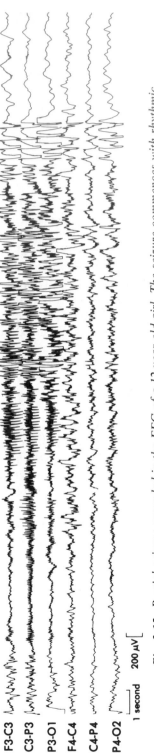

Fig. 2.15. Partial seizure recorded in the EEG of a 12-year-old girl. The seizure commences with rhythmic left-sided fast activity that increases in amplitude and becomes intermixed with slower elements, with some spread to the contralateral hemisphere. Slow waves with some associated spike discharges occur in the later part of the seizure, and this is followed by lower voltage, diffuse slow activity with a left-sided emphasis. Clinically, the seizure was characterized by clonic jerking of the right face and limbs, followed by unresponsiveness as slow activity became conspicuous in the later part of the trace.

exhibit intermittent focal sharp waves or spikes; continuous or paroxysmal focal slow activity; localized paroxysmal slow waves with associated spike discharges; or any combination of these features. Bilaterally synchronous spike and wave activity is an occasional finding; and unless it is markedly asymmetrical, has a focal onset, or is preceded by focal or lateralized discharges, it can be difficult to distinguish from the similar activity that is seen in patients with primary generalized epilepsy when it is presumed to relate to pathophysiologic changes in subcortical structures.

In patients with temporal lobe abnormalities, spike discharges may be confined to one hemisphere, may be found either independently or synchronously over both hemispheres, or may occur in the homologous region of both hemispheres with a consistent temporal relationship between the spikes. In the latter case it is presumed that the discharge originates from one side and spreads to the other via commissural connections such as the corpus callosum to produce a so-called mirror focus which eventually becomes independent of the original focus. Accordingly, it is sometimes impossible to localize the abnormality with any certainty. Jasper et al (1951), for example, found that in about 40 percent of cases lateralization was difficult or impossible.

Interictal abnormalities may be provoked by such harmless activation procedures as hyperventilation, sleep, or sleep deprivation (pp. 37–40), but flicker stimulation is unhelpful in most patients with partial epilepsy. When they arise in the anterior temporal region, they may only be recorded from nasopharyngeal or sphenoidal electrodes (p. 26). The site of focal interictal abnormalities does not necessarily correspond to the region in which seizures usually originate (Gloor, 1975), however, and this must be kept in mind when patients are being evaluated, as is discussed in Chapter 5. Moreover, the possibility of an underlying structural abnormality, such as a tumor, must also be remembered in patients with partial seizures.

In some patients, particularly those who have partial seizures with elementary symptomatology, the EEG shows no change during the ictal event. More commonly, however, the EEG shows local discharges (Fig. 2.15) or more diffuse changes during the ictal period. In some patients with complex partial seizures the ictal EEG shows a transient initial desynchronization which is either localized or diffuse and is followed by synchronous fast activity, while in others the initial flattening of the traces does not occur. In other cases rhythmic activity of variable frequency with or without associated sharp transients is seen during a seizure. The ictal discharge is often succeeded by a transient flattening of the traces, and then by slow activity which may have a localized distribution. If focal slow activity is present, the EEG examination may have to be repeated after several days to distinguish postictal slowing from that due to a structural lesion.

When partial seizures become generalized as a secondary phenomenon, patients usually go on to experience a tonic-clonic convulsion, and focal EEG abnormalities are then replaced by the more diffuse changes occurring during such seizures.

Status Epilepticus. In tonic-clonic status the EEG findings during the seizures are not substantially different from those seen during a single seizure, but the interictal background is usually—but not always—abnormal, with an excess of irregular, asynchronous, diffuse slow activity. In absence (petit mal) status, continuous or intermittent bursts of generalized, bilaterally symmetrical and synchronous slow wave and spike discharges are seen with a frontal emphasis. Their frequency is usually about 3 Hz, but they are sometimes much slower than this. The discharges may, however, be more irregular, and polyspikes rather than single spikes may be contained in the complexes.

Epilepsia partialis continua may be regarded as a variety of partial status epilepticus, and is characterized clinically by rhythmic clonic movements of a group of muscles. Thomas, Reagan, and Klass (1977) reported the EEG findings in 32 patients with this disorder, in 28 of whom at least one recording was made during the ictal activity. In 2 patients no abnormalities were detected, and others have also reported that the EEG may be normal. Epileptiform abnormalities may, however, have been obscured by the background rhythms, or by muscle or movement artifact; alternatively, they may not have been detected because they arose from infolded regions of the cortex and were therefore not picked up by the recording scalp electrodes. Focal EEG abnormalities, that were sometimes enhanced by hyperventilation, were present in 21 patients, and consisted of abnormal slow waves in 19, and/or sharp transients in 20. It was sometimes possible to identify a relationship between the EEG and muscle activity when the frequency of the jerking was slow (Fig. 2.16). In 25 patients the background activity was abnormally slow or asymmetric, and in 4 patients periodic lateralized epileptiform discharges were seen.

Radiotelemetry permits the EEG to be relayed by a small radio transmitter placed on the patient's scalp to recording equipment in the EEG laboratory.

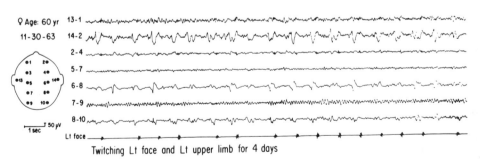

Fig. 2.16. EEG of 60-year-old woman with epilepsia partialis continua. Lowermost channel shows myogenic activity from clonic movements recorded by surface leads on left side of face. Sharp waves in EEG arise from right temporoparietal region and precede each of the muscle contractions, but occasional sharp waves occur without subsequent muscle contraction. Normal alpha rhythm is attenuated in the right parieto-occipital region (from Thomas, J. E., Reagan, T. J., and Klass, D. W. 1977. Arch. Neurol., 34, 266. Copyright 1977, American Medical Association).

The patient is allowed to move unrestricted about the ward but is continuously monitored by closed-circuit television while the EEG is recorded for prolonged periods. The technique can be helpful in determining whether a patient is experiencing attacks that are organic or functional in nature, in assessing the frequency of seizure activity, and in attempting to localize an epileptogenic source, but it is undertaken in only a few medical centers at the present time.

Value of EEG in Management of Patients with Epilepsy. In addition to the help that they provide in supporting a clinical diagnosis of epilepsy and excluding an underlying structural cause of the seizures, the EEG findings are useful in a number of other ways with regard to the management of patients with epilepsy. They are an important aid to the clinician who is attempting to classify the seizure disorder of individual patients, and may, therefore, influence the choice of anticonvulsant drugs that are prescribed. For example, difficulty sometimes arises in distinguishing clinically between certain types of partial seizure, petit mal attacks, and the so-called atypical absences that occur in patients with the Lennox-Gastaut syndrome, unless the EEG findings are taken into account. Again, the EEG may enable a focal or lateralized epileptogenic source to be identified, even when it is not apparent on clinical grounds, and this may be of prime importance when the etiology or surgical treatment of the disorder is under consideration. Further comment on this aspect is made in Chapter 5.

The EEG is particularly helpful in the diagnosis of absence (petit mal) and temporal lobe status epilepticus, and indeed it is often the only means that permits these diagnoses to be made with any confidence. In patients who are in tonic-clonic (grand mal) status, EEG monitoring can similarly be invaluable when there is clinical uncertainty as to whether or not seizure activity is continuing.

The EEG can provide a limited guide to the prognosis of patients with epilepsy. Thus, an EEG which is normal, and remains so following the standard activation procedures discussed earlier, generally implies a more favorable prognosis than otherwise, although this is not always supported by the outcome in individual cases. Again, in patients with absence attacks, slow spike and wave discharges suggest a poorer prognosis than bilaterally symmetrical and bisynchronous 3 Hz slow wave and spike activity, and the presence of abnormal background activity also implies a poor prognosis (Sato, Dreifuss, and Penry, 1976). The EEG findings have, however, proved to be disappointingly unreliable as a means of determining the prognosis for the subsequent development of seizures in children experiencing their first febrile convulsion, or in patients with head injuries. Considerable emphasis is sometimes placed on the EEG findings when the feasibility of withdrawing anticonvulsant drugs is under consideration after epileptic patients have been seizure-free for some years. However, the EEG provides no more than a guide to the outlook in such circumstances, and patients can certainly have further attacks after withdrawal of medication despite a normal EEG or, conversely, remain seizure-free despite a continuing EEG disturbance. Such decisions must, therefore, be based on clinical grounds, the context of individual cases being taken into account as well as the EEG findings.

Infections

In most of the acute meningitides and viral encephalitides, the EEG is characterized by diffuse slow activity, although focal abnormalities may sometimes be found as well. These findings are, therefore, not really helpful for diagnostic purposes, although they may be useful in following the course of the disorder, especially if the clinical features are relatively inconspicuous. The presence of focal abnormalities raises the possibility that an abscess is developing, although localized electrical abnormalities may also arise for other reasons, such as secondary vascular changes or scarring. In the chronic meningitides the EEG may show little change, although in other instances diffuse slowing is found. Again, the findings are sometimes helpful in following the course of the disorder.

In herpes simplex encephalitis the findings may be more specific, as was stressed particularly by Upton and Gumpert (1970). Superimposed on a generally slow background, repetitive slow wave complexes are seen over one or both hemispheres, particularly in the temporal regions, between the 2nd and 15th days of the illness. The interval between successive complexes is usually between 1 and 4 seconds, and the presence of such complexes bilaterally implies a more serious outlook. In time the amplitude of the repetitive complexes becomes less conspicuous until they can no longer be recognized, and as necrosis occurs the EEG becomes attenuated over the affected region. These changes may have considerable diagnostic value in suggesting the possibility of herpes simplex encephalitis when found during the course of an acute cerebral illness, and if not found initially the EEG examination should be repeated daily to allow their presence to be detected. They are not, however, an invariable finding (Illis and Taylor, 1972), and their absence does not exclude the possibility of this disorder.

Subacute Sclerosing Panencephalitis. Recurrent slow wave complexes, sometimes with associated sharp transients, occur in this disease (Fig. 2.17). The complexes usually last for up to 3 seconds (Cobb, 1966), but their form may show considerable variation in different patients or in the same patients at different times, as also may the interval—usually 4 to 14 seconds—between successive complexes. In most instances they have a generalized distribution and occur simultaneously over the two hemispheres, but in the early stages of the illness they are sometimes more conspicuous over one or the other side. Occasionally they seem to disappear for a time, but this is unusual except in the terminal stages of the illness (Markand and Panszi, 1975). When myoclonic jerking is a clinical feature of the patient's illness, the jerks are usually time-related to the periodic complexes, occurring just before or after them (Cobb, 1966; Markand and Panszi, 1975). Although the background EEG activity is sometimes relatively normal, it is generally characterized by reduction or loss

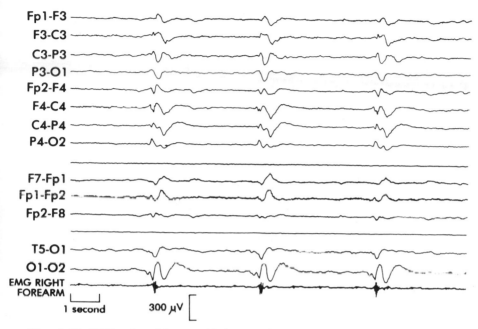

Fig. 2.17. EEG of a 16-year-old boy with SSPE of 8 months' duration. Generalized slow wave complexes are seen to occur approximately every 4 seconds, and last for up to 1 second. Each complex is accompanied by a brief EMG discharge from the right forearm extensor muscles.

of alpha rhythm, and the presence of diffuse slow activity. Randomly occurring spikes or sharp waves may be found, especially in the frontal regions, as may bilaterally synchronous spike and wave activity or rhythmic frontal delta activity (Markand and Panszi, 1975). Transient, relative quiescence of the background following a complex is an occasional finding.

Creutzfeldt-Jakob Disease. In this disorder the EEG is also characterized by periodic complexes occurring on a diffusely abnormal, slowed background (Fig. 2.18). The complexes are rather different from those occurring in subacute sclerosing panencephalitis, however, consisting of brief waves of rather variable—often triphasic—form and sharpened outline that recur about once every second and may show a temporal relationship to the myoclonic jerking that patients often exhibit. This periodic activity is usually present diffusely and is then bilaterally synchronous, but it may have a more restricted distribution in early stages of the disorder.

Abscess. In patients with cerebral abscess, the EEG is characterized by low frequency, high amplitude, polymorphic focal slow activity such as is shown in Figure 2.6. Depending on the degree to which consciousness is depressed, however, these changes are sometimes obscured by a more generalized slow wave disturbance.

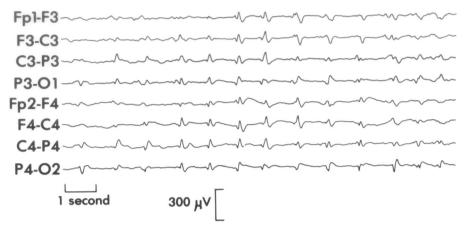

Fig. 2.18. *Repetitive complexes, often triphasic in form, occurring about once every second on a rather featureless background in the EEG of a 66-year-old patient with Creutzfeldt-Jakob disease.*

Vascular Lesions

In considering the changes that occur in patients with vascular lesions of the nervous system, it must be borne in mind that the findings at electroencephalography fail to provide a reliable means of distinguishing such lesions from other types of structural pathology, such as cerebral tumors, or even of distinguishing the underlying pathologic basis of the vascular disturbance, and this limits the utility of the technique. Only a brief description will, therefore, be provided, and the interested reader is referred to the recent review of Van Der Drift (1972) for more detailed information.

In patients with cerebral ischemia due to occlusive disease of major vessels, the normal background activity is often depressed in the affected portion of the hemisphere, and a slow (theta and/or delta) wave disturbance may be found, sometimes associated with sharp transients or PLEDs. Changes are usually most conspicuous in the ipsilateral mid-temporal and centroparietal region in cases with involvement of the middle cerebral or internal carotid artery, in the frontal region when the anterior cerebral artery is affected, and the occipital region when the posterior cerebral artery is occluded. The topographic extent of these changes varies in individual patients, however, depending on such factors as the site of the occlusion, the rapidity of its development, and the adequacy of the collateral circulation. The EEG may revert to normal with time despite a persisting clinical deficit, but sharp transients become more conspicuous in some cases. In patients with ischemia restricted to the internal capsule, the EEG is usually normal or shows only minor changes. Similarly in patients with vertebrobasilar ischemia, the EEG is often normal, although it may be of low voltage (Niedermeyer, 1963) and show other equivocal changes. In some cases of infarction of the lower brainstem (Fig. 2.19), however, activity in the alpha frequency range is more widely distributed than normal and fails to respond to sensory stimuli (Chase, Moretti, and Prensky, 1968). With involve-

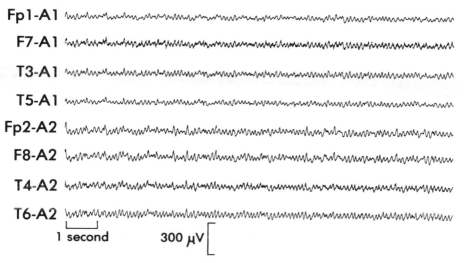

Fig. 2.19. *Generalized, rhythmic 9–10 Hz activity, unresponsive to sensory stimuli, in the EEG of a 68-year-old woman following cardiopulmonary arrest. Similar findings may also be encountered in patients with infarction of the lower brainstem.*

ment of more rostral brainstem regions and of the diencephalon, the EEG is characterized by predominant slow activity which is often organized into discrete, bilaterally synchronous runs without constant lateralization.

In patients with intracerebral hematomas, the extent of the EEG changes depends upon the site and size of the hematoma, and the rapidity of its development. Background activity is depressed over part or all of the affected side, and focal polymorphic delta activity is seen. Especially in the elderly, this slow activity is sometimes localized preferentially to the temporal region, irrespective of the site of the lesion. Sharp transients are seen more commonly than in patients with nonhemorrhagic vascular lesions, especially in the temporal region, and intermittent bilateral rhythmic delta activity may also be found, especially where there is secondary displacement of brainstem structures. EEG changes are often inconspicuous in patients with hemorrhage into the lower brainstem, but there may be widespread, nonreactive alpha-like activity. Cerebellar hemorrhage is associated with little—if any—change unless tonsillar herniation complicates the clinical picture, when diffuse slowing results.

The EEG findings in patients with cerebral venous or venous sinus thrombosis are similar to, but often more extensive than, those in patients with occlusive arterial disease. When the superior sagittal sinus is involved the changes are usually bilateral, often variable, and frequently asymmetrical (Van Der Drift, 1972).

Subarachnoid Hemorrhage. Although the EEG may be normal, diffuse slowing is a common finding, especially in patients with clouding of consciousness. Focal abnormalities may also be seen, and can relate either to the presence of a local hematoma, to the source of hemorrhage, especially when this is an angioma, or to secondary ischemia by arterial spasm.

Subdural Hematoma. The background activity is often either reduced in amplitude or virtually abolished over the affected hemisphere in patients with a chronic subdural hematoma (Fig. 2.20). In other instances, however, a focal ipsilateral slow wave disturbance is the most conspicuous abnormality, and there may be little suppression of background rhythms. In either case, generalized changes, such as intermittent frontal rhythmic delta activity, may be present as well, due to brainstem distortion. Repetitive periodic complexes have also been described in rare cases (Watson et al, 1958).

Since the EEG is sometimes normal in patients with a chronic subdural hematoma, the possibility of such a lesion cannot be excluded just because the electrical findings are unremarkable. Indeed, even when abnormalities are found, it can sometimes be difficult, if not impossible, to localize the lesion with any certainty, due to interplay of the various changes described above (Millar, 1959). Moreover, electroencephalography does not permit reliable distinction to be made between chronic subdural hematoma and other space-occupying lesions. In all instances, therefore, detailed neuroradiologic assessment is necessary if cases are to be managed correctly.

Intracranial Aneurysms and Arteriovenous Malformations. Focal slow activity is an occasional finding in patients with aneurysms, but in uncomplicated cases there is often little to find in the EEG. Following subarachnoid hemorrhage, focal or lateralized abnormalities are sometimes present and may provide a guide to the site of bleeding (Margerison, Binnie and McCaul, 1970).

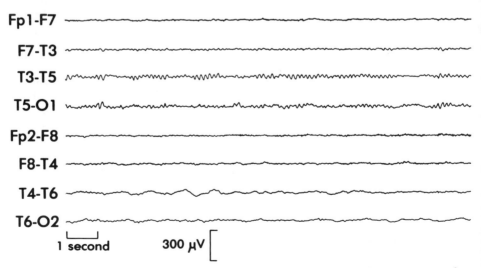

Fig. 2.20. Focal slowing in the right posterior quadrant and suppression of normal background rhythms over this side in the EEG of a patient with a suspected right subdural hematoma.

Focal slow and/or epileptiform activity may be found in the EEG of patients with intracranial angiomas.

Sturge-Weber Syndrome. Together with depression of normal background activity and of the responses to hyperventilation and photic stimulation, over the affected hemisphere, irregular slow activity and sharp transients are often seen (Brenner and Sharbrough, 1976). The reduction in background activity does not necessarily relate to the presence and degree of intracranial calcification. Abnormalities sometimes have a more generalized distribution that can be confusing, but in such circumstances they are commonly more conspicuous over the involved side.

Migraine

Electroencephalography has little relevance to the diagnosis of migraine, and in the author's view is probably best reserved for patients with migraine of late onset, those with headaches consistently localized to the same side, or those with other symptoms or signs that might be suggestive of an underlying structural lesion. In uncomplicated cases, the EEG is usually normal, or shows only minor nonspecific changes, between and during migrainous attacks. Focal or unilateral slow wave disturbances are not uncommon, however, particularly in patients developing lateralized aura or neurologic deficits in association with their attacks. Such localized abnormalities usually settle rapidly once the clinical disturbance has resolved, unless infarction has occurred or there is an underlying structural abnormality. Paroxysmal activity is sometimes found, but the proportion of cases with such a disturbance varies greatly in different series, as can be seen if the findings of Selby and Lance (1960) are compared with those of Hockaday and Whitty (1969). Its occurrence does not appear to be a secondary result of repeated attacks, but is thought to represent a primary phenomenon (Hockaday and Whitty, 1969).

Tumors

Tumors may affect the EEG by causing compression, displacement, or destruction of nervous tissue, by interfering with local blood supply, or by leading to an obstructive hydrocephalus. There is considerable variation in the presence, nature, and extent of abnormalities in different subjects, however, and this seems to depend, at least in part, upon the size and rate of growth of the tumor, and the age of the individual patient. An abnormal record is more likely to be found in patients with a supratentorial tumor than an infratentorial one, and in patients with a rapidly expanding tumor than a slowly growing lesion. Again, abnormalities are often more conspicuous in children than in adults. Even if the EEG is abnormal, however, the changes may be generalized rather than focal, so that they are not particularly helpful in the diagnosis or localization of the underlying neoplasm.

Diffuse abnormalities are common in all patients with cerebral tumors when conscious level is depressed, and in this context they are, therefore, particularly likely in patients with infratentorial lesions. In addition to diffuse slowing, intermittent bilateral rhythmic delta activity may be seen with a frontal emphasis in adults, or more posteriorly in children, and is indicative of brainstem dysfunction. In these circumstances, localization of the tumor on EEG grounds is often less feasible than at an earlier period in the natural history, although a gross asymmetry of such activity between the two hemispheres will raise the possibility of a lateralized hemispheric lesion. Earlier records sometimes permit more definite localization, but they may show only subtle changes that are easily missed.

Depression of electrical activity over a discrete region of the brain is a reliable local sign of an underlying cerebral lesion, but this may be masked by volume conduction of activity from adjacent areas. The presence of a focal slow wave disturbance (Fig. 2.21) is also important, although such an abnormality has less localizing significance when it is found over the temporal lobe. Focal ictal or interictal sharp activity is of some, but lesser, localizing value unless it is associated with an underlying focal slow wave disturbance. A number of other abnormalities have been described in patients with discrete cerebral lesions, including an asymmetry of drug-induced fast activity, a local increase in beta activity, or the presence of a mu rhythm, but these findings are of much lesser significance, and can anyway lead to difficulty in determining which of the two sides is the abnormal one.

In assessing the findings in patients with suspected brain tumors, it must be borne in mind that the main value of the EEG is in indicating which patients require more detailed investigation. Its value in this regard is limited, however, since a normal or equivocal EEG does not exclude the possibility of a tumor, and there are no abnormalities which will allow the differentiation of neoplastic

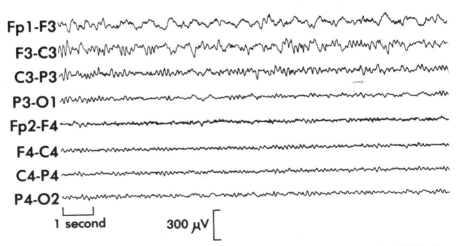

Fig. 2.21. Polymorphic slow activity in the left frontal region in the EEG of a 62-year-old man with a glioma.

lesions from other localized structural disorders, such as an abscess or infarct. Moreover, the EEG can provide no information about the nature of the tumor in individual cases, and the findings in patients with tumors of different histologic types or in different locations will not, therefore, be discussed. It is relevant to note, however, that deep-seated supratentorial tumors may produce no abnormalities whatsoever at an early stage, and that the EEG is likely to be normal in patients with pituitary tumors unless the lesion has extended beyond the pituitary fossa or has caused hormonal changes.

Tuberous Sclerosis

There are no pathognomonic EEG features of tuberous sclerosis, but epileptiform activity, or changes suggestive of space occupying lesion, may be found. The EEG is often normal in mild cases, but in others focal slow and/or sharp wave disturbances are seen. In more advanced cases a hypsarrhythmic pattern may be seen during infancy, while in older patients the record may contain generalized slow wave and spike activity, or independent multifocal spike discharges. Thus, focal or generalized changes may be found in this disorder.

Pseudotumor Cerebri

In benign intracranial hypertension the EEG is often normal, but abnormalities, consisting of a diffusely slowed background and bursts of activity in the alpha, theta, or delta frequency ranges, are sometimes found (Mani and Townsend, 1964).

Degenerative Disorders

The EEG abnormalities found in these disorders are of little diagnostic help, and will be considered only briefly.

Spinocerebellar Degeneration. The EEG is usually normal, but focal or generalized slowing sometimes occurs. In patients with an associated seizure disorder, epileptiform activity may also be found.

Parkinsonism. Mild nonspecific changes, consisting usually of background slowing that may or may not be lateralized, are an occasional finding, but in most patients the EEG is normal.

Paroxysmal Choreoathetosis. Epileptiform activity is not a feature of the electroencephalogram in patients with this disorder, records usually being normal or showing only an excess of generalized slow activity.

Huntington's Disease. Patients characteristically have a low voltage, featureless record (Hill, 1948), in which the predominant background activity is sometimes in the beta range. Irregular slow activity may be present in some cases, however, while in others the record is normal. Paroxysmal disturbances are an occasional finding. Despite early hopes to the contrary, the EEG findings seem to have no value in determining which of the apparently unaffected offspring of patients with this inherited disorder will go on to develop the disease.

Hepatolenticular Degeneration. The EEG is normal in most cases, but in some either generalized or paroxysmal slowing is found, sometimes together with spike discharges or sharp waves. In uncomplicated cases the presence of EEG abnormalities shows no clear correlation with the clinical or biochemical state, and patients with predominantly hepatic or neural involvement show similar changes (Hansotia, Harris, and Kennedy, 1969). Abnormalities are found most often when there are complications of the disease, and improve with clinical improvement.

Presenile and Senile Dementia. The EEG in early cases may be normal. As progression occurs, however, the amount and frequency of the alpha rhythm decline, and irregular theta and slower activity appears, sometimes with a focal or unilateral emphasis, especially in the temporal region. In patients with Alzheimer's disease, Letemendia and Pampiglione (1958) found during sleep that spindles were of low amplitude and K-complexes were seen only infrequently in response to sensory stimuli, and little fast activity developed in response to barbiturates. As a general rule, abnormalities occur earlier and are much more conspicuous in Alzheimer's disease than in Pick's disease. Indeed, in the latter disorder, the EEG is often normal (Gordon and Sim, 1967).

Metabolic Disorders

The EEG has been used to detect and monitor cerebral dysfunction in patients with a variety of metabolic disorders, and changes may certainly precede any alteration in clinical status. Diffuse—rather than focal—changes characteristically occur in such patients, unless there is a preexisting or concomitant structural lesion. Typically, there is desynchronization and slowing of the alpha rhythm, with subsequent appearance of theta, and then of delta, activity. These slower rhythms may initially be episodic or paroxysmal, and are enhanced by hyperventilation. Such changes have been described in hyper- or hypoglycemia, Addison's disease, hypopituitarism, pulmonary failure, and hyperparathyroidism. In hypoparathyroidism, similar changes are found in advanced cases, but spikes, sharp waves, and slow wave-spike discharges may also be seen. Myxedema is characterized by a low voltage record in which the alpha activity is classically preserved but slowed, and there may be some intermixed theta or slower elements; these changes may pass unrecognized, however, unless premorbid records are available for comparison. In hyperthyroidism, the alpha rhythm is usually diminished in amount but increased in frequency, beta activity is often conspicuous, and scattered theta elements may be present. The findings in Cushing's disease or pheochromocytoma are usually unremarkable. (Anoxic encephalopathy: see Ch. 17.)

The EEG shows progressive changes in patients with advancing hepatic encephalopathy, and in general there is good correlation between the clinical and electrical findings (MacGillivray, 1976). In early stages the alpha rhythm slows, gradually being replaced by theta and delta activity (Bickford and Butt, 1955), but in some instances it may coexist with this slow activity (Foley, Watson, and Adams, 1950; MacGillivray, 1976). As the disorder progresses, triphasic complexes, which consist of a major positive potential, preceded and followed by smaller negative waves, usually—but not invariably—occur symmetrically and synchronously over the two hemispheres, with a frontal emphasis (Fig. 2.22). Similar complexes have been found in other metabolic disturbances such as uremia, and the periodic complexes found in a number of other conditions (p. 36) may also take the form of triphasic waves. With further clinical deterioration, the EEG in patients with hepatic encephalopathy comes to consist of continuous triphasic and slow activity which shows a marked anterior emphasis and may be interrrupted by periods of relative quies-

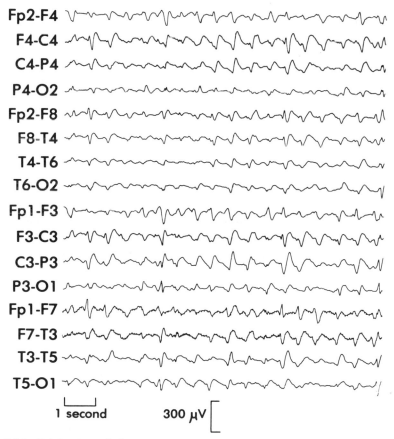

Fig. 2.22. Triphasic and slow wave activity in the EEG of a 79-year-old woman with hepatic encephalopathy.

cence. The amplitude of the slow activity gradually decreases as death approaches.

In patients with renal insufficiency the EEG may be normal initially, but the background eventually slows, theta and delta activity develop in increasing amounts and are sometimes paroxysmal, and ultimately the record is dominated by irregular slow activity that does not respond to external stimuli. Triphasic complexes are an occasional finding, but are not usually as well-formed as in hepatic encephalopathy. Spike and sharp wave discharges may also be seen in some patients. During hemodialysis, the EEG findings are often dramatic, even in patients who previously had a relatively normal record, consisting of bursts of generalized, high voltage rhythmic delta activity occurring on either a relatively normal or generally slowed background (Kennedy et al, 1963). In patients developing the progressive encephalopathy that sometimes occurs during chronic hemodialysis, the EEG contains diffuse slow activity interrupted by bilaterally synchronous complexes of slow, sharp, triphasic and spike waves (Mahurkar et al, 1973; Burks et al, 1974).

Multiple Sclerosis

Patients with multiple sclerosis not infrequently have abnormal EEGs. Focal or generalized activity in the theta and delta ranges may be found, as may diffuse or localized spike discharges. Focal changes are often evanescent, and probably relate to foci of acute demyelination. The findings are of no help in the diagnosis of the disorder, however, and usually bear little relationship to the clinical signs.

Trauma

Electroencephalography is generally undertaken to provide some guide as to the nature or severity of head injuries, the prognosis for recovery, and the likelihood of developing posttraumatic seizures. It is often also requested when patients with posttraumatic syndromes are being evaluated at a later stage, in the forlorn hope that it will provide a guide as to whether nonspecific symptoms have an organic basis, but its use in this regard has no rational basis.

There are no EEG abnormalities which develop specifically after head injury. In evaluating the findings at electroencephalography, it must be borne in mind that abnormalities may have existed prior to the injury, and also that the significance of any findings will depend in part on the time at which the study was undertaken in relation to the trauma. This is important because the correlation between clinical and electrical findings is often poor when the EEG is recorded three or more months after the injury was sustained.

The presence of a localized abnormality is often of particular concern because it may point to the existence of an intracerebral, subdural, or extradural hematoma. Unfortunately, there is no reliable way to distinguish electroencephalographically between surgically-remediable intracranial lesions—such as a subdural hematoma—and pathology that does not necessitate operative treatment. In such circumstances, of course, the judicious use of the CT scan will clearly facilitate the rational management of individual patients.

The electrical findings in individual cases depend in greater part on the patient's level of consciousness. The abnormalities that may be seen in comatose subjects will be discussed separately, and further comment on this aspect can also be found in Chapter 17. Other abnormalities that may be found following head trauma include local or generalized depression of normal activity; slowing of the alpha rhythm; focal or diffuse slow wave disturbances, especially in the temporal region in adults; and spike or paroxysmal discharges. These changes may develop progressively with time if serial recordings are undertaken. Focal abnormalities may relate directly to local injury, but may also occur as a sequel to such complications of cerebral trauma as ischemia or edema. They may initially be obscured by more generalized changes in the electroencephalogram, becoming conspicuous only as the latter diminish. Before pathologic implications can be attributed to a localized depression of electrocerebral activity, however, such extracerebral factors as subcutaneous edema or hemorrhage must be excluded by careful scrutiny of the patient. Localized or lateralized paroxysmal discharges are sometimes the sole evidence of a structural abnormality such as a hematoma, and indicate the need for further neuroradiologic investigations (Courjon and Scherzer, 1972).

Jennett and Van de Sande (1975) found that although abnormal records were more common in patients who developed seizures following head injury, the EEG findings did not improve the accuracy of predicting which patients were likely to go on to develop posttraumatic epilepsy. Patients with EEG abnormalities could remain seizure-free, while 20 percent of those who went on to develop posttraumatic epilepsy had at least one normal record in the three months following injury. Again, Courjon (1969) found that although the development of focal spike discharges was likely to be associated with the development of a posttraumatic seizure disorder, 25 percent of his patients had normal records at the time that their fits began.

Coma

Altered states of consciousness may result from many different types of disorder, and it is, therefore, hardly surprising that the EEG findings are very variable. Some of the changes that may be found have already been alluded to, and only brief reference will be made to them here. There are, however, a few general points that do require emphasis. In the first place, although the EEG changes are never specific to any particular disorder, they may certainly direct attention to diagnostic possibilities that might otherwise be overlooked. Secondly, in evaluting patients with depressed levels of consciousness, it is particularly important, both for prognostic purposes and for following the course of the disorder, that serial records are obtained. Finally, the responses evoked by external stimuli must be considered when the comatose patient is being evaluated or followed electrophysiologically. A change in electrical activity can be expected to occur following stimulation of a patient in a light coma, and this reactivity becomes inconstant, delayed, or lost as the depth of coma increases.

When consciousness is impaired the EEG becomes slowed, the degree of slowing often—but not always—corresponding to the extent to which consciousness is depressed. The slow activity may be episodic or continuous, and in the former instances often shows a frontal emphasis and bilateral synchronicity. As the depth of coma increases, the EEG becomes unresponsive to afferent stimuli, and its amplitude diminishes until eventually it becomes flat and featureless. Such a record should not be taken to indicate that irreversible brain death has occurred, because similar changes may be found in severe hypothermia or in coma due to barbiturate intoxication. Further discussion of this aspect may be found in Chapter 17. Records characterized by rhythmic generalized fast activity intermixed with slower rhythms are found in patients who have taken excessive quantities of certain drugs, particularly benzodiazepines or barbiturates (Cohn, Savage, and Raines, 1950), while in other patients the EEG may show a burst-suppression pattern (p. 535).

In some comatose patients, the EEG resembles that found during normal wakefulness, consisting predominantly of activity in the alpha frequency-range (Fig. 2.20). Such activity is distributed more widely than normal alpha rhythm, however, and unlike the latter is often unresponsive to sensory stimuli. This type of EEG has been reported particularly in patients with brainstem strokes or following cardiopulmonary arrest (Westmoreland et al, 1975), and is usually associated with a poor prognosis for survival although recovery has occurred in some instances (Chokroverty, 1975). In other instances, the EEG resembles that of stage 2 sleep, and even contains runs of 12 to 14 Hz activity resembling sleep spindles. These, however, are much more diffuse in distribution than normal sleep spindles (Courjon and Scherzer, 1972), and Chatrian, White, and Daly (1963), who described such findings in 11 comatose patients with severe head injuries, postulated that they related to functional derangement of the midbrain reticular formation.

The EEG may be diagnostically helpful in the evaluation of comatose patients. Electrographic seizure activity is sometimes found, or there may be localized changes in frequency and amplitude to suggest the presence of a structural supratentorial lesion. Repetitive complexes are seen in the EEGs of some comatose patients. The character and distribution of the complexes, the degree to which they exhibit a regular periodicity, and the interval between successive complexes may be helpful in suggesting the cause of the coma if the clinical circumstances surrounding the case are obscure. The findings in subacute sclerosing panencephalitis, Creutzfeldt-Jakob disease, herpes simplex encephalitis, and hepatic encephalopathy have already been referred to, and—as was also noted earlier—periodic complexes may be found in a number of other disorders including postanoxic coma. The burst-suppression pattern sometimes seen in the latter circumstance is considered further in Chapter 17, where the findings in de-efferented and persistent vegetative states are also discussed.

Psychiatric Disorders

Although a vast literature has accumulated on the EEG findings in patients with psychiatric disorders, there is little evidence that the EEG is of any use in the diagnosis and management of such patients, apart from when it suggests the possibility of an organic disturbance. Further comment on this subject will not, therefore, be made.

REFERENCES

Adams, A. (1959). Studies on the flat electroencephalogram in man. Electroencephalogr. Clin. Neurophysiol., *11*:35.

Adams, A. E. (1968). Frequenzanalyse des flachen EEG. Dtsch. Z. Nervenheilk, *193*:57.

Ajmone Marsan, C. and Lewis, W. R. (1960). Pathologic findings in patients with "centrencephalic" electroencephalographic patterns. Neurology, *10*:922.

Andersen, P. and Andersson, S. A. (1968). Physiological Basis of the Alpha Rhythm. Appleton-Century-Crofts, New York.

Anderson, P. and Andersson, S. A. (1974). Thalamic origin of cortical rhythmic activity. In: Handbook of Electroencephalography and Clinical Neurophysiology. Vol. 2C, Creutzfeldt, O., Ed., p. 90. Elsevier, Amsterdam.

Andersen, P., Andersson, S. A., and Lømo, T. (1967). Some factors involved in the thalamic control of spontaneous barbiturate spindles. J. Physiol., *192*:257.

Andersen, P. and Sears, T. A. (1964). The role of inhibition in the phasing of spontaneous thalamo-cortical discharge. J. Physiol., *173*:459.

Bickford, R. G. and Butt, H. R. 1955. Hepatic coma: the electroencephalographic pattern. J. Clin. Invest., *34*:790.

Bickford, R. G., Sem-Jacobsen, C. W., White, P. T., and Daly, D. (1952). Some observations on the mechanism of photic and photo-metrazol activation. Electroencephalogr. Clin. Neurophysiol., *4*:275.

Blume, W. T., David, R. B., and Gomez, M. R. (1973). Generalised sharp and slow wave complexes. Associated clinical features and long-term follow-up. Brain, *96*:289.

Bremer, F. (1935). Cerveau "isolé" et physiologie du sommeil. C. R. Soc. Biol. (Paris), *118*:1235.

Bremer, F. (1938). Effets de la déafférentation complète d'une région de l'écorce cérébrale sur son activité électrique spontanée. C. R. Soc. Biol. (Paris). *127*:355.

Brenner, R. P. and Sharbrough, F. W. (1976). Electroencephalographic evaluation in Sturge-Weber syndrome. Neurology, *26*:629.

Burks, J., Huddlestone, J., Lewin, E., Alfrey, A., and Rudolph, H. (1974). A progressive encephalopathy in chronic dialysis patients. Neurology, *24*:359.

Chase, T. N., Moretti, L., and Prensky, A. L. (1968). Clinical and electroencephalographic manifestations of vascular lesions of the pons. Neurology, *18*:357.

Chatrian, G. E., Shaw, C.-M. and Leffman, H. (1964). The significance of periodic lateralized epileptiform discharges in EEG: an electrographic, clinical and pathological study. Electroencephalogr. Clin. Neurophysiol., *17*:177.

Chatrian, G. E., White L. E., and Daly, D. (1963). Electroencephalographic patterns resembling those of sleep in certain comatose states after injuries to the head. Electroencephalogr. Clin. Neurophysiol., *15*:272.

Chokroverty, S. (1975). "Alpha like" rhythms in electroencephalograms in coma after cardiac arrest. Neurology, *25*:655.

Cobb, W. (1966). The periodic events of subacute sclerosing leucoencephalitis. Electroencephalogr. Clin. Neurophysiol., *21:*278.

Cobb, W. A. and Hill, D. (1950). Electroencephalogram in subacute progressive encephalitis. Brain, *73:*392.

Cohn, R., Savage, C., and Raines, G. N. (1950). Barbiturate intoxication: a clinical electroencephalographic study. Ann. Int. Med., *32:*1049.

Cooper, R., Osselton, J. W. and Shaw, J. C. (1974). EEG Technology. Butterworths, London.

Coull, B. M. and Pedley, T. A. (1978). Intermittent photic stimulation. Clinical usefulness of non-convulsive responses. Electroencephalogr. Clin. Neurophysiol., *44:*35.

Courjon, J. A. (1969). Post traumatic epilepsy in electroclinical practice. In: The Late Effects of Head Injury. Walker, A. E., Caveness, W. F. and Critchley, M., Eds., p. 215. C. C. Thomas, Springfield, Illinois.

Courjon, J. and Scherzer, E. (1972). Traumatic disorders. In: Handbook of Electroencephalography and Clinical Neurophysiology, Vol. 14B, Courjon, J., Ed., Elsevier, Amsterdam.

Currie, S., Heathfield, K. W. G., Henson, R. A., and Scott, D. F. (1971). Clinical course and prognosis of temporal lobe epilepsy. A survey of 666 patients. Brain, *94:*173.

Daly, D. D. (1968). The effect of sleep upon the electroencephalogram in patients with brain tumors. Electroencephalogr. Clin. Neurophysiol., *25:*521.

Dempsey, E. W. and Morison, R. S. (1942). The interaction of certain spontaneous and induced cortical potentials. Am. J. Physiol., *135:*301.

Finley, W. W. (1972). The effect of sleep stages on subclinical discharges during morning and afternoon naps. Clin. Electroencephalogr., *3:*45.

Foley, J. M., Watson, C. W., and Adams, R. D. (1950). Significance of the electroencephalographic changes in hepatic coma. Trans. Am. Neurol. Assoc., *75:*161.

Gastaut, H., Roger, J., Soulayrol, R., Tassinari, C. A., Régis, H., and Dravet, C. (1966). Childhood epileptic encephalopathy with diffuse slow spike-waves (otherwise known as "petit mal variant") or Lennox syndrome. Epilepsia, *7:*139.

Gloor, P. (1975). Contributions of electroencephalography and electrocorticography to the neurosurgical treatment of the epilepsies. In: Advances in Neurology, Vol. 8, Purpura, D. P., Penry, J. K., and Walter, R. D., Eds., p. 59, Raven Press, New York.

Gloor, P., Ball, G., and Schaul, N. (1977). Brain lesions that produce delta waves in the EEG. Neurology, *27:*326.

Gloor, P., Kalabay, O., and Giard, N. (1968). The electroencephalogram in diffuse encephalopathies: electroencephalographic correlates of grey and white matter lesions. Brain, *91:*779.

Gloor, P., Tsai, C., and Haddad, F. (1958). An assessment of the value of sleep-electroencephalography for the diagnosis of temporal lobe epilepsy. Electroencephalogr. Clin. Neurophysiol., *10:*633.

Gloor, P., Tsai, C., Haddad, F., and Jasper, H. H. (1957). The lack of necessity for sleep in the EEG or ECG diagnosis of temporal seizures. Electroencephalogr. Clin. Neurophysiol., *9:*393.

Gordon, E. B., and Sim, M. (1967). The EEG in presenile dementia. J. Neurol. Neurosurg. Psychiatry, *30:*285.

Green, R. L. and Wilson, W. P. (1961). Asymmetries of beta activity in epilepsy, brain tumor, and cerebrovascular disease. Electroencephalogr. Clin. Neurophysiol., *13:*75.

Hansotia, P., Harris, R., and Kennedy, J. (1969). EEG changes in Wilson's disease. Electroencephalogr. Clin. Neurophysiol., *27:*523.

Hill, D. (1948). Discussion on the electro-encephalogram in organic cerebral disease. Proc. R. Soc. Med., *41:*242.

Hirsch, J. F., Buisson-Ferey, J., Sachs, M., Hirsch, J. C., and Scherrer, J. (1966). Électrocorticogramme et activités unitaires lors de processus expansifs chez l'homme. Electroencephalogr. Clin. Neurophysiol., *21:*417.

Hockaday, J. M. and Whitty, C. W. M. (1969). Factors determining the electroencephalogram in migraine: a study of 560 patients, according to clinical type of migraine. Brain, *92:*769.

Illis, L. S. and Taylor, F. M. (1972). The electroencephalogram in herpes-simplex encephalitis. Lancet, *1:*718.

Jasper, H. (1949). Diffuse projection systems: the integrative action of the thalamic reticular system. Electroencephalogr. Clin. Neurophysiol., *1:*405.

Jasper, H. H. (1958). Report of the committee on methods of clinical examination in electroencephalography. Electroencephalogr. Clin. Neurophysiol., *10:*370.

Jasper, H., Pertuisset, B., and Flanigin, H. (1951). EEG and cortical electrograms in patients with temporal lobe seizures. Arch. Neurol. Psychiatry, *65:*272.

Jennett, B. and Van De Sande, J. (1975). EEG prediction of post-traumatic epilepsy. Epilepsia, *16:*251.

Kennedy, A. C., Linton, A. L., Luke, R. G., and Renfrew, S. (1963). Electroencephalographic changes during haemodialysis. Lancet, *1:*408.

Kiloh, L. G., McComas, A. J., and Osselton, J. W. (1974). Clinical electroencephalography. 3rd edn. Butterworths, London.

Klass, D. W. and Fischer-Williams, M. (1976). Sensory stimulation, sleep and sleep deprivation. In: Handbook of Electroencephalography and Clinical Neurophysiology, Vol. 3D, Naquet, R., Ed., p. 5. Elsevier, Amsterdam.

Kristiansen, K. and Courtois, G. (1949). Rhythmic electrical activity from isolated cerebral cortex. Electroencephalogr. Clin. Neurophysiol., *1:*265.

Letemendia, F. and Pampiglione, G. (1958). Clinical and electroencephalographic observations in Alzheimer's disease. J. Neurol. Neurosurg. Psychiatry, *21:*167.

Lugaresi, E., and Pazzaglia, P. (1975). Interictal electroencephalogram. In: Handbook of Electroencephalography and Clinical Neurophysiology, Vol. 13 A. Gastaut, H. and Tassinari, C. A., Eds., p. 7. Elsevier, Amsterdam.

MacGillivray, B. B. (1976). The EEG in liver disease. In: Handbook of Electroencephalography and Clinical Neurophysiology, Vol. 15C, Glaser, G. H., Ed., p. 26. Elsevier, Amsterdam.

Mahurkar, S. D., Dhar, S. K., Salta, R., Meyers, L., Smith, E. C., and Dunea, G. (1973). Dialysis dementia. Lancet, *1:*1412.

Mani, K. S. and Townsend, H. R. A. (1964). The EEG in benign intracranial hypertension. Electroencephalogr. Clin. Neurophysiol., *16:*604.

Margerison, J. H., Binnie, C. D., and McCaul, I. R. (1970). Electroencephalographic signs employed in the location of ruptured intracranial arterial aneurysms. Electroencephalogr. Clin. Neurophysiol., *28:*296.

Markand, O. N. (1977). Slow spike-wave activity in EEG and associated clinical features: often called 'Lennox' or 'Lennox-Gastaut' syndrome. Neurology, *27:*746.

Markand, O. N. and Daly, D. D. (1971). Pseudoperiodic lateralized paroxysmal discharges in electroencephalogram. Neurology, *21:*975.

Markand, O. N. and Panszi, J. G. (1975). The electroencephalogram in subacute sclerosing panencephalitis. Arch. Neurol., *32:*719.

Mattson, R. H., Pratt, K. L., and Calverley, J. R. (1965). Electroencephalograms of epileptics following sleep deprivation. Arch. Neurol., *13:*310.

Maulsby, R. L. (1971). Some guidelines for assessment of spikes and sharp waves in EEG tracings. Am J. EEG Technol., *11:*3.

Merlis, J. K., Grossman, C., and Henriksen, G. F. (1951). Comparative effectiveness of sleep and Metrazol-activated electroencephalography. Electroencephalogr. Clin. Neurophysiol., *3:*71.

Metrakos, K. and Metrakos, J. D. (1961). Is the centrencephalic EEG inherited as a dominant? Electroencephalogr. Clin. Neurophysiol., *13:*289.

Millar, J. H. D. (1959). The EEG in chronic subdural hematomata. Electroencephalogr. Clin. Neurophysiol., *11:*603.

Mundy-Castle, A. C. (1951). Theta and beta rhythm in the electroencephalograms of normal adults. Electroencephalogr. Clin. Neurophysiol., *3:*477.

Nakamura, Y. and Ohye, C. (1964). Delta wave production in neocortical EEG by acute lesions within thalamus and hypothalamus of the cat. Electroencephalogr. Clin. Neurophysiol., *17:*677.

Naquet, R., Louard, C., Rhodes, J., and Vigouroux, M. (1961). A propos de certaines décharges paroxystiques du carrefour temporo-pariéto-occipital. Leur activation par l'hypoxie. Rev. Neurol., *105:*203.

Niedermeyer, E. (1963). The electroencephalogram and vertebrobasilar artery insufficiency. Neurology, *13:*412.

Niedermeyer, E. (1966). Generalized seizure discharges and possible precipitating mechanisms. Epilepsia, *7:.*23.

Noriega-Sanchez, A. and Markand, O. N. (1976). Clinical and electroencephalographic correlations of independent multifocal spike discharges. Neurology, *26:*667.

Pampiglione, G. (1962). Electroencephalographic studies after cardiorespiratory resuscitation. Proc. R. Soc. Med., *55:*653.

Pratt, K. L., Mattson, R. H., Weikers, N. J., and Williams, R. (1968). EEG activation of epileptics following sleep deprivation: a prospective study of 114 cases. Electroencephalogr. Clin. Neurophysiol., *24:*11.

Rhee, R. S., Goldensohn, E. S., and Kim, R. C. (1975). EEG characteristics of solitary intracranial lesions in relationship to anatomical location. Electroencephalogr. Clin. Neurophysiol., *38:*553.

Ross, J. J., Johnson, L. C., and Walter R. D. (1966). Spike and wave discharges during stages of sleep. Arch. Neurol., *14:*399.

Sato, S., Dreifuss, F. E., and Penry, J. K. (1976). Prognostic factors in absence seizures. Neurology, *26:*788.

Selby, G. and Lance, J. W. (1960). Observations on 500 cases of migraine and allied vascular headache. J. Neurol. Neurosurg. Psychiatry, *23:*23.

Thomas, J. E., Reagan, T. J., and Klass, D. W. (1977). Epilepsia partialis continua. A review of 32 cases. Arch. Neurol., *34:*266.

Tükel, K. and Jasper, H. (1952). The electroencephalogram in parasagittal lesions. Electroencephalogr. Clin. Neurophysiol., *4:*481.

Upton, A. and Gumpert, J. (1970). Electroencephalography in diagnosis of herpes-simplex encephalitis. Lancet, *1:*650.

Van Der Drift, J. H. A. (1972). The EEG in cerebrovascular disease. In: Handbook of Clinical Neurology, Vinken, P. J. and Bruyn, G. W., Eds. Vol. 11, p. 267, North-Holland, Amsterdam.

Watson, C. W., Flynn, R. E., and Sullivan, J. F., (1958). A distinctive electroencephalographic change associated with subdural hematoma resembling changes which occur with hepatic encephalopathy. Electroencephalogr. Clin. Neurophysiol. *10:*780.

Westmoreland, B., Klass, D. W., Sharbrough, F. W., and Reagan, T. J. (1975). Alpha-coma. Electroencephalographic, clinical, pathologic, and etiologic correlations. Arch. Neurol., *32:*713.

Zappoli, R. (1959). Transient electroencephalographic pattern characteristic of subacute leuco-encephalitis in a case of acute head injury. Electroencephalogr. Clin. Neurophysiol., *11:*571.

Zivin, L. and Ajmone Marsan, C. (1968). Incidence and prognostic significance of "epileptiform" activity in the EEG of non-epileptic subjects. Brain, *91:*751.

3

Neonatal and Pediatric Electroencephalography

BARRY R. THARP

INTRODUCTION

The evaluation of a child with neurologic symptoms usually includes an electroencephalogram (EEG). EEGs are also used to monitor the progression of a disease and, less frequently, to determine the prognosis for recovery or the development of long-term sequelae. Many EEGs are obtained to "rule out organic disease" or simply to verify a diagnosis which has been well-established clinically. All too often little thought is given by the clinician to the potential value or yield of such a test. On the other hand, the EEG may be overinterpreted by the electroencephalographer (EEGer) with little pediatric experience or training. The clinician, faced with a report of an abnormal EEG, may then feel obliged to undertake other diagnostic tests, such as CT scanning, or even advise unnecessary therapy.

This chapter will not attempt to review all facets of pediatric electroencephalography. Most EEG abnormalities are nonspecific and, in the absence of a clinical history, are of little diagnostic value except to indicate the possibility of a pathologic process involving the CNS. Rather, the normal patterns seen during infancy and childhood will be discussed in detail, with emphasis on those that are often misinterpreted or "over-read." In addition, neurologic disorders which are often associated with specific and, in some cases, pathognomonic EEG patterns, will be indicated. It is hoped that this will give the reader an overview of pediatric EEG with particular emphasis on newborns and young infants, will illustrate its value even in the era of CT scanning, and will provide a source of references for those interested in a more detailed exposure of a particular disease or EEG pattern.

NEWBORN INFANTS

The EEG is an important adjunct to the neurologic evaluation of the sick newborn infant. It is only in recent years, however, that the EEG has been utilized routinely in this country for the evaluation of full-term newborns and premature infants. Improvements in the obstetric management of at-risk pregnancies and major advances in neonatal medicine have resulted in significantly decreased mortality and lessened morbidity of small premature infants. Stewart et al (1977) reported that 26 percent of the infants admitted to her nursery and weighing less than 1,000 g were long-term survivors. Of the 111 infants weighing up to 1,500 g admitted to the Stanford University Hospital Nurseries during 1977, 57 percent were discharged from the hospital. The neurologic evaluation of these small prematures is an important aspect of their overall assessment, particularly with reference to the quality of their long-term survival.

The major areas in which electroencephalography may provide unique information in the assessment of newborn full-term and premature infants are:

1. Diagnosis and therapy of seizures.
2. Prognosis of long-term neurologic outcome.
3. Evaluation of infants with compromised cerebral function due to primary neurologic disorders, as well as those with significant systemic disease (such as severe hyaline membrane disease, multiple congenital anomalies, or sepsis) but lacking clinical evidence of an encephalopathy.
4. Determination of specific neurologic entities such as intraventricular hemorrhage and congenital malformations.
5. Determination of conceptional age (CA).*

The EEG is also used in neonatal research concerned with the study of infant behavior and the assessment of physiologic functions which are dependent on the child's sleep state (Prechtl, 1974; Prechtl, Theorell and Blair, 1973).

---

* Conceptional age is the estimated gestational age (EGA) plus the legal age. The EGA is the age in weeks of the infant at birth as calculated from the 1st day of the mother's last menstrual period. Legal age is the age of the infant since birth.

Studies of neonatal apnea, for example, have demonstrated marked differences in the quantity and quality of apneas in active and quiet sleep (Ariagno, 1979). The clinical relevance of these studies is still under study and will not be discussed in this chapter.

In order to interpret neonatal EEGs, it is important to appreciate the rapid maturational changes which take place in the brain of the human newborn during the last trimester of fetal life; development which takes place in an extrauterine environment in the prematurely born infant. The brain's weight increases four-fold from 28 weeks to 40 weeks CA (Larroche, 1977). Its appearance changes from that of a simple structure at 28 weeks of age, when the major sulci make their appearance on the hitherto smooth surface of the cerebral hemispheres, to the complex brain of the full-term infant which resembles that of the older child (Larroche, 1977). Rapid maturational changes are also apparent in the histologic anatomy of the neuron, its projections, and the myelination of axons (Purpura, 1975; Yakovlev and Lecours, 1967).

Despite the apparent simplicity of the anatomy of the premature infant's brain, its repertoire of function is rather extensive. The premature infant of 28 weeks CA is capable of complex spontaneous motor activity, vigorous crying, and response to stimuli (Fenichel, 1978). Behavioral states are also relatively well-developed at this age. Active (REM) and quiet (nonREM) sleep can be easily identified in normal infants by 35 weeks CA and in many infants as early as 27 to 28 weeks CA (Fig. 3.1). The EEG patterns of the newborn infant are dependent, therefore, not only upon the conceptional age, but also upon the behavioral state(s) of the infant during the recording.

The neurologic disorders of newborn infants are often unique to this period of life (Larroche, 1977). Some neuropathologic conditions, such as germinal matrix hemorrhage, occur almost exclusively in small premature infants (younger than 32 weeks CA) and are uncommon in the term infant (Fedrick and Butler, 1970). Common metabolic encephalopathies such as hypoglycemia may cause transient EEG abnormalities yet permanently impair cerebral function. The EEG of the infant who suffers a severe anoxic-ischemic injury at birth may be quite abnormal during the first week of life, but often becomes normal over the next few weeks despite the presence of permanent cerebral damage which will ultimately result in mental retardation and cerebral palsy. The EEGer must be aware of the rapid maturational changes taking place in the brain of the normal premature infant in order to recognize significant deviations from normal. The transient nature of some EEG abnormalities must also be considered when a prognostic statement is being formulated.

Technical Considerations

There are many technical aspects of EEG recording which are unique to the newborn infant. It is beyond the scope of this chapter to detail the nuances of EEG recording in the newborn nursery. The reader should refer to the chapters devoted to neonatal EEG recording in a recent publication (Werner, Stockard, and Bickford, 1977). Table 3.1 is a summary of some major technical areas in

(A) KOS. CA 29w QUIET SLEEP

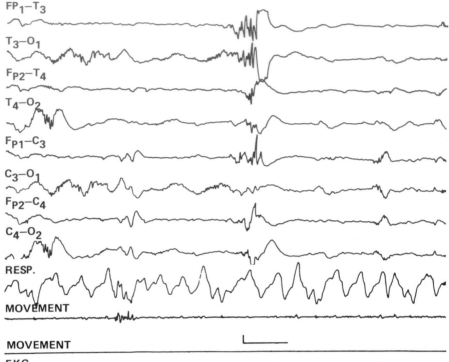

Fig. 3.1. (A) *Recording of quiet sleep of healthy premature infant (CA 29 weeks). Discontinuous background is associated with infrequent limb movements. Note burst of high amplitude theta in the left frontotemporal region. RESP—abdominal respiration. Upper "MOVEMENT" channel—movement monitor located under baby's body. Lower "MOVEMENT" channel—surface EMG on right leg. Calibration: 50 μV; 2 seconds.*

which neonatal EEG recording *differs* from that of older children and adults. The items listed in this table reflect the recording methods used in the author's laboratory and, for the sake of brevity, omit the many variations employed by others. This recording method is used for premature and full-term infants until approximately 1 to 2 months post-term.

The technologist will not only require additional training but should also become familiar with nursery procedures and develop a good rapport with the nursery staff. The technologist should become familiar with the normal and abnormal body and facial movements of newborn infants. This behavior should be noted on the record and will, in conjunction with the respirogram, extraoculogram, and EEG, provide the necessary data to determine the child's behavioral or sleep state. An EEG lacking such clinical observations and poly-

(B) KOS. CA 29w ACTIVE SLEEP

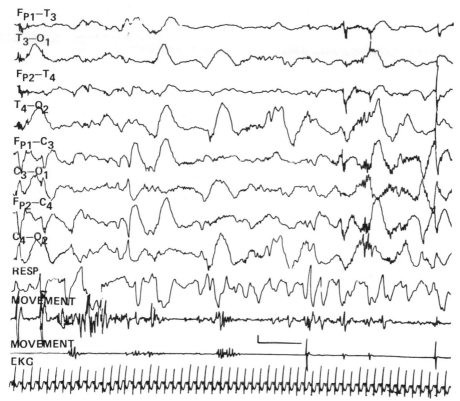

Fig. 3.1. (Continued) (B) Active sleep recorded in same infant. Continuous background associated with frequent body and limb movements. Bilateral brushes in the central regions are present in the right half of the tracing. Respirations are slightly more irregular than in Fig. 3.1A.

graphic (nonEEG) variables is extremely difficult if not impossible to interpret unless it is grossly abnormal.

Normal EEG

There is extensive literature on the normal cerebral electrical activity of the premature and full-term newborn to which the reader is referred (Werner et al, 1977), and only a summary of the salient characteristics of the normal EEG at each conceptional age will be given here.

The cerebral electrical activity of the healthy infant is dependent on the age of the brain and is independent of the number of days of extrauterine life. The EEG of a premature infant born at 30 weeks EGA whose legal age is 10 weeks (CA 40 weeks) is similar to that of a full-term infant (EGA 40 weeks). Recent studies have shown that there are some minor differences in the EEGs of premature infants of 40 weeks CA when compared to full-term newborns (EGA

Table 3.1. EEG RECORDING IN THE NEONATAL PERIOD

Recording Techniques	Comments
1. Electrodes and placement a. Paste or collodion attachment.	1. Electrodes and placement a. Needle electrodes never used; collodion may not be allowed in some nurseries.
b. Minimum 9 scalp electrodes applied in prematures and entire 10–20 array in term infants.	b. Small head limits electrode number to Fp, C, O, mid-temporal and Cz in prematures.
c. Fp1 and Fp2 placements replaced by Fp3 and Fp4 (halfway between 10–20 placements Fp and F)	c. Frontal sharp waves, delta and other activity of higher amplitude in prefrontal than fronto-polar region.
2. 16 channel recordings preferred.	2. Many nonEEG parameters must be measured; all brain areas must be monitored in one montage.
3. Single montage used for entire recording, particularly with 16 channel recording.	3. Generalized changes in background activity and state-related changes are more important than exact localization of focal abnormalities.
4. Paper speed—15 mm per second for entire record. Time constant—between 0.25 and 0.60 seconds.	4. Easier to recognize interhemispheric synchrony as well as slow background activity.
5. Polygraphic (nonEEG) variables recorded routinely—respiration (thoracic) (with or without nasal thermistor); extra-ocular movements (primarily in infants older than 36 weeks CA); and EKG.	5. These variables are critical in the determination of the behavior state (awake, active or quiet sleep).
6. Frequent notes made by the technologist of baby's body movement and, in small prematures, eye movement.	6. Valuable information for the determination of behavioral state.
7. Technologist attempts to record active and quiet sleep, particularly in older prematures and term infants. Duration of record may exceed 60 minutes.	7. Presence or absence of well developed sleep states is important for interpretation; some pathologic patterns seen primarily in quiet sleep; sleep onset usually active sleep.
8. Accurate notation of EGA, CA, recent drug administration, recent changes in blood gases.	8. Interpretation dependent on knowledge of conceptional age of infant. EEG very sensitive to abrupt changes in blood gases and certain drugs.

40 weeks) but these appear, at least at present, to be of little clinical significance (Nolte and Haas, 1978; Metcalf, 1969).

Before discussing the general features of the normal newborn EEG, various behavioral states will be defined. The full-term newborn has easily recognizable awake and sleeping behavior which is very similar to that of older children and adults. These states are generally classified as waking, quiet sleep (QS; non-REM sleep), active sleep (AS; REM sleep), and indeterminate sleep (a sleeping state which cannot be definitely classified as active or quiet sleep). Active sleep is most commonly the sleep-onset state in newborn infants, and remains so for the first 2 to 4 months of post-term life (Ellingson, 1975; Curzi-Dascalova, 1977); it constitutes approximately 50 percent of the sleeping time of term infants and somewhat more in the premature. The active sleep at onset is usually 10 to 20 minutes in duration but may exceed 30 to 40 minutes in the healthy newborn.

A normal child is considered awake if his eyes are open. His behavior may vary from quiet wakefulness to crying with vigorous motor activity. Transient eye closures may accompany crying and also occur during quiet wakefulness. If the child's eyes remain closed for an extended period of time (usually for more than 1 minute), he is considered asleep. (See Anders, Ende, and Parmelee, 1971, for the details of sleep scoring in infants.)

Active sleep is characterized by eye closure, bursts of rapid horizontal and vertical eye movements, irregular respirations, and frequent limb and body movements ranging from brief twitches of a limb to gross movements of one limb or the entire body, grimacing, smiling, frowning, and bursts of sucking.

Quiet sleep is characterized by the infant lying quietly with eyes closed, regular respiration, and the absence of rapid eye movements. Occasional gross body movements, characterized by brief stiffening of the trunk and limbs, may occur and may be associated with brief clonic jerks of the lower extremities (Anders et al, 1971; Prechtl, 1974).

EEG Patterns and Terminology. Certain waveforms that are common to the normal newborn EEG must now be considered, so that the normal EEG patterns of each conceptual age can be summarized. Figure 3.2 depicts some of these waveforms.

Brushes (Spindle-like Fast Rhythms). This pattern is most abundant in the EEG of the small premature with maximum expression between 32 and 35 weeks CA (Fig. 3.2). It consists of short bursts of 8 to 20 Hz rhythmic activity, often with a spindle morphology, superimposed on high amplitude slow waves. The amplitude of the spindles may range from 10 to 100 μV (usually 20 to 50 μV), and that of the 0.8 to 1.5 Hz slow waves from 25 to 200 μV. They occur primarily in the rolandic and occipital areas, with the former site predominating in very young prematures (less than 32 weeks CA) and the latter in older prematures. Brushes are more abundant in active sleep in younger infants (up to 33 weeks CA) and in quiet sleep in infants older than 33 weeks CA (Watanabe and Iwase, 1972; Lombroso, 1979). Lombroso (1979) counted the number of

NORMAL PATTERNS

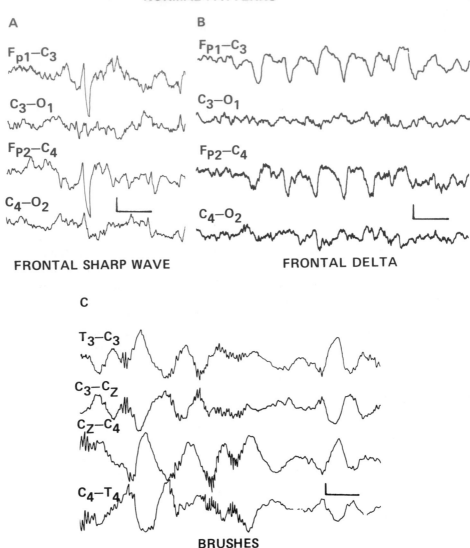

Fig. 3.2. *(A) Bilateral frontal sharp waves (encoches frontales) in healthy full term infant. (B) Anterior slow dysrhythmia in healthy pre-term infant. (C) Central brushes in healthy premature infant (CA 35 weeks). Calibration: 50 μV; 1 second.*

brushes during 5 minute epochs of well-established quiet and active sleep in a group of healthy infants between 31 and 43 weeks CA. At 33 to 34 weeks CA he found an average of 29 per epoch in quiet sleep and 22 per epoch in active sleep. The brushes decreased in number as the infant approached term, were infrequent during the quiet sleep of the term baby (0.8 per epoch), and were virtually absent in active sleep (0.1 per epoch). They disappeared during the first few weeks of post-term life.

Frontal Sharp Transients (*"Encoches Frontales"*). These are biphasic (usually negative-positive) sharp waves, often with a following slow wave, which are of maximal amplitude in the prefrontal regions (Fp3, Fp4), and occur during wakefulness and with increased incidence in sleep. They may appear bilaterally and synchronously, may be symmetric or asymmetric, or may be unilateral, shifting from one side to the other during the course of a single tracing. Typical encoches frontales appear at 35 weeks CA and persist until several weeks post-term (Fig. 3.2). Similar though less well-developed frontal sharp waves are also seen in younger prematures.

Anterior Slow Dysrhythmia. This consists of bursts and short runs of 2 to 4 Hz, 50 to 200 μV delta activity which is often monomorphic and of maximum amplitude in the frontal regions where it may be associated with encoches frontales (Fig. 3.2).

Synchrony. Synchrony is defined as the relatively simultaneous appearance in both hemispheres of bursts of cerebral activity during discontinuous portions of the tracing. Lombroso (1975, 1979) measured the degree of synchrony between interhemispheric burst activity during 5 consecutive minutes of discontinuous quiet sleep activity in normal infants. (Bursts were considered synchronous if they occurred within 2 seconds of each other.) He found that the percentage of synchronous bursts ranged from approximately 50 percent in infants under 30 weeks CA to near 100 percent at term.

Theta Bursts. Bursts of theta activity are commonly seen in the EEG of the very young premature, with maximal incidence between 29 and 31 weeks, and are rarely seen beyond 35 to 36 weeks. They consist of bursts of sharply contoured high amplitude (50 to 100 μV, occasionally 200 μV) 5 to 6 Hz activity which are maximum in the temporal areas, often diffuse, and frequently bilateral and synchronous.

Tracé Alternant. This is the discontinuous pattern which characterizes quiet sleep of the full-term newborn. It consists of 3 to 5 second bursts of high amplitude delta (1 to 3 Hz, 50 to 100 μV) admixed with lower amplitude beta and theta activity which occur at intervals of 3 to 10 seconds. The interburst background consists of diffuse moderate amplitude (25 to 50 μV) mixed frequency (usually 4 to 7 Hz) activity (Fig. 3.3).

Tracé Discontinu. This is the discontinuous pattern of quiet sleep in the normal pre-term infant. It differs from tracé alternant in that the interburst activity is lower in amplitude and may even be flat at standard amplification, the bursts are slightly less frequent, and the activity composing the bursts contains more monomorphic delta, fast activity, and brushes.

Pattern at 27 to 29 Weeks CA. The EEG is characterized by a discontinuous background of mixed frequency activity, primarily in the delta range, which is maximal in the occipital regions. There are periods during the tracing, often

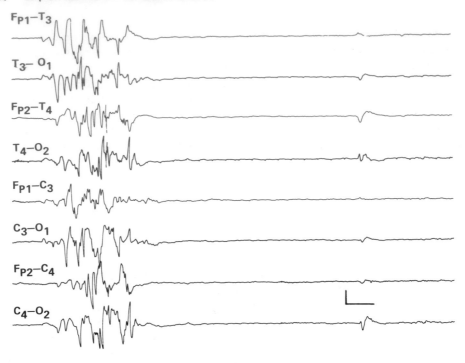

A   S. ♀ 57—66—49 FT 1D QUIET STATE

F_{P1}–T_3

T_3–O_1

F_{P2}–T_4

T_4–O_2

F_{P1}–C_3

C_3–O_1

F_{P2}–C_4

C_4–O_2

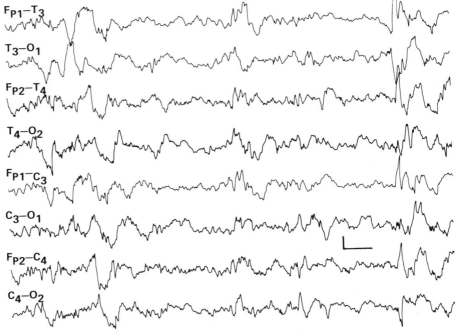

B   K ♂ 56—47—23 CA 38—40W QUIET SLEEP

F_{P1}–T_3

T_3–O_1

F_{P2}–T_4

T_4–O_2

F_{P1}–C_3

C_3–O_1

F_{P2}–C_4

C_4–O_2

Fig. 3.3. (A) *Paroxysmal pattern during quiet state in stuporous full term infant with severe ischemic-hypoxic encephalopathy.* (B) *Tracé alternant pattern in quiet sleep of healthy full term infant. Calibration: 50 μV; 1 second.*

exceeding 1 minute, when a continuous background is associated with REM and increased body activity consistent with active sleep. The infant tends to be more quiet during more discontinuous portions of the record. Brushes are present in the central (rolandic) regions. High voltage paroxysmal temporal theta is prominent. Interburst intervals are usually about 10 seconds but may exceed 30 seconds (Fig. 3.1).

Pattern at 30 to 32 Weeks CA. Two different types of background predominate at this age. A discontinuous background resembling that seen at an earlier age and consisting of 1 to 2 Hz, 25 to 100 μV occipitally dominant slow activity tends to appear during portions of the recording when the child is sleeping quietly. More continuous background often occurs with eye movements and more active body motility consistent with active sleep. Brushes are very abundant at this age, and are located in the occipital and rolandic regions with a higher incidence during the continuous or active sleep portions of the record. Synchrony approximates 50 to 70 percent during portions of the tracing with a discontinuous background (Lombroso, 1975, 1979). There is less paroxysmal temporal theta than at earlier ages.

Pattern at 33 to 35 Weeks CA. Sleep states are becoming more clearly defined with continuous background slow activity (primarily 1 to 2 Hz, 25 to 100 μV) which is maximal in the temporo-occipital and rolando-occipital regions and is more abundant during wakefulness and active sleep. Discontinuous activity is associated with quiet sleep. An increasing amount of lower voltage theta activity is also present. Brushes are still abundant but less than at an earlier age and are more frequent during quiet sleep. Synchrony approaches 75 to 90 percent at 35 weeks (Lombroso, 1975, 1979). Typical frontal sharp waves (encoches frontales) appear at 35 weeks.

Pattern at 36 to 38 Weeks CA. Three different EEG patterns predominate at this age. Continuous diffuse low voltage 4 to 6 Hz activity (usually less than 50 μV) admixed with 50 to 100 μV delta (2 to 4 Hz) characterizes wakefulness. A continuous slow wave pattern (1 to 3 Hz, 25 to 100 μV) of maximal amplitude over the posterior scalp regions is present during active sleep. A discontinuous pattern with bursts of mixed frequency slow activity and occasional brushes separated by low voltage background typifies quiet sleep (tracé discontinu). Encoches frontales and anterior slow dysrhythmia are still prominent. Synchrony approximates 80 to 90 percent during the discontinuous portions of the EEG (Lombroso, 1975, 1979).

Pattern at 38 to 40 Weeks CA (Full Term Newborn). Activité moyenne, continuous activity at 1 to 10 Hz (predominantly 4 to 7 Hz), and at 25 to 50 μV, characterizes wakefulness and active sleep, particularly when the latter follows a period of quiet sleep. Activité moyenne with superimposed delta (2 to 4 Hz, less than 100 μV) that appears as continuous activity or in short runs or bursts, characterizes active sleep, particularly at sleep onset. Diffuse continuous delta (0.5 to 2 Hz, 25 to 100 μV) is found at the beginning and end of quiet sleep periods and occasionally during long portions of such sleep, but tracé alternant is more characteristic of quiet sleep.

Brushes are infrequent in the EEG of the term infant and occur primarily in quiet sleep. Encoches frontales and anterior slow dysrhythmia are abundant, particularly during quiet sleep. The voltage of the background activity is relatively symmetric over the two hemispheres though transient asymmetries are frequent, particularly in the temporal regions. Interhemispheric synchrony during tracé alternant approaches 100 percent. Scattered sharp waves are common in the rolandic and temporal areas.

The inexperienced EEGer will often characterize the encoches frontales and anterior slow dysrhythmia of the older premature infant and the bursts of temporal theta of the very young infant as "epileptiform" or "paroxysmal." One must also distinguish the various discontinuous background patterns of the healthy premature from the abnormal paroxysmal patterns to be discussed in the next section. Significant transient interhemispheric voltage asymmetries are common at all age groups, as is asynchrony of the bursts during portions of the tracing with discontinuous background in the young premature. The abundant brushes in the EEG of the younger premature, particularly if slow paper speed is used, may also give the background a "spiky" or "paroxysmal" appearance. Multifocal sharp waves are also noted, particularly in the temporal and central regions of healthy infants.

Abnormal EEG

It is beyond the scope of this chapter to discuss all the deviations from normal encountered in the EEGs of newborn infants. We will concentrate, therefore, on those patterns which are associated with certain specific neurologic disorders and those that appear to be of prognostic value.

Seizures. Neonatal seizures are a common problem in the newborn nursery and can occur in infants at any conceptional age. The etiologies of neonatal seizures encompass virtually the entire spectrum of neurologic disorders of infancy (Rose and Lombroso, 1970; Lombroso, 1978; Dennis, 1978; Knauss and Marshall, 1977). The clinical spectrum of neonatal seizures is quite different from that of older children. Generalized convulsive seizures, particularly tonic-clonic or grand mal, are infrequent in the newborn, especially the premature. The most common seizure types are focal or multifocal clonic, fragmentary, tonic, myoclonic, and minimal or subtle (Lombroso, 1978).

The EEG is of particular diagnostic value in those infants whose seizures are subclinical, subtle, or easily confused with normal motor behavior. It can also be useful in the evaluation of jittery babies and those offspring of drug addicted mothers who have abnormal motor activity that is easily confused with seizures. Many infants with severely compromised pulmonary function or with persistent fetal circulation are now being treated with complete chemical neuromuscular blockade to improve the effectiveness of mechanical ventilatory support. Many of these infants have suffered a significant hypoxic-ischemic insult which may cause seizures, and we have been impressed by the large number of such infants in whom status epilepticus was concealed by the peripheral paralysis. The EEG must be relied upon to monitor CNS function in such babies and to determine the effectiveness of therapy.

In the EEG, neonatal seizures are usually focal with variable spread over the ipsilateral and contralateral hemispheres. The seizure is characterized by the progressive buildup of rhythmic activity at almost any frequency, or by repetitive sharp waves or spikes. Multifocal seizures are quite common in severe encephalopathies. Two seizures may appear concomitantly in the same hemisphere, or more commonly in opposite hemispheres, and progress independently. Figure 3.4 depicts some typical ictal patterns and Figure 3.5 illustrates some of the artifacts which may be confused with seizure discharges.

Interictal patterns are extremely variable and can range from normal background activity for the CA to isoelectric records. The interictal background reflects the severity of the underlying encephalopathy responsible for the seizures. The background activity may be transiently worsened by the hypoxia associated with a seizure, by intravenously administered anticonvulsant drugs, and by postictal changes.

The clinical and electrographic features of a seizure are related to the severity of the underlying encephalopathy which, in turn, determines the risk of permanent neurologic sequelae. Regardless of the type of interictal EEG background rhythms which coexist, typical clinical seizures which occur without concomitant ictal EEG activity are associated with a poor outcome, as are typical electrographic seizures that occur without clinical manifestations. The latter are infrequent in our experience. Close observation of the infant will usually reveal subtle clinical phenomena such as eye deviation, mouth or tongue movements, change in the respiratory pattern or brief apnea, or slight movement of an extremity.

Certain electrographic patterns may also be associated with a poor outcome. Multifocal ictal activity is more often followed by neurologic sequelae than unifocal seizure discharges, particularly if two or more focal seizures appear concomitantly in the same or opposite hemisphere and progress independently.

The interictal EEG patterns are most helpful in the prediction of the quality of long term survival, as is discussed below. These patterns reflect the severity of the encephalopathy and are of predictive value regardless of the presence or absence of neonatal seizures. Abnormal patterns, such as a paroxysmal background, may transiently appear immediately following a seizure, however, and the final interpretation of the EEG should, therefore, be made on the basis of the entire record, and particularly the pre-seizure background. If a seizure occurs in the early portions of the EEG, a prolonged recording session may be necessary to allow sufficient recovery from the postictal state that a judgment of the interictal background can be made.

Abnormal Background Patterns in Infants at or Near Term. Only the most common EEG abnormalities occurring in the neonatal EEG will be discussed in this section. Additional discussions of the prognostic value of the EEG in

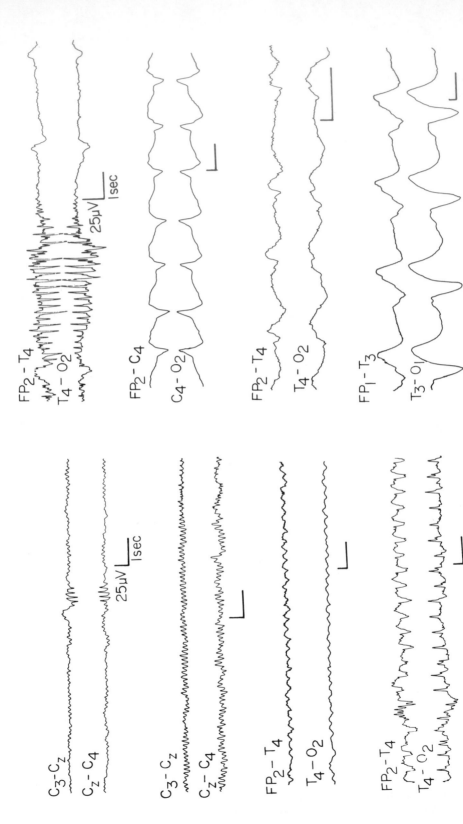

Fig. 3.4. *Typical ictal patterns in premature and full term infants. Except where otherwise indicated, calibration: 50 µV; 1 second.*

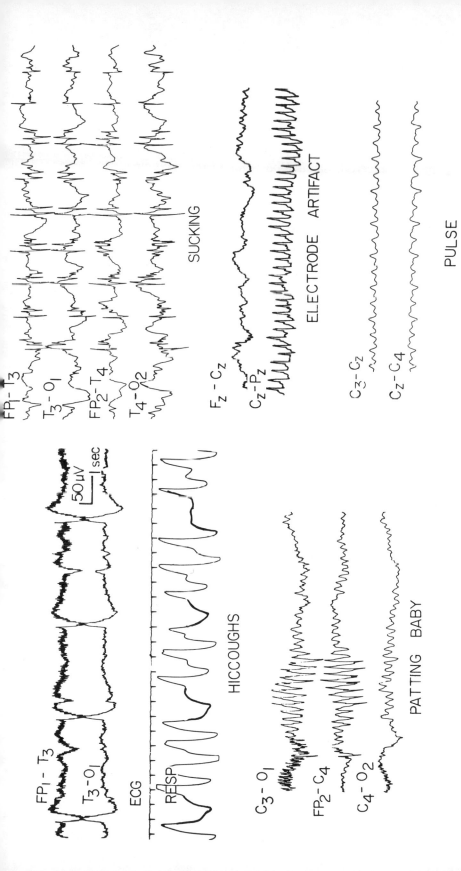

Fig. 3.5. *Rhythmic artifacts which can be confused with ictal patterns. Calibration: 50 µV; 1 second.*

full-term newborns can be found in the article by Monod, Pajot, and Guidasci (1972), and those by Rose and Lombroso (1970) and Lombroso (1979).

A poor neurologic outcome can be predicted if one of the following EEG patterns occurs in the EEG of a newborn infant at or near term, provided the infant has not received medication prior to the recording or experienced an acute change in metabolic status immediately preceding the EEG. The EEG may become transiently abnormal and even isoelectric if the respirator is removed or malfunctions during a recording and acute hypoxia ensues (Roberton, 1969). Intravenous diazepam may also cause an acute but reversible deterioration of the EEG (Werner et al, 1977). The numbers in parentheses following each type of EEG pattern are taken from the paper of Monod et al (1972). They represent the long-term neurologic outcome (relatively normal/severely abnormal) of all children whose neonatal EEGs included at least one tracing with that particular pattern. For example, *normal EEGs (102/6)* indicates that of the 108 infants with normal EEGs in the neonatal period, only 6 suffered significant neurologic sequelae.

Isoelectric (0/21). Though the majority of children with isoelectric EEGs will die in the neonatal period, some will survive with severe neurologic deficits. The isoelectric EEG is usually followed by other abnormal patterns, particularly diffusely slow backgrounds, but occasionally a flat EEG will persist for many months following the acute neurologic insult (Estivill, Monod, and Amiel-Tison, 1977). The same technical requirements for recording isoelectric records in adults are applied to infants.

Paroxysmal (1/44). This pattern (Fig. 3.3B) is characterized by an isoelectric background interrupted by aperiodic bursts of abnormal activity (delta and theta with admixed spikes and/or beta activity; less commonly, bursts or short runs of diffuse or focal alpha or theta activity, occasionally rhythmic). This abnormal pattern must be differentiated from the discontinuous patterns seen in the quiet sleep of normal infants. Normal discontinuous patterns may be affected by mild encephalopathies. The tracé alternant may manifest excessively long or low voltage interburst intervals and, less frequently, an intermittently discontinuous background may occur during active sleep. Such patterns have a less ominous prognosis and must be differentiated from the paroxysmal tracing which is invariant, minimally altered by stimuli, persists throughout all the sleep states (if they can be recognized) and lacks the normal background rhythms which are present during the bursts of an abnormal tracé alternant.

Diffusely Slow Activity (9/37). This pattern consists of diffuse amorphous delta activity that persists throughout the recording and is not significantly altered by sensory stimuli. The faster patterns in the theta and beta range, which are normally abundant in the EEG of term infants, are absent. This type of abnormal background must be distinguished from the high voltage slow-wave pattern which occurs during a portion of the normal quiet sleep of preterm and term infants and which gradually replaces the tracé alternant pattern during the first 4 to 6 weeks post-term (Watanabe, Iwase, and Hara, 1974).

Low Voltage Background with Theta Rhythms (0/31). This is a relatively common pattern and is characterized by a continuous low voltage background (5 to 25 μV) with superimposed bursts or runs of low voltage (5 to 15 μV) theta which may be diffuse but are more often focal or multifocal. There is no EEG reactivity to stimulation and usually sleep states cannot be recognized. This pattern is often the precursor of an isoelectric record.

Grossly Asynchronous Records (4/38). Monod et al (1972) classified a record as asynchronous if there was "gross asynergy and asynchrony between the activities of the two hemispheres." The majority of records with gross interhemispheric asynchrony have paroxysmal backgrounds (Fig. 3.6). Lombroso (1979) has described a technique for the more detailed analysis of interhemispheric synchrony. This technique has been applied to a small number of abnormal records (Lombroso, 1975), but there are no long-term follow-up studies of infants whose neonatal EEGs were excessively asynchronous for age according to this technique.

Low Voltage Record (21/50). This pattern was characterized by Monod et al (1972) as a low voltage background (5 to 15 μV during wakefulness, 10 to 25 μV in quiet sleep) which occurs frequently in newborns, is of little prognostic value when recorded in the first week of life (11/24), but is statistically associated with a poor prognosis if present in the third or fourth week post-term (3/14).

Spikes and Sharp Waves. These are commonly seen in neonatal EEGs and must be interpreted conservatively. Monod et al (1972) found fast transients in 38 percent of infants during the first month of life. They considered that spikes or sharp waves were more likely to be associated with a poor long-term prognosis if they exhibited a persistent and repetitive focality. Such spikes were often associated with focal slowing. A poor long-term prognosis was also indicated by spikes (of less than 150 msec duration) which persisted during quiet sleep in serial recordings. Rolandic spikes were excluded because they often occur during quiet sleep in normal infants and were not predictive of poor long-term outcome. Finally spikes in all locations, including rolandic, which occurred during wakefulness or active sleep after the second week of life were associated with a poor prognosis. It has been our experience, however, that spikes and sharp waves occurring in an otherwise normal record should be interpreted conservatively. Though the record may be interpreted as mildly abnormal solely on the basis of excessive numbers of spikes or the persistence of focal spikes or sharp waves, its value as a predictor of long-term neurologic outcome remains uncertain and awaits further study.

There are many abnormalities which in isolation are of little prognostic value but often accompany the severe abnormalities just discussed. They occur in children with mild hypoxic or metabolic encephalopathies, subarachnoid hemorrhage, or following complicated pregnancies or deliveries. As the abnormal clinical state resolves, the EEG returns rapidly to normal. These abnormalities are etiologically nonspecific and apparently have no predictive

A.N.♂S77–611 CA 39 QUIET SLEEP

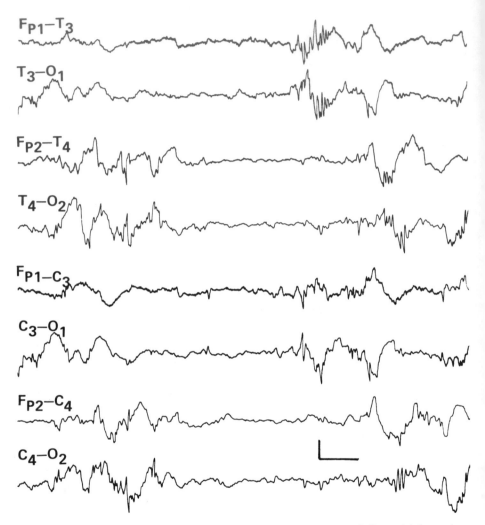

Fig. 3.6. *Excessive interhemispheric asynchrony. Premature infant with hypoxic encephalopathy and severe bronchopulmonary dysplasia. (EGA—28 weeks, legal age—11 weeks). The child exhibited severe developmental delay and seizures by the age of 16 months. Calibration: 50 μV; 1 second.*

value. They include the lack of well-developed active and quiet sleep; poor correlation (concordance) between the behavioral changes characterizing a particular state and the EEG (see Lombroso, 1979 for a study of the development of concordance in healthy premature infants); deviations from the normal percentages of specific behavioral states (e.g., increased percentage of active sleep in children born of diabetic mothers—Schulte et al, 1969); excessive amounts of anterior slow dysrhythmia and/or an increased incidence of encoches frontales; excessive amounts of fast background rhythms, particularly beta activity; excessively discontinuous tracé alternant and tracé discontinu patterns; and immature background activity (background patterns typical of a younger conceptional age or which contain certain waveforms that are more abundant in younger infants). Though it is suspected that immature background activity reflects significant brain damage, no long-term follow-up studies have been completed.

Abnormal Background Patterns in Premature Infants. There have been few comprehensive reports of the prognostic value of the EEG in premature infants. Ellingson, Dutch, and McIntire (1974) studied apparently normal premature and term infants by serial EEGs in the neonatal period. They were able to follow 57 percent of their population to 3 to 8 years of age. Minor deviations from the expected maturational changes of the EEG during the neonatal period could not be correlated with the ultimate neurologic outcome.

In a study of 82 infants with an EGA of less than 36 weeks, Tharp and colleagues (1977; and unpublished observations) found a number of patterns that occurred primarily in infants who died in the neonatal period or who developed long-term sequelae, although the number of children in each group was usually too small for statistical significance to be reached. The patterns included an isoelectric EEG; positive rolandic sharp waves; a paroxysmal disturbance distinct from the discontinuous pattern seen in normal small premature infants (Fig. 3.1); excessive interhemispheric asynchrony (Fig. 3.6); major (more than 50 percent) and persistent hemispheric voltage asymmetries, but excluding records with localized areas of voltage attenuation; and an excessively slow background of variable amplitude (10 to 100 μV) that was unresponsive to stimulation and was characterized by a paucity or absence of physiologic rhythms such as brushes (Fig. 3.7).

Other less severe EEG abnormalities were also encountered in this age group but were of no prognostic value. These included mild asymmetries, excessive asynchrony for the conceptional age, excessively discontinuous backgrounds, and alterations in the amount of background faster rhythms.

Several records were considered "immature for the conceptional age." These EEGs contained patterns more typical of a younger conceptional age, such as an excessive number of brushes, increased preponderance of occipital delta activity, or excessive discontinuity. This type of abnormality has been described by Lombroso (1975). It is often a transient abnormality related to a mild metabolic or hypoxic encephalopathy and has a good prognosis. Our observations of infants with persistently immature EEG activity suggest a poor prognosis, but a long-term study has not been completed.

It should be emphasized that the recording of *serial EEGs* is a very important aspect of the evaluation of premature infants. The EEG should be obtained at the time of acute neurologic deterioration and repeated 1 to 2 weeks later, particularly if the initial EEG is normal or only moderately abnormal. We have often been impressed by the development of a grossly abnormal EEG at a time

K.♂58–32–74 CA 34W SEMICOMATOSE–ANOXIA, S.A.H.

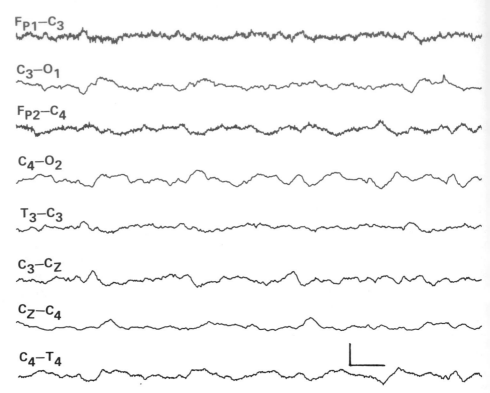

Fig. 3.7. *Diffusely slow background with absence of normal patterns for the conceptional age. Premature infant (EGA, CA—34 weeks) with hypoxic encephalopathy, severe respiratory distress syndrome and bloody CSF. The infant died on the 6th day of life, and autopsy revealed subarachnoid hemorrhage, cerebral edema, and widespread anoxic encephalopathy. Calibration: 50 μV; 1 second.*

when the child was stable or even improving clinically. In our series of 82 premature infants, an abnormal record following a normal EEG or a markedly abnormal EEG subsequent to a moderately abnormal record was seen in 41 percent of the children with major neurologic sequelae in contrast to 3 percent of children with normal development and 15 percent of those with minor sequelae.

Neonatal Neurologic Disorders with Characteristic EEG Patterns

The majority of the neurologic syndromes encountered in neonatal neurology are associated with nonspecific EEG abnormalities. The EEG changes are usually generalized and reflect the severity of the cerebral insult. A paroxysmal pattern, for example, can be caused by a severe meningitis, hypoxic encephalopathy or a subarachnoid hemorrhage. There is usually nothing about the EEG pattern per se which offers a clue to the etiology of the child's neurologic problem.

There are, however, a few specific neurologic disorders which may be associated with characteristic EEG abnormalities and which can allow the electroencephalographer to suggest certain etiologic considerations to the clinician.

Unexpected, Gross EEG Abnormalities. Abnormalities such as a paroxysmal background or gross interhemispheric asynchrony may be *unexpectedly recorded* in an infant who is relatively intact neurologically and whose birth history and early neonatal course are benign. A paroxysmal pattern is usually associated with a severely compromised neurologic status in infants with hypoxic-ischemic encephalopathy, meningo-encephalitis, subarachnoid hemorrhage, or traumatic encephalopathy. In contrast, many of the major CNS anomalies, such as holoprosencephaly, are relatively silent clinically in the neonatal period yet are often associated with major EEG abnormalities (Fig. 3.8) (DeMyer and White, 1964). Though these CNS anomalies are known to cause hypsarrhythmic EEG patterns later in the first year of life (Schimschock, Carlson, and Ojemann, 1969), little has been written about the characteristics of the neonatal EEG.

The rather characteristic EEG abnormalities caused by the holoprosencephalic brain are due to two distinct neuroanatomic features. The EEG is low voltage or isoelectric over the fluid-filled sac which overlies the most atrophic or underdeveloped brain. DeMyer and White (1964) found this isoelectric region to be most often posterior in location and to occur when the holotelencephalon was everted and reflected frontally. The EEG recorded from scalp regions overlying the portion of the anomaly with the largest tissue volume (frontally in the variation just mentioned) is grossly abnormal and manifests a variety of bizarre patterns, including a fast beta activity which probably represents subclinical seizures. In our experience, a typical patient with this anomaly is referred to the EEG laboratory because of a seizure or unexplained apnea. The infant may have external deformities, such as hypotelorism, cleft lip, or a nasal deformity, but relatively few abnormalities on neurologic examination except hypotonia. The EEG abnormalities are, therefore, "out of proportion" to the benign history and clinical state, and lead to the definitive diagnosis by CT scanning.

Another rare anomaly, Aicardi's syndrome, is associated with rather typical EEG abnormalities. This syndrome, first described by Aicardi (1969), occurs only in females and is characterized by the association of infantile spasms appearing during the first few months of life and multiple congenital anomalies. The major CNS anomalies consist of partial or complete agenesis of the corpus callosum, cortical heterotopias, and porencephalic cysts. The characteristic ocular lesions which often provide the initial clue to the diagnosis include a chorioretinopathy (bilateral footprint-shaped lacunae and multiple pigmented and atrophic lesions), staphyloma, coloboma of the optic papilla and microphthalmia. Other less common anomalies include dysplasia of the ribs and

B. ♀ S76–1781 FT 3d ARHINENCEPHALY

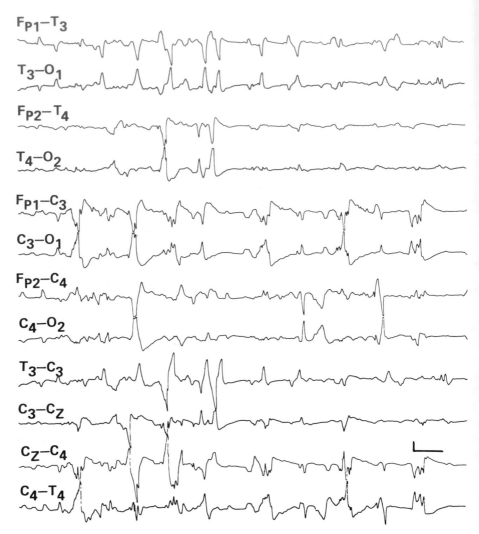

Fig. 3.8. *Multifocal sharp waves, absence of normal background rhythms and interhemispheric asynchrony in a full-term infant with seizures, a large head and ambiguous genitalia. At time of EEG baby was alert and vigorous with normal neurologic examination. Autopsy revealed absence of corpus callosum and septum pellucidum, and agenesis of the olfactory bulbs and olfactory tracts with a V-shaped bilobar cerebrum due to agenesis of posterior temporal and occipital lobes. Calibration: 50 μV; 1 second.*

vertebrae, hemivertebrae, scoliosis, and other osseous anomalies involving almost exclusively the ribs and vertebrae. Fariello et al (1977) reported the first cases from this country and emphasized the characteristic EEG features. They described a suppression-burst pattern which appeared completely asynchro-nously in the two hemispheres. This striking asynchrony was most prominent during the waking state and tended to disappear during sleep. A typical sus-tained hypsarrhythmia was not seen in Fariello's six cases. Aicardi (1969) described a case with hypsarrhythmia in one hemisphere and a completely independent suppression-burst pattern in the other. The characteristic asyn-chrony usually appears after 3 months of age but may be recorded as early as the first month post-term.

The rare inherited metabolic diseases of the newborn are associated with a variety of nonspecific EEG abnormalities. The EEGer may suspect one of these disorders, particularly an aminoacidopathy, when a grossly abnormal background such as a paroxysmal pattern occurs in an infant with a benign neonatal course who deteriorates following the initiation of protein feeds (Rosenberg, 1977). The absence of a history of intrauterine distress, neonatal hypoxia, signs of infection, or extracerebral anomalies would suggest that another etiology is responsible for the marked disturbance of cerebral electrical activity. We have recently studied a full-term infant whose EEGs contained, among other abnormalities, positive rolandic sharp waves; a CT scan documented low density white matter lesions and subsequent metabolic studies were consistent with proprionic acidemia. More detailed EEG studies in infants with the rare aminoacidurias are needed in order to determine the incidence of these rolandic sharp waves, as well as the presence of other specific patterns which may offer clues to the underlying etiology of the encephalopathy.

Intraventricular Hemorrhage. This is the most common primary neurologic disorder of infants under 32 weeks CA. These hemorrhages begin as small subependymal bleeds into the loose germinal matrix surrounding the head or body of the caudate nucleus. Intraventricular hemorrhages are usually as-sociated with a severe encephalopathy and a high mortality; however, the evaluation of large groups with CT scans has shown that hemorrhage may be clinically silent. Papile et al (1978) found hemorrhages in 43 percent of the 46 consecutive infants weighing less than 1,500 g that they studied with CT scans. Twenty-nine of these infants survived; subependymal or intraventricular hemorrhage was found in 9 (31 percent), only 2 of whom were suspected of having hemorrhage on clinical grounds.

Cukier et al (1972) described a characteristic EEG pattern consisting of positive rolandic sharp waves in infants with intraventricular hemorrhages that were confirmed at autopsy (26 cases) or were suspected clinically (acute neurologic deterioration, decrease in hematocrit, bloody spinal fluid, and hy-drocephalus). Our own unpublished study at Stanford has yielded only a 17 percent incidence of positive rolandic sharp waves (Fig. 3.9) in 29 prematures (11 infants with autopsy-proven intraventricular hemorrhage and 18 with in-traventricular or subependymal hemorrhage on CT scan). We have also seen

K.A. S79–303 CA 30W IVH

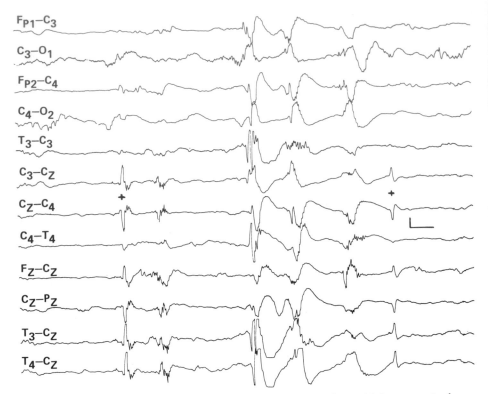

Fig. 3.9. Positive rolandic sharp waves in premature infant with intraventricular hemorrhage on CT scan. (+, positive sharp waves at Cz.) Calibration: 50 μV; 1 second.

positive rolandic sharp waves in two pre-term infants with leukomalacia and hydrocephalus, respectively.

Murat (1978) studied two groups of patients with suspected or autopsy-proven intraventricular hemorrhage. Group 1 consisted of 14 infants whose EEGs had abundant positive rolandic sharp waves (more than 1 per minute), while the EEGs of Group 2 infants contained these waves infrequently (less than 1 per minute). Group 1 infants had a high neonatal mortality or long-term morbidity and most had suffered an intraventricular hemorrhage. Eight infants died and such a hemorrhage was found at autopsy in seven, while leukomalacia and porencephaly were present in the eighth; five of the six survivors had significant neurologic sequelae and all had clinical signs in the neonatal period supporting the diagnosis. Group 2 infants fared somewhat better. Six died in the neonatal period. Four had autopsy-verified intraventricular hemorrhage, whereas two had evidence of minimal leukomalacia. Seven of the 10 survivors were neurologically normal at follow-up. Only 7 of the 16 infants in group 2 had clinical signs suggesting an intraventicular hemorrhage (as compared to 13 out of 14 in Group 1). The background EEG patterns were also more pathologic in the Group 1 infants.

Positive sharp waves occur unilaterally or bilaterally and synchronously in the rolandic area (C3 or C4) or are occasionally isolated to the central parasagittal region (Cz). The high amplitude (25 to 200 μV) positive component (100 to 500 msecs duration) is occasionally preceded but more often followed by a low amplitude negative wave. Low to moderate amplitude (10 to 60 μV) fast activity (8 to 30 Hz, usually 15 to 20 Hz) often occurs in the same location as the sharp waves, and is frequently superimposed on one phase of the sharp wave or immediately precedes or follows it.

Herpes Simplex Infection. This is one of the common fatal viral encephalitides encountered in the neonatal period. Herpes simplex encephalitis in older infants and adults is often associated with characterisitc periodic EEG patterns (Illis and Taylor, 1972) which typically appear in the temporal regions. The orbital frontal and temporal lobe predominance of the necrotizing lesion in older patients is not found in autopsies of neonates. The EEG is usually nonspecifically abnormal in neonates, but occasionally one sees a periodic pattern (Fig. 3.10) which may suggest the diagnosis (Estivill et al, 1977).

The periodic activity in the neonate consists of very slow monomorphic delta activity (.25 Hz) and slow sharp waves (repeating every 2 seconds) which are distributed widely over one hemisphere or localized to the central or temporal regions with minimal spread to homologous regions of the contralateral hemisphere. The fast repetitive sharp waves typical of the older child with herpes are not seen in the infant. (See, for example, Fig. 5 of Radermecker and Rabending, 1977.)

Focal Cerebral Pathology. This is relatively uncommon in the newborn, and is not as frequently associated with focal EEG abnormalities as in older children. Focal EEG abnormalities are not uncommon in the neonatal EEG but are usually associated with diffuse rather than focal encephalopathies. Occasionally marked focal EEG abnormalities, such as localized attenuation of the background rhythms, delta activity, or epileptiform discharges, will signal a focal intracerebral hemorrhage or a large subdural hematoma (Fig. 3.11). Focal EEG abnormalities occur more frequently in pre-term or term infants. Allemand, Monod, and Larroche (1977) studied 12 infants with subdural hematomas and found focal or unilateral EEG abnormalities in 2 and generalized EEG abnormalities in the rest. At autopsy, the EEG abnormalities were correlated with the severity of the cortical necrosis underlying the subdural rather than the size of the clot. We have recorded normal or mildly abnormal EEGs in several children with uni- or bilateral hematomas. These infants typically were neurologically intact, and it was speculated that the large clots were associated with little underlying cerebral damage. A term or preterm infant with a prominent focal EEG abnormality should probably be studied by CT scanning, even though the yield of focal pathology will be low.

N.W. 61–96–19 FT 3W HERPES ENCEPHALITIS

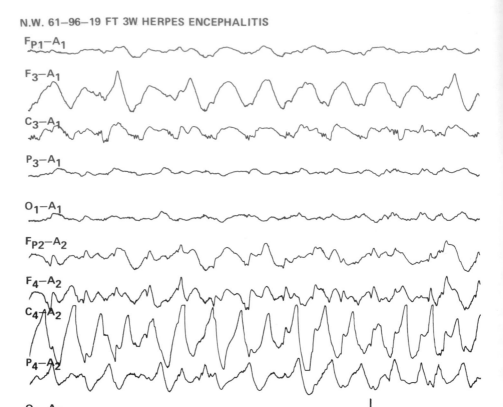

Fig. 3.10. *Herpes encephalitis in full term infant. Moderate amplitude periodic sharp waves in right central region and independent delta activity in left frontal region, which persisted throughout entire recording. Child died at 3 months of age with severe cortical atrophy. Calibration: 25 μV; 1 second.*

OLDER INFANTS AND CHILDREN

Normal Patterns During the First 2 Years

The brain grows rapidly during this period of life and significant maturational changes occur in the cerebral electrical patterns, though they are less dramatic than those encountered during the neonatal period. A brief summary of the more important maturational features will be given here, and several normal or questionably abnormal patterns which are often misinterpreted by the inexperienced EEGer will be discussed. The reader interested in a more comprehensive discussion of the normal EEG during the early years of life is referred to several excellent review articles (Kellaway and Fox, 1952; Hagne, 1968, 1972; Eeg-Olofsson, Petersén, and Selldén, 1971; Petersén and Eeg-Olofsson, 1971; Curzi-Dascalova, 1977; Pampiglione, 1977).

A.O. S79—546 FT 3D HEMORRHAGE R TEMP.

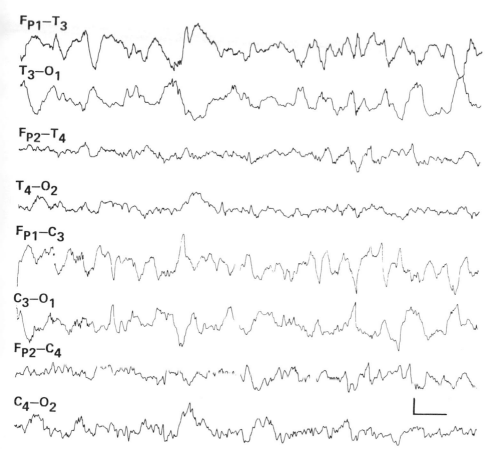

Fig. 3.11. Attenuation of the voltage of the background activity over the right hemisphere, maximal in the right temporal region, in a full term 3-day-old child who had occasional seizures, but was alert and without abnormality on neurologic examination. CT scan showed localized hemorrhage in the right temporal lobe, and carotid arteriogram suggested the presence of an arteriovenous malformation. Calibration: 50 μV; 1 second.

EEG During Wakefulness. An occipital rhythm, destined to become the alpha rhythm at 24 to 36 months of age, appears in normal infants at 3 to 6 months of age. This activity is of maximal amplitude in the midline occipital region (Oz) and appears when the child's eyes are gently and passively closed (Pampiglione, 1977). The frequency of this activity remains in the theta range until 24 to 30 months of age when it reaches 8 to 9 Hz in most normal children.

A rolandic theta rhythm which is usually 1 to 2 Hz faster than the occipital rhythm is present at 3 months of age, gradually increases in frequency to reach 8 to 9 Hz at 2 to 3 years of age. This activity is not attenuated by eye opening and probably represents the precursor of the mu rhythm. In addition to this, rhythmic theta activity may appear over the parieto-occipital and temporal regions during periods of crying. Runs of 4 Hz activity (50 to 100 μV) are also present in the temporal regions of many normal infants (Pampiglione, 1977).

Lambda activity may occur in healthy babies as early as the first few months of life (Fig. 3.12). A prominent driving response at the slower frequencies of photic stimulation is usually present in these tracings. High voltage sharp slow wave transients (often reaching 100 to 200 μV) with a triphasic morphology and located posteriorly may be seen following eye blinks in healthy children

K.B. S79–548 FT 2M AWAKE–EYES OPEN

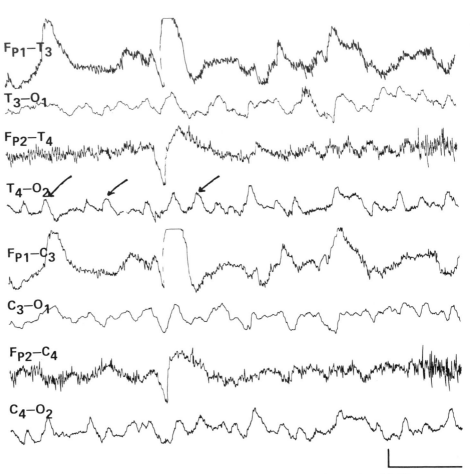

Fig. 3.12. Lambda activity in healthy full-term infant, 2 months old. There was respiratory distress during the neonatal period. The child's eyes were open and scanning the room during the EEG examination. Lambda waves are indicated by arrows. High voltage evoked responses to low frequency photic stimulation were present later in record. Calibration: 50 μV; 1 second.

(Westmoreland and Sharbrough, 1975). These transients are present between 6 months and 10 years of age with the peak incidence between 2 and 3 years. They should not be confused with epileptiform events.

EEG During Drowsiness. Drowsiness produces major interpretative problems for most electroencephalographers. The EEG patterns of drowsiness are often seen when the child appears awake with eyes open. This is noted particularly after arousal from a long period of sleep, when sedating drugs are administered or following a prolonged period of vigorous crying. Most healthy full-term infants have definite EEG changes during drowsiness which are usually characterized by an increase in the amplitude and a slowing of the frequency of the background rhythms. Drowsiness is often difficult to identify in the full-term newborn and during the first few months of life, as it may be admixed with active (REM) sleep activity. At 4 to 6 months of age, hypnagogic hypersynchrony (Kellaway and Fox, 1952) characterizes drowsiness. This pattern consists of runs lasting seconds to many minutes of high amplitude (100 to 200 μV) rhythmic 2 to 5 Hz activity. It is characterized during the first year of life by the gradual appearance during drowsiness of rhythmic activity in the parieto-occipital and temporal regions. During the second year of life, the drowsy state is often ushered in by a gradual decrease in amplitude of the background activity, which is then interrupted by bursts of high amplitude theta that are most conspicuous in the central areas, with preferential spread to the frontal regions. This paroxysmal pattern occurs most commonly in children between 3 to 6 years of age but may still be present at 12 years of age.

Paroxysmal hypnagogic hypersynchrony is often admixed with sharp waves and occasionally with random spikes, which lead to an "epileptiform" morphology. These bursts of high amplitude theta are often interpreted as abnormal and represent one of the most difficult interpretative areas in pediatric EEG (Fig. 3.13). We have been conservative in our interpretation of all paroxysmal activity which is confined to the transition between waking and sleep. We classify such activity as normal if it occurs only in drowsiness, disappears when typical sleep complexes such as vertex waves and spindles appear, and when the spikes or sharp waves have a random temporal relationship to the theta waves.

EEG During Sleep. As mentioned earlier, active (REM) sleep characterizes sleep onset in newborns. This REM onset persists in the EEG laboratory setting until approximately 3 months of age, at which time the adult quiet (nonREM) pattern of sleep onset appears (Curzi-Dascalova, 1977). Studies of normal infants in their home environment have revealed the persistence of REM sleep onset in some subjects until 22 weeks of age (Kligman, Smyrl, and Emde, 1975). Within the first few months of life, several typical patterns of quiet (nonREM) sleep make their appearance. The *12 to 14 Hz spindles* which characterize stages 2 and 3 sleep in older children and adults can be seen in the quiet sleep of some infants as early as the second month of life and are present throughout quiet sleep in the majority of infants by 3 to 4 months of age

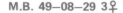

M.B. 49–08–29 3♀

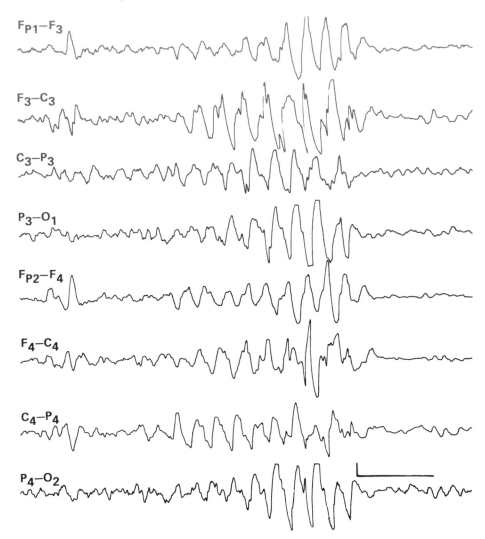

Fig. 3.13. *Hypnagogic hypersynchrony during drowsiness in a healthy 3-year-old female. Time constant, 0.035 seconds. Calibration: 50 μV; 1 second.*

(Curzi-Dascalova, 1977; Lenard, 1970; Metcalf, 1970). Spindles are usually present symmetrically over the central regions but are characteristically asynchronous. This asynchrony may persist until 2 years of age and is often seen in older children during the early stages of nonREM sleep. Spindles in the first year of life have a monophasic and frequently "spiky" morphology and may exceed 10 seconds in duration. The longest spindles appear at 3 to 4 months of age. As the child enters the second year of life the duration of the sleep spindles decreases, the interval between the spindles increases, and the incidence decreases. The incidence during nonREM sleep remains low until an increase occurs at 4 to 5 years of age (Tanguay et al, 1975). It is not uncommon, therefore, for sleep spindles to be sparse or absent in very light sleep of older infants, whereas their absence in infants between 5 and 12 months is unusual and considered abnormal by many electroencephalographers. Hypothyroid infants have a striking reduction of spindles (Schultz et al, 1968). In a few normal infants, sleep spindles may be more abundant over one hemisphere during the entire tracing. Only major and persistent voltage asymmetries or an absence of spindles during quiet sleep in the second half of the first year should be considered abnormal.

Vertex sharp waves can usually be identified during nonREM sleep after the fifth month of life (Metcalf, Mondale, and Butler, 1971). Their voltage field is more diffuse in infants and they often blend into the background activity, making identification difficult. Curzi-Dascalova (1977) has identified repetitive sharp waves, confined to the central parasagittal regions (Cz), in infants during the first month of life. She believes that these focal sharp waves are the precursors of vertex waves. Vertex waves consist primarily of monophasic negative sharp waves during the first 2 years of life. In older children there is a tendency for vertex activity to consist of bursts and runs of repetitive, high amplitude sharp waves, which are frequently admixed with sleep spindles. The repetition may occur 3 to 9 times within 1 to 3 seconds (Metcalf et al, 1971). One must be careful not to classify high amplitude, short duration, and repetitive vertex waves as epileptiform. Vertex waves are usually symmetrical and synchronous but transient voltage asymmetries do occur, and not infrequently a series of vertex waves will appear unilaterally for several seconds over one hemisphere. In our experience, typical *K-complexes* do not appear until 2 to 3 years of age.

REM sleep is often recorded during the first year of life, but is rarely seen thereafter in routine clinical EEGs. The low to moderate amplitude mixed frequency slow background is usually easily distinguishable from nonREM sleep. Rhythmic sharp 3 to 6 Hz activity occurring in bursts or runs may be seen in the posterior head regions. These sharp waves are confined to the midline occipital electrode (Oz) until 4 months of age, after which they can be recorded from more widespread areas posteriorly. This activity is often temporally associated with the rapid eye movements. It should be considered an entirely normal pattern.

Normal Patterns After the First 2 Years

No attempt will be made here to cover all the various patterns encountered in normal children as the EEG evolves to its adult form. Rather, discussion will be centered on those areas which, in our experience, present the most difficult interpretative problems for the EEGer. The reader interested in a detailed discussion of the normal EEG patterns of childhood and adolescence should refer to the articles by Petersén, Selldén, and Eeg-Olofsson (1975); Petersén and Eeg-Olofsson (1971); and Eeg-Olofsson et al (1971).

Occipital slow activity in the delta and theta range is common in children of all ages. There are no definite guidelines as to what constitutes excessive posterior slowing. Each EEGer must develop his or her own normative range. A conservative approach is suggested. Many EEGs are overread because of an exaggerated concern for slightly excessive theta activity during the waking recording. In many instances the slowing is caused by drowsiness. For this reason technologists should alert all cooperative children for at least a portion of the record by engaging the patient in conversation and attempting to record the waking EEG prior to sleep. Several varieties of slow activity may be encountered.

Occipital slow waves (''slow-fused transients'') consist of single, high amplitude delta waves which are admixed with the ongoing alpha (Kellaway, Crawley, and Kagawa, 1959). The alpha wave immediately preceding the slow transient is often of higher amplitude than the preceding alpha and, in conjunction with the slow wave, creates a sharp-slow wave complex which is not infrequently referred to as epileptiform by the inexperienced reader.

Rhythmic 2.5 to 4.5 Hz activity in the temporo-occipital regions is common in children (25 percent, according to Petersén and Eeg-Olofsson, 1971) and reaches maximal expression at 5 to 7 years of age. This activity may have a sharp morphology, particularly when it is admixed with the alpha activity, and usually appears in short runs or bursts.

Doose and his colleagues (Gerken and Doose, 1972; Doose, Gerken, and Völzke, 1972) have studied the genetics of two varieties of posterior slowing— parietal theta (4 to 6 Hz), and occipital delta (2 to 4 Hz). The EEGs of children with centrencephalic seizures are more likely to contain these patterns. The normal siblings of epileptic children with parietal theta have a higher incidence of this pattern (13 percent) than siblings of epileptic children without parietal theta (3.2 percent), or a control group of normal children (5.6 percent).

Bursts and runs of occipital delta are commonly seen in children with petit mal epilepsy (Aird and Gastaut, 1959). The delta in epileptic children usually occurs in high amplitude bursts and is frequently admixed with spikes forming a typical 3/sec spike and wave complex. Doose et al (1972) found similar occipital delta activity without the accompanying spikes in 6.8 percent of normal control subjects. This rhythm often appears in short runs immediately following eye closure and should be interpreted conservatively unless other abnormalities coexist.

A mu rhythm is occasionally seen in young children and the incidence increases progressively with age. A typical 7 to 11 Hz central rhythm with a comb-like form was found by Petersén and Eeg-Olofsson (1971) in 7.1 percent of normal children. If one accepts all centrally located 7 to 11 Hz rhythms that are not attenuated by eye opening, the incidence of mu exceeds 7 percent. Monophasic sharply contoured mu often occurs unilaterally in the central regions where it may be misinterpreted as an abnormal pattern.

Hyperventilation usually provokes a buildup of high amplitude mixed delta and theta activity in normal children at all ages. This response most commonly consists of an increase in the pre-existing posterior slow activity, such as the slow-fused transients, or a buildup of posteriorly dominant or diffuse slow activity. Less commonly, and usually in older children, frontally dominant delta and theta activity will be provoked. A buildup with hyperventilation is abnormal only if persistently focal slow activity or epileptiform potentials appear, generalized spike and slow wave activity is activated, or the buildup is markedly asymmetrical. In the latter situation the hemisphere which manifests the lower voltage slowing or fails to respond to the hyperventilation is often more involved pathologically. A generalized buildup of delta, even if it has a "paroxysmal appearance" should be considered normal, unless definite spikes are admixed with the slow waves. The admixture of a high amplitude alpha and a prominent buildup of occipital delta often leads to the appearance of sharp-slow wave complexes which can easily be misinterpreted as epileptiform.

Intermittent photic stimulation is routinely performed in most clinical laboratories. The main value of this technique is to provoke epileptiform activity (photoconvulsive response). It is well-known that paroxysmal responses may be provoked in normal children. Eeg-Olofsson et al (1971) found an "abnormal" response in 8.9 percent of their normal population. In approximately half of these children, the response was characterized by bursts of high voltage slow activity, often with admixed spikes; and in the remainder the response was characterized by a bitemporo-occipital sharp-slow wave or spike-slow wave response. Their results were similar to those of Doose et al (1969), who found photoconvulsive responses in 6.8 percent of a control population. They emphasized the genetic features of the response, which occurred more frequently in the siblings of epileptic children with a photoconvulsive response than in the control population.

Occipital spikes may be provoked in a very small number of nonepileptic children in the absence of a photoconvulsive response by photic stimulation, using a photo stimulator with a fine grid pattern (Maheshwari and Jeavons, 1975). These spikes, which are confined to the parieto-occipital regions, gradually increase in amplitude as the stimulus is continued. They occur in a wide variety of nonepileptic disorders and are of doubtful pathologic significance.

Colon et al (1979) have recently described an "off-response" in infants with a variety of neonatal conditions, particularly the respiratory distress syndrome. The pathologic significance of this spike complex which immediately follows the cessation of photic stimulation must await further studies.

Drowsiness and sleep present as many interpretative problems in older children as they do in the first 2 years of life. High voltage paroxysmal "hypnagogic hypersynchrony," which in our experience is maximally expressed between 3 and 5 years of age, is still encountered in the EEGs of children up to 12 years of age (Fig. 3.13). Drowsiness in children is usually characterized by the gradual disappearance of the alpha rhythm, an increase in the amount of fronto-central beta activity, and the appearance of rhythmic posterior 2.5 to 6 Hz activity. Artifact from slow horizontal eye movements may be noted in the lateral frontal leads. More anterior rhythms are noted in children beyond 10 to 12 years of age.

During light sleep, runs of high voltage repetitive sharp vertex waves are common and frequently admix with central spindles leading to complexes which are often classified as epileptiform. Sleep spindles may appear to have spiky harmonic components when recorded with bipolar montages (Fig. 3.14). A referential montage will reveal the benign morphology of this paroxysmal sleep activity.

14 and 6 Hz positive spikes are commonly recorded in the EEGs of adolescents and are considered a normal pattern by most EEGers. Schwartz and Lombroso (1968) found an incidence of 55 percent in a group of healthy schoolchildren between 8 and 16 years, and Lombroso et al (1966) reported 14 and 6 Hz positive spikes in the EEGs of 58 percent of a group of 155 boys aged 13 to 15 years. Eeg-Olofsson (1971), on the other hand, found them in only 14.6 percent of a group of healthy adolescents. Some authors believe that 14 and 6 Hz positive spikes can be correlated with autonomic ("vegetative") dysfunction, behavior disorders, and abdominal epilepsy (Hughes, 1965).

Yamada, Young, and Kimura (1977) have observed a high incidence of positive spike bursts in a group of children with Reye's syndrome. This activity appeared during deep stages of coma, in some instances only following auditory or tactile stimulation. The bursts disappeared or were less abundant as the children recovered. Fourteen and six per second positive spikes have also been reported in adults during hepatic coma (Silverman, 1964). The significance of these observations is still unclear.

Psychomotor variant discharge was first described by Gibbs, Rich, and Gibbs (1963). They found that the highest incidence of this rhythmic sharp temporal theta was in adolescents between the ages of 15 and 19 years. Ten percent of their patients were younger than 10 years. Lipman and Hughes

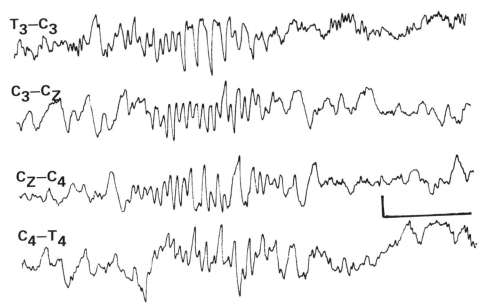

Fig. 3.14. *Sleep spindle (sigma) and vertex waves in a healthy 3-year-old female (same child as in Fig. 3.13). Calibration: 50 μV; 1 second.*

(1969) found this pattern, which they called "rhythmic mid-temporal discharge," in 0.3 percent of their laboratory population. Thirteen percent of their patients were under 20 years of age (3.6 percent were younger than 10). Both of these groups considered the pattern abnormal and associated it with vegetative and psychiatric disorders and seizures, particularly psychomotor attacks.

Eeg-Olofsson et al (1971), on the other hand, found this pattern in 6 normal children between the ages of 6 and 14 years (0.8 percent of their total population of normal children). The pathologic significance of this rare pattern is still uncertain. It is our opinion that the psychomotor variant discharge has not been established as an epileptiform disturbance and should be interpreted conservatively.

Abnormal EEGs in Infants and Children

The EEG has wide use in pediatric neurology and can be of value in evaluating children with a variety of proven or suspected neurologic disorders. In most instances, the EEG is used to verify the organic nature of a particular neurologic disturbance, confirm a clinical suspicion as to the location of a particular lesion, follow the progression of a disease and the response to therapy, investigate the possibility that episodic behavioral or motor phenomena are epileptic in nature, or provide data which will help the clinician classify a seizure disorder and develop rational therapy. In this section we will briefly discuss some of the EEG patterns seen in children after the age of 1 month which are relatively specific for certain diseases, contribute significantly to the therapy of the patient, assist in reaching a diagnosis, or are of prognostic value.

Epilepsy. The EEG is a valuable diagnostic test in the evaluation of children with episodic disturbances of behavior. However, the episodic nature of the problem results in a significant number of nondiagnostic EEGs. In order to increase the yield of abnormal records, the clinician should be familiar with the factors which may provoke the appearance of epileptiform activity. These factors include adequate waking and sleeping recordings obtained at a time of day when the child is more likely to be having seizures; activating procedures such as hyperventilation, photic stimulation, and sleep deprivation (in older children); the use of nasopharyngeal electrodes in older children and adolescents; and the recording of an EEG in close proximity to a seizure, particularly if a previous EEG was normal or nonspecifically abnormal (Ajmone Marsan and Zivin, 1970; Knight, Le Portz, and Harper, 1977). Occasionally, anticonvulsant drugs should be discontinued, particularly if the diagnosis of epilepsy is uncertain or if the patient is being evaluated for surgical excision of a focal epileptogenic area. During and immediately after anticonvulsant drug withdrawal, bursts of generalized spike and wave activity may transiently appear in the EEGs of patients with focal epileptogenic lesions as well as in nonepileptic patients who are withdrawing from short-acting barbiturate drugs (Ludwig and Ajmone Marsan, 1975). In the former situation the record should not be interpreted as indicative of a focal *and* generalized epileptic disturbance until the drug withdrawal effect is dissipated. In the case of the adolescent with the sudden onset of generalized seizures whose EEG contains generalized, usually 4 to 6 per second spike and wave activity, a urine and serum sample should be screened for illicit drugs.

The EEG findings in patients with various types of seizure disorders, defined according to the International Classification of Epilepsy (Gastaut, 1970), are summarized in Chapter 2, but certain additional aspects that relate particularly to the pediatrician will be discussed here.

Petit Mal Epilepsy. The EEG is only rarely normal (approximately 5 percent of cases) in children with untreated petit mal epilepsy (Gibbs and Gibbs, 1952). Repeatedly normal EEGs in a child with absence attacks is, therefore, more consistent with a focal seizure disorder. Long-term monitoring of children with untreated petit mal has shown that there are often periods during the day when a child may be free of clinical seizures and the EEG relatively devoid of epileptiform discharges. It is important, therefore, to determine prior to the EEG if such a seizure-free period is recognized by the family, and to arrange the EEG for some other time of the day.

The morphology of the 3 per second spike and wave discharge is modified by sleep (Niedermeyer, 1965). The bursts during nonREM sleep are shorter in duration and more irregular in morphology with generalized polyspike and polyspike and wave discharges, replacing the typical 3 per second spike and wave burst. This polyspike activity does not appear to predict the concurrence or future appearance of generalized motor seizures. It must not be confused with the slow spike and wave activity of the Lennox-Gastaut syndrome.

Generalized atypical spike and slow wave activity occasionally appears in the EEG of a normal child. These bursts are noted particularly during hyperventilation (0.3 percent) and drowsiness (7 percent) (Petersén and Eeg-Olofsson, 1971). Typical 3 per second spike and slow wave activity may be seen in the normal nonepileptic siblings of children with clinical petit mal seizures.

The EEG is also of value in formulating a long-term prognosis for a child with petit mal. Sato, Dreifuss, and Penry (1976) prospectively studied a group of children with petit mal epilepsy of whom over 50 percent also had generalized tonic-clonic seizures and a few had focal attacks. They found three variables that were statistically correlated with the ultimate outcome of all types of seizures. A negative history of generalized tonic-clonic seizures, an I.Q. greater than 90, and a negative family history of seizures were associated with the ultimate disappearance of all types of seizures. A normal EEG background at the time of the initial evaluation and an I.Q. above 90 were significant factors for the cessation of absence seizures. Cessation of absence seizures occurred in 87.5 percent of children who satisfied such criteria.

Secondary Generalized Epilepsy. There are three major electroencephalographic syndromes that occur in children with static or progressive encephalopathies: hypsarrhythmia, Lennox-Gastaut syndrome, and the independent multifocal spike foci pattern. These syndromes were developed primarily on the basis of specific EEG abnormalities and are associated with a heterogeneous group of diseases. They are the electrographic expression of a diffuse encephalopathy and any neurologic disorder which is associated with a generalized involvement of the neocortex may manifest one or all of these EEG patterns. In this section we will discuss the salient features of each syndrome and emphasize, particularly, the more recent observations in the literature.

Hypsarrhythmia is characterized by a diffusely abnormal background comprised of high amplitude delta activity with admixed multifocal spikes and sharp waves (Gibbs and Gibbs, 1952). This pattern is usually associated with the clinical syndrome of infantile spasms (Lacy and Penry, 1976). Hypsarrhythmia is the electroencephalographic expression of a diffuse encephalopathy, occurring primarily in the first year of life due to any diffuse insult to the developing brain. It is expressed clinically by infantile spasms, delay of developmental milestones, abnormalities of the neurologic examination, and a very poor prognosis for ultimate intellectual development. Infantile spasms can be the result of a specific disease entity such as viral encephalitis, or the sequelae of a severe neonatal insult such as an anoxic-ischemic encephalopathy. Approximately 60 percent of cases can be placed in this symptomatic group (Lacy and Penry, 1976). The remainder are cryptogenic, the syndrome appearing de novo in a previously healthy child. Normal intellectual development is more common following recovery in this latter group.

Infants in the symptomatic group are often neurologically abnormal in the neonatal period, and have abnormal EEGs. In many cases, however, the EEG and the neurologic examination become normal during the first few months of life. Subsequently, minor abnormalities, such as focal sharp waves, will gradually appear in the EEG and evolve into a pattern of full-blown hypsarrhythmia (Watanabe, Iwase, and Hara, 1973).

It should be emphasized that not all children with hypsarrhythmia have infantile spasms. In the series of children with hypsarrhythmia reported by Friedman and Pampiglione (1971), 26 percent did not have spasms during their illness, though some children had other types of seizures. Children with hypsarrhythmia and seizures other than infantile spasms had a poorer prognosis than those with spasms alone.

On the other hand, children with the clinical syndrome of infantile spasms may have EEG abnormalities other than typical hypsarrhythmia. These nonhypsarrhythmic abnormalities include focal or multifocal sharp waves or spikes and suppression-burst patterns, as well as other periodic patterns (so-called modified hypsarrhythmia). A small number of infants may develop hypsarrhythmia only during sleep. Others develop infantile spasms before the appearance of the typical EEG abnormalities. Unilateral hypsarrhythmia has been reported in some rare congenital malformations of the brain (Aicardi et al, 1969; Tjiam et al, 1978).

Lombroso and Fejerman (1977) described a group of children aged 3 to 8 months, who developed a disorder characterized by infantile spasms but whose EEGs were entirely normal and whose recovery was complete.

Moreover, these children did not manifest the regression or arrest of development typical of the classical infantile spasms syndrome.

The EEG is of little value in formulating a prognosis for ultimate intellectual development. There is a tendency for full recovery in those infants whose initial EEGs are less severely abnormal (i.e. lacking hypsarrhythmia), but many exceptions occur. The syndrome reported by Lombroso and Fejerman (1977) appears to have an uniformly good prognosis. Jeavons, Bower, and Dimitrakoudi (1973) discuss the many clinical factors which can be correlated with the outcome.

The Lennox-Gastaut syndrome includes a heterogeneous group of static and progressive encephalopathies which are grouped together on the basis of the presence of slow spike and slow wave discharges on the EEG. The EEG pattern is commonly recorded during the first two decades of life, but seizure onset is most frequently between 6 months and 3 years of age. Occasional patients have had the onset of seizures in the teens. Gastaut et al (1966) described the clinical spectrum which accompanies this particular EEG pattern: mental retardation, high incidence of abnormalities on neurologic examination, and the frequent occurrence of tonic, akinetic, atypical absence, and generalized tonic-clonic seizures which are characteristically refractory to anticonvulsant drugs. The pathology underlying the syndrome may range from a postanoxic encephalopathy dating from the neonatal period to a progressive form of Batten's disease. Markand (1977) found a close relationship between the EEG patterns of this syndrome and hypsarrhythmia, whereas Blume, David, and Gomez (1973) reported a lower incidence of infantile spasms preceding the slow spike-wave syndrome in his patient population. Markand (1977) also described a subpopulation of children whose waking EEG had little or no epileptiform activity but whose sleeping recording contained abundant and often continuous generalized spike and slow wave activity. Despite the striking enhancement of epileptiform activity by sleep, these children had a better prognosis for intellectual development than the group as a whole.

Blume et al (1973) reported a long-term follow-up study of 84 children whose initial EEG contained slow spike and wave discharges. Only 14 of the 68 patients included in the follow-up were attending regular classes in school or working at independent jobs. Forty-six percent of the patients for whom sufficient follow-up data existed were dead or in institutions. The mean duration of follow-up was 12 years 3 months. Only one-third of the survivors were seizure free at follow-up. The prognosis for intellectual development was unfavorable in those patients whose seizures began before the age of 2, those who had tonic seizures, and those with an abnormal neurologic or ophthalmologic examination at the time of the initial evaluation or whose EEG at any time showed a slow spike-wave pattern with a repetition rate less than 1.5 per second.

The *multiple spike foci pattern* is not infrequently seen in children with a prior history of hypsarrhythmia or the Lennox-Gastaut syndrome. This pattern is defined as "epileptiform discharges (spikes, sharp waves, or both) which, on any single recording, arise from at least three noncontiguous electrode positions with at least one focus in each hemisphere" (Blume, 1978). The majority of patients with this EEG pattern are in the first two decades of life. Most (84 percent) of the children with this EEG pattern have seizures (Blume, 1978), and the majority of those with seizures have more than one type, with generalized tonic-clonic attacks being the most common. Almost half the patients reported by Blume (1978) and by Noriega-Sanchez and Markand (1976) experienced daily attacks. Many patients are intellectually subnormal, particularly if seizures started before the age of 2, and have abnormal neurologic examinations. Blume (1978) described three EEG variables that appeared to reflect the severity of the encephalopathy and, in turn, the degree of intellectual impairment and the severity of the epilepsy: spike incidence, number of spike foci, and the normality of the background activity. If the EEG contained 10 or more foci, more than 1 spike per 10 seconds, and an excessive amount of background delta activity, the child was almost always intellectually impaired.

These three patterns appear to represent the electroencephalographic expression of severe, diffuse encephalopathies. Some infants will manifest a progression from hypsarrhythmia in the first year of life, through the Lennox-Gastaut syndrome during the next few years of life, to multiple independent spike foci. It should be reemphasized that these patterns are caused by a wide variety of static and progressive neurologic disorders and are not diagnostic of any particular pathologic entity.

Benign focal epilepsy of childhood (rolandic epilepsy) has received so much attention in the literature over the last decade that it will be discussed only briefly. Bancaud, Colomb, and Dell (1958) and Nayrac and Beaussart (1958) first described the clinical and electrographic features of this syndrome, and Bray and Wiser (1964) described the genetic aspects of focal spikes in mid-temporal and rolandic areas. Subsequent studies have clearly delineated a syndrome which is characterized clinically by the occurrence of seizures in a healthy child between the ages of 5 and 12. The seizures are typically focal (usually hemifacial) when they occur during waking hours, and have a tendency to generalize during sleep (Lerman and Livity, 1975). The EEG features biphasic sharp waves in the centrotemporal regions and a normal background (Lombroso, 1967). These epileptiform transients are often bilateral and asynchronous and may be markedly increased in frequency during sleep. Long-term follow-up studies reveal that 50 to 100 percent of infants will become seizure free in their mid-teens (Lerman and Livity, 1975; Beaussart and Faou, 1978). There is rarely any demonstrable focal pathology and diagnostic radiologic procedures are usually not indicated. An autosomal dominant gene with age-dependent penetrance is responsible for the EEG trait (Heijbel, Blom, and Rasmuson, 1975). Focal centrotemporal spikes are, therefore, quite common in siblings of children with this syndrome and can also occur in normal children with negative family histories for epilepsy (1.1 percent of the series of 743 children studied by Eeg-Olofsson et al, 1971).

Other Benign Epileptiform Syndromes. Occipital foci occur frequently in nonepileptic children, particularly those with ocular or visual abnormalities

(Smith and Kellaway, 1964). Foci in this area are seen in the EEGs of children at all ages and are usually not associated with neurologic or intellectual abnormalities. In our experience, however, they are more likely to be associated with significant underlying pathology when occurring in the neonatal period and during the first 2 years of life.

Benign epileptiform transients of sleep or small sharp spikes are commonly seen in the normal population, particularly if nasopharyngeal electrodes are used (White, Langston, and Pedley, 1977). These sleep activated spikes have a high incidence in adults but can occur in teenagers. In a recent study of 120 normal subjects between the ages of 10 and 80 years, they were recorded in 24 percent (White et al, 1977). They were present in 10 percent of individuals between 10 and 20 years of age. The youngest patient to be reported with this paroxysmal pattern is a child aged 9 years (White, J.; personal communication).

Loiseau and Orgogozo (1978) described a syndrome of benign focal epilepsy in teenagers which they differentiated from benign rolandic epilepsy. They retrospectively selected a group of patients between the ages of 10 and 20 who had experienced a single focal motor, sensorimotor, or sensory seizure, or a flurry of such seizures, and whose ultimate course was benign. Seventy-two percent of the patients were males, there was an absence of a family history of seizures, the neurologic examination was normal, and the EEG was normal or contained nonspecific slowing. Recurrent seizures did not occur even when therapy was withheld.

Febrile Seizures. The EEG is of little value in the evaluation of children with febrile seizures. Approximately one-third of children with febrile seizures have abnormal EEGs during the first post-seizure week, characterized by excessive posterior slowing (Frantzen, Lennox-Buchthal, and Nygaard, 1968; Lennox-Buchthal, 1973). Paroxysmal activity rarely occurs in the immediate post-seizure period, and another etiology must be considered if abundant spikes or generalized paroxysmal epileptiform activity are present at such a time.

Paroxysmal activity subsequently develops in a significant number of children with febrile seizures. It did so in 29 percent in the study of Lennox-Buchthal (1973). This activity consisted primarily of generalized spike and wave activity and focal spikes, usually temporal or occipital in location. Children who developed these paroxysmal abnormalities did not have a higher risk for the development of nonfebrile seizures when compared with children whose EEGs lacked paroxysmal activity. Schiottz-Christensen and Hammerberg (1975) confirmed these findings in a follow-up study of 59 pairs of twins of the same sex. The incidence of paroxysmal EEG abnormalities was significantly higher in the twin who had had a febrile seizure than in the normal sibling.

The EEG does not appear to be of value in predicting which child will have future febrile seizures or will develop epilepsy. Risk factors for epilepsy after febrile seizures are clinical: family history of febrile seizures, pre-existing neurologic abnormality and a complicated initial seizure (more than 15 minutes duration; more than 1 seizure in 24 hours; focal features) (Nelson and Ellenberg, 1976, 1978).

We do not suggest that an EEG be routinely obtained on a child who has had a febrile seizure unless there is evidence of an underlying neurologic disorder. It is also the EEGer's responsibility to comment about the possible relationship between an unexpected paroxysmal event in the EEG of an older child and a history of febrile seizures. A burst of spike and slow wave activity in the EEG of a 6-year-old child with dyslexia may be the genetic "marker" of a previous febrile seizure disorder, rather than being in any way related to the child's present complaint.

Convulsive Aphasia. This is an uncommon disorder, first described by Landau and Kleffner (1957), characterized by the appearance of a progressive aphasia in a previously healthy child. The EEG is characterized by relatively continuous generalized slow spike and slow wave discharges which are of higher amplitude over the temporal or posterior head regions. The degree of aphasia appears to roughly parallel the EEG abnormalities (Shoumaker et al, 1974). Seizures frequently occur after onset of the aphasia but are easily treated with anticonvulsant medication. Treatment has no effect on the aphasia which disappears partially or completely over a period of years. The etiology is unknown.

Infectious Diseases. The electroencephalographic abnormalities in children with CNS infections are usually nonspecific. Localized slowing or epileptiform activity may indicate focal pathology such as abscesses or subdural empyemas, and a unilateral attenuation of the voltage of the background activity may suggest a subdural effusion. As a rule, however, the EEG has not been of particular value in the detection of subdural effusions (Rabe, 1967) and has been replaced in many situations by CT scanning. This discussion will, therefore, be limited to two infectious illnesses which are associated with EEG patterns that are relatively specific and may allow the EEGer to suggest the proper diagnosis.

Subacute Sclerosing Panencephalitis (Dawson's Encephalitis; SSPE). The periodic EEG complexes which characterize this rare chronic, progressive disease of the CNS consist of relatively stereotyped, bilaterally simultaneous bursts of slow activity and sharp waves with a periodicity approximating 3 to 10 seconds (occasionally as long as 90 seconds), which are usually accompanied clinically by myoclonic jerks. They can occur early in the illness and may be associated with normal waking and sleep activity. They may be asymmetric and, even more infrequently, asynchronous (Markand and Panszi, 1975; Ibrahim and Jeavons, 1974). Occasionally the periodic activity is focal, in which case it usually consists of repetitive sharp slow waves which have a less complex morphology than the more generalized complexes (Fig. 3.15). The complexes occasionally appear only during sleep, with normal or nonspecifically abnormal waking tracings (Westmoreland, Gomez, and Blume, 1977). Prominent epileptiform activity in the form of spikes, sharp waves, or spike and slow wave discharges may accompany the bursts. This activity may assume a pattern

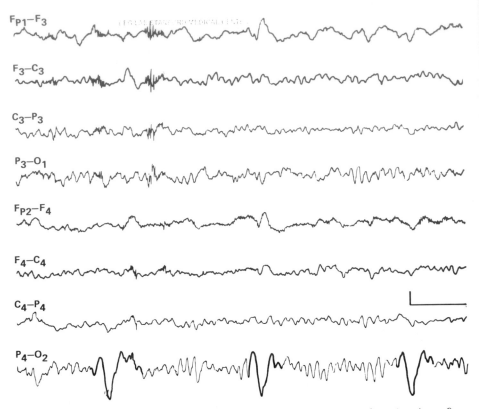

Fig. 3.15. *Focal periodic sharp slow waves in right occipital region in a 9-year-old boy with biopsy-proven SSPE. Note preservation of alpha rhythm. (Periodic complexes retouched for clarity.) Calibration: 50 μV; 1 second.*

resembling that seen in the Lennox-Gastaut syndrome (Westmoreland, Blume, and Gomez, 1976). Patients have been described with prolonged runs of generalized epileptiform activity and a clinical state resembling petit mal status. The typical periodic pattern may appear after the epileptiform activity is suppressed by intravenous diazepam (Lombroso, 1968). Lombroso (1968) described one child presenting with the clinical and electrographic features of epilepsia partialis continua who never developed a periodic EEG pattern. On rare occasions, the repetitive myoclonic jerks will occur during the waking state without the accompanying EEG complexes. More commonly the EEG complexes persist during sleep after disappearance of the clinical myoclonus.

Periodic complexes resembling those of SSPE have been reported in other forms of encephalitis (Ibrahim and Jeavons, 1974). Chronic progressive rubella encephalitis, which may clinically resemble SSPE, does not appear to manifest periodic EEG complexes (Weil et al, 1975). Townsend et al (1975) described the EEG findings in one of their cases (Case 2) as "generalized periodic low amplitude polyspike complexes that were closely related to myoclonic movements." A comparison to the periodic complexes of SSPE was not made.

Unfortunately, detailed EEG studies of this rare syndrome have not been published.

Periodic complexes resembling those of SSPE may occur in other neurologic disorders. We have reported a similar pattern during the post-ictal state in a child with seizures arising from the orbitofrontal region (Tharp, 1972). Unusual periodic discharges resembling those of SSPE have been reported in phencyclidine (PCP) intoxication (Fariello and Black, 1978).

Herpes Simplex Encephalitis. This disorder is often associated with a rather characteristic EEG pattern. Though this periodic pattern has been described more frequently in adults, it has been reported in children as young as a few days of age (Smith et al, 1975; Radermecker and Rabending, 1977; Estivill et al, 1977; Ch'ien et al, 1977). The periodic activity consists of high amplitude mono- or biphasic sharp slow waves that recur every 2 to 4 seconds. These complexes appear focally, primarily in the frontotemporal area, or diffusely over one hemisphere with variable spread to the contralateral side. The early recognition of herpes encephalitis has assumed more importance since the report that adenine arabinoside may be an effective therapy in this illness (Whitley et al, 1977).

Reye's Syndrome. This syndrome represents one of the most common and often fatal encephalopathies of childhood. Although there is multisystem involvement in Reye's syndrome, the CNS impairment is responsible for the mortality and long morbidity. Most cases are preceded by a prodromal illness, usually viral in nature, which rapidly progresses to an encephalopathy of variable severity associated with chemical evidence of severe hepatic disease and hyperammonemia. The cause of the encephalopathy is unknown, but it does not appear to be secondary to the hyperammonemia or to any single metabolic disturbance. There is often severe cerebral edema, and death is not infrequently caused by tentorial herniation and brainstem compression. Aoki and Lombroso (1973) developed an EEG scoring system which reflected the severity of the encephalopathy and could be correlated with the ultimate outcome. Their EEG categories 4 and 5 were associated with 100 percent mortality, while approximately 50 percent of infants with group 3 EEGs and 100 percent with groups 1 and 2 survived. Subsequent authors have confirmed these findings and even stated that the EEGs obtained prior to therapy were excellent predictors of outcome despite the prompt institution of therapy (van Caillie et al, 1977). Continuous intracranial pressure monitoring has been shown to be particularly helpful in treatment. The vigorous and prompt use of dehydrating agents has been followed by the survival of infants with severely abnormal EEGs (Kindt et al, 1975).

Continuous EEG monitoring has been advocated as a guide to the effectiveness of therapy. Trauner, Stockard, and Sweetman (1977) were able to correlate alterations in the EEG activity and serum organic acid concentrations. They suggested that elevations of the serum levels of short-chain fatty acids may be responsible at least in part for the encephalopathy.

We have discussed in a previous section the reported appearance of positive spike bursts in Reye's syndrome (Yamada et al, 1977). The specificity of this activity to the encephalopathy of Reye's syndrome is still uncertain.

Progressive Neurologic Syndromes. The EEG abnormalities accompanying most of the progressive neurologic syndromes of childhood are nonspecific and consist of variably slowed background activity, and focal or generalized epileptiform discharges. In the early phases of the diffuse encephalopathies, a distinction can sometimes be made between a primary grey or white matter disorder on the basis of the EEG pattern (Gloor, Kalabay, and Giard, 1968). Continuous nonparoxysmal polymorphous delta activity is more commonly associated with the leukoencephalopathies, whereas multifocal cortical or generalized epileptiform activity in association with bilateral paroxysmal slow activity is more consistent with neuronal disease including cortical and subcortical grey matter. As the disease progresses this distinction becomes less prominent (Blom and Hagberg, 1967).

There are several neurodegenerative disorders with EEG abnormalities that are sufficiently characteristic to warrant discussion.

Neuronal Ceroid Lipofuscinosis. Zeman and Dyken (1969) introduced the term "neuronal ceroid lipofuscinosis" as a neuropathologic description for all forms of amaurotic familial idiocy except Tay-Sachs disease. Among the many clinical and pathologic subgroups in this disease, three have been reported with peculiar EEG abnormalities.

In the late infantile form (Bielschowsky type), a characteristic high voltage response to low rates of photic stimulation has been reported (Harden, Pampiglione, and Picton-Robinson, 1973; Pampiglione and Harden, 1973). High voltage visual evoked potentials (VEP) and a low voltage or absent electroretinogram (ERG) are also typical. This disease begins at 2 to 4 years of age, usually with seizures.

Santavuori, Haltia, and Rapola (1974) described a type of ceroid lipofuscinosis with onset in the first 2 years of life, and characterized clinically by a regression of developmental milestones followed by myoclonus. Serial EEGs in this early infantile form revealed a progressive diminution in amplitude, culminating in isoelectricity. The rapid development of a flat EEG in conjunction with a gradual loss of the ERG and VEP is not seen in other forms of neuronal storage disease.

The EEG features of a third variety of ceroid lipofuscinosis (Spielmeyer type) were described by Pampiglione and Harden (1977). The main clinical feature of this variant is progressive visual loss beginning at 4 to 7 years of age. The EEGs contain runs of high amplitude slow wave and spike activity. The ERG disappears at an early stage of the illness and the VEP gradually becomes of low amplitude.

Menkes' Disease. This is a rare sex-linked metabolic disease which has been called "kinky hair disease" or "steely hair disease" because of the characteristic malformed hair found in patients with it. These infants have been found to have deficiencies of serum copper and ceruloplasmin. Friedman et al (1978) described unusual EEG features appearing during the first few months of life and consisting of runs of high voltage multifocal sharp waves which recurred in different regions at different times. Independent of the discharges were intermittent multifocal areas of diminished amplitude of background activity.

Cherry Red Spot-Myoclonus Syndrome. This is a rare metabolic disorder occurring in the first few decades of life which is due to a deficiency of a specific lysosomal neuroaminidase. These patients suffer from severe myoclonus and visual impairment and are noted to have cherry-red spots on the macula. We have recently investigated a young woman with this syndrome who also had a peripheral neuropathy (Steinman et al, in preparation). Engel, Rapin, and Giblin (1977) described two patients with this syndrome whose EEGs contained unusual low voltage fast activity with 10 to 20 Hz vertex positive spikes that correlated with the myoclonus.

Neuroaxonal Dystrophy. This is a progressive neurodegenerative disorder which is characterized pathologically by accumulations of dystrophic axonal swellings or spheroids. Ferriss, Happel, and Duncan (1977) described a characteristic EEG pattern of high voltage unreactive 16 to 24 Hz rhythms and an absence of responses to a variety of sensory stimuli. We have reported two brothers with this disorder whose EEGs lacked this striking beta activity and were characteristic of a myoclonic epilepsy (Dorfman et al, 1978). The EEG and evoked potential alterations were similar to those described in other progressive myoclonic encephalopathies (Charlton, 1975).

Traumatic Disorders. The abnormalities resulting from head trauma are nonspecific, but tend to be more pronounced in children than adults. Generalized epileptiform activity may occur after head injury, usually disappears within 6 months, and is not accompanied or followed by clinical seizures (Courjon and Scherzer, 1972). The EEG appears to be of little value in the prediction of post-traumatic epilepsy (Jennett and van de Sande, 1975).

Minimal Cerebral Dysfunction and Hyperactivity. There is an extensive literature on the EEG changes in children with behavioral, language, motorical, or social maladaptation syndromes (Dongier et al, 1974). In most instances the EEG "abnormalities" consist of "excessive" amounts of normal background slow activity, "exaggerated" build-ups to hyperventilation, 14 and 6 Hz positive spikes, or occipital sharp waves which in most cases appear to be the admixture of a sharp alpha wave and a slow fused transient. Most studies lack the critical feature of a true "blind" review of the data. Certain specific EEG patterns have been reported in children with minimal cerebral dysfunction but these appear to be quite rare (White and Tharp, 1974).

The major factor which limits the validity of many of these studies is the heterogeneity of the patient population (Rie, 1975). The definition of EEG "abnormality" is often vague and many of the patterns considered abnormal by some investigators would be rejected by others. It is this author's opinion that the EEG has little to offer in the evaluation of children with learning disorders, dyslexia, and the like.

REFERENCES

Aicardi, J., Chevrie, J.-J., and Rousselie, F. (1969). Le syndrome spasmes en flexion, agenesie calleuse, anomalies chorio-retiniennes. Arch. Fr. Pediatr., *26:*1103.

Aird, R. and Gastaut, Y. (1959). Occipital and posterior electroencephalographic rhythms. Electroencephalogr. Clin. Neurophysiol., *11:*637.

Ajmone Marsan, C. and Zivin, L. (1970). Factors related to the occurrence of typical paroxysmal abnormalities in the EEG records of epileptic patients. Epilepsia, *11:*361.

Allemand, F., Monod, N., and Larroche, J. Cl. (1977). L' Électro-encéphalogramme dans les hémorragies sous-durales du nouveau-né. Rev. Electroencephalogr. Neurophysiol., *7:*365.

Anders, T., Emde, R., and Parmelee, A., Eds. (1971). A manual of standardized terminology, technique and criteria for scoring states of sleep and wakefulness in newborn infants. UCLA Brain Information Service/BRI Publications Office, NINDS Neurological Information Network.

Aoki, Y. and Lombroso, C. (1973). Prognostic value of electroencephalography in Reye's syndrome. Neurology, *23:*333.

Ariagno, R. (1979). Development of respiratory control. In: Advances in Perinatal Neurology, Vol. 1, Korobkin, R., and Guilleminault, C., Eds., p. 249, Spectrum, New York.

Bancaud, J., Colomb, D., and Dell, M. B. (1958). Les pointes rolandiques "un symptôme E.E.G. propre a l'enfant." Rev. Neurol., *99:*206.

Beaussart, M. and Faou, R. (1978). Evolution of epilepsy with rolandic paroxysmal foci: a study of 324 cases. Epilepsia, *19:*337.

Blom, S. and Hagberg, B. (1967). EEG findings in late infantile metachromatic and globoid cell leucodystrophy. Electroencephalogr. Clin. Neurophysiol., *22:*253.

Blume, W. (1978). Clinical and electroencephalographic correlates of the multiple independent spike foci pattern in children. Arch. Neurol., *4:*541.

Blume, W., David, R., and Gomez, M. (1973). Generalized sharp and slow wave complexes. Brain, *96:*289.

Bray, P. and Wiser, W. (1964). Evidence for a genetic etiology of temporal-central abnormalities in focal epilepsy. N. Engl. J. Med., *271:*926.

Charlton, M., Ed. (1975). Myoclonic seizures. Excerpta Medica, Princeton, N.J.

Ch'ien, L., Boehm, R., Robinson, H., Liu, C., and Frenkel, L. (1977). Characteristic early electroencephalographic changes in herpes simplex encephalitis. Arch. Neurol., *34:*361.

Colon, E., Vingerhoets, H., Notermans, S., and Krijgsman, J. (1979). Off-response: its clinical incidence in very young children. Electroencephalogr. Clin. Neurophysiol., *46:*601.

Courjon, J. and Scherzer, E. (1972). Traumatic disorders. In: Handbook of Electroencephalography and Clinical Neurophysiology, Vol. 14,B, Courjon, J. B., Ed., Elsevier, Amsterdam.

Cukier, F., André, M., Monod, N., and Dreyfus-Brisac, C. (1972). Apport de l'EEG au diagnostic des hémorragies intra-ventriculaires du prématuré. Rev. Electroencephalogr. Neurophysiol., *2:*318.

Curzi-Dascalova, L. (1977). EEG de vielle et de sommeil du nourrisson normal avant 6 mois d'age. Rev. Electroencephalogr., *7:*316.
DeMyer, W. and White, P. (1964). EEG in holoprosencephaly (arhinencephaly). Arch. Neurol., *11:*507.
Dennis, J. (1978). Neonatal convulsions: aetiology, late neonatal status and long-term outcome. Develop. Med. Child Neurol., *20:*143.
Dongier, M., Harding, G., Lairy, G., McCallum, W. and Small, J. (1974). Mental diseases. In: Handbook of Electroencephalography and Clinical Neurophysiology, Vol. 13,B, Dongier, M., Ed., Elsevier, Amsterdam.
Doose, H., Gerken, H., Hien-Völpel, K., and Völzke, E. (1969). Genetics of photosensitive epilepsy. Neuropädiatrie, *1:*56.
Doose, H., Gerken, H., and Völzke, E. (1972). On the genetics of EEG-anomalies in childhood. I. Abnormal theta rhythms. Neuropädiatrie, *3:*386.
Dorfman, L., Pedley, T., Tharp, B., and Scheithauer, B. (1978). Juvenile neuroaxonal dystrophy: clinical, electrophysiological, and neuropathological features. Ann. Neurol., *3:*419.
Eeg-Olofsson, O. (1971). The development of the EEG in normal children from the ages of 1 to 15 years: 14- and 6-per-second positive spike phenomenon. Neuropädiatrie, *4:*405.
Eeg-Olofsson, O., Petersén, I., and Selldén, U. (1971). The development of the electroencephalogram in normal children from the age of 1 through 15 years. Paroxysmal activity. Neuropädiatrie, *2:*375.
Ellingson, R. (1975). Ontogenesis of sleep in the human. In: Experimental Study of Human Sleep: Methodological Problems. Lairy, G., and Salzarulo, P., Eds., p. 129, Elsevier, Amsterdam.
Ellingson, R., Dutch, S., and McIntire, M. (1974). EEGs of prematures: 3–8 year follow-up study. Dev. Psychobiol., *7:*529.
Engel, J., Rapin, I., and Giblin, D. (1977). Electrophysiological studies in two patients with cherry red spot-myoclonus syndrome. Epilepsia, *18:*73.
Estivill, E., Monod, N., and Amiel-Tison, C. (1977). Étude électro-encéphalographique d'un cas d'encéphalite herpétique néo-natale. Rev. Electroencephalogr. Neurophysiol., *7:*380.
Fariello, R. and Black, J. (1978). Pseudoperiodic bilateral EEG paroxysms in a case of phencyclidine intoxication. J. Clin. Psychiatry, *39:*579.
Fariello, R., Chun, R., Doro, J., Buncle, J., and Prichard, J. (1977). EEG recognition of Aicardi's syndrome. Arch. Neurol., *34:*563.
Fedrick, J. and Butler, N. (1970). Certain causes of neonatal death. II. Intraventricular haemorrhage. Biol. Neonate, *15:*257.
Fenichel, G. (1978). Neurological assessment of the 25- to 30-week premature infant. Ann. Neurol., *4:*92.
Ferriss, G., Happel, L., and Duncan, M. (1977). Cerebral cortical isolation in infantile neuroaxonal dystrophy. Electroencephalogr. Clin. Neurophysiol., *43:*168.
Frantzen, E., Lennox-Buchthal, M., and Nygaard, A. (1968). Longitudinal EEG and clinical study of children with febrile convulsions. Electroencephalogr. Clin. Neurophysiol., *24:*197.
Friedman, E. and Pampiglione, G. (1971). Prognostic implications of electroencephalographic findings of hypsarrhythmia in first year of life. Br. Med. J., *4:*323.
Friedman, E., Harden, A., Koivikko, M., and Pampiglione, G. (1978). Menkes disease: neurophysiological aspects. J. Neurol. Neurosurg. Psychiatry, *41:*505.
Gastaut, H. (1970). Clinical and electroencephalographic classification of epileptic seizures. Epilepsia, *11:*102.
Gastaut, H., Roger, J., Soulayrol, R., Tassinari, C., Régis, H., and Dravet, C. (1966). Childhood epileptic encephalopathy with diffuse slow spike-waves (otherwise known as "petit mal variant") or Lennox syndrome. Epilepsia, *7:*139.

Gerken, H., and Doose, H. (1972). On the genetics of EEG-anomalies in childhood. II. Occipital 2-4/s rhythms. Neuropädiatrie, *3:*437.

Gibbs, F. and Gibbs, E. (1952). Atlas of Electroencephalography, Vol. 2 (Epilepsy). Addison-Wesley, Cambridge, Mass.

Gibbs, F., Rich, C., and Gibbs, E. (1963). Psychomotor variant type of seizure discharge. Neurology, *13:*991.

Gloor, P., Kalabay, O., and Giard, N. (1968). The electroencephalogram in diffuse encephalopathies: electroencephalographic correlates of grey and white matter diseases. Brain, *91:*779.

Hagne, I. (1968). Development of the waking EEG in normal infants during the first year of life. In: Clinical Electroencephalography of Children. Kellaway, P., and Petersen, I., Eds., p. 97, Almquist and Wilksell, Stockholm.

Hagne, I. (1972). Development of the sleep EEG in normal infant during the first year of life. Acta Paediat. Scand. Suppl. *232:*25.

Harden, A., Pampiglione, G., and Picton-Robinson, N. (1973). Electroretinogram and visual evoked response in a form of 'neuronal lipidosis' with diagnostic EEG features. J. Neurol. Neurosurg. Psychiatry, *36:*61.

Heijbel, J., Blom, S., and Rasmuson, M. (1975). Benign epilepsy of childhood with centrotemporal EEG foci: a genetic study. Epilepsia, *16:*285.

Hughes, J. (1965). A review of the positive spike phenomenon. In: Applications of Electroencephalography in Psychiatry, Wilson, W., Ed., p. 54, Duke University Press, Durham, N.C.

Ibrahim, M. and Jeavons, P. (1974). The value of electroencephalography in the diagnosis of subacute sclerosing panencephalitis. Dev. Med. Child Neurol., *16:* 295.

Illis, L. and Taylor, F. (1972). The electroencephalogram in herpes-simplex encephalitis. Lancet, *1:*718.

Jeavons, P., Bower, B., and Dimitrakoudi, M. (1973). Long-term prognosis of 150 cases of "West Syndrome." Epilepsia, *14:*153.

Jennett, B. and van de Sande, J. (1975). EEG prediction of post-traumatic epilepsy. Epilepsia, *16:*251.

Kellaway, P. and Fox, B. (1952). Electroencephalographic diagnosis of cerebral pathology in infants during sleep. I. Rationale, technique and the characteristics of normal sleep in infants. J. Pediatr., *41:*262.

Kellaway, P., Crawley, J., and Kagawa, N. (1959). A specific electroencephalographic correlate of convulsive equivalent disorders in children. J. Pediatr., *55:*582.

Kindt, G., Waldman, J., Kohl, S., Baublis, J., and Tucker, R. (1975). Intracranial pressure in Reye syndrome. Monitoring and control. JAMA *231:*822.

Kligman, D., Smyrl, R., and Emde, R. (1975). A "nonintrusive" longitudinal study of infant sleep. Psychosom. Med., *37:*448.

Knauss, T. and Marshall, R. (1977). Seizures in a neonatal intensive care unit. Dev. Med. Child Neurol., *19:*719.

Knight, D., Le Portz, M., and Harper, J. (1977). Natural sleep as an aid to electroencephalographic diagnosis in young children. Dev. Med. Child Neurol., *19:*503.

Lacy, J. and Penry, J. (1976). Infantile Spasms. Raven Press, New York.

Landau, W. and Kleffner, F. (1957). Syndrome of acquired aphasia with convulsive disorder in children. Neurology, *7:*523.

Larroche, J. (1977). Developmental Pathology of the Neonate. Excerpta Medica, Amsterdam.

Lenard, H. (1970). The development of sleep spindles in the EEG during the first two years of life. Neuropädiatrie, *1:*264.

Lennox-Buchthal, M. (1973). Febrile convulsions. A reappraisal. Electroencephalogr. Clin. Neurophysiol., Suppl. 32.

Lerman, P. and Livity, S. (1975). Benign focal epilepsy of childhood. A follow-up study of 100 recovered patients. Arch. Neurol., *32:*261.

Lipman, I. and Hughes, J. (1969). Rhythmic mid-temporal discharges. An electroclinical study. Electroencephalogr. Clin. Neurophysiol., *27:*43.

Loiseau, P. and Orgogozo, J. (1978). An unrecognized syndrome of benign focal epileptic seizures in teenagers. Lancet, *2:*1070.

Lombroso, C. (1967). Sylvian seizures and midtemporal spike foci in children. Arch. Neurol., *17:*52.

Lombroso, C. (1968). Remarks on the EEG and movement disorder in SSPE. Neurology, *18:*60.

Lombroso, C. (1975). Neurophysiological observations in diseased newborns. Biol. Psychiatry, *10:*527.

Lombroso, C., (1978). Convulsive disorders in newborns. In: Pediatric Neurology and Neurosurgery, Thomson, R. and Green, J., Eds. p. 202, Spectrum, New York.

Lombroso, C. (1979). Quantified electrographic scales on 10 pre-term healthy newborns followed up to 40–43 weeks of conceptional age by serial polygraphic recordings. Electroencephalogr. Clin. Neurophysiol., *46:*460.

Lombroso, C. and Fejerman, N. (1977). Benign myoclonus of early infancy. Ann. Neurol., *1:*138.

Lombroso, C., Schwartz, I., Clark, D., Muench, H., and Barry, U. (1966). Ctenoids in healthy youths. Controlled study of 14- and 6-per-second positive spiking. Neurology, *16:*1152.

Ludwig, B. and Ajmone Marsan, C. (1975). EEG changes after withdrawal of medication in epileptic patients. Electroencephalogr. Clin. Neurophysiol., *39:*173.

Maheshwari, M. and Jeavons, P. (1975). The clinical significance of occipital spikes as a sole response to intermittent photic stimulation. Electroencephalogr. Clin. Neurophysiol., *39:*93.

Markand, O. (1977). Slow spike-wave activity in EEG and associated clinical features. Often called 'Lennox' or 'Lennox-Gastaut' syndrome. Neurology, *27:*746.

Markand, O. and Panszi, J. G. (1975). The electroencephalogram in subacute sclerosing panencephalitis. Arch. Neurol., *32:*719.

Metcalf, D. (1969). The effect of extrauterine experience on the ontogenesis of EEG sleep spindles. Psychosom. Med., *31:*393.

Metcalf, D. (1970). EEG sleep spindle ontogenesis. Neuropädiatrie, *1:*428.

Metcalf, D., Mondale, J., and Butler, F. (1971). Ontogenesis of spontaneous K-complexes. Psychophysiol., *8:*340.

Monod, N., Pajot, N., and Guidasci, S. (1972). The neonatal EEG: statistical studies and prognostic value in full-term and pre-term babies. Electroencephalogr. Clin. Neurophysiol., *32:*529.

Murat, I. (1978). Interet discriminatif des pointes positives rolandiques. These pour le doctorat en medecine. Academie de Paris, Universite Rene Descartes.

Nayrac, P. and Beaussart, M. (1958). Les pointes-ondes prérolandiques. Expression EEG très particulière. Etude électroclinique de 21 cas. Rev. Neurol., *99:*201.

Nelson, K. and Ellenberg, J. (1976). Predictors of epilepsy in children who have experienced febrile seizures. N. Engl. J. Med., *295:*1029.

Nelson, K. and Ellenberg, J. (1978). Prognosis in children with febrile seizures. Pediatr., *61:*720.

Niedermeyer, E. (1965). Sleep electroencephalogram in petit mal. Arch. Neurol., *12:*625.

Nolte, R. and Haas, G. (1978). A polygraphic study of bioelectrical brain maturation in preterm infants. Dev. Med. Child Neurol., *20:*167.

Noriega-Sanchez, A. and Markand, O. (1976). Clinical and electroencephalographic correlation of independent multifocal spike discharge. Neurology, *26:*667.

Pampiglione, G. (1977). Development of rhythmic EEG activities in infancy. (Waking state.) Rev. Electroencephalogr. Neurophysiol., *7:*327.

Pampiglione, G. and Harden, A. (1973). Neurophysiological identification of a late infantile form of 'neuronal lipidosis.' J. Neurol. Neurosurg. Psychiatry, *36:*68.

Pampiglione, G. and Harden, A. (1977). So-called neuronal ceroid lipofuscinosis. J. Neurol. Neurosurg. Psychiatry, *40:*323.

Papile, L., Burstein, J., Burstein, R., and Koffler, H. (1978). Incidence and evolution of subependymal and intraventricular hemorrhage: a study of infants with birth weights less than 1,500 gm. J. Pediatr., *92:*529.

Petersén, I. and Eeg-Olofsson, O. (1971). The development of the electroencephalogram in normal children from the age of 1 through 15 years. Non-paroxysmal activity. Neuropädiatrie, *2:*247.

Petersén, I., Selldén, U., and Eeg-Olofsson, O. (1975). The evolution of the EEG in normal children and adolescents from 1 to 21 years. In: Handbook of Electroencephalography and Clinical Neurophysiology, Vol. 6, B, Lairy, G., Ed., p. 31. Elsevier, Amsterdam.

Prechtl, H. (1974). The behavioural states of the newborn infant (A Review). Brain Research, *76:*185.

Prechtl, H., Theorell, K., and Blair, A. (1973). Behavioral state cycles in abnormal infants. Dev. Med. Child Neurol., *15:*606.

Purpura, D. (1975). Morphogenesis of visual cortex in the preterm infant. In: Growth and Development of the Brain, Brazier, M., Ed., p. 33, Raven Press, New York.

Rabe, E. (1967). Subdural effusions in infants. Ped. Clin. of North Amer., *14:*831.

Radermecker, F. and Rabending, G. (1977). Encephalitis predominant in the basal cortex (acute necrotizing encephalitis, herpes simplex encephalitis). In: Handbook of Electroencephalography and Clinical Neurophysiology, Vol. 15, A, Radermecker, F. Ed., p. 23. Elsevier, Amsterdam.

Rie, H. (1975). Hyperactivity in children. Am. J. Dis. Child., *129:*783.

Roberton, N. (1969). Effect of acute hypoxia on blood pressure and electroencephalogram of newborn babies. Arch. Dis. Child., *44:*719.

Rose, A. and Lombroso, C. (1970). Neonatal seizure states. Pediatr., *45:*404.

Rosenberg, L. (1977). Inherited metabolic disorders of the newborn. In: Topics in Child Neurology, Blaw, M., Rapin, I., and Kinsbourne, M., Eds., p. 85. Spectrum, New York.

Santavuori, P., Haltia, M., and Rapola, J. (1974). Infantile type of so-called neuronal ceroid-lipofuscinosis. Develop. Med. Child Neurol., *16:*644.

Sato, S., Dreifuss, F., and Penry, J. (1976). Prognostic factors in absence seizures. Neurology, *26:*788.

Schimschock, J., Carlson, C., and Ojemann, L. (1969). Massive spasms associated with holoprosencephaly. Am. J. Dis. Child., *118:*520.

Schiottz-Christensen, E. and Hammerberg, P. (1975). EEG in twins with febrile convulsions. Follow-up on 59 pairs of the same sex. Neuropädiatrie, *6:*142.

Schulte, F., Lasson, U., Parl, U., Nolte, R., and Jürgens, U. (1969). Brain and behavioural maturation in newborn infants of diabetic mothers. Neuropädiatrie, *1:*36.

Schultz, M., Schulte, F., Akiyama, Y., and Parmelee, A. (1968). Development of electroencephalographic sleep phenomena in hypothyroid infants. Electroencephalogr. Clin. Neurophysiol., *25:*351.

Schwartz, L. and Lombroso, C. (1968). 14 and 6/second positive spiking (ctenoids) in the electroencephalogram of primary school pupils. J. Pediatr., *72:*678.

Shoumaker, R., Bennett, D., Bray, P., and Curless, R. (1974). Clinical and EEG manifestations of an unusual aphasic syndrome in children. Neurology, *24:*10.

Silverman, D. (1964). Fourteen-and-six-per-second positive spike pattern in a patient with hepatic coma. Electroencephalogr. Clin. Neurophysiol., *16:*395.

Smith, J. and Kellaway, P. (1964). The natural history and clinical correlates of occipital foci in children. In: Neurological and Electroencephalographic Correlative Studies in Infancy, Kellaway, P. and Petersén, I., Eds., p. 230. Grune and Stratton, New York.

Smith, J., Westmoreland, B., Regan, T., and Sandok, B. (1975). A distinctive clinical EEG profile in herpes simplex encephalitis. Mayo Clin. Proc., *50:*460.

Steinman, L., Dorfman, L., Tharp, B., Forno, L., and Sogg, P., in preparation. Cherry red spot myoclonic syndrome. A case with peripheral neuropathy.

Stewart, A., Turcan, D., Rawlings, G. and Reynolds, E. (1977). Prognosis for infants weighing 1000g or less at birth. Arch. Dis. Child., *52:*97.

Tanguay, P., Ornitz, E., Kaplan, A., and Bozzo, E. (1975). Evolution of sleep spindles in childhood. Electroencephalogr. Clin. Neurophysiol., *38:*175.

Tharp, B. (1972). Orbital frontal seizures. An unique electroencephalographic and clinical syndrome. Epilepsia, *13:*627.

Tharp, B., Cukier, F., and Monod, N. (1977). Valeur prognostique de l'EEG du prématuré. Rev. Electroencephalogr. Neurophysiol., *7:*386.

Tjiam, A., Stefanko, S., Schenk, V., and de Vlieger, M. (1978). Infantile spasms associated with hemihypsarrhythmia and hemimegalencephaly. Dev. Med. Child Neurol., *20:*779.

Townsend, J., Baringer, J., Wolinsky, J., Malamud, N., Mednick, J., Panitch, H., Scott, R., Oshiro, I., and Cremer, N. (1975). Progressive rubella panencephalitis. Late onset after congenital rubella. N. Engl. J. Med., *292:*990.

Trauner, D., Stockard, J., and Sweetman, L. (1977). EEG correlations with biochemical abnormalities in Reye syndrome. Arch. Neurol., *34:*116.

Van Caillie, M., Morin, C., Roy, C., Geoffrcy, G., and McLaughlin, G. (1977). Reye's syndrome: relapses and neurological sequelae. Pediatr., *59:*244.

Watanabe, K. and Iwase, K. (1972). Spindle-like fast rhythms in the EEGs of low birthweight infants. Dev. Med. Child Neurol., *14:*373.

Watanabe, K., Iwase, K., and Hara, K. (1973). The evolution of EEG features in infantile spasms: a prospective study. Dev. Med. Child Neurol., *15:*584.

Watanabe, K., Iwase, K., and Hara, K. (1974). Development of slow-wave sleep in low birthweight infants. Dev. Med. Child Neurol., *16:*23.

Weil, M., Itabashi, H., Cremer, N., Oshiro, L., Lennette, E., and Carnay, L. (1975). Chronic progressive panencephalitis due to rubella virus simulating subacute sclerosing panencephalitis. N. Engl. J. Med., *292:*994.

Werner, S., Stockard, J., and Bickford, R. (1977). Atlas of Neonatal Encephalography, Raven Press, New York.

Westmoreland, B. and Sharbrough, F. (1975). Posterior slow wave transients associated with eye blinks in children. Am. J. EEG Technol., *15:*14.

Westmoreland, B., Blume, W., and Gomez, M. (1976). Generalized sharp and slow wave and electrodecremental seizure pattern in subacute sclerosing panencephalitis. Mayo Clin. Proc., *51:*107.

Westmoreland, B., Gomez, M., and Blume, W. (1977). Activation of periodic complexes of subacute sclerosing panencephalitis by sleep. Ann. Neurol., *1:*185.

White, J. and Tharp, B. (1974). An arousal pattern in children with organic cerebral dysfunction. Electroencephalogr. Clin. Neurophysiol., *37:*265.

White, J., Langston, W., and Pedley, T. (1977). Benign epileptiform transients of sleep. Neurology, *27:*1061.

Whitley, R., Soong, S., Dolin, R., Galasso, G., Ch'ien, L., Alford, C., and the collaborative study group (1977). Adenine arabinoside therapy of biopsy-proven herpes simplex encephalitis. N. Engl. J. Med., *297:*289.

Yakovlev, P. and Lecours, A. (1967). The myelogenetic cycles of regional maturation of the brain. In: Regional Development of the Brain in Early Life, p. 3, Blackwell, Oxford.

Yamada, T., Young, S., and Kimura, J. (1977). Significance of positive spike bursts in Reye syndrome. Arch. Neurol., *34:*376.

Zeman, W. and Dyken, P. (1969). Neuronal ceroid-lipofuscinosis (Batten's disease): relationship to amaurotic familial idiocy. Pediatr., *44:*570.

4

Quantitative Aspects of Electroencephalography

A. S. GEVINS

INTRODUCTION

This chapter will discuss the limitations of the conventional method of EEG interpretation and the steps necessary to substitute more objective quantitative techniques. The application of such quantitative techniques to several clinically important problems will also be considered. Two points must, however, be stressed at the outset. First, performance and economic considerations do not generally justify the substitution of automated analyses for human interpretation of the wide variety of EEGs obtained in routine clinical practice. Second, the potential utility of quantitative analyses is in narrowly defined clinical problems in which there is sufficient medical justification to incur the high costs of development.

In order to render comprehensible the ensuing review of current research, techniques of digital signal processing and pattern recognition as applied to the EEG will be briefly summarized, with emphasis on the most common forms of analysis, namely power spectral (frequency) analysis and transient (paroxysmal waveform) detection, and on the methods by which the findings so obtained have been validated. The ambiguities caused by extracerebral artifact and drowsiness will be discussed, and some initial solutions to the problem of automatic artifact rejection will be presented. The remainder of the chapter will be concerned with several areas in which significant developments have taken place. Research applications in psychiatry, including quantification of the EEG correlates of psychotropic medication (Itil, 1974; Dolce and Decker, 1975; Fink, 1977), will not be considered. The technical aspects of the special purpose devices and quantitative algorithms applied to the EEG have previously been extensively reviewed (Walter and Brazier, 1968; Cox, Nolle, and Arthur, 1972; Matoušek, 1973; Kellaway and Petersen, 1973, 1976; Gevins et al, 1975; Dolce and Kunkel, 1975; Matějček and Schenk, 1975; Remond, 1977; John, 1977) and will likewise not be discussed here.

Difficulty of Quantifying the EEG

The desirability of standardized recording procedures and interpretation has inspired efforts towards quantified analysis almost since the inception of electroencephalography. There has traditionally been the hope that with a more powerful computer, or a more complicated form of analysis, Hans Berger's original dream that the EEG would be a "window on the mind" might be fulfilled. Every promising new technology, from analog band pass filtering to multivariate pattern recognition technology, has been applied to the EEG, with varying success. As long ago as 1938, Grass and Gibbs wrote: "After having made transforms of 300 electroencephalograms, we are convinced that the system not only expresses data in a manner more useful and concise than is possible by present methods, but that in many cases it indicates important changes in the electroencephalogram which would otherwise remain hidden." Although 40 years old, this summary of the first Fourier analysis of an EEG could very well have been used *verbatim* in any one of a number of recent studies.

The EEG is one of the last of the standard clinical tests to be quantified. Factors contributing to this delay include the relatively low volume of EEG examinations performed, the complexity of the EEG signal, the lack of knowledge concerning the anatomic and physiologic basic of the EEG, the fact that the EEG findings are corroborative rather than diagnostic per se, the subjective method of polygraph interpretation, and the application of quantitative methodologies without adequate consideration of the idiosyncracies of the EEG.

The considerable efforts made towards quantification have not substantially altered the daily practice of clinical electroencephalography. The reasons for this will be considered below, as well as possible solutions to this impasse.

Limitations of the Traditional Method of EEG Polygraph Interpretation

Complexity of Visual Assessment. Electroencephalographers (EEGers) employ complex, subjective techniques to reduce the polygraph recording to a few interpretive statements (Gibbs and Gibbs, 1951, 1952, 1964; Walter, 1963;

Hill and Parr, 1963; Kooi, 1971; Kiloh, McComas, and Osselton, 1972). Electrocerebral activity is characterized by its frequency, amplitude, and wave morphology, and by its spatial and temporal distribution. Patterns of activity are either considered to constitute a background continuum or are regarded as transients, such as are the paroxysmal sharp transient wave forms (sharp waves and spikes) associated with the epilepsies (Jasper, Ward, and Pope, 1969; Kooi, 1971). Interchannel comparisons aimed at discovering major discrepancies in amplitude, frequency, and wave morphology (e.g. hemispheric asymmetries and focal patterns) are central to the interpretive process, since these abnormalities may be associated with various pathologic conditions, but an evaluation of the total *gestalt* of the multi-channel tracing is also essential. Since wave features vary with recording conditions, and no *precise* definitions of most wave properties exist, electroencephalographic decisions and recommendations are made largely on a contextual basis. In complex records, the analysis and identification of the individual components are often so difficult that specific analysis must be neglected in favor of a general interpretation of the overall pattern. Few of these methods are directly amenable to quantification, or to precise definition. Efforts made by the International Terminology Committee (Jasper, 1958) to standardize commonly used terms have resulted in official definitions which are too vague to directly embody in computer algorithms.

Intrarater Reliability and Interrater Validity. Surprisingly few studies have been concerned with the intrarater reliability (reproducibility) and interrater validity (agreement) of subjective assessments of EEG polygraphs. Blum (1954) reported poor agreement on the interpretation of 10 test records by five experienced EEGers. The shortcomings of this study motivated Houfek and Ellingson (1959) to conduct a study of differences in interpretation between two EEGers on 140 consecutive clinical EEGs. There was good agreement in 123 cases in distinguishing normal from abnormal records. Of the 17 disagreements, 13 concerned borderline cases showing minimal abnormal activity, but there was a greater amount of disagreement as to degree, type, and location of abnormality. Little and Raffel (1962) further improved experimental procedures by ensuring that neither of two EEGers had access to the patient's clinical data when each interpreted a series of 50 randomly chosen EEGs. They found 85 percent agreement in classifying cases as normal or abnormal.

More recently Volavka et al (1973) compared the interpretations of seven EEGers on 98 recordings when the only available clinical information was the patients' ages. A structured report was used for the interpretation, and very good agreement was found as to overall normality or abnormality of the traces. In a comprehensive and methodologically rigorous study, Rose et al (1973) tested the reliability of assessment of two EEGers on 200 EEGs from children with possible seizure disorders. Reliability in the overall decision of normal vs. abnormal was 88 percent. There was greater agreement in the detection of paroxysmal spike and wave activity than in characterizing the background activity as slow or fast.

Interrater validity studies have also been conducted in connection with the development of computer algorithms to detect specific EEG patterns, including sharp transient paroxysmal activity associated with the seizure disorders (Gose, Werner, and Bickford, 1974), extracerebral artifact (Gevins et al, 1977a), and EEG signs of drowsiness (Gevins et al, 1977b). In summary, while there is good overall agreement as to presence and type of abnormality, there are large interrater variations in the characterization of individual elements of the EEG. This presents an obstacle to the development of quantitative analyses.

METHODOLOGIC CONSIDERATIONS

Standardizing Assessment of the Polygraph

There have been many methods for standardizing the assessment of the EEG. The Mayo system of classification (Yeager, 1937; Bickford and Klass, 1976), which was the prototype, classifies an EEG according to its pattern class (normal, asymmetry, dysrhythmia, delta, etc.), intensity (Grades, I, II, and III), location of the abnormality, wave description (spike, spike and wave, etc.) and additional descriptors. Classification of an EEG according to this system is routinely included with the EEG report. The various categories and descriptors are defined in terms of voltage or percentages. The system provides a summary that is more meaningful than the conventional report for nonEEGers, allows for computer storage and retrieval, and helps to standardize interpretation (Bickford and Klass, 1976).

Assessment systems of this sort call for the extraction of such basic features of the EEG as dominant frequency, amplitude, and interchannel relations. A checklist is often used for this purpose, and judgments are then drawn from it. These procedures are collectively referred to as structured methods of EEG interpretation. The use of such methods is essential to the evaluation and validation of quantitative methods of analysis. In this regard, structured reports of several types have been described by Volavka et al (1973); Rose et al (1973); Gotman, Gloor, and Ray (1975); and by Gotman, Gloor and Schaul (1978).

One such structured method of polygraph assessment, which has the virtue of attempting to concisely classify the wide variety of routinely occurring clinical EEGs (Gevins et al, 1976a; Yeager, Gevins, and Henderson, 1977), will be briefly described (Fig. 4.1), attention being confined to its application to the analysis of the EEG recorded while the patient is lying quietly with his eyes closed. The EEG is first classified into normal, borderline, or abnormal categories. Normal EEGs are then classified as dominant or minimal alpha activity types. Borderline EEGs are those which show only minimal changes from the normal. Abnormal EEGs are subdivided in turn into nonparoxysmal, paroxysmal, or mixed categories. Nonparoxysmal EEGs are further subclassified as slow, fast, or mixed types, while paroxysmal EEGs are divided into sharp transient, burst patterns, or mixed types. Decisions concerning localization and severity (the latter based on a three-point ordinal scale) are reached

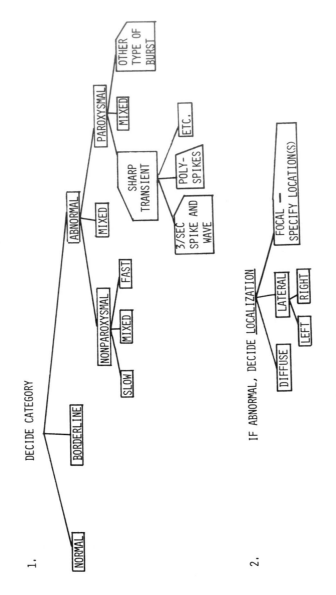

Fig. 4.1. Outline of a concise method of EEG polygraph interpretation. For clarity, only the major categories are shown. By using such a method, inter- and intrarater variability is reduced, and a more standardized interpretation of the characteristics of the polygraph is achieved. Such standardization is necessary for developing and validating a method of quantified EEG analysis. See text for details.

using semiobjective criteria. Initially, these final judgments may be reached via an intermediate detailed checklist, such as the one presented by Rose et al (1973), but with experience the method may be applied directly to the polygraph.

While such a structured method of EEG assessment seems reasonable *a priori,* its actual utility cannot be known until studies of interrater validity and intrarater retest reliability have determined that the method is sufficiently explicit and the results obtained with it are consistent. The degree of agreement between two EEG raters on the independent application of this concise method to 307 routine clinical EEG recordings was, therefore, studied. The recordings were obtained from patients in one or other of four diagnostic categories, namely metabolic disorders (73); psychiatric disorders (23); space occupying lesions (143); and seizure disorders (68). Twelve EEG channels (bipolar parasagittal and temporal montage) were recorded for subsequent computer analysis. The two raters worked independently, and did not have access to the traditional descriptive clinical EEG reports. Interpretations were performed in two stages, each of which had an associated form. The first was a checklist which allowed for a detailed description of the frequency, amplitude, quantity, rhythmicity, and topography of the background EEG for each of the four traditional frequency bands. From these items a concise summary was formed for *Category* (normal, borderline, abnormal slow, etc.), *Location* (diffuse, lateralized, or focal), and *Degree* of abnormality (slight, moderate, or marked) as shown in Figure 4.2.

The decision of the two raters as to category is shown in Table 4.1. There was high overall agreement concerning records placed in the normal, abnormal slow, and abnormal paroxysmal categories, while the number of records placed in the borderline and fast categories was too few to permit any definite conclusions to be reached. Agreement on the degree of severity is shown in Table 4.2.

Table 4.1. AGREEMENT OF TWO RATERS ON CATEGORY
Using a method of concise clinical EEG classification (N = 307)

Rater 1 \ Rater 2	Normal	Border- line	Abnormal slow	Abnormal fast	Abnormal paroxysmal	Subtotals	
Normal	95	7	15	2	4	123	40.1%
Border- line	1	2	5			8	2.6%
Abnormal slow	9	5	126		1	141	46.0%
Abnormal fast				3			0.9%
Abnormal paroxysmal			8		24	32	10.4%
Subtotals:	105	14	154	5	29		
	34.2%	4.6%	50.2%	1.6%	9.4%		

EEG SYSTEMS LAB - CONCISE EEG Coding Form

EEG'ers Initials:

PT ID	AGE	HAND	DATE	STATES	ARTIFACT	NORMAL	ABNORMAL/DEGREE	TOPOGRAPHY	COMMENTS
		L		EC	E 1 - 2 - 3	N	Slow 1 - 2 - 3	Dif LA RA	
		R		EO	M 1 - 2 - 3	NM	Fast 1 - 2 - 3	Lef LP RP	
				SLP	P 1 - 2 - 3	NR	Sharp T 1 - 2 - 3	Rit LT RT	
				PHV	D 1 - 2 - 3	NSLP	Burst 1 - 2 - 3		
				PHO		NB	Suppr 1 - 2 - 3		
				EC	E 1 - 2 - 3	N	Slow 1 - 2 - 3	Dif LA RA	
				EO	M 1 - 2 - 3	NM	Fast 1 - 2 - 3	Lef LP RP	
				SLP	P 1 - 2 - 3	NR	Sharp T 1 - 2 - 3	Rit LT RT	
				PHV	D 1 - 2 - 3	NSLP	Burst 1 - 2 - 3		
				PHO		NB	Suppr 1 - 2 - 3		
				EC	E 1 - 2 - 3	N	Slow 1 - 2 - 3	Dif LA RA	
				EO	M 1 - 2 - 3	NM	Fast 1 - 2 - 3	Lef LP RP	
				SLP	P 1 - 2 - 3	NR	Sharp T 1 - 2 - 3	Rit LT RT	
				PHV	D 1 - 2 - 3	NSLP	Burst 1 - 2 - 3		
				PHO		NB	Suppr 1 - 2 - 3		
				EC	E 1 - 2 - 3	N	Slow 1 - 2 - 3	Dif LA RA	
				EO	M 1 - 2 - 3	NM	Fast 1 - 2 - 3	Lef LP RP	
				SLP	P 1 - 2 - 3	NR	Sharp T 1 - 2 - 3	Rit LT RT	
				PHV	D 1 - 2 - 3	NSLP	Burst 1 - 2 - 3		
				PHO		NB	Suppr 1 - 2 - 3		
				EC	E 1 - 2 - 3	N	Slow 1 - 2 - 3	Dif LA RA	
				EO	M 1 - 2 - 3	NM	Fast 1 - 2 - 3	Lef LP RP	
				SLP	P 1 - 2 - 3	NR	Sharp T 1 - 2 - 3	Rit LT RT	
				PHV	D 1 - 2 - 3	NSLP	Burst 1 - 2 - 3		
				PHO		NB	Suppr 1 - 2 - 3		
				EC	E 1 - 2 - 3	N	Slow 1 - 2 - 3	Dif LA RA	
				EO	M 1 - 2 - 3	NM	Fast 1 - 2 - 3	Lef LP RP	
				SLP	P 1 - 2 - 3	NR	Sharp T 1 - 2 - 3	Rit LT RT	
				PHV	D 1 - 2 - 3	NSLP	Burst 1 - 2 - 3		
				PHO		NB	Suppr 1 - 2 - 3		
				EC	E 1 - 2 - 3	N	Slow 1 - 2 - 3	Dif LA RA	
				EO	M 1 - 2 - 3	NM	Fast 1 - 2 - 3	Lef LP RP	
				SLP	P 1 - 2 - 3	NR	Sharp T 1 - 2 - 3	Rit LT RT	
				PHV	D 1 - 2 - 3	NSLP	Burst 1 - 2 - 3		
				PHO		NB	Suppr 1 - 2 - 3		
				EC	E 1 - 2 - 3	N	Slow 1 - 2 - 3	Dif LA RA	
				EO	M 1 - 2 - 3	NM	Fast 1 - 2 - 3	Lef LP RP	
				SLP	P 1 - 2 - 3	NR	Sharp T 1 - 2 - 3	Rit LT RT	
				PHV	D 1 - 2 - 3	NSLP	Burst 1 - 2 - 3		
				PHO		NB	Suppr 1 - 2 - 3		

Fig. 4.2. Coding form used in applying our concise method of EEG polygraph assessment. Use of such forms facilitates and standardizes application of the method. EC, eyes closed; EO, eyes open: SLP, sleep; PHV, posthyperventilation; PHO, Photic stimulation; N, normal; NM, normal with minimal sleep; NR, normal with responsive alpha; NSLP, normal sleep; NB, borderline normal; Dif. diffuse; Lef, left side; Rit, right side; L, left; R, right; A, anterior; P, posterior; T, temporal.

Table 4.2. AGREEMENT OF TWO RATERS
ON DEGREE OF SEVERITY
Using a method of concise clinical EEG classification (N = 307)

Rater 1 \ Rater 2	Normal	Slight	Moderate	Marked	Subtotals	
Normal	88	8	17	1	114	37.1%
Slight	13	11	26	1	51	16.6%
Moderate	5	2	75	9	91	29.7%
Marked	3	1	10	37	51	16.6%
Subtotals:	109	22	128	48		
	35.5%	7.2%	41.7%	15.8%		

There was good overall agreement as to which records were judged normal, moderately abnormal, or markedly abnormal, but more discrepancies as to which were regarded as slightly abnormal. The final comparison of the two raters dealt with the overall disagreement concerning category and location (Table 4.3). The number of disagreements as to category and location of abnormality were coded into a four-point ordinal scale. The "no disagreement" listing was the most frequent, while there were relatively few moderate or marked disagreements.

In summary, comparison on category, location, and degree of abnormality indicated that all records with distinct features were appraised in very nearly the same way by both raters. As the categories became less distinct or mixed, the location less circumscribed, and the degree less demarcated, the number of discrepancies increased. Thus, use of this concise method seems to provide

Table 4.3. COMPARISON OF
TWO RATERS ON OVERALL
DISAGREEMENT
Using a method of concise
clinical EEG classification
(N = 307)

	Category	Location
None	208	219
	67.8%	71.3%
Slight	55	37
	17.9%	12.0%
Moderate	18	23
	5.8%	7.5%
Marked	26	28
	8.5%	9.2%

more standardized data for validation of quantified analyses than does the purely intuitive evaluation of the EEG, and further refinement of the method therefore appears to be justified.

Digital Signal Processing and Pattern Recognition

Techniques for quantifying the EEG are collectively known to electrical engineers, computer scientists, and statisticians as methods of digital (and analog) signal processing and pattern recognition. Analog methods are mostly used for prefiltering or other signal processing functions prior to digitization.

Figure 4.3 is a simplified diagram of a complete EEG analysis. Five major steps are shown in the figure, namely: (1) signal conditioning and digitization, (2) primary analysis, (3) feature extraction, (4) classification and/or decision, and (5) validation.

Signal Conditioning. During signal conditioning the signals from the EEG amplifiers are prepared for sampling by the computer. This typically consists of attenuating the high (above 50 Hz) and low (below 1 Hz) frequency components by passing the signals through filters with strong attenuation (24 dB per octave or more). In most circumstances this is necessary because the filters incorporated in commercial electroencephalographs do not attenuate strongly enough for efficient computer analysis. Signal conditioning is followed by digitization, in which the analog EEG signals are sampled by the computer, converted to a digital representation, and stored in the computer's memory.

Primary Analysis. Following signal conditioning and digitization, one or both of two different classes of primary analysis are performed, namely frequency analysis and transient detection.

Frequency Analysis. During frequency analysis, which may be performed in a variety of different ways (Matoušek, 1973), the EEG is broken down into its constituent components. In electrical engineering, frequency analysis is referred to as spectral analysis, which makes clear the analogy to a prism breaking down white light into a spectrum. Frequency analysis generally results in the separation of activity into groups based on frequency, that is, delta (less than 4 Hz), theta (4 to 7 Hz), alpha (8 to 13 Hz), beta (14 to 22 Hz), and higher frequency activity (from 22 to 35 or 50 Hz).

The most popular current way of applying this analysis to EEGs is on a digital computer using the Fast Fourier Transform algorithm (Dumermuth and Fluhler, 1967; Johnson et al, 1969; Dumermuth et al, 1970; Bickford, Fleming, and Billinger, 1971; Bickford et al, 1973; Gevins and Yeager, 1972; Gotman et al, 1973, 1975). Other methods are likely to become available in the near future, however, as a result of developments in integrated electronics (charge coupled devices) and computer science (number theoretic transforms).

Another common form of frequency analysis is period-amplitude analysis (Saltzberg and Burch, 1959; Leader et al, 1967; Leggewie and Probst, 1969;

Carrie and Frost, 1971; Homma et al, 1973; Schenk, 1976; Harner, 1977). In general, this method extracts frequency information by tabulating properties of the individual waves, such as the time between zero crosses. While in principle this method is more computationally efficient than spectral analysis, it may be subject to various practical problems, including distortions due to low amplitude, high frequency signal components. Because of space limitations, other forms of time domain analysis (Barlow and Brazier, 1956; Remond, 1966; Hjorth, 1970; Remond, Baillon, and Bienenfeld, 1975; Schenk and Ruegg, 1975; Schenk, 1976; Harner and Ostergren, 1976) will not be discussed here.

COMPLETE EEG ANALYSIS

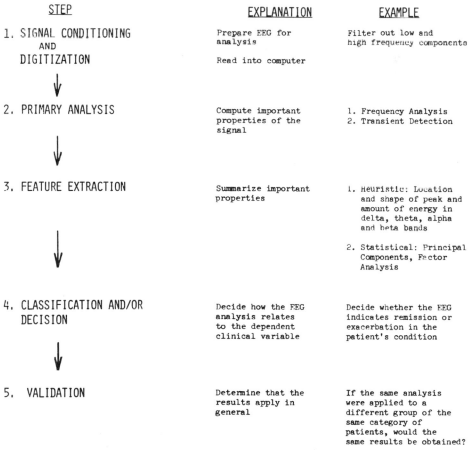

STEP	EXPLANATION	EXAMPLE
1. SIGNAL CONDITIONING AND DIGITIZATION	Prepare EEG for analysis Read into computer	Filter out low and high frequency components
2. PRIMARY ANALYSIS	Compute important properties of the signal	1. Frequency Analysis 2. Transient Detection
3. FEATURE EXTRACTION	Summarize important properties	1. Heuristic: Location and shape of peak and amount of energy in delta, theta, alpha and beta bands 2. Statistical: Principal Components, Factor Analysis
4. CLASSIFICATION AND/OR DECISION	Decide how the EEG analysis relates to the dependent clinical variable	Decide whether the EEG indicates remission or exacerbation in the patient's condition
5. VALIDATION	Determine that the results apply in general	If the same analysis were applied to a different group of the same category of patients, would the same results be obtained?

Fig. 4.3. Steps for a complete quantitative analysis of the EEG. Completion of all five steps is necessary in order to determine the validity and utility of any particular quantitative method. It is then no longer necessary to routinely perform the fifth step.

The results of frequency analysis may be expressed as numerical tabulations of the amount of energy or activity in each frequency band, as a histogram or line graph, in an abstract form (Gotman et al, 1973), or as a compressed spectral array (CSA) (Joy, 1968; Bickford et al, 1971). This latter form of display is currently very popular. It simply consists of displaying the successive results of frequency analysis, performed on short segments of data, as a series of vertically arranged graphs. For example, Figure 4.4 shows the CSAs of a patient with uncontrolled complex partial seizures prior to (upper half of figure) and following (lower half) surgical resection of the left temporal lobe. In each case, six EEG channels are shown, namely the left and right frontal (F3 and F4), temporal (T3 and T4), and occipital (O1 and O2). Within each channel, the abscissa represents frequency in Hertz (Hz), extending from 1 to 16 Hz. The height of each line is the spectral intensity (proportional to the square of voltage) expressed in microvolts squared per Hz. In this instance, each successive line represents 4 seconds of EEG (the average of 4 one-second analyses). Time is increasing from the bottom up, so that the 32 lines in each box represent a total of 2 minutes and 8 seconds of EEG. Large, abnormal 1 to 6 Hz peaks can be seen in the graphs prior to surgery, while following surgery these peaks are reduced, and asymmetrical alpha peaks (8 to 11 Hz) are evident over the occipital electrode placements.

Although it was originally thought that the interpretation of CSAs, in conjunction with transient detection, might routinely replace the interpretation of the polygraph, there is currently some doubt about this (Matoušek, 1977) (see p. 134). Nevertheless, the CSA is a useful means of examining the results of primary analysis, prior to further feature extraction and multivariate analysis. The CSA in the form of somnograms is also being used to study EEG changes during sleep (Bickford, 1977).

Transient Detection. As shown in Figure 4.3, the other major type of primary analysis is the detection of transient, infrequent but clinically important EEG events. The most familiar examples of such events are the paroxysmal waveforms (spikes, polyspikes, spike and wave discharges, etc.) associated with seizure disorders. Because a single isolated transient may have too little energy to stand out from the averaged background, or because transient events may have the same frequency distribution as other kinds of EEG activity, frequency analysis may not be sensitive to their occurrence. Moreover, in applying frequency analysis, information about individual wave morphology, crucial for the detection and characterization of transients, is lost. Since formal analytic solutions are not generally applicable to the detection of specific EEG transients, many different methods have been tried in the attempt to accurately detect transient waveforms, as is discussed below (p. 146).

Feature Extraction. The third step in a complete analysis of the EEG is feature extraction (Fig. 4.3.). The purpose of this step is to reduce the amount of data generated from the primary analysis by forming summary indices which

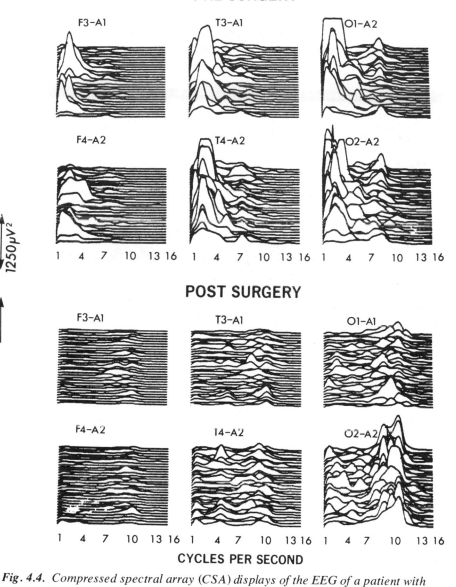

PRE SURGERY

F3–A1   T3–A1   O1–A2

F4–A2   T4–A2   O2–A2

1 4 7 10 13 16 1 4 7 10 13 16 1 4 7 10 13 16

POST SURGERY

F3–A1   T3–A1   O1–A1

F4–A2   T4–A2   O2–A2

1 4 7 10 13 16 1 4 7 10 13 16 1 4 7 10 13 16

CYCLES PER SECOND

22 mm / 1250 μV^2

TIME

Fig. 4.4. *Compressed spectral array (CSA) displays of the EEG of a patient with uncontrolled complex partial seizures, prior to (upper) and following (lower) surgery. The abscissa represents frequency in Hz or cycles per second. The height of each individual line represents intensity (proportional to the square of voltage). Each successive line starting at the bottom is the average of the magnitude of the next 4 one-second Fourier Transforms. A total of about 128 seconds of EEG is displayed for each condition. For each condition, six channels are depicted—the top three are the left frontal, temporal, and occipital placements, while the bottom three are the homologous right-sided placements. Prior to surgery, note the large, abnormal 1 to 6 Hz peaks corresponding with frequent paroxysmal activity on the polygraph. Following surgery (lower), these peaks are reduced, and asymmetrical alpha peaks (8 to 11 Hz) are evident over the occipital electrode placements.*

characterize important properties of the EEG. There are both ad-hoc (heuristic) and formal (statistical) procedures for performing feature extraction.

Heuristic Methods. A variety of indices may be formed based upon the traditional visual assessment of the polygraph. For example, by combining the individual 1 Hz frequency bins into bands, and by taking the ratio between homologous left- and right-sided placements, an index sensitive to the amount of asymmetry may be formed. One can derive such simple indices to characterize asynchronies, amount of abnormal slowing, recovery from hyperventilation, reaction to photic stimulation, etc. It must be noted, however, that such indices, while intuitively appealing, may not necessarily correspond with the visually assessed characteristics of the EEG polygraph. To determine the correlation of an index and a characteristic such as asymmetry, validation studies are necessary. Furthermore, before such indices can be submitted to statistical hypothesis-testing, study of their distribution must be undertaken; and, if needed, one of a variety of normalizing transforms must be applied.

Statistical Methods. The other type of feature extraction is formally defined and does not make use of *a priori* knowledge of the EEG. The purpose of this type of feature extraction is the same as the heuristic type, namely to efficiently reduce the amount of data generated by the primary analysis. The most familiar example of such a procedure is principal components factor analysis, a technique well known to statisticians and experimental psychologists (Harman, 1967). This procedure simply forms a linear combination of a large set of variables (e.g. the results of frequency analysis) such that the resulting smaller set of variables both account for a large amount of the variance of the original data, and are maximally uncorrelated with each other. Although computationally time-consuming, this procedure has proven to be a valuable step in the analysis of the background EEG (Dymond and Coger, 1975; John et al, 1977). Heuristic and statistical feature extraction may be used as sequential steps in the analysis (Doyle, personal communication).

Classification. The fourth and most important step in the analysis of the EEG is the final classification or decision (Fig. 4.3). This simply involves reaching a decision as to the relevance to the individual patient (or class of patients) of the results of the EEG analysis. This may be accomplished manually or with further computation, depending on circumstances. Sometimes the results of feature extraction are obvious, and further computation is not required. For example, an index of the number and duration of 3 per second spike and wave discharges could be compared before and after alterations of an anticonvulsant drug regime, to determine whether a reduction of absence seizures had been achieved. (Of course, standards for such changes must previously have been compiled from a large group of patients in order to determine whether the observed change was significant.)

In many instances, the results of primary analysis and feature extraction are not obviously related to the clinical condition under investigation. For example, in attempting to predict the onset of a grand mal seizure 10 minutes or more prior to its occurrence, no simple relations between the results of feature extraction and the subsequent seizure onset are apparent. In this instance, it is necessary to employ one of a number of methods of multivariate statistical analyses (Rao, 1952, 1965; Anderson, 1958; Harris, 1975). Since this subject is itself quite complex, mention will be made here of only one class of such analyses, namely multivariate pattern recognition (Nilsson, 1965; Andrews, 1972; Meisel, 1972; Chen, 1973). The most familiar and widely available type of multivariate pattern recognition is stepwise linear discriminant analysis. By examining many examples of EEGs from each of several different clinical categories, discriminant analysis can determine a mathematical rule (if one exists) to correctly classify the EEG with the associated clinical category. The value of such a mathematical decision rule is that it may then be used to classify an unknown EEG sample into the associated clinical condition. In the example given above, one may use this type of analysis to attempt to predict, from the EEG, if a grand mal seizure will occur in 10 or so minutes. The difficulty encountered in the practical application of multivariate pattern recognition is that it is generally quite difficult to gather an adequate sample of data for each of the clinical categories to be discriminated. The result of computing a decision rule on insufficient data is that when a previously unclassified EEG sample is presented, classification is likely to be incorrect because the actual invariant EEG patterns (if such exist) related to the clinical category may not have been extracted.

Validation. The fifth step of a complete analysis of the EEG, validation (Fig. 4.3), is of paramount importance if practical application is to be made of the results of a study. Since this step is crucial, an entire section will be devoted to it.

ADIEEG—A Computer System for a Complete Analysis of the EEG

Efficient analysis of a multichannel, complex signal, such as the EEG, must be based on a high degree of integration among computer hardware, analysis algorithms, and program code. Operation of the complex system must also be simple enough to avoid interference with the routine of clinical or research EEG examinations. Since the same single system must typically be used for a variety of clinical and experimental applications, it must also be flexible enough to rapidly allow alteration of analysis paradigms.

The ADIEEG system (Fig. 4.5) is the first integrated, interactive computing system dedicated to performing a complete multichannel analysis of the EEG as outlined above. Since it has been detailed elsewhere (Gevins et al, 1975, 1979b), only a brief outline of its functions will be presented here. The following functions are performed: (1) automatic calibration of detection thresholds to each patient's EEG, (2) continuous spectral analysis using the Fast Fourier Transform to produce estimates of auto- and cross-spectral intensity and coherence on up to 16 EEG channels in real time, (3) parallel (simultaneous) time-domain analysis to detect sharp transients that may be significant in patients with epilepsy, (4) several forms of interactive graphics, including CSAs, reconstructed EEG, and transient histograms, (5) rejection of physiologic and instrumental artifact and data contaminated by drowiness, (6) statistical and heuristic extraction of summary EEG indices, (7) data subset selection (outlier pruning) to form ensembles of relatively homogeneous segments of EEG, (8) within-subjects normalization of data, (9) a variety of uni-

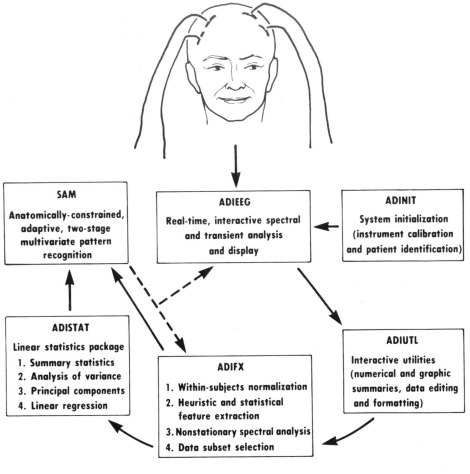

ADIEEG INTERACTIVE EEG ANALYSIS SYSTEM
(each box is a discrete software subsystem)

Fig. 4.5. Block diagram of major software subsystems comprising the ADIEEG system. The ADIEEG system is an integrated, interactive system designed to perform a complete analysis of the EEG. Acronyms are names of subsystems. It is implemented in a dedicated minicomputer (PD15-76) (from Gevins, A. S., Zeitlin, G. M., Yingling, C. D., Doyle, J. C., Dedon, M. F., Henderson, J. H., Schaffer, R. E., Roumasset, J. T., and Yeager, C. L. 1979. Electroencephalogr. Clin. Neurophysiol., in press).

variate and linear multivariate statistical procedures, and (10) anatomically constrained, adaptive, two-layered multivariate pattern recognition to calculate decision rules which classify electrophysiologic data into appropriate clinical or experimental categories.

Validation of Quantified Analyses

A crucial, but often underemphasized step in the introduction of a quantitative method into clinical medicine is the validation phase. During this phase, the new method must be compared with the method it is to supplement or replace. For quantitative EEG methods, this usually entails the tedious process of comparing the new procedure with assessments previously derived from the polygraph. Unfortunately, one immediately encounters the problem that the polygraph assessment is itself subject to the limitations listed previously, so a method of standardizing the polygraph interpretation to a reasonable degree is prerequisite to this type of validation. However, even when an adequate degree of standardization has been achieved, a difficult problem remains, not unlike the attempt to compare apples and oranges. The results of structured EEG assessment generally consist of several dichotomous or discrete categories (e.g. normal vs abnormal), while the results of quantitative analyses are numerical. It is obvious that to make comparisons, the two methods must be expressed in the same language. Since it is not possible to meaningfully transform subjective assessments into precise numerical quantities, the results of quantitative analyses must be formulated in dichotomous or discrete categories, and this is accomplished during the classification or decision step of the analysis (Fig. 4.3).

Surprisingly, there are only a few instances of this sort of validation in the EEG literature. The premier work is by Jean Gotman and associates of the Montreal Neurologic Institute (1973, 1975, 1978). In their research on the quantification of EEG slow wave patterns associated with supratentorial lesions, they used a structured EEG interpretation form to reduce the visual assessment into a judgment concerning the location (in one of four quadrants) and severity (mild, moderate, severe) of the abnormality. The computer graphs were then similarly interpreted, and the two methods compared. This method was also applied by Gotman and associates to the results of transient detection (p. 146). In our own studies, we have made consistent use of this method to evaluate the performance of computer algorithms to detect extracerebral artifacts and drowsiness (p. 136), and the sharp transient activity associated with the epilepsies (p. 146).

A similar method of validation was used by Isaksson and Wennberg (1975) to compare several spectral parameters derived from an autoregressive model of the EEG with visual assessment of the amount of slow activity on the polygraph. In 65 adult controls it was found that the results of computer analysis corresponded in a predictable manner with the amount of visually evaluated slow activity.

Matoušek, Petersen and associates (1973) have dealt with this aspect of validation in a novel manner by implementing computer algorithms to translate the results of quantified analysis into English language summaries similar to those generated by an EEGer (p. 141). Similar procedures have also been used by MacGillivray (1977) and John (1977) (p. 142).

Another method of validation is direct comparison of the results of quantitative analysis with a dependent clinical variable. This is the only method possible when visual assessment of the polygraph is equivocal, such as in determining the EEG correlates of psychotropic medication (Itil, 1974). Application of this method of validation to the EEG is performed using standard statistical techniques of hypothesis testing (Matějček and Devos, 1976; Dolce and Decker, 1975).

In order to emphasize the importance of obtaining adequate validation of quantitative methods of analyzing the EEG, the results of a personal study of the usefulness of the compressed spectral array (CSA) technique can briefly be discussed. The study was designed to determine whether similar interpretations could be drawn from the CSA as are routinely drawn from the polygraph in a variety of clinical EEGs. 138 cases were randomly selected from our clinical EEG data base for a comparison of three different methods of visual assessment of polygraphs and one method of interpretation of the CSA. Approximately 50 percent of the cases were from patients with space-occupying lesions, 25 percent from patients with seizure disorders, and the rest were from either normal subjects or patients in other diagnostic categories. The four types of assessment were: (1) the traditional, descriptive clinical EEG report; (2) a structured polygraph interpretation form, similar to the ones described earlier, and consisting essentially of descriptors for each frequency band; (3) a structured CSA interpretation form, which was similarly composed; and (4) direct classification from the polygraph into the six summary descriptive categories described below. Detailed instructions were written for the application of each of the procedures. Separate raters applied each method, except for the structured polygraph and structured CSA interpretations, which were performed by the same person but on separate occasions so that he could not associate a polygraph with the corresponding CSA.

These four types of assessment were then contrasted in six summary descriptive categories. Their ability to distinguish normal from abnormal were first compared. Among the abnormal records, comparisons were then made of their ability to discriminate type of abnormal activity (slow, fast, sharp transient, other paroxysmal burst, or mixed); continuous vs intermittent abnormality; severity of the abnormality based on a 3-point ordinal scale; location of the abnormality (diffuse vs lateralized or focal); and location of a focal abnormality. A chi-square test was applied to test the hypothesis that the four methods of interpretation were different from each other for each of these six descriptive categories (Table 4.4). The results indicated that, except for the category of location, the four methods were all significantly different from each other. Since interpretation of the CSA was consistently different from the other three methods, further analyses were performed with these data omitted. As is clear from Table 4.4, the three remaining methods of interpretation, all based on the

Table 4.4. COMPARISON OF FOUR METHODS OF INTERPRETING THE EEG
(Three methods based on polygraph, one method based on compressed spectral array)

	Chi-square test that the four methods are different	
	All four methods	**Three methods (Structured compressed spectral array omitted)**
Normal vs abnormal	9.18 *	0.18
Type (slow, fast, sharp transient, or other paroxysmal)	37.70 ‡	11.21 *
Continuous vs intermittent	24.34 ‡	10.26 †
Severity (mild, moderate, or marked)	17.04 †	6.88
Diffuse vs lateralized or focal	44.96 ‡	2.75
Location of abnormality	10.20	3.74 §

* p ≤ .05
† p ≤ .01
‡ p ≤ .001
§ For this analysis the concise method of classification was omitted (too few patients), instead of the structured compressed spectral array.

polygraph and all independently performed by different persons, were not significantly different from each other for the categories of normal vs abnormal, severity of abnormality, and location of abnormality. Moreover, there was a marked reduction in the significance of the difference between these methods of interpreting the polygraph with regard to type of abnormality, and whether the abnormality was continuous or intermittent. Since the rater was experienced in interpreting CSAs, these results are probably due to (1) excessive prominence given in CSAs to low-amplitude, continuous slow activity, (2) lack of sensitivity of spectral analyses to transient events; and (3) high inter- and intrasubject variability in such factors as state of alertness. In visually interpreting the polygraphs, considerations of individual wave morphology allow, in most instances, these distinctions to be drawn.

Although this preliminary study cannot be regarded as methodologically rigorous, it was adequate to conclude that until further studies are performed, it would not be advisable to rely upon displays of spectral analysis to form the sort of clinical judgments which are currently made from the polygraph.

Artifact Rejection

It is not possible to routinely apply quantitative methods to the analysis of the EEG without objective control of artifacts. Contamination or distortion of scalp-recorded brain potentials can be caused by a wide variety of physiologic and instrumental sources, the most common of which include intermittent electrode contacts, body movement, muscle activity, and eye movement. In this context, gross changes in the subject's state of arousal, such as drowsiness, may also be considered a form of artifact.

In most studies employing quantitative EEG, the usual practice has been to visually select a short segment of data (i.e. 10 to 60 seconds) for computer analysis. Such procedures obviously introduce an element of subjective bias. Additionally, in many instances such short segments of data do not take into account the often large intrasubject variation of electrophysiologic parameters. In obtaining long segments of data (i.e. 1 to 18 hours), simple behavioral controls of arousal and visual rejection of artifact are not practical procedures.

Our efforts over the last several years have, therefore, been directed at automating electrophysiologic data screening and selection, and various artifact and drowsiness-detecting algorithms (Gevins et al, 1977a, 1977b) have been implemented as program modules in the ADIEEG system (Fig. 4.5). From a short artifact-free segment of EEG, thresholds are automatically calibrated for each patient for each of three major classes of artifact: (1) head and body movements, perspiration, and low frequency instrumental artifact (under 1 Hz); (2) high frequency artifact including gross EMG (34 to 50 Hz); and (3) EOG (under 3 Hz, frontal channels). Following calibration, EEG data exceeding any of the thresholds are automatically discarded. The performance of these simple algorithms was evaluated on 35 (15 normal, 20 abnormal) 3-minute, 8-channel, artifact-contaminated EEG recordings. One hundred forty-nine events were found (65 percent of the total number of events found by at least two of three scorers). Eighty events were missed (35 percent of the total events found by the consensus of scorers). Seventy-one events were detected which had not been marked as artifact by any of the scorers (27 percent of the total number of event detections were false positives). The cases with the greatest number of misses had low-amplitude, low-frequency, eye-movement artifact, while the cases with the greatest number of false detections all had high-amplitude paroxysmal activity of cortical origin which did not occur during the calibration period. Surprisingly, this performance did not differ significantly (.05 level) from that of the "average" scorer.

Similar algorithms are used to detect EEG changes due to drowsiness. From a short segment of waking data, thresholds are set for each patient based upon ratios of delta-to-alpha and theta-to-alpha spectral intensity. Following calibration, the occurrence of drowsiness is detected by comparison to these thresholds and the use of additional heuristic criteria. To test the method, 31 (17 normal and 14 abnormal) recordings obtained from drowsy subjects were scored for drowsiness individually by five expert scorers; only those periods marked by a consensus of three or more were considered further in the study. On twenty validation recordings a total of 70 episodes were found (84 percent of the events found by the consensus); 13 were missed (16 percent). Ten of the 11 false identifications (13 percent) were of episodes found by one or two scorers, or of episodes which bordered on periods of drowsiness.

Figure 4.6 (upper) is a polygraph excerpt from a 75-year-old patient (MM) with a left-sided cerebral vascular accident. Figure 4.6 (middle) are CSAs of the data from the same patient without removal of artifact and drowsiness contaminated data, while Figure 4.6 (lower) is the same data following automatic removal of these contaminants. While these algorithms obviously need further refinements, they are useful in their current form for initial automatic data screening. Further editing is then performed interactively on the computer graphics terminal.

APPLICATIONS OF QUANTIFIED EEG

Structural Supratentorial Lesions

The single most relevant EEG feature associated with supratentorial tumors is the presence, extent, morphologic character, and distribution of focal slow (theta, and especially delta) activity (Daly, 1958; Decker and Knott, 1972). Until the development and widespread use of computerized axial tomography, much research was concerned with quantifying the EEG correlates of space-occupying lesions. There is now much less impetus to this approach, however, and the excellent work which was performed in this area is mostly of historical importance. It will not, therefore, be discussed here, but the interested reader should consult the original papers (Gotman et al, 1973, 1975; Matousek and Petersen, 1973a) for more detailed information. Similar techniques have been used to develop EEG indices of acute cerebral vascular accidents (Cohen, Bravo-Fernandez, and Sances, 1976, 1977; John, 1977).

Figure 4.7 is an example of quantified EEG correlates of a patient's response to brain tumor chemotherapy (Spire, Renaudin, and Gevins, 1975). Changes are shown over approximately 4 months in the power and thresholded coherence spectra of a 44-year-old man who underwent a subtotal removal of a right parietal occipital glioblastoma five months before entering a chemotherapy treatment protocol in July, 1972. On 12/18/72, the clinical examination showed much deterioration, the patient having become dysarthric and partially blind in the interval. Four months later, the patient had further deteriorated clinically, and was now almost completely blind, dysarthric, and hemiparetic. In Figure 4.7, the anatomically arranged CSAs each represent 2.5 minutes of EEG recorded on 12/18/72, 2/13/73, and 4/4/73 respectively. The frequency scale extends from 1 to 14 Hz. A marked progressive increase in asymmetric activity is evident on the CSAs, with the largest peaks being in the right frontocentral and centroparietal electrodes. Changes in the thresholded coherence spectra (Figure 4.7, lower right) also parallel the progressive clinical deterioration.

Automated Clinical EEG Assessment

The utility of routine computer analyses of the wide variety of clinical EEGs is not currently known. While displays of frequency analysis, such as the CSA, present the background information contained in the traditional polygraph in a compact manner that is simpler to interpret, the loss of information about wave

A

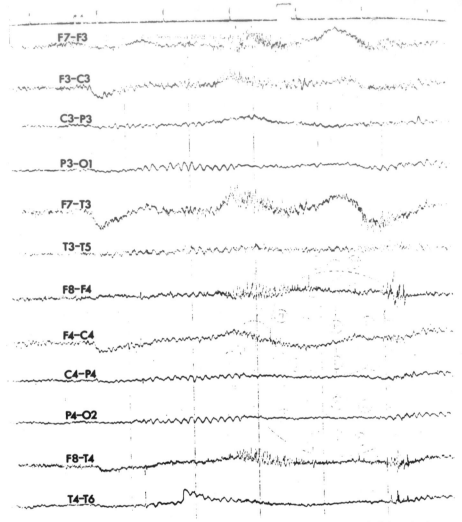

F7–F3

F3–C3

C3–P3

P3–O1

F7–T3

T3–T5

F8–F4

F4–C4

C4–P4

P4–O2

F8–T4

T4–T6

Fig. 4.6. (A) *Polygraph excerpt from a 75-year-old woman with a left hemisphere cerebrovascular accident. Recording is contaminated by eye movement, muscle potential, drowsiness, and other artifact.* (B) *CSAs of the same patient. The abscissa represents frequency from 1 to approximately 25 Hz (the higher frequencies are combined), while the ordinate represents spectral intensity (the height of individual lines) and ongoing time (each successive line is the ensemble average of the next ten 1-second data epochs). The height of any of the alphanumeric characters is equal to 6 μV^2 per Hz on the spectral intensity graphs. From behavioral observation and the polygraph recording, there was evidence of drowsiness and eye movement and muscle potential artifact. These are apparent on the spectral graphs as intermittent low frequency peaks, especially prominent in the frontal area, and as breaks in the 8 Hz peaks which can more clearly be seen in the centro-parieto-occipital derivations.* (C) *The same data analyzed with automatic rejection of data contaminated by artifact and drowsiness. The remaining data are relatively free of contamination, and are now in agreement with the clinical EEG report which described an "essentially normal" recording. A few low intensity, low frequency peaks still remain because a forward and backward refractory period was not used to purge data surrounding detected artifact. (Figure continues on next page.)*

B 9/2/76 M.M. ADIEEG WITHOUT ARTIFACT REJECTION
SQRT INTENSITY SPECTRUM I=1.3 UV/SQRT HZ 10FFT AVERAGING PAGE 0 00:00:
00

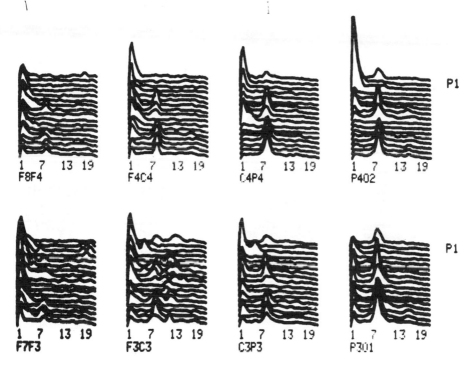

C 9/2/76 M.M. ADIEEG WITH ARTIFACT REJECTION
SQRT INTENSITY SPECTRUM I=1.3 UV/SQRT HZ 10FFT AVERAGING PAGE 0 00:00:
00

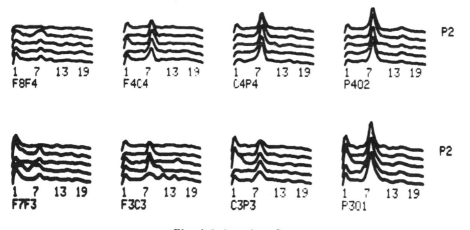

Fig. 4.6. (*continued*)

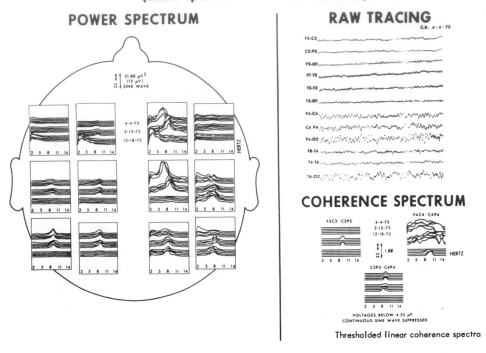

RIGHT PARIETAL GLIOMA
(each spectral line is 30 seconds)

POWER SPECTRUM

RAW TRACING

COHERENCE SPECTRUM

Thresholded linear coherence spectra

Fig. 4.7. *Polygraph excerpt and processed EEG from a patient with a right parietal glioma. The EEG excerpt (6 sec) of 4/4/73 reveals an asymmetry with maximal voltage in the right frontal and parietal regions (F4-C4 and C4-P4). The CSA shows 2.5 minutes analyzed on each of three successive occasions spanning a period of about 3.5 months. The activity is clearly localized in the right fronto-central and centro-parietal regions. The thresholded linear coherence spectra reveal both the locus of abnormal activity and the electrophysiologic trends which corresponded to a deterioration in the patient's condition.*

morphology in such methods may limit their applications. Such information is necessary to differentiate various pathologic transients (PLEDs, rhythmic delta, the variety of sharp transients, etc.), artifacts, and drowsiness. While it has been thought that less subjective judgment would be required to interpret displays of frequency analysis than the conventional polygraph, controlled validation studies on unselected clinical EEGs will be necessary to determine whether this is the case. Indeed, it even remains uncertain whether the same conclusions would be drawn from such computer displays as routinely follow from interpretation of the polygraph (p. 134).

An alternative approach to routine clinical application involves statistical comparison of the results of frequency analysis with numerical standards computed from appropriate patient and control populations (Matoušek and Petersen, 1973a, b; John et al, 1977). Current numerical standards are adequate for automatically forming the determination that a particular EEG pattern is grossly abnormal. However, prior to the determination of more subtle abnormalities, more extensive normative data will be needed, since the range of normal variation of the EEG characteristics of children and adults is rather large.

Because of the above difficulties, there has generally been a shift in research during the last several years from emphasis on automated interpretation of the wide variety of EEGs obtained in routine clinical practice, to quantification of the EEG in connection with specific, more narrowly circumscribed pathologic conditions. This shift in emphasis is no doubt also partly attributable to the increasing use of computerized axial tomography for the diagnosis and evaluation of intracranial space-occupying lesions.

Four laboratories have recently reported the results of large projects concerned with EEG automation. The pioneers of the modern phase of this research are M. Matoušek, I. Petersen, and associates at the Sahlgren Hospital in Göteborg, Sweden (Matoušek, 1968; Matoušek and Petersen, 1973a, b; Friberg et al, 1976; Matoušek, 1977). The current state of development of their system is quite advanced, achieving a correct automatic interpretation of EEG background activity in approximately 90 percent of 106 randomly selected routine EEGs (Friberg et al, 1976; Matoušek, 1977). The results of the analysis are automatically expressed in conventional EEG terminology (Fig. 4.8). These computer-generated verbal assessments can be used by the referring clinician without change in about half of the cases. In about 30 percent of the cases, it is necessary to change 1 to 10 words. Broader use of the system is hampered by the need for improved automatic selection of data to be analyzed, improved automatic artifact rejection, and incorporation of methods for the detection and analysis of transient activity.

In Japan, a consortium of medical and industrial investigators has developed an integrated minicomputer system for the analysis of routine EEGs (Homma et al, 1973; Ebe et al, 1973; Ogawa et al, 1974). Every 10 seconds a decision is made concerning state of arousal, abnormal asymmetry, abnormal slowing, abnormal distribution of amplitude, and extent of abnormal paroxysmal patterns. In a sample of randomly selected adult EEGs, correct decisions

EEG 1974-11-04

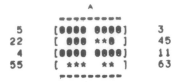

Alpha activity with a frequency of 8 c/s and with an
amplitude of about 30 microvolts is prominent . Moderate amount
of delta activity which is more pronounced in the fronto-temporal
region on both sides and in the central and temporal region
on the left side .

CONCLUSION:

Very severe abnormality diffusely located with maximum in
the central and temporal region on the left side and in the
fronto-temporal region bilaterally .

*Fig. 4.8. Output of the automatic clinical EEG interpretation system developed
by Matoušek, Petersen, and associates at the Sahlgren Hospital in Göteborg,
Sweden. English language summary and conclusion were generated automatically by the computer, based upon results of frequency analysis and computation of age-dependent quotients. The degree of abnormality is indicated by the
number of 0's, while the numerical values placed to the left and right of the
schematic outline of the head are the age-dependent quotients for each region.
On unselected routine clinical EEG's the system is correct as to the decision of
normality or abnormality about 80 percent of the time (with the courtesy of M.
Matoušek, Sahlgren Hospital, Göteborg, Sweden).*

concerning normality or abnormality were made in about 85 percent of the
cases. Recent reports have not appeared in the English language literature on
further development or clinical application of the device.

In England, MacGillivray and associates (MacGillivray and Wadbrook,
1975; MacGillivray, 1977) have developed a system for automatically analyzing
and interpreting routine clinical EEGs. Easy-to-read numerical summaries are
produced for the energy in each frequency band, as well as for spikes and
asymmetries. An extensive English language summary of the findings is then
automatically created, similar in kind to that of Matousek and Petersen described above. Evaluation of the system's performance on unselected clinical
EEGs is awaited.

Recently, E. Roy John and associates (John, 1977; John et al, 1977) at New York University announced the completion of a system for the collection and analysis of EEGs. Small minicomputers are to be placed in each laboratory for the presentation of stimuli and collection of data, while the analysis is to be performed on larger computers at regionally distributed centers. Designed into the system at the outset were computer programs to present a "neurometric battery," a systematic series of stimuli and tasks designed to assess the integrity of functioning of sensory, perceptual and, to a limited extent, cognitive processes. Both background EEG and sensory-evoked potentials are recorded during the battery. An advanced degree of integration of research in many areas has obviously been achieved. Figure 4.9, which is a preliminary version of the automatically generated output from this system for a child with a seizure disorder, is self-explanatory. Formal clinical evaluation of this system will both determine the limits of its accuracy and the extent of its utility in diagnosis and evaluation of treatment.

Metabolic Disorders

Quantitative EEG indices of uremic encephalopathy may provide a noninvasive assessment of the adequacy of dialysis and other forms of treatment of renal patients (Ginn et al, 1975; Teschan et al, 1975). An anatomically diffuse increase of spectral intensity of low frequency EEG components is the major quantitative EEG pattern associated with increased renal insufficiency. In a series of studies in a nondialyzed patient population with renal failure, Bourne and associates (Bourne et al, 1975a, b) determined that EEG slowing was highly correlated with increased creatinine concentrations (Fig. 4.10). With dialysis, the intensity of low frequency components decreased. In subsequent studies (Bowling and Bourne, 1978), multivariate discriminant analysis was used to form an optimal combination of EEG spectral intensity measurements to separate renal patients from normal controls. Previously unanalyzed EEGs (validation data) from 19 patients and controls were correctly classified as to clinical category in 95 percent of cases. Discrimination of EEG patterns associated with renal failure from those associated with light sleep is the aim of ongoing research (Sur et al, 1975). Confirmatory results have been reported by Spehr et al (1977), who performed computer analysis of EEGs from 20 patients with renal failure before and after dialysis. Before dialysis, EEG slowing was most strongly associated with creatinine concentration. After dialysis, the percentage of slow activity decreased; and the ratio of theta to alpha band activity correlated significantly with the clinical state of the patient.

It is apparent that quantitative EEG indices are reliably correlated with the level of biochemical abnormalities before dialysis, and with the metabolic and clinical results of dialysis. If ongoing research is successful, use of quantitative EEG techniques in monitoring renal patients will shortly enter the phase of clinical testing.

Subject: Birth Date: Project: Site: Operator:

Test Date: Report written by: Date:

A neurometric clinical evaluation was conducted on the portion of the brain electrical activity related to the resting state of the subject when his or her eyes were closed. This consisted of frequency and symmetry analyses carried out on the resting EEG from bilateral central (C3-Cz and C4-Cz), temporal (T3-T5 and T4-T6), parieto-occipital (P3-O1 and P4-O2), and fronto-temporal (F7-T3 and F8-T4) regions.

Average evoked potentials were computed from all derivations using a blank flash and patterned visual stimuli consisting of checkerboard grids with 27 lines/inch and 7 lines/inch. Average evoked response to click stimuli was also computed.

The waveshape symmetry of average evoked potentials was assessed by computing the cross-correlation coefficient between bilateral derivations, while asymmetries were assessed by computing the 't'-test difference of the amplitude at each of 10 msec time point after stimulus presentation.

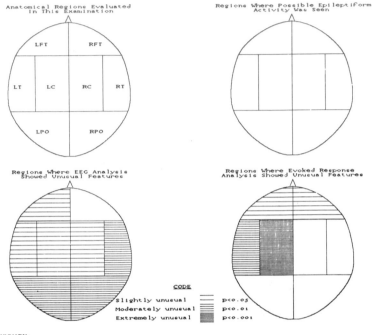

CODE

Slightly unusual ≡ p<0.05
Moderately unusual ≣ p<0.01
Extremely unusual ▓ p<0.001

SUMMARY:

This is a severely abnormal record.

Indications of hypersensitivity to visual stimulation were seen in the following regions: Frontal derivations.

Excessive slow waves were present.

Significant asymmetries were found in both the EEG and evoked potentials.

A conventional EEG examination is recommended.

IMPLICATIONS:

The following implications are based on the literature regarding the consequences of organic brain pathology and our clinical experience to date. These conclusions are not invariant and depend on a number of factors such as age of onset of dysfunction, degree of remediative compensation as well as idiosyncratic factors. Bearing in mind these qualifications the following deficiencies (in processing are expected):

There was no evidence of spikes or sharp waves in the EEG. However, excessive beta activity was present. Such a condition is sometimes associated with an epileptic condition. A conventional EEG is recommended if behavioral symptoms warrant.

Features of the activity evoked in certain regions by presentation of some stimuli suggest that this patient may have sub-clinical seizure sensitivity.

Such activity was elicited by visual stimuli in the following regions:

Frontal derivations.

Widespread theta activity is often associated with attention difficulties including a short attention span and/or hyperdistractability.

There is a moderate probability that abnormal neurometric values in the parietal and posterior regions will be associated with letter and word perception problems. This may include reading problems with a history of letter reversals.

There is a moderate probability that abnormal neurometric values in the temporal regions will be associated with problems with language skills and the memory of complex auditory sequences.

There is a moderate probability that abnormal neurometric values in the central regions will be associated with skilled motor movement problems which may include gross body clumsiness, poor hand writing, and/or difficulties in the pronunciation of polysyllabic words. Problems in short term memory may also be encountered.

Fig. 4.9. *Preliminary version of the automatically generated output from the Neurometrics System of E. R. John at the New York University. The report summarizes analysis of the EEG and averaged evoked reponse recorded from a child with a seizure disorder. The decision as to degree of abnormality is made by comparison with normative values derived from a substantial data base (with the courtesy of E. R. John, Brain Research Laboratories, New York University, New York).*

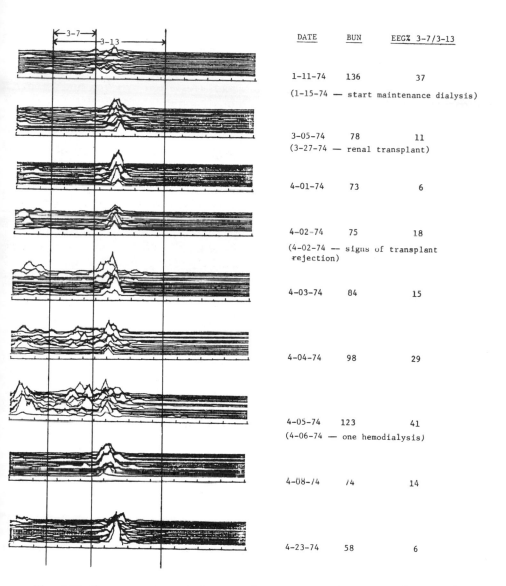

DATE	BUN	EEG% 3-7/3-13
1-11-74	136	37
(1-15-74 — start maintenance dialysis)		
3-05-74	78	11
(3-27-74 — renal transplant)		
4-01-74	73	6
4-02-74	75	18
(4-02-74 — signs of transplant rejection)		
4-03-74	84	15
4-04-74	98	29
4-05-74	123	41
(4-06-74 — one hemodialysis)		
4-08-74	74	14
4-23-74	58	6

Fig. 4.10. Compressed spectral arrays from a pre- and posttransplant renal patient. BUN, blood urea nitrogen, EEG percent, the percentage of spectral power between 3 and 7 Hz referred to a total bandwidth of 3 to 13 Hz. Maintenance dialysis was begun on 1/15/74. Renal transplant was performed on 3/27/74. Rejection of the implant began on 4/2/74. Immunosuppressive treatment was increased on 4/2/74 and tapered after 4/8/74. The degree of EEG slowing clearly parallels the patient's clinical history (from Bourne, J. R., Ward, J. W., Teschan, P. E., Musso, M., Johnston, H. B., Jr., and Ginn, H. E. 1975a. Electroencephalogr. Clin. Neurophysiol., 39, 377).

Anesthesia Level

Previous research, dating back to the work of Gibbs, Gibbs, and Lennox (1937), suggested that the EEG could be used to monitor the depth of anesthesia for a wide variety of anesthetic agents (reviewed by Clark and Rosner, 1973). It was suggested by Martin, Faulkoner, and Bickford (1959) that a dose-dependent relation existed between many common anesthetic agents and a stereotyped sequence of EEG changes. McEwen and associates (1975) noted that progress in quantifying these relations has been impeded by lack of precise definition of anesthesia levels, lack of adequate understanding of the specific relation between EEG patterns and anesthesia level, high intra- and interrater variability in EEG polygraph interpretation, and variations in EEG patterns associated with different anesthetic agents. In order to overcome these problems, they investigated the relation between various EEG measurements and five physiologically and behaviorally defined levels of halothane-nitrous oxide anesthesia. Using measures based on either frequency or time-domain analysis, 51 percent correct classification of anesthesia level was obtained using validation data from 15 patients. These results were deemed adequate to undertake the development of a compact monitoring instrument for use in the operating room. Ongoing research is focused on the detection of artifact, the characterization of EEG patterns related to other anesthetic agents, and on improving EEG feature extraction and pattern recognition.

Investigating this latter issue, Gersch (1978) applied advanced forms of analysis to the set of data collected by McEwan and associates. These procedures (which used autoregressive modeling for the primary analysis and the Kullback Leibler nearest neighbor rule for classification) have the advantage of eliminating the arbitrary use of ad-hoc procedures at every step in the analysis. Eighty-five percent correct replication classification was obtained of anesthesia levels 1 and 3. Unfortunately, since all five anesthesia levels were not analyzed, direct comparison with the results of McEwan and associates (1975) is not possible.

Seizure Disorders

Computer analysis of the EEG is of greatest potential clinical utility in the seizure disorders. In this context, there are several areas in which research has proceeded to such an extent that routine clinical application is likely within the next few years.

Sharp Transient Detection. Many reports have been published of computer algorithms and special-purpose devices designed to detect paroxysmal EEG events (Bickford, 1959; Buckley et al, 1968; Carrie, 1972; Goldberg, Sampson-Dollfus, and Gremy, 1973; Homma et al, 1973; Zetterberg, 1973; Hill and Townsend, 1973, 1974; Smith, 1974; Ktonas and Smith, 1974; Gevins et al, 1975, 1976, 1978; Luders et al, 1976; Ehrenberg and Penry, 1976; Ma, Celesia, and Birkemeier, 1976; Gotman and Gloor, 1976; Carrie and Frost, 1977; Mac-

Gillivray, 1977; Birkemeier et al, 1978; Gotman et al, 1978). However, adequate validation of detection performance by comparison with the *consensus* of clinical judgment has only been reported in a few instances (Gevins et al, 1975, 1976; Ehrenberg and Penry, 1976; Carrie, 1976; Carrie and Frost, 1977; Gotman et al, 1978).

Computerized detection of sharp transients would be simplified if parameters of such waveforms were even approximately known. Quantitative studies by Celesia and Chen (1976) are of paramount importance in this regard. Studying the parameters of 600 spikes in 100 epileptic patients, they found that 88 percent of spikes were surface negative, that 98 percent of these spikes were at least 30 percent greater in amplitude than the background, and that 75 percent were followed by a "slow wave" lasting 130 to 200 msec. Mean duration of spikes was 45 msec, with a range of 9 to 200 msec. Ktonas and Smith (1974) confirmed Kooi's (1966) observation that spikes have a slope above $2 \mu V$ per msec, and additionally noted that, since a spike is not symmetrical, it cannot be modeled by an isosceles triangle.

Because of both technical and clinical considerations, results of automated EEG screening to detect rarely occurring iterictal spikes must be cautiously interpreted. Technically, detection accuracy has not yet achieved a sufficiently high level to obviate the need for human review. Computer reconstruction of detected events (Fig. 4.11) is useful for this purpose. Since it is generally true that false detections are made more often than events are missed, the first generation of imperfect detectors may reasonably be used to screen very long EEG recordings for epochs in which clinically significant paroxysmal activity is likely to be present, and the final decision could then be made by the EEGer.

Clinically, it must be kept in mind that instances are common in which there is no simple relation between interictal paroxysmal EEG activity, blood level of anticonvulsant drug, and number and duration of clinical seizures (see below, and Stevens, Lonsbury, and Goel, 1972; Stevens, 1976). In these instances computed quantities, such as the number or duration of paroxysms, are not currently known to be correlated with clinically relevant variables.

Absences of Petit Mal Type. There is a paroxysmal waveform (3 per second generalized spike-wave discharge, or GSWD) whose occurrence may be taken as a sign of a clinical seizure. Such seizures are often too frequent, too brief in duration, and too minor in their behavioral manifestations to quantify clinically. In a pioneering study which developed the methodology for future research, Penry, Porter, and Dreifuss (1972, 1975) studied in 18 patients the relation between oral dose, plasma level of anticonvulsants, the number and length of GSWDs, and a composite index of absence seizures derived from clinical observation. Using telemetered EEG recordings, it was determined that the greatest response to ethosuximide occurred within 48 hours of the initiation of medication. Figure 4.12 is an example, from a single patient, of the relationship between time of day, behavioral activity, and seizures (Sato, Penry, and Dreifuss, 1976). Using the same experimental procedures, Dreifuss et al (1975) investigated serum clonazepam concentrations in 10 children with absence sei-

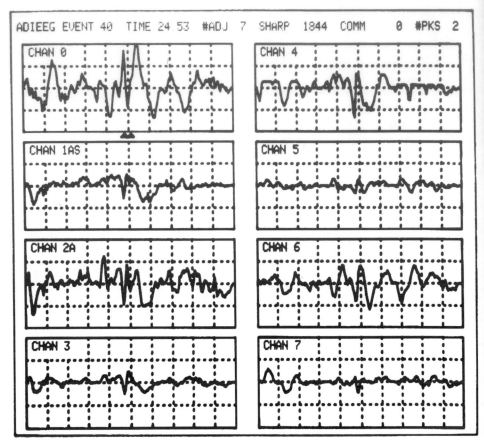

Fig. 4.11. *Computer-reconstructed EEG surrounding the detection of sharp-transient event number 40 (bracketed by marks under channel 0—Fp1-F3). The letter A next to channels 1 (Fp2-F4) and 2 (F3-C3) indicates the detection of a near simultaneous sharp-transient event on an anatomically adjacent channel. The recordings in the other channels were 3, F4-C4; 4, C3-P3; 5, C4-P4; 6, P3-O1; 7, P4-O2. Information across top of page gives time (24.53), sharpness (1844), and number of peaks (2), of event number 40. With such displays, it is possible to unambiguously verify that the computer's detection of a particular transient event in the EEG corresponds with expert judgment.*

zures. As determined both from 12-hour telemetered EEG recordings, and from the composite seizure index, 8 of the 10 patients showed a significant decrease in seizure frequency with serum levels ranging from 13 to 72 ng per ml. Current research in this area is concentrating on the development of computer algorithms with sufficient accuracy for dedicated use in clinical trials of new anticonvulsants.

Only a few studies have been concerned specifically with accurate detection of GSWDs (Carrie, 1972; Carrie and Frost, 1977; Ehrenberg and Penry, 1976; Gevins et al, 1978). During an exhaustive evaluation of the detection accuracy

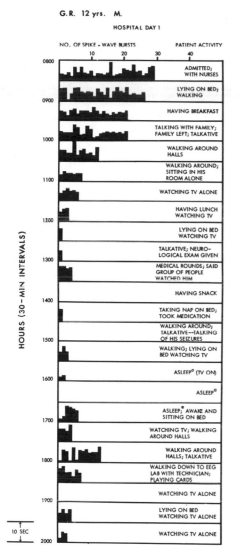

G.R. 12 yrs. M.

aDURING SLEEP, MANY SHORT ASYNCHRONOUS DISCHARGES WERE OBSERVED, AS WE HAVE REPORTED ELSEWHERE.

Fig. 4.12. Frequency and duration of generalized 3 per second spike and wave discharges (GSWDs) in a 12-year-old patient with intractable absence seizures. The relationship between time of day (at 30 minute intervals), behavioral activity, and seizures (as determined from clinical observation and telemetered EEG) is shown. Seizures occurred most frequently in the morning (from Sato, S., Penry, J. K., and Dreifuss, F. E. 1976. In: Quantitative Analytic Studies in Epilepsy, Kellaway, P. and Petersen, I., Eds., pp. 237–251. Raven Press, New York).

of a simple computer algorithm for the detection of GSWDs, Ehrenberg and Penry (1976) examined 12-hour telemetered, daytime EEG recordings from 7 patients with absence seizures. Of 609 discharges found by all three scorers, the computer algorithm detected 85 percent. Approximately as many isolated detections were made by the algorithm as by any of the three scorers. The performance of this system was not deemed adequate for routine use. Using active filters and computer algorithms improved in several respects from those used in their earlier research, Carrie and Frost (1971, 1977) analyzed 10 to 12 hour, 1 channel waking recordings from each of 5 patients with absence seizures. Ninety-five percent of those seizures rated by two EEGers as lasting more than 3 seconds were detected, but only 30 percent of those seizures lasting between 1 and 3 seconds were picked up.

More complex forms of analysis have been applied to this problem. Using a combination of linear prediction and double differentiation, Birkemeier et al (1978) reported detection of 53 of 65 GSWDs (81 percent) found by an EEGer on single channel recordings from 5 patients. There were 17 false detections. Since these complex algorithms are sensitive to extracerebral artifact and EEG changes related to changes in mental or physical state, additional heuristic or statistical algorithms must still be employed to obtain an acceptably high level of GSWD detection accuracy. Recently, Gevins and associates (1978) reported a preliminary evaluation of complex, second-generation computer algorithms specifically designed to detect 3 per second GSWDs from patients with absence seizures. All 27 GSWDs occurring during 900 seconds on 4-channel EEG excerpts from 8 patients with absence seizures were detected. There were no false detections arising from physiologic or instrumental artifact, or other sources. If this performance is maintained during a more extensive evaluation, it would be adequate to eventually replace human judgment in the routine recognition and tabulation of GSWDs. Even so, clinical review of computer results would still be advisable.

Seizure-Anticonvulsant-EEG Relations. In a unique study (Carrie, 1976), a computer-assisted method for detecting and quantifying sharp transients was applied to serial overnight sleep EEG recordings of a patient with a cerebellar stimulator implanted to control generalized tonic-clonic seizures. When the serum diphenylhydantoin (DPH) level fell into the subtherapeutic range and the number of seizures increased, the frequency of interictal transients decreased; while when the serum anticonvulsant level was elevated, interictal transients increased in frequency and seizures occurred less often. These findings are consistent with reports indicating that the anticonvulsant action of DPH is mainly due to the prevention of seizure spread, rather than to suppression of abnormal activity at the epileptogenic focus. Carrie, noting that different patterns of correlation between these three variables had been found in preliminary studies from other patients, stressed the need for further research to determine how the relation between EEG and clinical patterns varies with the type of seizure and the anticonvulsant agent.

Seizure Onset Prediction. Viglione, Ordon, and Risch (1970) and Viglione (1974) reported the results of an 8-year project to determine the feasibility of predicting generalized tonic-clonic seizures 10 minutes or so in advance of their onset in ambulatory patients with poorly controlled seizure disorders. Figure 4.13 shows a patient being instrumented for this study. In the validation phase of the study, very large EEG samples (18 hours a day for at least 12 days) were collected by telemetry from each of 13 patients. The behavior of 7 patients was recorded on video tape. Based upon seizure characteristics and extensive computer analysis of this vast body of data (approximately 250 seizures were recorded on tape, and over 2,000 hours of EEG were analyzed!), miniature seizure-warning systems, that could be worn, were developed for each patient. Each system continuously monitored 2 to 4 EEG channels, performed a frequency analysis, and decided whether each 15-second sample represented a preseizure, baseline, or artifact episode. Seizure prediction was based, not upon changes in the pattern of occurrence of paroxysmal events, but rather on subtle, slowly varying changes in the frequency of the background EEG activity. In 6 of the 13 subjects, the systems predicted more than half of the clinical seizures. There were an unacceptably high number of false alarms, arising from a variety of sources including artifacts and subclinical seizures. A composite system had zero or one false alarms on 3 of 4 nonepileptic controls. It is likely that further development will lead to a reduction in the number of false alarms, but a number of practical problems still remain to be solved.

Localization of Epileptogenic Foci. Another area of potential application of quantitative EEG is in the spatial localization of the onset of paroxysmal activity, the measurement of its anatomic propagation, and the determination of the time of their occurrence during the day. This would be particularly important for patients with uncontrolled complex partial seizures who are candidates for unilateral temporal lobe resection (reviewed by Tailairach and Bancaud, 1974; Klass, 1975; and Rasmussen, 1975). The advantage of quantitative techniques in this area would derive principally from the resultant capability of routinely examining long recordings. The possibility of computing the depth location of a focus, at which an electrode had not been implanted, is also of long-term interest. Localization has been attempted using scalp, depth, and simultaneous scalp and depth recordings.

Brazier and colleagues (Brazier, 1972) have undertaken spectral analysis of the EEG recorded from the depths of the brain. By comparing patterns of spectral coherence from interictal and ictal recordings, she concluded that seizures propagate through both normally used and normally unused pathways (rather than by volume conduction). It also was apparent that scalp electrodes were only sensitive to seizures that had spread to the cortex.

Gersch and Tharp (1976) demonstrated the application of advanced algorithms to the problem of the depth localization of a seizure focus in a patient with uncontrolled complex partial seizures. Spectral regression was used to lateralize the epileptogenic source, while a measure of the amount of informa-

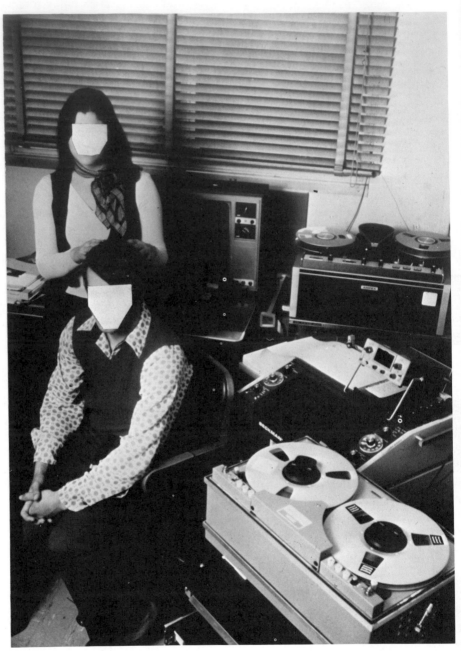

Fig. 4.13. *Epileptic patient being instrumented with experimental seizure warning system. System attempted to predict onset of uncontrolled tonic clonic seizure 10 minutes prior to its occurrence (from Viglione, S. S. 1974. McDonnell Douglas Astronautics Company, Huntington Beach, Calif., MDAC Paper APA 74133, Dec. 1974).*

tion was used to compute the exact location. Such elegant techniques eliminate the use of ad-hoc judgments at various points during the analysis. Gotman and associates (Gotman and Gloor, 1976; Gotman et al, 1978) have developed and evaluated an automatic method for quantifying interictal sharp transient paroxysmal activity in the scalp-recorded EEG. The method incorporates several tests designed to isolate the characteristic morphologic properties of sharp transients. Results of analysis are presented in an attractive, anatomically arranged display (Fig. 4.14). A study was undertaken to compare independent interpretation, by two EEGers, of these computer displays with interpretation of the polygraph. In each case, a structured report was used to summarize conclusions about localization and degree of abnormality. While the average

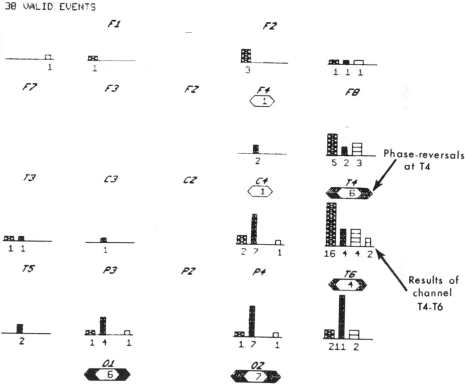

Fig. 4.14. Anatomically arranged, sixteen-channel histograms of interictal sharp transient event detections during 3 minutes of EEG recording from a patient with a right temporal focus of paroxysmal activity. When sharp transient events have been detected at a particular location, from 1 to 4 vertical bars are drawn with their height proportional to the number of detections. From left to right these bars correspond to four classes of sharp transient events, namely those which are large and sharp, small and sharp, large and less sharp, and small and less sharp. The number of phase reversals at an electrode is indicated under the electrode (from Gotman, J., and Gloor, P. 1976. Electroencephalogr. Clin. Neurophysiol., 41, 513).

correlation between conclusions drawn from the polygraph and from the computer display was only about 60 percent, correlation between the two EEGers' conclusions was higher for the computer display than the polygraph (84 percent vs 72 percent).

The problem of quantitatively relating EEG patterns recorded at the scalp to paroxysmal activity in the depths of the brain is an intriguing one. If such relationships could reliably be found, they would have immediate clinical application in the diagnosis and management of patients with a wide variety of seizure disorders, and would obviate the need to implant depth electrodes. Over the years, Saltzberg and associates (Saltzberg, Lusrick, and Heath, 1971; Saltzberg, 1976) have investigated matched digital filtering and cepstral (higher order spectral) analysis in this regard. The major problem encountered in their studies was that without the presence of simultaneously recorded depth activity to serve as a reference, it was not possible to unambiguously determine that scalp-detected patterns corresponded to paroxysmal activity within the brain.

Lopes da Silva et al (1977) applied autoregressive filtering to detect nonstationarities (changes) in EEGs simultaneously recorded from the scalp and depth. In some instances, although paroxysmal events were not visible at scalp sites, events detected at the scalp corresponded temporally with paroxysmal events at depth sites (Fig. 4.15). In four patients, localization of paroxysmal activity by this method was the same as localization derived from interpretation of the polygraph. Clinical application of this elegant method awaits the development of algorithms which can distinguish nonstationarities attributable to changes in behavioral state (e.g. eye-opening, level of arousal, or extracerebral artifact) from those attributable to paroxysmal activity associated with seizure disorders.

Lieb et al (1978) used a relatively simple computer algorithm to quantify sharp transient paroxysmal activity originating in medial temporal lobe sites. In 14 patients whose complex partial seizures were refractory to anticonvulsant medication, the maximum rate and consistency of paroxysmal activity was found by this method to be the same temporal lobe as was chosen by polygraph interpretation to be the likely site of seizure origination (Fig. 4.16). No simple relation was found between time of clinical seizure onset and parameters of depth spike occurrence. The authors concluded that computer analysis of depth recordings of interictal paroxysmal activity may prove useful in determining the suitability of individual patients for surgery.

Higher Cortical Functions

In an attempt to fulfill Hans Berger's original dream that the EEG could be used as a "window on the mind," over the last 40 years signal processing technologies of all sorts have been applied to the EEG (Gevins and Schaffer, 1979). In each instance, early enthusiasm has been dampened when subsequent controlled studies revealed the problem to be far more difficult than originally thought. This is certainly not surprising, for the theories of neural mass action advanced by Lashley (1937), elaborated more recently by Bartlett and John

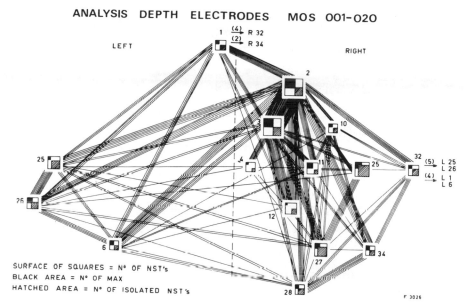

ANALYSIS DEPTH ELECTRODES   MOS 001–020

SURFACE OF SQUARES = N° OF NST's
BLACK AREA = N° OF MAX
HATCHED AREA = N° OF ISOLATED NST's

Fig. 4.15. *Spatial map of the results of analysis of a 100 second EEG epoch from 15 depth-electrodes from a patient with intractable seizures. The number of events detected is indicated by the size of the squares. Lines indicate the number of times events have been detected at the same time in the two channels connected by the lines. Isolated events are indicated by hatched squares. Electrodes R2 and R3 (fronto-orbital) have the largest number of events and the most simultaneous detections. A number of events detected at scalp sites by this method, although not corresponding with visible sharp transients on the polygraph, coincide with sharp transient events in depth locations (from Lopes da Silva, F. H., Van Hulten, K., Lommen, J. G., Storm van Leeuwen, W., Van Veelen, C. W. M. and Vliegenthart, W. 1977. Electroencephalogr. Clin. Neurophysiol., 43, 1).*

(1973), and further developed and quantified by Freeman (1975), are among the few theoretical studies supporting research in this area.

In practice, the search for EEG correlates of higher cortical functions is conducted by recording the EEG as a subject or patient engages in problem-solving tasks of one sort or another. For the most part, only nonspecific task-related desynchronization of the EEG can be seen on the polygraph during the performance of such tasks (for an exception, see Fig. 4.17). Accordingly, more detailed information can be obtained only by effective computer analysis. In the pioneer studies of the current era, D. O. Walter, W. R. Adey and associates (Walter et al, 1966; Walter, Rhodes, and Adey, 1967, summarized in Adey, 1969) at the UCLA Brain Research Institute automatically classified into appropriate behavioral condition the multichannel EEG features computed from frequency analysis. Such an approach necessitates rather extensive data processing, but John and associates (1977) have used similar quantitative tech-

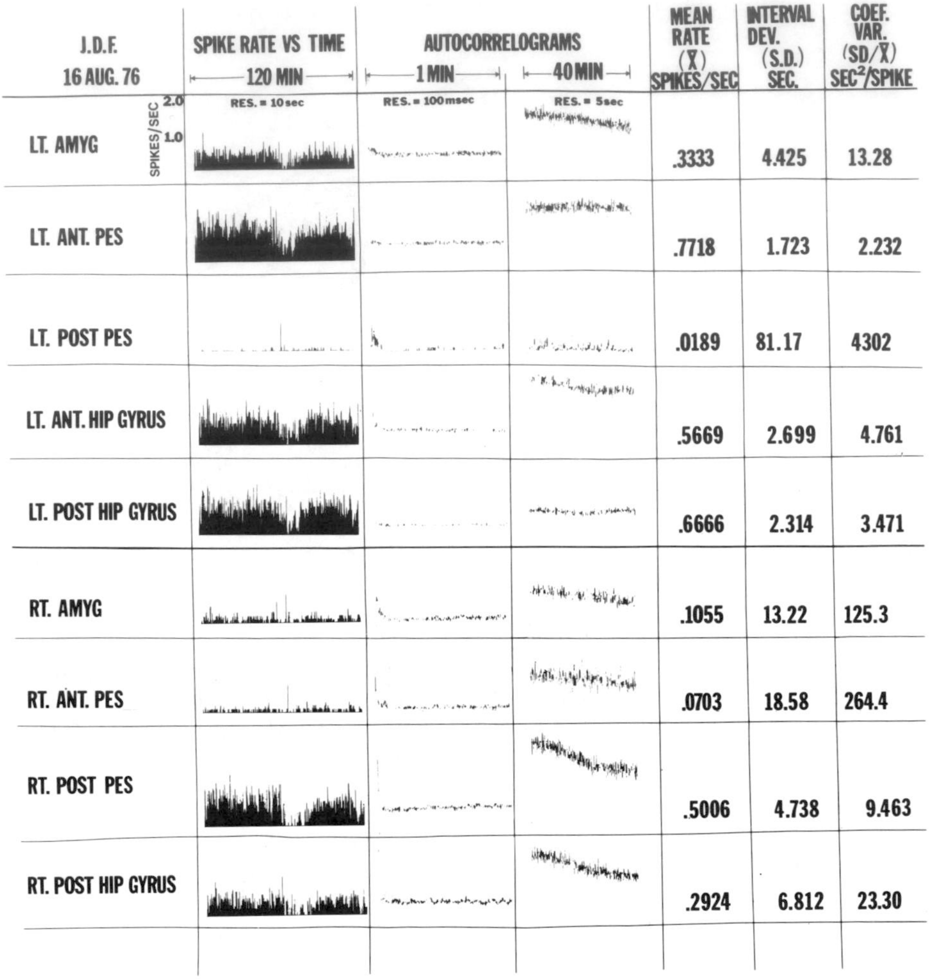

J.D.F. 16 AUG. 76	SPIKE RATE VS TIME ← 120 MIN →	AUTOCORRELOGRAMS ← 1 MIN → ← 40 MIN →		MEAN RATE ($\bar{X}$) SPIKES/SEC	INTERVAL DEV. (S.D.) SEC.	COEF. VAR. (SD/$\bar{X}$) SEC²/SPIKE
LT. AMYG	RES. = 10 sec	RES. = 100 msec	RES. = 5 sec	.3333	4.425	13.28
LT. ANT. PES				.7718	1.723	2.232
LT. POST PES				.0189	81.17	4302
LT. ANT. HIP GYRUS				.5669	2.699	4.761
LT. POST HIP GYRUS				.6666	2.314	3.471
RT. AMYG				.1055	13.22	125.3
RT. ANT. PES				.0703	18.58	264.4
RT. POST PES				.5006	4.738	9.463
RT. POST HIP GYRUS				.2924	6.812	23.30

Fig. 4.16. A depth-spike analysis of a patient with uncontrolled complex partial seizures. The most active site was the left anterior pes hippocampi. This site also displayed the lowest standard deviation of interspike intervals as well as the lowest coefficient of variation. No periodicities in spike occurrence were uncovered by either the 1 or 40 minute autocorrelograms. Each vertical scale indicates 10 counts (from Lieb, J. P., Woods. S. C., Siccardi, A., Crandall, P. H., Walter, D. O., and Leake, B. 1978. Electroencephalogr. Clin. Neurophysiol., 44, 641).

niques to categorize differences in EEGs between several patient populations (see p. 142).

In the most recent series of studies relating the background EEG to higher cortical functions, interhemispheric asymmetries, notably in the alpha (8 to 13 Hz) band, have been related to differences between "cognitive" tasks (Galin and Ornstein, 1972; McKee, Humphrey, and McAdam, 1973; Butler and Glass, 1974; Doyle, Ornstein, and Galin, 1974; Morgan, Macdonald, and Hilgard,

1974; Dumas and Morgan, 1975; Rebert and Low, 1978; critically reviewed by Donchin et al, 1977, and by Gevins and Schaffer, 1979). These results have been viewed as supporting popular concepts of the functional specialization of the left and right cerebral hemispheres respectively for "verbal" and "spatial" cognitive processes. In these studies, interhemispheric EEG asymmetries were often the only effects studied, with the implication that asymmetries were the

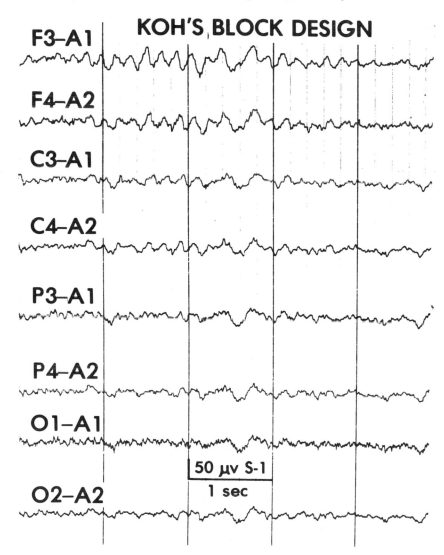

Fig. 4.17. *Polygraph excerpts during performance of Koh's block design. A singular example of bursts of theta band activity, maximal over the frontal region, during performance of the block design task is shown. (Data obviously contaminated by muscle action potential artifact did not enter into the analysis.) The functional significance of this pattern is not currently known.*

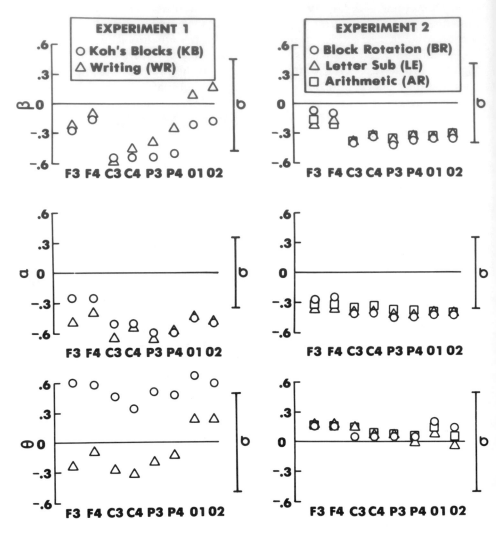

Fig. 4.18. Means over more than 20 subjects of EEG spectral intensities recorded during performance of several "cognitive" tasks. EEG observations associated with tasks were first grouped with EEG observations of EO (eye-opening) and standard scores computed (ordinate). Upper, middle, and lower sets of graphs are for spectral intensities in the beta, alpha, and theta bands. Abscissa is scalp electrode placements. Tasks of Experiment 1 (left) were 1 minute long and involved limb movements, and uncontrolled sensory and performance differences. Tasks of Experiment 2 (right) were less than 15 seconds long and required no motion of the limbs; sensory stimulation and performance were relatively controlled. With these controls, there are no appreciable differences between tasks (from Gevins, A. S., Zeitlin, G. M., Doyle, J. C., Yingling, C. D., Schaffer, R. E., Callaway, E., and Yeager, C. L. 1979. Science, 203, 665. Copyright 1979 by the American Association for the Advancement of Science).

most prominent EEG patterns associated with the tasks. Most importantly for potential clinical application of these findings, in assessing subtle patterns of cortical dysfunction, it has not been established that the EEG asymmetries found were attributable to the cognitive components of the experimental tasks employed. Such tasks were unduly complex and lengthy, and involved different patterns of sensory stimulation, limb movements, and performance levels.

We have, therefore, investigated these issues using the ADIEEG analysis system (Gevins et al, 1979a, b). In a series of two experiments, we have found that asymmetries associated with some commonly employed "verbal" and "spatial" tasks are quite weak in comparison to other task-related EEG patterns. Moreover, when movement of the limbs was not required during the performance of a task, and when stimuli and performance-related differences between tasks were relatively controlled, strong task-related EEG patterns were not found. With these controls, only weak intertask EEG differences were found, and these only by resort to a powerful analytical technique—multivariate nonlinear pattern recognition. Figure 4.18 summarizes the essential results of these studies. From these results, it is clear that proposed clinical application of measurements derived from the background EEG for the assessment of subtle patterns of cortical dysfunction must await further research.

ACKNOWLEDGEMENTS

I would like to express my gratitude to my mentor and colleague, Dr. Charles L. Yeager, and to acknowledge the collaboration of Dr. J. P. Spire in some of the original experimental work described here. I am grateful also for financial support under Grant NS-10471 from the National Institutes of Neurologic and Communicative Diseases and Strokes. Supplementary support has also been received from United States Public Health Service Research Support Grant RR-05755 to the Langley Porter Institute, and from the Epilepsy Foundation of America.

REFERENCES

Adey, W. R. (1969). Spectral analysis of EEG data from animals and man during alerting, orienting and discriminating responses. In: Attention in Neurophysiology, Mulholland, T., and Evans, C., Eds. Butterworth, London.

Anderson, T. W. (1958). An Introduction to Multivariate Statistical Analysis. Wiley, New York.

Andrews, H. C. (1972). Introduction to Mathematical Techniques in Pattern Recognition. Wiley, New York.

Barlow, J. S. and Brazier, M. A. B. (1956). Some applications of correlation analysis to clinical problems in electroencephalography. Electroencephalogr. Clin. Neurophysiol., 8:325.

Bartlett, F. and John, E. R. (1973). Equipotentiality quantified: The anatomical distribution of the engram. Science, 181:764.

Bickford, R. G. (1959). An automatic recognition system for spike-and-wave with simultaneous testing of motor response. Electroencephalogr. Clin. Neurophysiol., *11:*397.

Bickford, R. G. (1977). Computer Analysis of Background Activity. In: EEG Informatics. A Didactic Review of Methods and Applications of EEG Data Processing, Remond, A., Ed., p. 215. Elsevier, Amsterdam.

Bickford, R. G. and Klass, D. W. (1976) Electroencephalography. In: Clinical Examinations in Neurology, Mayo Clinic and Mayo Foundation. Saunders, Philadelphia.

Bickford, R. G., Fleming, N. I., and Billinger, T. W. (1971). Compression of EEG data by isometric power spectral plots. Electroencephalogr. Clin. Neurophysiol., *31:*632.

Bickford, R. G., Brimm, J., Berger, L., and Aung, M. (1973). Application of compressed spectral array in clinical EEG. In: Automation of Clinical Electroencephalography, Kellaway, P. and Petersen, I., Eds., p. 55. Raven Press, New York.

Birkemeier, W. P., Fontaine, A. B., Celesia, G. G., and Ma, K. M. (1978). Pattern recognition techniques for the detection of epileptic transients in EEG. IEEE Trans. Biomed. Eng., *BME-25:*213.

Blum, R. H. (1954). A note on the reliability of electroencephalographic judgments. Neurology, *4:*143.

Bourne, J. R., Miezin, F. M., Ward, J. W., and Teschan, P. E. (1975b). Computer quantification of electroencephalographic data recorded from renal patients. Comput. Biomed. Res., *8:*461.

Bourne, J. R., Ward, J. W., Teschan, P. E., Musso, M., Johnston, H. B., Jr., and Ginn, H. E. (1975a). Quantitative assessment of the electroencephalogram in renal disease. Electroencephalogr. Clin. Neurophysiol., *39:*377.

Bowling, P. S. and Bourne, J. R. (1978). Discriminant analysis of electroencephalograms recorded from renal patients. IEEE Trans. Biomed. Eng., *BME-25:*12.

Brazier, Mary A. B. (1972). Interactions of deep structures during seizures in man. In: Synchronization of EEG Activity in Epilepsies, A Symposium organized by the Austrian Academy of Sciences, Vienna, Austria, September 12–13, 1971. Petsche, H., and Brazier, Mary A. B., Eds., p. 409. Springer-Verlag, Wien.

Buckley, J. K., Saltzberg, B., and Heath, R. G. (1968). Decision criteria and detection circuitry for multiple channel EEG correlation. In: 1968 IEEE Region 3 Conv. Rec., vol. 26, p. 1.

Butler, S. and Glass, A. (1974). Asymmetries in the electroencephalogram associated with cerebral dominance. Electroencephalogr. Clin. Neurophysiol., *36:*481.

Carrie, J. R. G. (1972). A hybrid computer system for detecting and quantifying spike and wave EEG patterns. Electroencephalogr. Clin. Neurophysiol., *33:*339.

Carrie, J. R. G. (1976). Computer-assisted EEG sharp-transient detection and quantification during overnight recordings in an epileptic patient. In: Quantitative Analytic Studies in Epilepsy, Kellaway, P., and Petersen, I., Eds., p. *225.* Raven Press, New York.

Carrie, J. R. G. and Frost, J. D., Jr. (1971). A small computer system for EEG wavelength amplitude profile analysis. Biomed. Comput., *2:*251–263.

Carrie, J. R. G. and Frost, J. D., Jr. (1977). Clinical evaluation of a method for quantification of generalized spike-wave EEG patterns by computer during prolonged recordings. Comput. Biomed. Res., *10:*449.

Celesia, G. G. and Chen, R. (1976). Parameters of spikes in human epilepsy. Dis. Nerv. Syst., *37:*277.

Chen, C. (1973). Statistical Pattern Recognition. Spartan, Rochelle Park, New Jersey.

Clark, D. L. and Rosner, B. S. (1973). Neurophysiological effects of general anesthetics: the electroencephalogram and sensory evoked responses in man. Anesthesiology, *38:*564.

Cohen, B. A., Bravo-Fernandez, E. J., and Sances, A., Jr. (1976). Quantification of computer analyzed serial EEGs from stroke patients. Electroencephalogr. Clin. Neurophysiol., *41:*379.

Cohen, B. A., Bravo-Fernandez, E. J., and Sances, A., Jr. (1977). Automated electroencephalographic analysis as a prognostic indicator in stroke. Med. Biol. Eng. Comput., *15:*431.

Cox, J. R., Jr., Nolle, F. M., and Arthur, R. M. (1972). Digital analysis of the electroencephalogram, the blood pressure wave, and the electrocardiogram. Proc. IEEE *60:*1137.

Daly, D. (1958). Sequential alterations in the EEGs of patients with brain tumors. Electroencephalogr. Clin. Neurophysiol., *10:*395.

Decker, D. A. and Knott, R. (1972). The EEG in intrinsic supratentorial brain tumors. Electroencephalogr. Clin. Neurophysiol., *33:*303.

Dolce, G. and Decker, H. (1975). Application of multivariate statistical methods in analysis of spectral values of the EEG. In: CEAN Computerized EEG Analysis, Dolce, G., and Kunkel, H., Eds., p. 157. Gustav Fischer Verlag, Stuttgart.

Dolce, G. and Kunkel, H., Eds. (1975). CEAN Computerized EEG Analysis. Gustav Fischer Verlag, Stuttgart.

Donchin, E., Kutas, M., and McCarthy, G. (1977). Electrocortical indices of hemispheric utilization. In: Lateralization in the Nervous System. Harnad, S., Ed., p. 339. Academic Press, New York.

Doyle, J., Ornstein, R., and Galin, D. (1974). Lateral specialization of cognitive mode: II. EEG frequency analysis. Psychophysiology, *11:*567.

Dreifuss, F. E., Penry, J. K., Rose, S. W., Kupferberg, H. J., Dyken, P., and Sato, S. (1975). Serum clonazepam concentrations in children with absence seizures. Neurology, *25:*255.

Dumas, R. and Morgan, A. (1975). EEG asymmetry as a function of occupation, task, and task difficulty. Neuropsychologia, *13:*219.

Dumermuth, G. and Fluhler, H. (1967). Some modern aspects in numerical spectrum analysis of multichannel electroencephalographic data. Med. Biol. Eng. Comput., *5:*319.

Dumermuth, G., Huber, P. J., Kleiner, B., and Gasser, T. (1970). Numerical analysis of elctroencephalographic data. IEEE Trans. Audio Electroacoust., *AU-18:*404.

Dymond, A. M., Coger, R. W. and Serafetinides, E. A. (1975). Extension to three psychiatric populations of a factor analysis grouping of ongoing EEG. 28th ACEMB, Sept. 1975.

Ebe, M., Homma, I., Ogawa, T., Schiono, H., Ishiyama, Y., Nakamura, T., Suzuki, T., and Abe, Z. (1973). Automatic analysis of clinical information in EEG. Electroencephalogr. Clin. Neurophysiol., *34:*706.

Ehrenberg, B. L. and Penry, J. K. (1976). Computer recognition of generalized spikewave discharges. Electroencephalogr. Clin. Neurophysiol., *41:*25.

Fink, M. (1977). Quantitative EEG analysis and psychopharmacology. In: EEG Informatics. A Didactic Review of Methods and Applications of EEG Data Processing, Remond, A., Ed., p. 301. Elsevier, Amsterdam.

Freeman, W. J. (1975). Mass Action in the Nervous System, Academic Press, New York.

Friberg, S., Magnusson, R. I., Matoušek, M., and Petersen, I. (1976). Automatic EEG diagnosis by means of digital signal processing. In: Quantitative Analytic Studies in Epilepsy, Kellaway, P., and Petersen, I., Eds., p. 289. Raven Press, New York.

Galin, D. and Ornstein, R. (1972). Lateral specialization of cognitive mode: an EEG study. Psychophysiology, *9:*412.

Gersch, W. (1978). Kullback Leibler number cluster/classification analysis of stationary time series. In: Proc. 4th Intnl Pattern Recognition Conf Japan November 1978.

Gersch, W. and Tharp, B. R. (1976). Spectral regression-amount of information analysis of seizures in humans. In: Quantititative Analytic Studies in Epilepsy, Kellaway, P., and Petersen, I., Eds., p. 509. Raven Press, New York.

Gevins, A. S. and Schaffer, R. E. (1979). A critical review of studies of EEG correlates of higher cortical functions, CRC Critical Reviews in Bioengineering, in press.

Gevins, A. S. and Yeager, C. L. (1972). EEG spectral analysis in real time. In: 1972 DECUS Spring Proc., p. 71.

Gevins, A., Blackburn, J., and Dedon, M. (1978). Very accurate computer recognition of generalized spike and wave discharges (GSWD's). Epilepsy International Symposium, Vancouver, Canada, September 10–14.

Gevins, A. S., Yeager, C. L., Spire, J. P., and Henderson, J. H. (1976a). Database for clinical EEG quantification. Proc. 30th Ann. Meeting American EEG Society.

Gevins, A. S., Zeitlin, G. M., Ancoli, S., and Yeager, C. L. (1977b). Computer rejection of EEG artifact. II. Contamination by drowsiness. Electroencephalogr. Clin. Neurophysiology, *42:*31.

Gevins, A. S., Yeager, C. L., Zeitlin, G. M., Ancoli, S., and Dedon, M. F. (1977a). On-line computer rejection of EEG artifact. Electroencephalogr. Clin. Neurophysiol., *42:*267.

Gevins, A. S., Yeager, C. L., Diamond, S. L., Spire, J., Zeitlin, G. M., and Gevins, A. H. (1975). Automated analysis of the electrical activity of the human brain (EEG): A progress report. Proc. IEEE, *63:*1382.

Gevins, A. S., Yeager, C. L., Diamond, S. L., Zeitlin, G. M., Spire, J. P., and Gevins, A. H. (1976). Sharp-transient analysis and thresholded linear coherence spectra of paroxysmal EEGs. In: Quantitative Analytic Studies in Epilepsy, Kellaway, P., and Petersen, I., Eds., p. 463. Raven Press, New York.

Gevins, A. S., Zeitlin, G. M., Doyle, J. C., Yingling, C. D., Schaffer, R. E., Callaway, E. and Yeager, C. L. (1979a). Electroencephalogram correlates of higher cortical functions. Science, *203:* 665.

Gevins, A., Zeitlin, G., Yingling, C., Doyle, J., Dedon, M., Schaffer, R., Roumasett, J., Callaway, E. and Yeager, C. (1979b). EEG during "cognitive" tasks, parts 1 and 2, Electroencephalogr. Clin. Neurophysiol., in press.

Gibbs, F. A. and Gibbs, E. L., Atlas of Electroencephalography, vol. 1, Methodology and Controls, (1951). vol. 2, Epilepsy (1952). Vol. 3, Neurological and Psychiatric Disorders (1964). Addison-Wesley, Reading, Mass.

Gibbs, F. A., Gibbs, E. L., and Lennox, W. G. (1937). Effect on the electroencephalogram of certain drugs which influence nervous activity. Arch. Intern. Med., *60:*154.

Ginn, H. E., Teschan, P. E., Walker, P. J., Bourne, J. R., Fristoe, M., Ward, J. W., McLain, L. W., Johnston, H. B., Jr., and Hamel, B. (1975). Neurotoxicity in uremia. Kidney Int., *7:*S–357.

Goldberg, P., Samson-Dollfus, D., and Gremy, F. (1973). An approach to automatic recognition of the electroencephalogram: background rhythm and paroxysmal elements. Math. Inform. Med., *12:*155.

Gose, E. E., Werner, S., and Bickford, R. G. (1974). Computerized spike detection. In: Proc. 13th Ann. San Diego Biomedical Symp.

Gotman, J. and Gloor, P. (1976). Automatic recognition and quantification of interictal epileptic activity in the human scalp EEG. Electroencephalogr. Clin. Neurophysiol., *41:*513.

Gotman, J., Gloor, P., and Ray, W. F. (1975). A quantitative comparison of traditional reading of the EEG and interpretation of computer-extracted features in patients with supratentorial brain lesions. Electroencephalogr. Clin. Neurophysiol., *38:*623.

Gotman, J., Gloor, P., and Schaul, N. (1978). Comparison of traditional reading of the EEG and automatic recognition of interictal epileptic activity. Electroencephalogr. Clin. Neurophysiol., *44:*48.

Gotman, J., Skuce, D., Thompson, C., Gloor, P., Ives, J., and Ray, W. (1973). Clinical application of spectral analysis and extraction of features from electroencephalograms with slow waves in adult patients. Electroencephalogr. Clin. Neurophysiol., *35:*225.

Grass, A. M., and Gibbs, F. A. (1938). A Fourier transform of the electroencephalogram. J. Neurophysiol., *1:*521.

Harman, H. H. (1967). Modern Factor Analysis, 2nd edn, University of Chicago Press.

Harner, R. N. (1977). EEG analysis in the time domain. In: EEG Informatics. A Didactic Review of Methods and Applications of EEG Data Processing, Remond, A. Ed., p. 57. Elsevier, Amsterdam.

Harner, R. N. and Ostergren, K. A. (1976). Sequential analysis of quasi-stable and paroxysmal EEG activity. In: Quantitative Analytic Studies in Epilepsy, Kellaway, P., and Petersen, I., Eds., p. 343. Raven Press, New York.

Harris, R. J. (1975). A Primer of Multivariate Statistics. Academic Press, New York.

Hill, D. and Parr, G., eds. (1963). Electroencephalography, a Symposium on Its Various Aspects. Macdonald, London.

Hill, A. G. and Townsend, H. R. A. (1973). The automatic estimation of epileptic spike activity. Biomed. Comput., *4:*149.

Hill, A. G. and Townsend, H. R. A. (1974). Determining the patterns of epileptic spikes despite inefficient recognition. In: 1974 Medinfo Proc., p. 731.

Hjorth, B. (1970). EEG analysis based on time domain properties. Electroencephalogr. Clin. Neurophysiol., *29:*306.

Homma, I., Ogawa, T., Ebe, M., Shiono, H., Ishiyama, Y., Nakamura, T., Suzuki, T., and Abe, Z. (1973). Automatic analyzer of clinical EEG in 12 channels—recording. In: Digest of the 10th International Conference on Medical and Biological Engineering—Dresden, p. 121.

Houfek, E. E. and Ellingson, R. J. (1959). On the reliability of clinical EEG interpretation. J. Nerv. Ment. Dis., *128:*425.

Isaksson, A. and Wennberg, A. (1975). Visual evaluation and computer analysis of the EEG—a comparison. Electroencephalogr. Clin. Neurophysiol., *38:*79.

Itil, T. M., Ed. (1974). Psychotropic Drugs and the Human EEG. Karger, New York.

Jasper, H. H. (1958). Report of the committee on methods of clinical examination in electroencephalography. Electroencephalogr. Clin. Neurophysiol., *10:*370.

Jasper, H. H., Ward, A. A., Jr., and Pope, A., Eds. (1969). Basic Mechanisms of the Epilepsies. Little, Brown, Boston.

John, E. R. (1977). Functional Neuroscience, Vol. II. Lawrence Erlbaum Associates, Hillsdale.

John, E. R., Karmel, B. Z., Corning, W. C., Easton, P., Brown, D., Ahn, H., John, M., Harmony, T., Prichep, L., Toro, A., Gerson, I., Bartlett, F., Thatcher, R., Kaye, H., Valdes, P., Schwartz, E. (1977). Neurometrics: numerical taxonomy identifies different profiles of brain functions within groups of behaviorally similar people. Science, *196:*1393.

Johnson, L., Lubin, A., Naitoh, P., Nute, C., Austin, M. (1969). Spectral analysis of the EEG of dominant and nondominant alpha subjects during waking and sleeping. Electroencephalogr. Clin. Neurophysiol., *26:*361.

Joy, R. M. (1968). The use of time series analysis in the comparison of the effects of a series of Benzodiazepines upon the EEG. Neuropharmacologist, *10:*161.

Kellaway, P. and Petersen, I., Eds. (1973). Automation of Clinical Electroencephalography. Raven Press, New York.

Kellaway, P. and Petersen, I., Eds. (1976). Quantitative Analytic Studies in Epilepsy. Raven Press, New York.

Kiloh, L. G., McComas, A. J., and Osselton, J. W. (1972). Clinical Electroencephalography, 3rd edn. Butterworth, London.

Klass, D. W. (1975). Electroencephalographic Manifestations of Complex Partial Seizures. In: Advances in Neurology, Volume II: Complex Partial Seizures and Their Treatment, Penry, J. K., and Daly, D. D., Eds., p. 113. Raven Press, New York.

Kooi, K. A. (1966). Voltage-time characteristics of spikes and other rapid electroencephalographic transients. Neurology, *16:*59.

Kooi, K. A. (1971). Fundamentals of Electroencephalography. Harper and Row, New York.

Ktonas, P. Y. and Smith, J. R. (1974). Quantification of abnormal EEG spike characteristics. Comput. Biol. Med., *4:*157.

Lashley, K. S. (1937). Functional determinants of cerebral localization. Arch. Neurol. Psychiatry, *38:*371.

Leader, H. S., Cohen, R., Weihrer, A. L., and Caceres, C. A. (1967). Pattern reading of the clinical electroencephalogram with a digital computer. Electroencephalogr. Clin. Neurophysiol., *23:*566.

Leggewie, H. and Probst, W. (1969). On-line analysis of EEG with a small computer (period-amplitude analysis). Electroencephalogr. Clin. Neurophysiol., *27:*533.

Lieb, J. P., Woods, S. C., Siccardi, A., Crandall, P. H., Walter, D. O., and Leake, B. (1978). Quantitative analysis of depth spiking in relation to seizure foci in patients with temporal lobe epilepsy. Electroencephalogr. Clin. Neurophysiol., *44:*641.

Little, S. C. and Raffel, S. C. (1962). Intra-rater reliability of EEG interpretation. J. Nerv. Ment. Dis., *135:*77.

Lopes da Silva, F. H., Van Hulten, K., Lommen, J. G., Storm van Leeuwen, W., Van Veelen, C. W. M. and Vliegenthart, W. (1977). Automatic detection and localization of epileptic foci. Electroencephalogr. Clin. Neurophysiol., *43:*1.

Luders, H., Daube, J. R., Taylor, W. F., and Klass, D. W. (1976). A computer system for statistical analysis of EEG transients. In: Quantitative Analytic Studies in Epilepsy, Kellaway, P., and Petersen, I., Eds., p. 403. Raven Press, New York.

Ma, K. M., Celesia, G. G., and Birkemeier, W. P. (1976). Cluster analysis and spike detection in EEG. In: Proc. 7th Internat. Symp. on Epilepsy, Janz, D., Ed., p. 386. Thieme, Stuttgart.

MacGillivray, B. (1977). Application of automated EEG analysis to the diagnosis of epilepsy. In: EEG Informatics. A Didactic Review of Methods and Applications of EEG Data Processing, Remond, A., Ed., p. 243. Elsevier. Amsterdam.

MacGillivray, B. B. and Wadbrook, D. G. (1975). A system for extracting a diagnosis from the clinical EEG. In: CEAN Computerized EEG Analysis, Symposium of Merck'sche Gesellschaft fur Kunst und Wissenschaft, Kronberg/Taunus, April 8th–10th, 1974, Dolce, G., and Kunkel, H., Eds., p. 344. Gustav Fischer Verlag, Stuttgart.

Martin, J. T., Faulkoner, A., Jr., and Bickford, R. G. (1959). Electroencephalography in anesthesiology. Anesthesiology, *20:*359.

Matějček, M., and Devos, J. E. (1976). Selected methods of quantitative EEG analysis and their applications in psychotropic drug research. In: Quantitative Analytic Studies in Epilepsy, Kellaway, P. and Petersen, I., Eds., p. 183. Raven Press, New York.

Matějček, M. and Schenk, G. K., Eds. (1975). Quantitative Analysis of the EEG: Methods and Applications. Proceedings of 2nd Symposium of the Study Group for EEG Methodology, held under the auspices of the Swiss Association for EEG and Clinical Neurophysiology, Jongny sur Vevey, Switzerland, April 31–May 4, 1975. Printed by AEG-TELEFUNKEN, EDP-Division, Konstanz.

Matoušek, M. (1968). Frequency analysis in routine electroencephalography. Electroencephalogr. Clin. Neurophysiol., *24:*365.

Matoušek, M., Ed. (1973). Frequency and Correlation Analysis. Handbook of Electroencephalography and Clinical Neurophysiology, vol. 5 A. Elsevier, Amsterdam.

Matoušek, M. (1977). Clinical application of EEG analysis: Presentation of EEG results and dialogue with the clinician. In: EEG Informatics. A Didactic Review of Methods and Applications of EEG Data Processing, Remond, A., Ed., p. 233. Elsevier, Amsterdam.

Matoušek, M., and Petersen, I. (1973a). Frequency analysis of the EEG in normal children and adolescents. In: Automation of Clinical Electroencephalography, Kellaway, P., and Petersen, I., Eds. Raven Press, New York.

Matoušek, M., and Petersen, I. (1973b). Automatic evaluation of EEG background activity by means of age-dependent quotients. Electroencephalogr. Clin. Neurophysiol., *35:*603.

McEwen, J. A., Anderson, G. B., Low, M. D., and Jenkins, L. C. (1975). Monitoring the level of anesthesia by automatic analysis of spontaneous EEG activity. IEEE Trans. Biomed. Eng., BME-22:299.

McKee, G., Humphrey, B., and McAdam, D. (1973). Scaled lateralization of alpha activity during linguistic and musical tasks. Psychophysiology, *10:*441.

Meisel, W. S. (1972). Computer-Oriented Approaches to Pattern Recognition. Academic Press, New York.

Morgan, A., MacDonald, H., and Hilgard, E. (1974). EEG alpha: lateral asymmetry related to task, and hypnotizability. Psychophysiology, *11:*275.

Nilsson, N. J. (1965). Learning Machines. McGraw-Hill, New York.

Ogawa, T., Homma, I., Ebe, M., Shiono, H., Ishiyama, Y., Nakamura, T., Suzuki, T., Abe, Z. (1974). EEG automatic analyzer. In: 27th ACEMB, vol. 16, p. 142.

Penry, J. K., Porter, R. J., and Dreifuss, F. E. (1972). Ethosuximide: Relation of plasma levels to clinical control. In: Antiepileptic Drugs, Woodbury, D. M., Penry, J. K., and Schmidt, R. P., Eds., p. 431. Raven Press, New York.

Penry, J. K., Porter, R. J., and Dreifuss, F. E. (1975). Simultaneous recording of absence seizures with video tape and electroencephalography. Brain, *98:*427.

Rao, C. R. (1952). Advanced Statistical Methods in Biometric Research. Wiley, New York.

Rao, C. R. (1965). Linear Statistical Inference and Its Applications. Wiley, New York.

Rasmussen, T. (1975). Surgical treatment of patients with complex partial seizures. In: Advances in Neurology, Vol. 11: Complex Partial Seizures and Their Treatment, Penry, J. K., and Daly, D. D., Eds., p. 415. Raven Press, New York.

Rebert, C. and Low, D. (1978). Differential hemispheric activation during complex visuomotor performance. Electroencephalogr. Clin. Neurophysiol., *44:*724.

Remond, A. (1966). The importance of topographic data in EEG phenomena, and an electrical model to reproduce them. Electroencephalogr. Clin. Neurophysiol., Suppl. *27:*29.

Remond, A., Ed. (1977). EEG Informatics. A Didactic Review of Methods and Applications of EEG Data Processing. Elsevier, Amsterdam.

Remond, A., Baillon, J. F., Bienenfeld, G. (1975). Time domain analysis of EEG waves and bursts. In: Quantitative Analysis of the EEG, Methods and Applications, Matějček, M., and Schenk, G. K., Eds., p. 321. Proceedings of the 2nd Symposium of the Study Group for EEG-Methodology, Jongny sur Vevey, May 1975, Printed by AEG-TELEFUNKEN, EDP Division, Konstanz.

Rose, S. W., Penry, J. K., White, B. G., and Sato, S. (1973). Reliability and validity of visual EEG assessment in third grade children. Clin. Electroencephalogr., *4:*197.

Saltzberg, B. (1976). A model for relating ripples in the EEG power spectral density to transient patterns of brain electrical activity induced by subcortial spiking. IEEE Trans. Biomed. Eng., BME-23:355.

Saltzberg, B. and Burch, N. R. (1959). A rapidly convergent orthogonal representation for EEG time series and related methods of automatic analysis. In: IRE Wescon Conv. Rec., vol. 8, p. 35.

Saltzberg, B., Lustick, L. S., and Heath, R. G. (1971). Detection of focal depth spiking in the scalp EEG of monkeys. Electroencephalogr. Clin. Neurophysiol., *31:*327.

Sato, S., Penry, J. K., and Dreifuss, F. E. (1976). Electroencephalographic monitoring of generalized spike-wave paroxysms in the hospital and at home. In: Quantitative Analytic Studies in Epilepsy, Kellaway, P., and Petersen, I., Eds., p. 237. Raven Press, New York.

Schenk, G. K. (1976). The pattern-oriented aspect of EEG quantification. Model and clinical basis of the iterative time-domain approach. In: Quantitative Analytic Studies in Epilepsy, Kellaway, P., and Peterson, I., Eds., p. 431. Raven Press, New York.

Schenk, G. K. and Ruegg, T. (1975). A geometric model for the analysis of antagonistic activation and deactivation in electroencephalograms. In: Quantitative Analysis of the EEG, Methods and Applications, Proceedings of the 2nd Symposium of the

Study Group for EEG-Methodology, Jongny sur Vevey, May 1975, Matějček, M., and Schenk, G. K., Eds., p. 337. Printed by AEG-TELEFUNKEN, EDP-Division, Konstanz.

Smith, J. R. (1974). Automatic analysis and detection of EEG spikes. IEEE Trans. Biomed. Eng., BME-21:1.

Spehr, W., Sartorius, H., Berglund, K., Hjorth, B., Kablitz, C., Plog, U., Wiedemann, P. H., and Zapf, K. (1977). EEG and haemodialysis. A structural survey of EEG spectral analysis, Hjorth's EEG descriptors, blood variables and psychological data. Electroencephalogr. Clin. Neurophysiol., *43:*787.

Spire, J. P., Renaudin, J., and Gevins, A. S. (1975). EEG as an indicator of response to brain tumor chemotheraphy. Electroencephalogr. Clin. Neurophysiol., *38:*548.

Stevens, J. R. (1976). "All that spikes is not fits," Presidential Address to the American EEG Society, Seattle, Washington, July, 1974.

Stevens, J. R., Lonsbury, B. L., and Goel, S. L. (1972). Seizure occurrence and interspike interval, telemetered electroencephalogram studies. Arch. Neurol., *26:*409.

Sur, M., Bourne, J., Ward, J., and Teschan, P. (1975). Quantification of EEG slowing in renal disease: the influence of arousal. In: 28th ACEMB, vol. 17.

Tailairach, J. and Bancaud, J. (1974). Approche nouvelle de la neurochirurgie de l'epilepsie. Methodologie stereotaxique et resultats therapeutiques. Neurochirurgie, 20, suppl. 1. Masson, Paris.

Teschan, P. E., Ginn, H. E., Bourne, J. R., Walker, P. J., and Ward, J. W. (1975). Quantitative neurobehavioral responses to renal failure and maintenance dialysis. Trans. Amer. Soc. Artif. Int. Organs, *21:*448–491.

Viglione, S. S. (1974). Validation of epilepsy seizure warning system, McDonnell Douglas Astronautics Company, Huntington Beach, Calif., MDAC Paper APA 74133, Dec. 1974.

Viglione, S. S., Ordon, V. A., and Risch, F. (1970). A methodology for detecting ongoing changes in the EEG prior to clinical seizures. McDonnell Douglas Astronautics Co., West Huntington Beach, Calif., MDAC Paper WD 1399 (A), Feb. 1970.

Volavka, J., Matoušek, M., Feldstein, S., Roubicek, J., Prior, P., Scott, D. F., Brazinova, V., and Synek, V. (1973). Die Zuverlässigkeit der EEG-Beurteilung. Z. EEG-EMG, *4:*123–130.

Walter, D. O. and Brazier, M. A. B., Eds. (1968). Advances in EEG analysis. Electroencephalogr. Clin. Neurophysiol. Suppl. *27.*

Walter, D. O., Rhodes, J. M., and Adey, W. R. (1967). Discriminating among states of consciousness by EEG measurements; a study of four subjects. Electroencephalogr. Clin. Neurophysiol., *22:*22.

Walter, D. O., Rhodes, J. M., Brown, B. S., and Adey, W. R. (1966). Comprehensive spectral analysis of human EEG generators in posterior cerebral regions. Electroencephalogr. Clin. Neurophysiol., *20:*224.

Walter, W. G. (1963). Technique-interpretation. In: Electroencephalography, a Symposium on Its Various Aspects, Hill, D., and Parr, G., Eds., p. 65. Macdonald, London.

Yeager, Charles L. (1937). A Method for Electroencephalographic Classification. Mayo Clinic, Rochester, Minn. Unpublished manuscript.

Yeager, C. L., Gevins, A. S., and Henderson, J. H. (1977). A concise method of EEG classification for compiling a clinical EEG data base. Electroencephalogr. Clin. Neurophysiol., *43:*459.

Zetterberg, L. H. (1973). Spike detection by computer and by analog equipment. In: Automation of Clinical Electroencephalography, Kellaway, P., and Petersen, I., Eds., p. 227. Raven Press, New York.

5

Depth Electrography and Electrocorticography

C. AJMONE MARSAN

DEPTH ELECTROGRAPHY

Depth electrography is an electrophysiologic procedure which is almost exclusively of neurosurgical interest. Not only is it dependent upon a close collaboration between neurophysiologist and neurosurgeon, but its application as a diagnostic help should be considered only in those clinical situations in which surgical treatment is either seriously contemplated or about to be performed.

The general term *depth electrography* refers to a diagnostic procedure which utilizes the implantation of a number of electrodes within the cranial cavity for the acute (a few hours) or chronic (up to 10 or 15 days) recording from different cortical and subcortical brain structures. The same electrodes may also be used for electrical stimulation. When the electrodes are implanted by means of stereotactic techniques, this form of functional exploration is commonly referred to as stereo-electroencephalography (Bancaud et al, 1965, 1973; Talairach et al, 1974). It is worth emphasizing that, regardless of whether stereotactic techniques are employed or not, and regardless of whether "needle" electrodes alone, or both these and "flap" electrodes, are used, direct recording from the cortical surface should always be included as a most important part of the investigative procedure.

Indications and Limitations

Ever since the pioneer studies of depth electrography (Symposium 1953), and from the data which have accumulated in the last 20 years, it has become abundantly clear that a considerable amount of information is lost in routine scalp tracings. This has been repeatedly demonstrated not only by the comparison of such tracings with activities recorded simultaneously from a number of deeply located brain structures, but also by comparing scalp with subdural—or even extradural—recordings. Indeed, the substantial signal attenuation (and distortion) produced by the interposition of relatively inactive tissue, such as dura, skull, and skin, between the source of the signal itself and the recording leads had already been demonstrated at the very beginning of EEG by direct cortical recording in the course of surgical exposure of the brain. After the early observations by Berger, and on the basis of the subsequent neurosurgical experience, it became generally accepted that the amplitude of an average signal at the cortical level would undergo a decrease of about ten times when the same signal is recorded at the scalp level (Penfield and Jasper, 1954). Actually, subsequent studies utilizing a more direct, simultaneous comparison of the same signals at the two (cortical and scalp) levels showed that the ratio between them could be much higher than 10-to-1. Such ratio may reach 60-to-1 and also varies, somewhat capriciously, within a few seconds and under apparently similar conditions, differing according to morphology, duration, and frequency of the signal itself, and in relation to its topographic distribution and size of area involved (Abraham and Ajmone Marsan, 1958).

It is, therefore, obvious that a large number of electrical events will not be recognized at the scalp level, while others will appear there greatly attenuated or distorted. It is particularly, if not exclusively, in the field of seizure disorders that the discrepancy between scalp and depth or surface cortical recording is often very striking and may have practical, diagnostic consequences. Indeed, in many such cases, a large amount of typical high voltage epileptiform discharges can be seen from electrodes located within certain brain structures, but only a small percentage of these discharges is reflected in the scalp tracing (Fig. 5.7).

Use of the technique of recording from chronically implanted electrodes has also been suggested for another, somewhat related, motive. In the electrographic diagnostic localization of the point of origin of the seizures in any individual, it had been traditional to attribute a sound localizing value to the discrete, interictal manifestations, which, in the form of epileptiform discharges (spikes, sharp waves), can generally be detected in relatively large number in the EEGs of epileptic patients in their seizure-free intervals. The logical assumption had always been that, whenever a clinical seizure occurs, the electrographic correlates of such an ictal episode would develop from the same neuronal aggregate(s) giving rise to the sporadic, isolated, interictal discharges. Such an assumption is in fact supported by a wealth of experimental evidence, indicating a very close functional and topographic relationship between interictal and ictal events, and is correlated by data on the basic mechanisms for the transition from one to the other at the single neuron level (Masumoto and Ajmone Marsan, 1964). The situation is, however, less clear in the human epileptic brain. Whereas in many cases the electrographic events are indicative or strongly supportive of a close topographic identity between interictal and ictal phonomena, cases are not uncommon in which the location (or even lateralization) of these two phenomena are quite different. Whenever this happens, a problem of interpretation faces the electroencephalographer. Although the question has not been settled definitively (see below), there is general agreement among epileptologists interested in partial (or focal) epilepsy and in its surgical treatment, that the most reliable EEG phenomena for a correct localization of the site or origin of a seizure disorder are the electrical correlates of the seizure itself. The abovementioned limitations of scalp EEG, therefore, become particularly evident in the case of organized ictal activity, especially when this consists of low voltage rhythms of relatively high frequency. Furthermore, in this situation, the problem is often complicated by the occurrence of electrical phenomena of extracerebral origin (such as movement and muscle potentials) which tend to obscure any trace of cortical or subcortical activity that might appear at the scalp level. In fact the number of negative or useless scalp EEGs recorded in the course of clinical seizures is discouragingly high; this is true especially in the case of partial seizures where electrographic information is often crucial for the correct localization of the epileptogenic source and its possible surgical therapy. With implanted electrodes the recording of an ictal episode is generally free of artifacts and, even more importantly, the localizing feature of its electrographic correlates are fully preserved. Thus, it is often possible to observe exquisitely focal activations at the onset of an ictal episode and to follow their preferential spread in the course of its development (Figs. 5.3 and 5.6; see also case RG in Ajmone Marsan and Abraham, 1960).

In view of the serious limitations of the scalp-recorded EEG, the use of chronically implanted electrodes can be considered when it is important to obtain an accurate localizing diagnosis of the epileptogenic process. However, it is still necessary to justify the use of this procedure, which is not entirely harmless.

General criteria to be followed for the decision to employ such a procedure have been provided by a number of investigators, including Crandall, Walter, and Rand (1963), and, more recently, Walter (1973). These criteria are summarized below. As a first principle, and as already mentioned, it is safe to state that the use of chronically implanted electrodes should be considered only in those patients with epilepsy who are potential candiates for surgical treatment. Excluding patients in whom surgery is contemplated because of the nature of the underlying pathology (e.g. an expanding lesion), such candidates are cases in which (a) the number and severity of seizures have such a serious socioeconomic impact as to preclude any useful activity on the part of the patient, and (b) the condition has proven refractory to any form of appropriate and systematically delivered medical therapy. (Walter, 1973, also includes the patient's age and mental status among the criteria to be taken into consideration.)

Whenever these two main criteria do not apply, the question of surgical intervention should not arise and the correct classification of the seizure disorder and, in particular, the exact localization of the epileptogenic process become primarily a matter of academic rather than practical interest.* In such circumstances there is no real justification for depth electrography and its necessity can hardly be defended on ethical grounds.

On the other hand, when all medical treatments have failed and the clinical and socioeconomic situation suggests the possibility or strong advisability of surgical intervention, the diagnostic and localization workup of the case assumes an obviously important role. Any attempt should be made to determine the side and precise location of the epileptogenic process, and if this information cannot be provided by the routine methods of examination, implantation of electrodes is justified and should be given serious consideration.

The specific instances in which depth electrography can be of some help, and is, therefore, indicated, will now be considered. A first major field of application of this technique is in the investigation of patients with so-called temporal lobe epilepsy ("partial seizures with complex symptomatology").

A rather wide range of "indications" for depth electrography in this context have been advanced on the basis of the material published by different investigators. For instance, it is of interest to consider why implanted electrodes were used in the individual cases—with sufficient information—included in the 1965 monograph by Bancaud et al. In 7 patients (JLRe, JS, NL, NCh, GeL, HuDe, BeBo), on the basis of clinical ictal pattern and scalp EEG, the diagnostic conclusions appeared to be fairly clear-cut for both location (antero-mid-temporal) and side (right hemisphere in 4 and left in 3 cases) of the epileptogenic process. Yet, the investigators point out that, in spite of this information, it was not possible to determine whether the "focus" was exclusively in the lateral surface of the temporal cortex or whether it involved also (or mainly) deep limbic structures (in 5 cases) or insular cortex (in 2 cases). In 1 additional patient (Fde), the problem was similar but there was also pneumoencephalographic evidence for a localized, expanding lesion.

The electrode implantation was bilateral in 4 of these 8 patients, and probably unilateral in 1, while in the remaining 3 cases there was no mention as to whether the studies were carried out on one or both sides. Surgical therapy had been considered advisable and an excision was eventually carried out in all these patients. Thus, strictly speaking, one can find some justification for the preoperative use of depth electrography in such patients. On the other hand, since the lateralization and general localization of the main epileptogenic process seemed to be sufficiently well established in all cases, one can question the practical usefulness of whatever additional information this procedure would—and did—provide. For instance, the necessity of a bilateral implantation is not immediately obvious, particularly in those cases in which neither the

---

* Current medical treatment does not yet appear to be specifically dependent upon—and selectively different for—the different forms of partial epilepsy. At least it does not seem to be crucially related to the subtle topographic differences in localization or lateralization which depth electrography generally provides. A possible exception bearing on the medical therapeutic conduct may be found in the rare instances in which the differential diagnosis is between a form of primary generalized versus partial seizure disorder.

clinical nor the scalp EEG signs had suggested the possibility of contralateral involvement.

As additional support for the justification of depth electrography in one case (BeBo) of this group, it should be mentioned that, upon establishing that the main focus was in the amygdala, a local destruction by means of radioactive isotope was carried out—with sparing of the lateral surface and other structures of the involved temporal lobe—and this procedure allegedly resulted in a cessation of the seizures. This would seem to be a fairly strong argument in favor of depth electrography. Unfortunately, the authors do not provide any information on the duration of the postoperative follow-up. A temporary remission of seizures is a rather common finding after surgery in epileptics, but a follow-up of at least 3 years—and preferably 5 in our experience (Van Buren et al, 1975b)—is necessary before one can accept the results of an excision as totally successful. The same comments and arguments apply to another case of Bancaud's series (AnSu) in which, however, there was an obvious justification for additional localizing studies since the scalp EEG interictal findings were positive but somewhat equivocal and the ictal electrographic changes were noncontributory. In this patient it was possible to localize the epileptogenic process in the left parahippocampal gyrus and a local destruction of this structure and of the nearby amygdala, by means of radioactive yttrium, eventually resulted in the cessation of seizures. In the remaining 5 cases which were reported in some detail (AnMa, AnMi, SeLo, EtLa, JPT), the use of depth electrography appeared to be unquestionably justified since either the clinical seizure patterns or the scalp EEG or both suggested the possibility of multiple or bilateral foci within the temporopararhinal structures. In some of these cases the implanted electrode findings confirmed the complex nature of the epileptogenic process and, on the basis of such findings, surgical treatment was considered inadvisable. In others, it was possible to demonstrate the existence of a prominent—or single—focus which was eventually excised.

In the overall group of temporal lobe patients described by Bancaud et al in the same study, there were several in whom the results of depth electrography were interpreted to indicate an exclusively cortical involvement with no paroxysmal discharges arising primarily from rhinencephalic structures. In such cases, very good therapeutic results were apparently obtained following a limited excision of the cortical lateral surface of the temporal lobe with sparing of deep structures. As in the abovementioned instance, however, these cases suffer from lack of information concerning duration of postoperative follow-up and subsequent systematic observation. In any case, even if the validity of such therapeutic results is accepted, the discrepancy with the experience of other investigators in this field cannot be disregarded. The surgical excision of limited portions of the temporal lobe, either partial gyrectomies sparing mesial structures or selective destructions of the latter with preservation of temporal cortex, has yielded disappointingly poor results, according to most neurosurgeons. This has also been our own experience, recently confirmed in a review of 124 cases of temporal lobe seizures with a postoperative follow-up of from 4 to 16 years (Van Buren et al, 1975b). This point is emphasized here because of its important implications with regard to the use of depth electrography. It is obvious that if it were indeed possible to treat this type of seizure disorder with limited excisions, the preoperative investigation with depth electrography would assume a most crucial role and become a mandatory procedure in practically all cases which are considered for surgical treatment. At present, this important question remains unsettled, but even if the promising therapeutic results claimed by Bancaud et al are not confirmed, we can conclude that there was generally a justified indication for a thorough investigation by means of implanted electrodes in the temporal lobe patients reported in their study, with some minor reservation as to the use of bilateral implantation in a few cases.

There is another major field of seizure disorders in which clinical data and the findings derived from scalp EEG are at times inadequate to reach a reliable diagnostic classification and correct localization of the epileptogenic process. This encompasses cases of apparently generalized seizures in which there may be some feature suggestive of a focal onset and in which the electrographic data raise the problem of a differential diagnosis between a primary generalized seizure disorder (or what used to be described as ''centrencephalic'' epilepsy) and bilateral synchrony secondary to a focal cortical process. Dynamic investigations, with the help of pharmacologic agents, as advocated by Rovit, Gloor, and Rasmussen (1961) and Gloor et al (1964), may sometimes provide a partial answer to the problem (for instance by confirming that the disorder is not a typical idiopathic form of epilepsy and/or by indicating the side affected by the epileptogenic process). As a rule, however, these are complex situations (see Ajmone Marsan and Laskowski, 1962 and the several cases reported by Bancaud et al, 1965, 1973) with clinical and EEG features that are difficult to interpret. It is often not possible to classify such cases and any projected surgical treatment has to be abandoned.

Somewhat similar to these are certain cases of partial seizures with a presumed focal process of uncertain location in the cerebral convexity above the Sylvian fissure. The clinical ictal episodes in such cases are characterized by motor patterns which may be clearly lateralized, but generally consist of complex tonic features without the specific localizing value of, for instance, a Jacksonian march (Ajmone Marsan and Goldhammer, 1973). Occasionlly even the lateralization of their onset may be in question, and the motor phenomena may be accompanied by autonomic components and/or episodes of automatic behavior which further complicate the diagnostic interpretation. The corresponding EEG findings in these patients are frequently noncontributory, with nonspecific abnormalities or diffuse and/or bilateral discharges. In certain cases, even when apparently focal paroxysms are present, it is not possible to pinpoint—by means of scalp EEG—the exact area primarily involved by the epileptogenic process and, for instance, to distinguish between pre- and postcentral, or between motor and premotor area involvement. Other potentially epileptogenic regions, such as the mesial and orbital surface of the frontal lobe, or the mesial face of the occipital lobe, are inaccessible to scalp electrodes and the existence of foci in such locations can only be indirectly presumed on the basis of rather empirical electrographic criteria of questionable validity.

In all these cases, when the seizures are frequent and/or severe enough to interfere with the patient's social and economic activities and when medical treatment fails, there is a reasonable indication for additional investigations by means of implanted electrodes. Several examples of such cases, each presenting with a different individual diagnostic problem are available in the literature, for instance in the recent papers by Crandall (1973), and Ludwig, Ajmone Marsan, and Van Buren (1975, 1976), and, again, in the publications of Bancaud et al (1965, 1973). The latter monographs include a number of case reports representative of complex diagnostic situations in which the epileptogenic process was apparently located in, respectively, the intermediate frontal, supplementary motor area, temporoparieto-occipital trigone, and mesial occipital region.

According to Bancaud et al (1965), the use of implanted electrodes may also be indicated in cases of apparently typical Jacksonian epilepsy, and they provide an illustrative example in which the differential diagnostic localization involved the parietal, rolandic, and parasagittal regions as well as the thalamus. The advisability of implanting electrodes in the latter structure, as part of routine depth electrography in epileptics, can be questioned, since all studies published in the last 20 years have failed to demonstrate in any convincing way the primary or exclusive involvement of thalamic nuclei in the epileptogenic process. Our experience on this aspect is equally negative. The pathophysiologic mechanisms involving the thalamus in such a process have been mainly hypothetical, and are still so at the present time. In fact, in most cases of Bancaud et al, the thalamic implantation—and related negative findings—have been used essentially to challenge the original concept of "centrencephalic" epilepsy. The clinical and electrographic features in all of their cases were already sufficiently atypical to make such a diagnosis rather unlikely, thus weakening the validity of their critique. The fact remains, however, that there is little positive information to be gained by thalamic leads in epileptics who are being considered for surgical treatment, and the advisability of using such a site of implantation should be carefully weighed in each individual case.

In our experience of close to 100 cases of partial seizures, the decision to employ chronically implanted electrodes before attempting a surgical excision has been generally based on one or several of the following criteria or situations:

1. Scalp (and/or nasopharyngeal) EEG evidence of bilateral temporal independent involvement, with only questionable or moderate one-sided predominance.
2. Discrepancy in scalp EEG lateralization between interictal and ictal phenomena.
3. Discrepancy in localization and/or lateralization between interictal EEG findings and clinical seizure pattern(s), with questionable or unavailable EEG ictal phenomena.
4. Equivocal localizing EEG findings or strong EEG evidence of both supra- and infrasylvian involvement (especially frontotemporal).

5. Need to determine the exact extent of the epileptogenic process prior to the excision of essential structures. For instance, in cases of scalp EEG evidence of central (Rolandic) involvement or of predominant involvement of posterior temporal regions in the dominant hemisphere.
6. Determination of a possible primary focus (superficial or subcortical) in cases with scalp EEG evidence of multifocal involvement.
7. Absence of clearly paroxysmal discharges in scalp EEG in cases of unquestionable epileptic disorder with focal seizure patterns clinically.

These are, in our experience, the most common situations but there are, of course, other specific and rather unique problems which might justify the use of depth electrography. For instance in their 1973 monograph, Bancaud et al advocate such use, with stereotactic techniques, in the topographic delimitation of cerebral expanding lesions.

All our seizure cases in which depth electrography was eventually carried out, and the large majority of similar cases reported in the literature, have two important aspects in common: (a) they are all cases in which the diagnosis of epilepsy had been previously established beyond any reasonable doubt, and (b) they all had abnormal scalp EEG with—but for rare exceptions—clearly paroxysmal discharges. In other words, the use of implanted electrodes is not indicated for the primary purpose of diagnosing the (epileptic) nature of episodic disorders of questionable interpretation, especially if such episodes occur in subjects with a totally normal scalp EEG; and we are not aware of any report of this particular application of depth electrography by a reliable investigator. One should hardly need to emphasize this point, since seldom, if ever, do cases in question meet the above-described criteria for possible surgical treatment. It is, however, an important negative indication which deserves mentioning to caution against an irrational and ethically unjustified application of depth electrography.

Technique

It is not the purpose of this chapter to outline in detail the various technical aspects of electrode implantation for direct cortical and subcortical recording. Especially for an accurate stereotactic approach, sophisticated equipment and radiologic procedures are involved, and the reader should refer to appropriate publications (Bancaud et al, 1973, 1975; Talairach et al, 1974; Van Buren, 1965; Van Buren, Ajmone Marsan, and Mutsuga, 1975a; Leksell, 1957; Spiegel, Wycis, and Goode, 1956). Equipment and techniques are seldom standardized in fields which are highly specialized, and stereoelectroencephalography is no exception to this rule. Indeed, most teams of investigators favor the use of "homemade" apparatus which generally incorporates features of pre-existing models with a number of more or less important modifications. According to Van Buren (1965), an ideal stereotactic instrument should be designed in such a way as to: (a) be usable without the need of special X-ray equipment, (b) permit full head movement for fractional pneumography and full surgical draping, (c) permit graduated alignment of the stereotaxic planes to intracerebral axes and full three-planes graduated movement, (d) allow entry of the skull at any point without recomputation or use of phantom target points, (e) permit precise realignment for staged procedures.

The type of pick-up electrodes also varies among different investigators but the sets which are most commonly employed are obviously based on similar general principles. Some investigators use exclusively needle electrode sets with multiple contacts (usually 4 to 10), either rigid or, more frequently, flexible. Several of these (an average of 10 in the case material of Talairach et al, 1974) are generally introduced, by means of a stereotactically guided probe, into different cerebral structures toward predetermined targets. Other investigators combine the use of such depth electrode sets with several multicontact flap electrodes for simultaneous cortical surface recording (epidural or, exceptionally, subdural). In our experience, the latter type of superficial electrodes is particularly useful, and is actually better suited than the needle electrode, to monitor the electrical activity of certain cortical regions (such as the orbital surface or the mesial parasagittal and cingulate areas). The type of flap electrode used in our laboratory has three or four platinum-iridium contacts, at 1 cm intervals, embedded in segmented polyurethane (Lycra). These flaps are slipped into the epidural space with a probe inserted into a pocket on the dorsal surface of the flap to guide it under the calvarium. Except in the case of the abovementioned special cortical regions where an epidural position cannot be used, it is preferable to avoid the direct surface cortical placement, since this can produce hyperemia and a reaction of the cortex to the foreign material, and may thereby create a potentially epileptogenic lesion. In spite of some distortion and attenuation of the signals and their less precise localization, an extradural electrode set will still yield useful information that is far superior to that provided by scalp electrodes. It should be kept in mind, however, that extradural leads cannot be used for stimulation purposes: this represents their main limitation in comparison with subdural or needle electrodes.

There is no standard target for electrode implantation. Such targets are generally "customed-tailored" to each individual case, their selection being determined on the basis of both clinical seizure pattern(s) and the evidence obtained from scalp EEG data. This general rule applies particularly in the case of potentially epileptogenic processes presumably located above the Sylvian fissure. In cases of partial seizures with complex manifestations and probable involvement of temporal and pararhinencephalic structures, the targets are still individually selected but their location can be relatively stereotyped since one should always attempt to monitor at least the activity of both the temporal convexity and the hippocampal-amygdaloid complex. A large number of examples of multiple, different targets in a variety of temporal and extratemporal situations are illustrated in great detail in the two monographs by Bancaud et al (1973) and Talairach et al (1974), which should be consulted by any interested reader.

The number of electrode sets and actual electrode contacts to be used for a reliable topographic localization of an epileptogenic process, and for its delimitation, is also variable and depends on the specific problem presented by the individual case under investigation. In theory, the larger the number of leads, the greater the amount of useful information that would be obtained, not only about location and limits of the "focus" but also about the structures which are secondarily involved in the multidirectional spread of the ictal discharge. In practice, however, there are obvious limitations since the number of needle insertions—and related lesional tracks—should be kept to a minimum within cerebral tissue which will not be excised. Although the study of "normal" formations which might be progressively invaded by seizure activity originating elsewhere may be of considerable scientific interest, it contributes little to the decision on the main surgical target. Perhaps even more important than these ethical considerations are the practical limitations dictated by the nature of the electrical phenomenon under study, its anatomophysiologic substrate and the size of electrodes used. Any given EEG signal which is recorded by electrodes with a relatively large area of contact (i.e. by macro- rather than micro-electrodes), reflects the summated activity of neuronal aggregates. The number and extension of these aggregates and the degree of synchronization of their activities will determine the amplitude of the signal. In practice, a detectable signal involves a minimum of several cubic millimeters of cerebral tissue and, even when discretely localized in its origin, volume conduction phenomena can often cause it to appear up to several centimeters away, with identical characteristic of form and even amplitude. In view of this situation it is obvious that there is a limit beyond which an increase in the number of closely spaced electrode contacts will not provide any additional information (Fig. 5.1).

The above considerations are primarily dictated by the necessity of minimizing the risk of complications inherent in the procedure. In fact, potential complications, such as hemorrhages, have been rather rare (three intracerebral hematomata in 560 patients according to Talairach et al, 1974, and one subdural hematoma in our series of about 100 patients). No cases of infection had been reported in the past, but Bernoulli et al (1977) have recently published in a letter to the editor of Lancet their unfortunate experience of transmission of Creutzfeldt-Jakob disease in two epileptic patients—2½ years after depth electrographic exploration performed with silver electrodes that had been previously (respectively about 2 and 3 months) implanted in a patient with that disease.

Recording methods are essentially similar to those employed in conventional scalp EEG. Montages are preferentially bipolar although referential runs, using for instance the contralateral ear or a noncephalic lead such as a neck band, provide rather good localization information. The main differences in recording technique are represented by the much larger number of input leads in depth electrography and the consequent greater amount of data derived from different sources within the brain. Since it is always preferable to record simultaneously from these numerous inputs, one should use recording equipment with a large number of channels (at least 16 and preferably more). In practice, however, it remains rather difficult to obtain a simultaneous record from some 50 to 100 electrode contacts and a compromise becomes necessary. In such cases one generally surveys the activity from all these electrodes in separate steps in the first two or three recording sessions and then limits the monitoring to those regions which appear to yield epileptiform activity most consistently, in the subsequent sessions. This survey can be facilitated by the use of a special master switch which permits a quick selection and change of montages simultaneously from 16 or more of the available leads, or to shift from recording to stimulation on any electrode pair (Bancaud et al, 1975). It should also be kept in mind that, whereas oscilloscopic recording has little practical application in scalp EEG, it can provide useful information in depth electrography, often making it possible to distinguish the original from the projected event between two apparently synchronous phenomena.

As mentioned above, one of the main purposes of recording from chronically implanted electrodes in epileptic patients is to observe and monitor the electrical development of at least one, and preferably several, spontaneous seizures. For this reason long recording sessions should be planned. Radiotelemetry, possibly combined with a closed circuit videotape monitoring of the patient's ictal pattern, is a useful adjunct in this situation (see "Intensive Monitoring" in Penry, 1977). The chances to record an ictal episode in the course of such sessions remain, however, rather small and in a certain number of patients none will occur spontaneously. In such cases the advisability of inducing a seizure, either by local electrical stimulation or by systemic administration of a convulsant agent, can be considered. Neither of these two techniques, however, is totally satisfactory, and the interpretation of their effects requires particular caution. In the case of pharmacologic activation (e.g. by intravenous injection of pentylenetetrazol or of Megimide), the main interpretation problem arises from the nonspecific phenomena which are commonly induced by the drug (Ajmone Marsan and Ralston, 1957) and the necessity of distinguishing them from the possible (but unfortunately much less frequent) specific activation of a pre-existing epileptogenic process. This task is relatively easy in the case of scalp EEG where the electrographic survey covers wide areas of both cerebral hemispheres—a situation which permits the immediate recognition of the diffuse and bilaterally synchronous events characteristic of those effects which are considered as nonspecific. On the other hand, the correct identification of such events may be rather difficult when recording with implanted electrodes since, in spite of a large number of contacts, the total area surveyed often corresponds to a limited portion of one hemisphere or to a single lobe. It is, of course, possible to improve this situation by sacrificing some potentially important sites and extending the number of homologous regions surveyed on both hemispheres in the same montage and/or by combining the recording from implanted leads with the simultaneous scalp recording from other cortical areas which are not involved in depth electrography, whenever such a pharmacologic activation is planned (Ajmone Marsan and Abraham, 1960). But in spite of these obvious precautions, the interpretation of its electrographic effects will still present some difficulty, especially when the activation procedure fails to reproduce a clinical ictal pattern suggestively similiar to those occurring spontaneously in the same subject.

In the diagnostic investigation of epileptic patients, electrical stimulation is generally performed through pairs of electrode contacts for the main purpose of reproducing an aura and/or inducing an electroclinical ictal pattern. The occasional occurrence of an electrical after-discharge localized at the point of stimulation has little diagnostic value since this generally reflects an intrinsically low excitation threshold of a given neuronal population rather than being a true sign of local epileptogenicity. Stimulation parameters consist of brief trains of 0.5 to 5 msec square pulses at 40 to 60 Hz. Duration of the train (2 to 10 seconds) and intensity of individual pulses (2 to 10 mA) should be adjusted to individual cases and specific structures, preferably beginning with subthreshold intensity and progressively increasing it until the required effect is obtained (Ajmone Marsan, 1972; Ajmone Marsan and O'Connor, 1973). Results of local electrical stimulation should be interpreted with caution and, for a reliable localization of a presumed "focus," they should be easily reproducible. This technique has been employed with apparent success by Bancaud and collaborators, and a number of illustrative examples of its possibilities are available in their above mentioned monographs (see also Bancaud et al, 1966).

The same technique of local electrical stimulation may be occasionally used—with slightly different parameters (lower intensity and shorter pulse duration)—to confirm the electrode location and to identify the structure involved by eliciting appropriate physiologic (generally local motor or sensory) responses characteristic of that structure.

Information That Can Be Derived From Implanted Electrodes

A systematization of findings provided by this technique is obviously not possible since each implantation is designed for a specific problem and the number of electrode contacts and type of structures surveyed vary according to the problem under investigation. Moreover, since it is almost exclusively the most complex and atypical cases which are investigated with implanted electrodes, eventual conclusions on the pathophysiologic nature of the underlying disorder remain exquisitely individual and are only applicable to the case in question. Thus, the use of depth electrography seldom permits conclusive generalizations to be reached concerning particular aspects of the seizure disorders, and we consider at least premature any suggestion of nosologic subclassifications of the epilepsies on the basis of anatomoelectrographic criteria derived exclusively from such a technique. It is worth noting that an attempt in this direction by Bancaud et al in their early study (1965) was eventually abandoned in their later contribution (1973).

As a rule the records obtained from implanted electrodes are totally free of artifacts (especially of those which are commonly present in scalp EEG, such as EMG and oculogram), and the recognition of typical epileptiform activity presents no problem (see below). The interpretation of other, nonparoxysmal patterns, such as slow rhythms or transients, depression of activity, and asymmetries, is somewhat less reliable and the pathologic significance of such patterns is often open to question. For instance, it is not uncommon to observe a large amount of slow waves from some of the implanted leads, especially in records obtained early, in the first few days after implantation, but this slow activity tends to decrease or totally disappear in later records. Even though, strictly speaking, such an activity is "abnormal," it simply reflects transitory pathologic changes probably related to the trauma of electrode insertion and has no direct bearing on the possible presence of true structural pathology. Since traumatic and lesional factors, albeit modest (Angeleri, Ferro Milone, and Parigi, 1964; Dodge et al, 1955; Rand, Crandall, and Walter, 1964), are always associated with the procedure of electrode implantation, the correct evaluation of slow activity, which is almost always appreciable in greater or lesser amounts and variable amplitude at some of the leads, is generally difficult and requires great caution (Walter, 1973). A number of examples which, in our opinion, confirm this point, are illustrated in the monograph by Bancaud et al (1973). This includes a series of cases with cerebral expanding lesions investigated by depth electrography and in which the presence of polymorphic delta and other slow rhythms is utilized for the delimitation of the tumor. Several of such examples (e.g. case De.D., Fig. 64, and case Ca.A., Fig. 90 in Bancaud et al, 1973) also show that some "slow" waves probably are, in reality, the reflection of projected or larval epileptiform discharges (see also Figs. 5.2, 5.3, 5.4, 5.5).

Another finding, the interpretation of which also requires the greatest caution, is the local depression of activity or so-called "electrical silence." It has long been recognized that brain tumors, in themselves, are electrically inactive (Foerster and Altenburger, 1935; Scarff and Rahm, 1941); thus, one would expect to see a flat record when both electrodes are placed on tumoral surface (while the characteristic irregular delta activity would arise from altered neuronal elements within cerebral tissue at the periphery of the expanding lesion). A true localized electrical silence is seldom observed in scalp EEG where volume conduction of the activity from surrounding regions tends to mask the local depression. On the other hand, needle electrodes, with closely spaced contacts, inserted within the tumoral mass, appear ideal to detect such a depression. This is in fact the case, as illustrated in Figure 5.6 and in several convincing examples in the monograph by Bancaud et al (1973). But, as these authors themselves point out, it would be dangerous to accept the finding of a localized electrical silence as definite evidence of tumor. In fact, it is fair to say that in the majority of cases such a finding is probably meaningless, especially when derived from a pair of closely spaced (0.5 to 1 cm) leads. Equipotentiality of the two equally active contacts results in a flat record, and the same is seen when both leads are within the white matter or in one ventricle, and whenever they are shunted by surrounding fluid. Modification of montages and different couplings of the suspected lead(s), as well as the combined use of referential electrodes generally help in the correct interpretation of such a finding. But the fact remains that too many spurious factors can play a role in its appearance and weaken its practical significance as a useful diagnostic sign.

Whereas depth electrography seems to be a valuable tool in the investigation of intracranial expanding lesions in the hands of Bancaud et al (1973), all other investigators agree that the main, if not exclusive, field of application of this technique is the field of seizure disorders. As mentioned before, the electrographic correlates of such disorders are easily identifiable. Furthermore, these characteristic paroxysmal patterns are almost exclusively observed in epileptic patients. It is obviously impossible to rule out their occasional occurrence in other conditions, but our experience in this regard is based on the comparison of electrographic findings in patients affected by seizure disorders with those obtained in a relatively large group of patients with various types of involuntary movements in which depth electrodes had been implanted stereotactically to produce electrolytic lesions within certain thalamic nuclei. In this latter group of cases, recording from multiple contacts prior to the passage of coagulating current never showed a pattern which could be defined as "epileptiform." Similarly negative in this respect—at least in our opinion— are the scattered reports of depth recording in different psychiatric patients. Thus, the various types of interictal patterns can be safely considered pathognomonic, but they still need to be correctly interpreted to provide a reliable identification and outline of the main epileptogenic process. This task is often complicated since one is faced with an excess of abnormal discharges with variable and multiple locations (Fig. 5.1).

As already mentioned, the patients selected for investigation with this technique generally present very complex problems, their seizure disorder often resulting from multiple, independent epileptogenic processes. In this situation such multiplicity of foci is commonly confirmed and it is not always possible to identify a primary focus; as a consequence, therapeutic conduct will be dictated by other considerations or the idea of surgery may be completely abandoned. In other cases it is instead possible to demonstrate a site of clearly predominant abnormalities. The criteria for this demonstration are somewhat empirical and should be based on both interictal and ictal phenomena. As stated before, the majority of investigators attribute the greatest significance to the latter, and some (Bancaud et al, 1973; Walter, 1973) are of the opinion that only those findings which are obtained during the occurrence of a spontaneous clinical seizure are sufficiently reliable to permit the identification of the site of origin of the seizure itself. For this reason it is suggested (Walter, 1973) that at least three (preferably spontaneous) ictal episodes in every subject be monitored and analyzed in their electrographic manifestations before reaching a decision on the localization and lateralization of the epileptogenic process, and Bancaud et al (1973) claim to have studied over 10,000 of such ictal episodes in about 400 patients. Other investigators (Rossi, 1973) attribute comparable significance to the information derived from both ictal and interictal events and, in our experience, it would be a mistake to totally ignore the latter. Of interest in this regard is one of the cases reported by Rossi (1973). In his Case 4, focal ictal activity was observed to arise from the right temporal lobe, the left temporal lobe, and the frontal regions respectively in the course of three different seizures (Metrazol-induced), whereas the interictal activity was consistently predominant in the right temporal region (Ammon's horn). Because of the multifocal characteristics of the electrographic seizure patterns, surgery was not

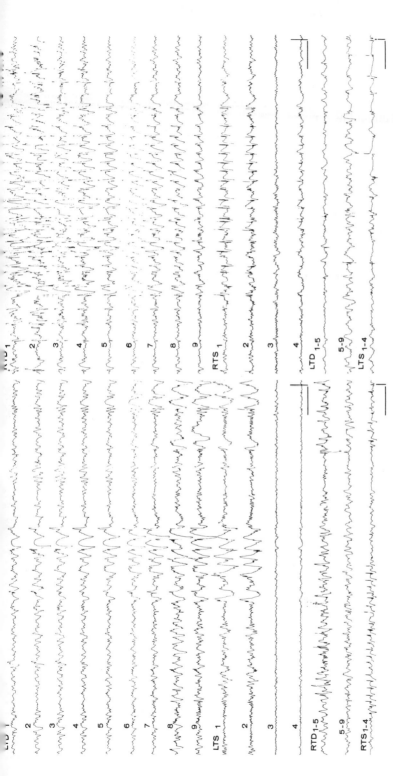

Fig. 5.1. Electrodes implanted bilaterally on and within the temporal regions. On each side there is one 9-contact needle electrode set (LTD and RTD) and one 4-contact flap electrode set (LTS and RTS). The flap electrodes are over the second temporal convolution with contact 1 about 1 cm from the tip of the temporal fossa, and contact 4 about 4 cm from it. Contacts for the two needles are: 1,2,3: amygdala; 4,5: deep temporal white; 6,7: mid-temporal white; 8,9: superficial temporal white (T2). The placements are fairly symmetrical. Recording is partly bipolar (bottom 3 channels) and partly in reference to the ipsilateral ear (top 13 channels). (Two different montages are shown.) See Fig. 5.2. for further details. Calibrations: 2 sec.; 200 μV.

considered indicated and the patient was discharged. A few months later, she was readmitted comatose following prolonged status epilepticus and died within a few hours. An autopsy demonstrated a large and old lesion within the tip of the right temporal lobe, i.e. in the same region as the maximal *interictal* discharges. It should also be kept in mind that although an ictal episode can be characterized by exquisitely focal features, it often tends to involve different structures in a quasi-simultaneous way. In such cases the identification of its site of origin is not always easy and may require sophisticated techniques (see Brazier, 1973; Brazier and Crandall, 1978). Fortunately, in the majority of cases there seems to be a fairly good agreement between the localization suggested by interictal phenomena and that derived from ictal episodes (see Case 3 of Rossi, 1973; also Figs. 5.3 and 5.6) and, as already stated, it is only when the two sets of data are in conflict that one should attribute greater significance to the latter.

The morphologic characteristics of the various types of interictal patterns are essentially similar to those described in scalp EEG and corticography (Penfield and Jasper, 1954) with the expected differences in amplitude (much greater) and duration (often very short in typical spikes). Numerous examples of such patterns are displayed in the specialized monographs mentioned earlier, as well as in previous publications (Ajmone Marsan and Van Buren, 1958; Ajmone Marsan and Abraham, 1966) and a few are illustrated here: rhythmic spike and wave complexes which generally predominate in records from the cortical surface or from the most superficial contacts of the needle electrodes (Figs. 5.1 and 5.6); relatively small amplitude, rhythmically recurring spikes (Figs. 5.1, 5.2, and 5.4); multiphasic sharp waves, isolated or in rhythmic trains of variable duration (Figs. 5.1, 5.2, 5.3, 5.6 and 5.7); and typical, large amplitude, very brief duration spikes (Figs. 5.2 and 5.5).

The criteria for evaluating the localizing significance of these various interictal patterns are also similar, in principle, to those utilized in scalp EEG and remain rather empirical in both situations. It is especially the presence of multiple discharges of different morphology and different or variable localization that adds to the complexity of the problem and to the difficulty of interpretation. In some of these cases, the temporal relationship of one to other related discharges (earlier), its relative amplitude (greater), and its duration (briefer) should be reasonably interpreted to indicate that the discharge in question is probably the closest one to the presumed epileptogenic process. In other cases, where there is no temporal or morphologic relationship between two or several interictal phenomena which arise independently from different structures, the relative localizing significance of individual discharges can be reliably evaluated according to criteria similar to those outlined by Rossi (1973). These emphasize the following points: (a) "intensity" of interictal discharges, i.e. their rate and amount; (b) their regularity or stability; and (c) the pattern and characteristics of the background from which they arise. Concerning the first point, it is commonly recognized that the structure (or side) in which the interictal discharges are most numerous is more likely to be the site of the main epileptogenic process. The above-quoted Case 4 of Rossi appears to be a con-

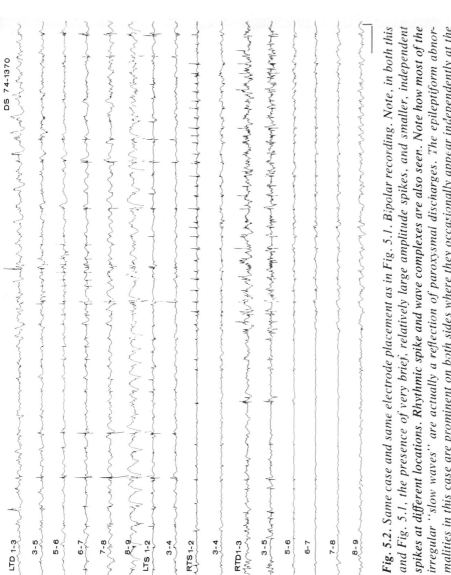

DS 74-1370

LTD 1-3
3-5
5-6
6-7
7-8
8-9
LTS 1-2
3-4
RTS 1-2
3-4
RTD 1-3
3-5
5-6
6-7
7-8
8-9

Fig. 5.2. Same case and same electrode placement as in Fig. 5.1. Bipolar recording. Note, in both this and Fig. 5.1, the presence of very brief, relatively large amplitude spikes, and smaller, independent spikes at different locations. Rhythmic spike and wave complexes are also seen. Note how most of the irregular "slow waves" are actually a reflection of paroxysmal discharges. The epileptiform abnormalities in this case are prominent on both sides where they occasionally appear independently at the cortical and subcortical levels (especially on the left). Calibrations: 2 sec.; 200 μV.

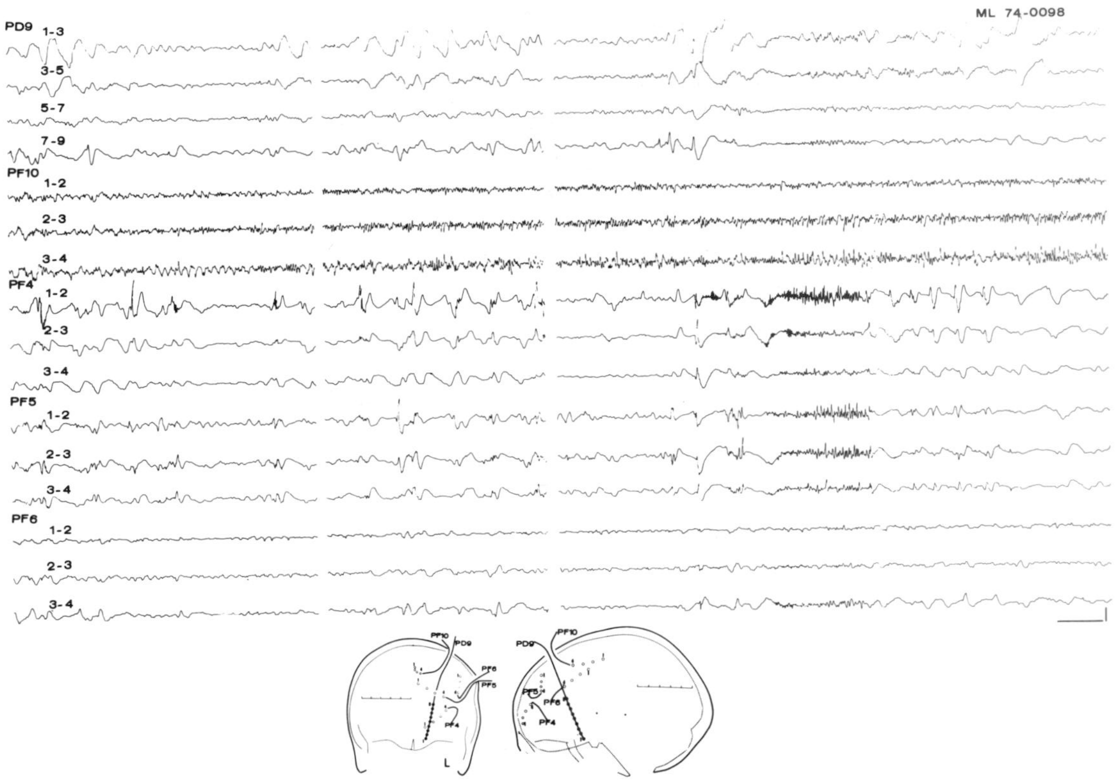

Fig. 5.3. Electrodes implanted on the left side only, on and within the frontal lobe. There are 4 flap electrode sets (PF4, PF5, PF6, PF10) with 4 contacts each and 1 needle (PD9) with 9 contacts. Placements of these electrodes as indicated at the bottom of the illustration. Recording is bipolar. Maximal interictal epileptiform activity is seen over the lateral frontal surface (PF4 and PF5) and a brief subclinical ictal episode displays a similar distribution. Calibrations: 1 sec., 200 μV.

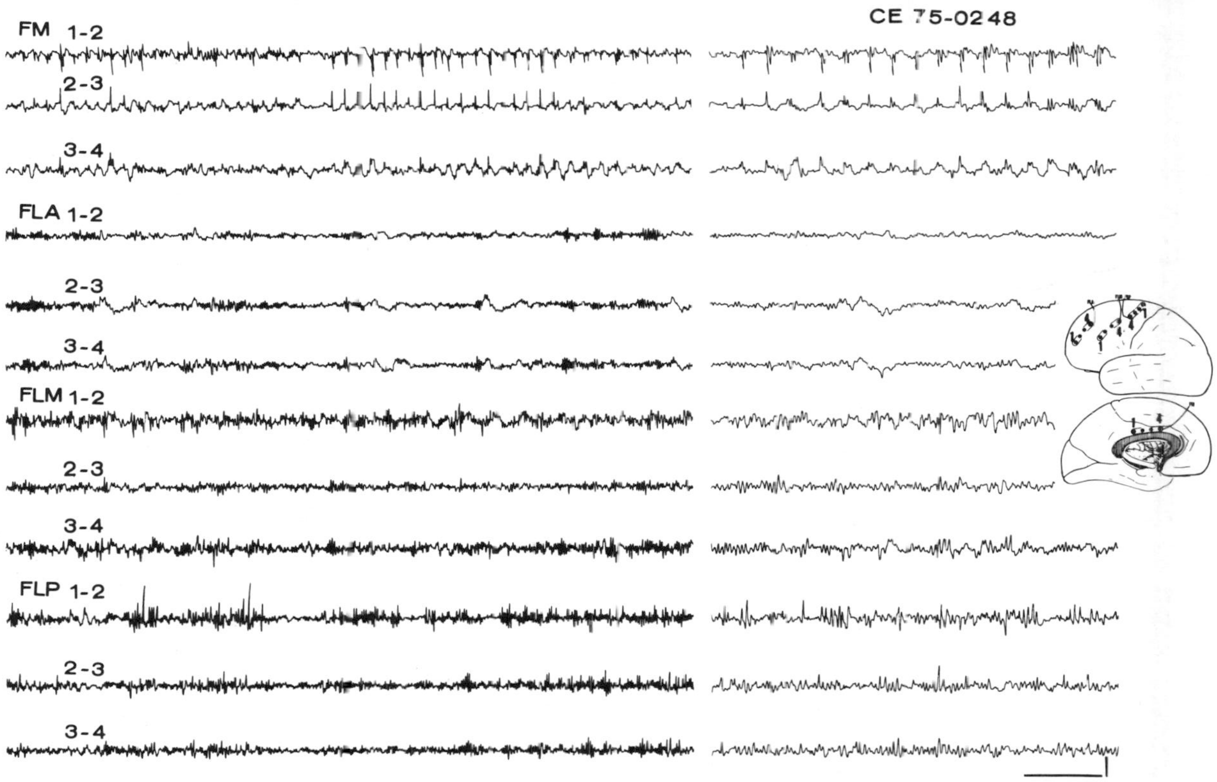

Fig. 5.4. Electrodes implanted on the left side only, on the cingulate cortex (FM) and lateral (FLA, FLM, FLP) frontal cortex. Each flap has 4 contacts as indicated on the brain map. Rhythmically recurring, small amplitude spikes are present exclusively in the mesial cortex. Normal activity is seen from the other leads. Bipolar recording. Calibrations: 2 sec. (left tracing) and 1 sec. (right tracing); 100 μV.

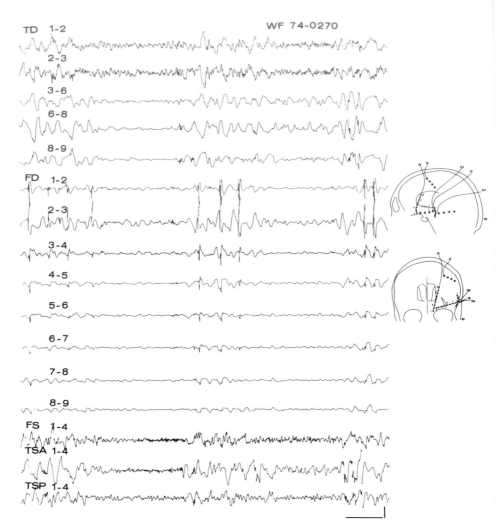

Fig. 5.5. *Electrodes implanted on the left side only, on and within frontal and temporal structures. There are 3 flaps (with 4 contacts each), two on the third temporal gyrus (TSA, TSP) and one on the frontal cortex (FS) as indicated on the schematic drawing. Of the two needles electrodes with 9 contacts each, one (FD) is directed toward the frontal orbital cortex and overlying white (contacts 1,2), passing through the lower margin of the lateral projections of the genu of corpus callosum (3), the frontal white anterior to head of caudate (4,5,6) and deep and mid frontal white matter (7,8,9). The other (TD) is directed to lateral amygdala and ventricle (contacts 1,2) through temporal white (3–9). Bipolar recording. Note large amplitude, spikes, and spike and wave complexes primarily localized in proximity to the frontal orbital surface. Calibrations: 2 sec.; 200 μV.*

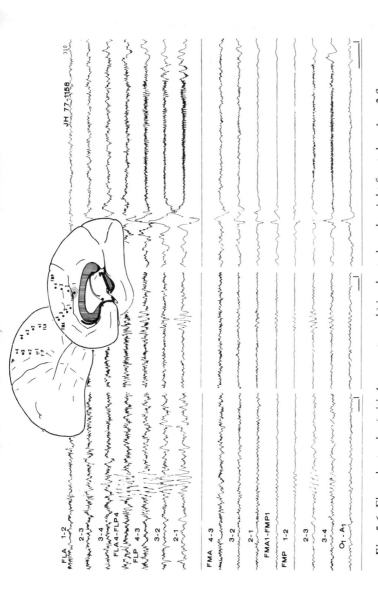

Fig. 5.6. *Flap electrodes (with 4 contacts each) implanted on the right frontal region: 2 flaps are on the lateral surface (FLA, FLP) and 2 on the mesial surface (FMA, FMP) as outlined in the schematic brain map. A lesion was found at operation (astrocytoma) at the junction of the mesial frontal and cingulate regions (grey area close to contacts FMA 1 and FMP 1). Bottom channel is from scalp EEG. Bipolar recording. Note depression of activity from the electrodes which are presumably overlying the small tumor. Interictal and ictal epileptiform activity arises from the same electrode pairs (FLP and contacts 3,4 of FMP). Calibrations: 1 sec.; 200 μV.*

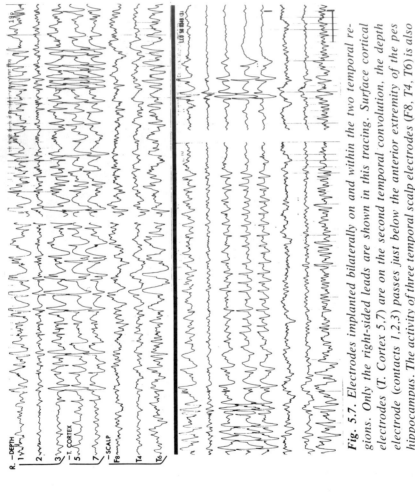

Fig. 5.7. *Electrodes implanted bilaterally on and within the two temporal regions. Only the right-sided leads are shown in this tracing. Surface cortical electrodes (T. Cortex 5,7) are on the second temporal convolution, the depth electrode (contacts 1,2,3) passes just below the anterior extremity of the pes hippocampus. The activity of three temporal scalp electrodes (F8, T4, T6) is also shown. Recording is "monopolar" with reference to a neck band electrode. Note large amount of rhythmically recurring biphasic sharp waves from implanted leads, maximally from temporal cortex. Also note how most of these discharges fail to appear at the scalp level. Calibrations: 1 sec.; 50 µV (scalp) and 100 µV (implanted electrodes).*

vincing example in support of this point of view (although exceptions to it are not uncommon). In relation to the second point, Rossi is probably the first investigator to draw attention to the rather interesting observation that the interictal discharges which are generated in close proximity to the epileptogenic zone tend to fire with a certain regularity and stability, independently of the patient's condition or other factors. For instance, the firing pattern of the "primary" discharges does not seem to be significantly influenced by—and remains quite active during—wakefulness, slow wave sleep, or even REM sleep, whereas the discharges in other structures (presumably not directly involved in the epileptogenic process) may be totally absent during waking and REM sleep states to become activated mainly during stage 2 sleep (Fig. 12 in Rossi, 1973). In analogy to these findings, anticonvulsant medication would tend to affect the primary discharges less than those recorded from other parts of the brain (Fig. 13 in Rossi, 1973). The third point refers to the possible significance of slow (nonepileptiform) activity already discussed in the first part of this section. Keeping in mind the often questionable nature of this activity, its continous occurrence at the site of maximal interictal discharges may occasionally represent a valuable confirmatory sign for the presence of a lesion (Bancaud et al, 1973; Walter, 1973).

On the basis of these criteria, it is thus generally possible to reach a reasonably reliable conclusion on the most likely site of the main epileptogenic focus, but—as repeatedly pointed out—this should always be confirmed by the observation of at least one, and preferably several, clinical seizures and the determination of the site of origin of their electrographic correlates. Occasionally a rhythmically organized ictal discharge is seen either in the absence of any obvious clinical sign or in relationship to some subjective sensations (aura) which do not proceed to a fully developed seizure (Figs. 5.3 and 5.6.) It seems reasonable to attribute to such episodes a localizing significance comparable to that of those which are associated with clinical manifestations. A large number of examples of seizure patterns from various cortical and subcortical regions are illustrated in the monographs of Bancaud et al (1965 and 1973); most of these examples are provided with a detailed description of the specific case and clinical problem under investigation and these data should be directly consulted.

Conclusions

In this brief compendium on depth electrography, we have attempted to emphasize the main indications and contraindications for this technique, and have outlined its most important possibilities and limitations. We have repeatedly referred the reader to illustrative examples included in various specialized and detailed publications, since the nature of the procedure and the complexity and variability of its results do not lend themselves to generalizations or systematizations but are better understood through an iconographic display of different individual situations.

A correct and totally satisfactory interpretation of the data provided by the procedure can be very difficult. However, from a practical point of view, useful information on diagnostic localization is often obtained in individual cases, thus helping the neurosurgeon in his decision on whether to proceed with the operation and on which structure(s) to excise. On the other hand, very few problems of a physiopathogenetic nature in the field of seizure disorders are likely to be solved by this technique and, in this respect, our impression remains essentially similar to that expressed 20 years ago (Ajmone Marsan and Van Buren, 1958) on the basis of a much more limited experience. In most situations to which depth electrography is applied, the data provided by this procedure not only tend to confirm the complexity of the problem but will probably demonstrate that this is in reality greater than one might have originally suspected.

ELECTROCORTICOGRAPHY

Electrocorticography (ECoG) is the term used in reference to the electrophysiologic technique of recording directly from the cortex. Although this term applies to both humans and experimental animals and to both acute and chronic conditions, this section deals exclusively with the clinical applications of the technique under acute conditions, in the course of surgical exposure of the human cortex. As we have already seen in the preceding section on depth electrography, direct cortical recording also represents an important part of that neurophysiologic technique and provides useful information, though of a somewhat different nature, and in an obviously different situation.

Applications and Limitations

The most common, and practically the exclusive, field of application of ECoG is in seizure disorders and specifically in those patients who have been selected for surgical treatment of medically intractable partial seizures. The main purpose of this technique is: (a) to confirm and outline the actual site and extent of the epileptogenic process which had been diagnosed and provisionally localized by means of clinical, radiologic, scalp EEG and, often, depth electrographic criteria in the preoperative workup of the case; and (b) to check for the persistence of potentially epileptogenic tissue after the excision of the main focus.

In spite of the fact that ECoG can be now considered a routine procedure, it is carried out almost exclusively in the few centers specializing in the surgical treatment of seizure disorders. Since the early 1950's, when the technique began to be widely employed and was eventually perfected by Penfield and Jasper at the Montreal Neurological Institute, there has been relatively little change in its methodology, in the indications for its use, or in general aspects of its interpretation. For this reason it is not necessary to repeat in this chapter the historical background and the various major technical and interpretative details which are available in the literature and to which the reader is referred (Penfield and Jasper, 1954; Ajmone Marsan and O'Connor, 1973). Instead, attention will be directed here to the general aspects of this procedure and to a discussion of some of its more specific points.

Although both scalp EEG and ECoG record essentially the same phenomena, there are obvious differences inherent in the two techniques and, consequently, in the type of data that they provide. Thus, the extent of the electrographic survey is always necessarily limited by the size of the exposed area in ECoG, whereas in scalp EEG most of the lateral surface of both hemispheres can be monitored simultaneously. In analogy to the similar situation already discussed in depth electrography, this obvious fact should always be kept in mind when interpreting ECoG findings since any apparently "focal" electrographic event on the basis of this technique could actually be bilateral and/or involve other regions which are outside the exposed cortical surface. Possible misinterpretations in relation to this situation are not uncommon, in the course of "activating" procedures of a systemic nature such as hyperventilation or intravenous injections of Metrazol. These procedures can induce changes which are easily recognizable as nonspecific in scalp EEG because of their bilateral distribution, but may appear as "local" if all the electrodes are concentrated within a relatively restricted area of one hemisphere as in ECoG. On the other hand, with the latter procedure, the characteristic patterns of the recorded electrical phenomena are not distorted or attenuated by the interposition of inert tissue as is invariably the case in scalp EEG. This is especially true for the discretely localized, short duration, spike-like events characteristic of an epileptogenic process which often may be totally unappreciable at the scalp level (Abraham and Ajmone Marsan, 1958). It is also true for many types of ictal patterns, particularly those characterized by relatively low voltage rhythmic activity restricted to a small area. Other differences between the two procedures reflect the obviously different conditions in which the records are obtained (patient relaxed and comfortable in the EEG laboratory, while in a stressful situation and often under the effects of several drugs in the operating room), or the different nature and general purpose of the examination in the two situations.

Scalp EEG is generally a non-emergency diagnostic procedure which, especially in seizure disorders, may require repeated examinations to confirm questionable findings and is susceptible to discussion, consultations, and provisional (i.e. modifiable) opinions before the electroencephalographer reaches what can be considered the final interpretation leading to the classification of the case under investigation. In the surgical room, on the other hand, time is a very important factor and ECoG becomes an emergency procedure which requires an immediate and definitive interpretation with consequences which are often irreversible, since it will influence and guide the decision of the neurosurgeon.

The specific purpose of ECoG in the surgical treatment of seizure disorders has been briefly mentioned above. The usefulness of this procedure stems in part from the limitations of scalp EEG and its inadequacy in providing a truly accurate localization of the epileptogenic process. With the latter technique, and in the most favorable situations, it is generally only possible to circumscribe the presumed site of origin of any "focal" electrographic phonomenon, either interictal or ictal, to a cortical area of at least several square centimeters. In most cases crucial differences in topography, such as the separation between pre- and postcentral region or between supra- and infrasylvian areas, cannot be reliably provided by scalp EEG or by the relatively "blind" procedure of depth electrography. On the other hand, the placement of electrodes on the cortical surface under direct visual inspection enables one to pinpoint the exact location of epileptiform discharges within a few square millimeters of cortical tissue. But besides yielding a much more accurate localization of the electrical manifestations of a presumed epileptogenic process, ECoG plays an important role in determining the neurosurgical decision and in the overall subsequent surgical conduct. This point deserves some elaboration.

A well-known characteristic feature of epileptiform phenomena is their random, somewhat capricious appearance. In the routine preoperative workup of any individual case, such phenomena may be quite numerous in one or several EEG's but may often be totally absent in other EEG's, even in the course of protracted recording sessions. Thus, it is not surprising that they may also be absent during the ECoG examination, especially since the subject is often heavily sedated and/or under obvious stress, and the recording cannot be extended for too long, seldom exceeding one hour. Such a situation is fortunately not too common, but whenever it occurs, and if the negative findings persist despite achieving better relaxation of the subject and the use of some mild activating procedure, the neurosurgeon is faced with a difficult decision. The main point to keep in mind is that if one decides to proceed with the excision (on the basis of clinical and preoperative scalp EEG findings), there will be no reliable way to control for its completeness in the immediate postexcision record, inasmuch as the absence of epileptiform potentials in the remaining cortical tissue will simply reflect the general lack of such activity already noted in the pre-excision tracing. For this reason it has been the general practice in our Institute to postpone the main excision in such cases in which ECoG fails to demonstrate the presence of clearly epileptiform abnormalities, and to reschedule the operation after a few days' delay. This practice, in our opinion, should be followed in all similar situations, and it is definitely indicated when the neurosurgical procedure depends on the accurate detection of focal "active" pathology for the treatment of seizure disorders originating from cortical regions *outside* the temporal lobe.

In the case of temporal lobe epilepsy, the situation is somewhat different. This type of epilepsy, at variance from other forms of partial seizures in which the epileptogenic process is commonly localized at the cortical level, may originate from any portion of the pararhinencephalic system within the depth of the temporal lobe, beside involving the cortex of its three main convolutions. Actually, a purely cortical epileptogenic lesion is rather exceptional in this form of epilepsy, even when its characteristic electrographic manifestations appear to be very prominent at the temporal cortex level. Furthermore, in relation to its surgical treatment, an extensive experience has shown that partial, selective ablations of discrete cortical regions or of small portions of the lobe seldom produce satisfactory results, even in those situations in which both pathologic and electrographic evidence is suggestively indicative of a discrete focus at the temporal surface or within one of its deep structures. As already mentioned in the preceding section, there is at the present time a rather general agreement that the best therapeutic results are obtained with a partial lobectomy, i.e. with a more or less standard excision of the anterior two-thirds of the involved temporal lobe (up to about 9 cm from its tip—or less if in the dominant hemisphere—and including its mesial deep structures). In view of this situation there are certain neurosurgeons, and in particular Falconer (1958), who feel that this excision can be carried out without any need for ECoG control and simply on the basis of preoperative scalp EEG studies. The problem with this "blind" approach is the impossibility to check for coexisting extratemporal, potentially epileptogenic abnormalities, to evaluate the extent of the epileptogenic process, especially toward the posterior portions of the temporal lobe and, more important, to confirm the completeness of excision. Residual tissue yielding paroxysmal activity is commonly present at the borders of the main, standard temporal ablation and if these regions of "electrically" abnormal tissue are left in place, a therapeutic failure will often result. In fact, it is our experience (Ajmone Marsan and Baldwin, 1958; Van Buren et al, 1975b) that a recurrence of seizures after temporal excision is due, in the large majority of cases, to persisting epileptiform abnormalities in areas adjacent to the main excision rather than to the presence of an independent epileptogenic process in the opposite temporal lobe.

Normal and Abnormal Activities in ECoG

These activities are essentially the same as in scalp EEG and only the difference in the two recording situations may present some problems as to their individualization and correct interpretation. The characteristic distribution of normal rhythms over the scalp of the two cerebral hemispheres is not immediately evident in ECoG where all the recording electrodes are crowded over a relatively small area of one hemisphere and generally monitor the activity of a few gyri or portions of one lobe. In this situation, however, the normal background rhythms during (relaxed) wakefulness will tend to reflect the specific region(s) under investigation in a much clearer way than with scalp EEG. If the exposure involves the cortex of parieto-occipital or posterior temporal areas the dominant rhythms of these regions will consist of characteristic regular patterns in the alpha frequency range. Typical activity noted around the Rolandic fissure, and especially in the motor and premotor areas, is in the beta frequency range. The prominence of this fast activity and the sharp demarcation of its distribution may be so striking as to permit the identification and outline of anatomic functional regions. For instance, the distinction between first temporal convolution and the lower portions of the precentral gyrus is often possible and topographic distribution of beta rhytms is not infrequently a more reliable criterion than the simple visual inspection for the identification of supra versus infrasylvian regions since this characteristic fast activity is not present on the temporal convolutions. It should be pointed out, however, that this is true only in relation to the "physiologic" beta activity. Activities in the same general frequency range which are induced by various drugs (barbiturates, Diazepam, etc.), have a rather diffuse distribution and actually the electrographic individual characteristics of the different cortical regions tend to be attenuated or are totally lost under the effect of such drugs.

Alpha and beta activities in the ECoG of relaxed, awake patients, and in the absence of obvious medication or anesthesia effects, are considered to be normal rhythms. But in the practical application of ECoG and its interpretation, the concept of "normality" versus "abnormality" is somewhat relative and the criteria for evaluating a record are different from those used in scalp EEG. Specifically, one should keep in mind the following points: (a) ECoG is seldom if ever performed on a "normal" brain. (b) Exposure of the cortex and its manipulations can, and often do, produce electrographic changes which are, strictly speaking, abnormal; yet they are simply an expression of contingent (acute traumatic or hypoxic) local factors rather than being indicative of a pre-existing pathologic process. (c) ECoG is performed not so much to determine whether the record is normal or abnormal but, as already mentioned, to confirm the presence of a previously established epileptogenic process, determine its accurate localization and circumscribe it within a given region of cerebral cortex, and, after excision of the main site of involvement, to check for possible persistence of potentially epileptogenic tissue. (d) The presence of abnormal electrographic patterns of a nonspecific nature (such as local slow waves or areas of amplitude depression), even when these are clearly associated with visible cortical pathology, is seldom a reliable indication of the actual site of the epileptogenic process. The latter, or at least its electrographic expression, is generally located at the periphery of the main lesion, within cortical tissue which might appear normal at visual inspection.

From what precedes it is obvious that the main emphasis in ECoG is the detection, identification, and localization of typical epileptiform discharges. As in the case of depth electrography the practical value of other nonspecific abnormalities is relatively small, and it is rather exceptional for cerebral tissue to be excised only on the basis of such electrographic phenomena. The type and characteristic features of epileptiform events are essentially similar to those described and illustrated in the preceding section on depth electrography. Also identical in the two situations is the problem which generally arises in the identification and distinction of interictal and ictal events and, more important, in the correct evaluation of their respective significance in the topographic diagnosis of the site of the epileptogenic process. The occurrence of an ictal activation, often accompanied by overt clinical manifestations, is less common in ECoG than in chronic depth electrography as might have been expected from the great differences in recording conditions and available recording time between the two situations. Actually, in the surgical room, with the brain exposed, one hopes to avoid such an occurrence because of the potential risks for the patient, especially if the seizure consists of violent automatic movements or of a generalized tonic-clonic convulsion. But occasionally a spontaneous ictal episode occurs during the ECoG examination and in such cases the electrographic changes and, specifically, their location provide a useful confirmation—or a correction—of the site of the epileptogenic process which had been presumed on the basis of interictal phenomena. Possible conflicts between the two sets of data are not as prominent as in scalp EEG or depth electrography in view of the relatively small area available for survey, and the correction of the original diagnosis is generally minor.

REFERENCES

Abraham, K. and Ajmone Marsan, C. (1958). Patterns of cortical discharges and their relation to routine scalp electroencephalography. Electroencephalogr. Clin. Neurophysiol., *10:*447.

Ajmone Marsan, C. (1972). Focal electrical stimulation. In: Experimental Models of Epilepsy, Purpura, D. P., Penry, J. K., Tower, D. B., Woodbury, D. M. and Walter, R. D., Eds., p. 147. Raven Press, New York.

Ajmone Marsan, C. and Abraham, K. (1960). A Seizure Atlas. Electroencephalogr. Clin. Neurophysiol., Suppl. 15.

Ajmone Marsan, C. and Abraham, L. (1966). Considerations on the use of chronically implanted electrodes in seizure disorders. Confin. Neurol., *27:*95.

Ajmone Marsan, C. and Baldwin, M. (1958). Electrocorticography. In: Temporal Lobe Epilepsy, Baldwin, M. and Bailey, P., Eds., p. 368. C. C. Thomas, Springfield, Ill.

Ajmone Marsan, C. and Goldhammer, L. (1973). Clinical ictal patterns and electrographic data in cases of partial seizures of frontal-central-parietal origin. In: Epilepsy: Its Phenomena in Man, Brazier, M.A.B., Ed., p. 236. Academic Press, New York.

Ajmone Marsan, C. and Laskowski, E. (1962). Callosal effects and excitability changes in the human epileptic cortex. Electroencephalogr. Clin. Neurophysiol., *14:*303.

Ajmone Marsan, C. and O'Connor, M. (1973). Electrocorticography. Handbook of Electroencephalography and Clinical Neurophysiology, Vol. 10 C, Ajmone Marsan, C., Ed. Elsevier, Amsterdam.

Ajmone Marsan, C. and Ralston, B. (1957). The Epileptic Seizure. Its Functional Morphology and Diagnostic Significance. C. C. Thomas, Springfield, Ill.

Ajmone Marsan, C. and Van Buren, J. (1958). Epileptiform activity in cortical and subcortical structures in the temporal lobe of man. In: Temporal Lobe Epilepsy, Baldwin, M. and Bailey, P., Eds., p. 78. C. C. Thomas, Springfield, Ill.

Angeleri, F., Ferro Milone, F. and Parigi, S. (1964). Electrical activity and reactivity of the rhinencephalic, pararhinencephalic and thalamic structures: prolonged implantation of electrodes in man. Electroencephalogr. Clin. Neurophysiol., *16:*100.

Bancaud, J., Albe-Fessard, D., Rayport, M. and Talairach, J. (1975). Stereoelectroencephalography In: Handbook of Electroencephalography and Clinical Neurophysiology, Vol. 10 B, Bancaud, J., Ed., p. 1. Elsevier, Amsterdam.

Bancaud, J., Talairach, J., Geier, S. and Scarabin, J. M. (1973). EEG et SEEG dans les Tumeurs Cérébrales et l'Epilepsie. Esifor, Paris.

Bancaud, J., Talairach, J., Morel, P., and Bresson, M. (1966) La corne d'Ammon et le noyau amygdalien: effects cliniques et éléctriques de leur stimulation chez l'homme. Rev. Neurol., *115:*329.

Bancaud, J., Talairach, J., Bonis, A., Schaub, G., Morel, P. and Bordas-Ferrer, M. (1965). La Stéréo-électroencéphalographie dans l'Epilepsie. Masson, Paris.

Bernoulli, C., Siegfried, J., Baumgartner, G., Regli, F., Rabinowicz, T., Gajdusek, D. C. and Gibbs, C. J. Jr. (1977). Danger of accidental person-to-person transmission of Creutzfeldt-Jakob disease by surgery. Lancet, *1:*478.

Brazier, M.A.B. (1973). Electrical seizure discharges within the human brain: the problem of spread. In: Epilepsy: Its Phenomena in Man, Brazier, M. A. B., Ed., p. 153. Academic Press, New York.

Brazier, M. A. B. and Crandall, P. H. (1978). Tests of predictive value of EEG recording from within the brain in the partial epilepsies. Electroencephalogr. Clin. Neurophysiol., Suppl. *34,* 83.

Crandall, P. H. (1973). Developments in direct recordings from epileptogenic regions in the surgical treatment of partial epilepsies. In: Epilepsy: Its Phenomena in Man, Brazier, M. A. B., Ed., p. 287. Academic Press, New York.

Crandall, P. H., Walter, R. D. and Rand, R. W. (1963). Clinical applications of studies on stereotactically implanted electrodes in temporal lobe epilepsy. J. Neurosurg., *20:*827.

Dodge, H. W. Jr., Petersen, M. C., Sem-Jacobsen, C. W., Sayre, G. P. and Bickford, R. G. (1955). The paucity of demonstrable brain damage following intracerebral electrography: Report of the case. Proc. Staff Meet. Mayo Clinic, *30:*215.

Falconer, M. A. (1958). Discussion. In: Temporal Lobe Epilepsy, Baldwin, M. and Bailey, P., Eds., p. 483. C. C. Thomas, Springfield, Ill.

Foerster, O. and Altenburger, H. (1935). Electrobiologische Vorgänge an der menslichen Hirnrinde. Dtsch. Z. Nervenkr., *135:*277.

Gloor, P., Rasmussen, T., Garretson H. and Maroun, F. (1964). Fractionized intracarotid Metrazol injection: A new diagnostic method in electroencephalography. Electroencephalogr. Clin. Neurophysiol., *17:*322.

Leksell, L. (1957). Gezielte Hirnoperationen. In: Handbuch der Neurochirurgie, Olivecrona, H. and Tonnis, W., Eds., vol. 6, p. 178. Springer, Berlin.

Ludwig, B., Ajmone Marsan, C. and Van Buren, J. M. (1975). Cerebral seizures of probable orbito-frontal origin. Epilepsia, *16:*141.

Ludwig, B., Ajmone Marsan, C. and Van Buren, J. (1976). Depth and direct cortical recording in seizure disorders of extratemporal origin. Neurology *26:*1085.

Matsumoto, H. and Ajmone Marsan, C. (1964). Cortical cellular phenomena in experimental epilepsy: ictal manifestations. Exp. Neurol., *9:*305.

Penfield, W. and Jasper, H. H. (1954). Epilepsy and the Functional Anatomy of the Human Brain. Little, Brown, Boston.

Penry, J. K., Ed. (1977). Epilepsy. The Eighth International Symposium. p. 95. Raven Press, New York.

Rand, R. W., Crandall, P. H. and Walter, R. D. (1964). Chronic stereotactic implantation of depth electrodes for psychomotor epilepsy. Acta Neurochir. (Wien), *11:*609.

Rossi, G. F. (1973). Problems of analysis and interpretation of electrocerebral signals in human epilepsy. A neurosurgeon's view. In: Epilepsy: Its Phenomena in Man, Brazier, M. A. B., Ed., p. 259. Academic Press, New York.

Rovit, R., Gloor, P. and Rasmussen, T. (1961). Intracarotic amobarbital in epilepsy. Arch. Neurol., *5:*606.

Scarff, J. E. and Rahm, W. E. (1941). The human electro-corticogram. A report of spontaneous electrical potentials obtained from the exposed human brain. J. Neurophysiol., *4:*418.

Spiegel, E. A., Wycis, H. T. and Goode, R. (1956). Studies in stereoencephalotomy. V.A. universal stereoencephalotome (model V) for use in man and experimental animals. J. Neurosurg., *13:*305.

Symposium on intracerebral electrography. (1953). Proc. Staff Meet. Mayo Clinic, *28:*145.

Talairach, J., Bancaud, J., Szikla, G., Bonis, A., Geier, S., Vedrenne C. et al (1974). Approche nouvelle de la neurochirurgie de l'épilepsie. Méthodologie stéréotaxique et résultats thérapeutiques. Neurochirurgie, *20,* Suppl. 1, 1.

Van Buren, J. M. (1965). A stereotaxic instrument for man. Electroencephalogr. Clin. Neurophysiol., *19:*398.

Van Buren, J. M., Ajmone Marsan, C. and Mutsuga, N. (1975a). Temporal-lobe seizures with additional foci treated by resection. J. Neurosurg., *43:*596.

Van Buren, J. M., Ajmone Marsan, C., Mutsuga, N. and Sadowsky, D. (1975b). Surgery of temporal lobe epilepsy. In: Neurosurgical Management of the Epilepsies. Purpura, D. P., Penry, J. K. and Walter, R. D., Eds., p. 155. Raven Press, New York.

Walter, R. D. (1973). Tactical considerations leading to surgical treatment of limbic epilepsy. In: Epilepsy: Its Phenomena in Man. Brazier, M. A. B., Ed., p. 99. Academic Press, New York.

6
Electromyography

M. J. AMINOFF

INTRODUCTION

The term *electromyography* refers to methods of studying the electrical activity of muscle, and over the years such methods have come to be recognized as an invaluable aid to neurologic diagnosis. They have been used to detect and characterize disease processes affecting the motor units, and are particularly helpful when clinical evaluation is difficult or equivocal. The findings often permit the underlying lesion to be localized to the neural, muscular, or junctional component of the motor units in question. Indeed, when the neural component is involved, the nature and distribution of electromyographic abnormalities may permit the lesion to be localized to the level of the cell bodies of the lower motor neurons or to their axons as they transverse a spinal root, nerve plexus, or peripheral nerve. The electromyographic findings *per se* are never pathognomonic of specific diseases and cannot provide a definitive diagnosis, although they may justifiably be used to support or refute a diagnosis advanced on clinical or other grounds.

Electromyography is also used in conjunction with nerve conduction studies to obtain information of prognostic significance in the management of patients with peripheral nerve lesions. For example, electromyographic evidence of denervation implies a less favorable prognosis than otherwise, in patients with a compressive or entrapment neuropathy. Again, evidence that some motor units remain under voluntary control after a traumatic peripheral nerve lesion implies a more favorable outlook than otherwise for ultimate recovery, indicating as it does that the nerve remains in functional continuity, at least in part.

Over the years, the activity of individual muscles in the maintenance of posture, and during normal or abnormal movement, has also been studied by electromyography. Although such studies are of considerable academic interest they are of little clinical or diagnostic relevance at the present time, and will therefore receive no further consideration here.

PRACTICAL ASPECTS

The electrical activity of muscle is best studied for diagnostic purposes by inserting a recording electrode directly into the muscle to be examined. The bioelectric potentials that are picked up by this electrode are amplified, and then displayed on a cathode ray oscilloscope for visual analysis and fed through a loudspeaker system so that they can be monitored acoustically. A permanent photographic record of the oscilloscope trace can be made if desired, or the amplified bioelectric signals can be recorded on magnetic tape for retrieval at a later date.

The concentric needle electrode (Adrian and Bronk, 1929) is probably the most convenient recording electrode for clinical purposes. It consists of a pointed steel cannula within which runs a fine silver, steel, or platinum wire that is insulated except at its tip. The potential difference between the outer cannula and inner wire is recorded, while the patient is grounded by a separate surface electrode. An electrode exhibits some opposition or impedance to the flow of an electric current, and it is therefore important that the amplifier to which it is connected should have a relatively high input impedance to prevent loss of the signal. The amplifier—and the recording system to which it is connected—should have a frequency response of 2 to 10,000 Hz so that signals within this frequency spectrum are amplified uniformly without distortion. The frequency response of the amplifier can, however, be altered when necessary by the use of filters, which usually consists of variable resistance-capacitance circuits. This allows the attenuation of noise or interference signals that have a different frequency to that of the potentials under study.

Noise, which appears as a random fluctuation of the baseline, is generated within the amplifier and by movement of the recording electrodes or their leads, and can obscure the bioelectric signals to be studied, as also may any unwanted interference signals that are picked up by the recording apparatus. Interference signals are usually generated by the AC power line, appliances such as radios, or paging systems, but occasionally are biologic in origin. Attention was directed by Guld, Rosenfalck, and Willison (1970) to various technical and safety factors that are important when the electrical activity of muscle is to be recorded, and to the various technical problems which those undertaking such studies might face, and the reader is referred to their paper for a detailed account of this aspect.

Procedure

The patient is examined in a warm, quiet room. Muscles are selected for examination on the basis of the patient's symptoms and signs, and the diagnostic problem that they raise. A ground lead is attached to the same limb as the muscles that are to be examined. A concentric needle electrode is inserted into the muscle while it is relaxed, so that the presence and extent of any insertion activity can be noted, and the muscle is explored systematically with the electrode for the presence of any spontaneous activity. The parameters of individual motor unit potentials are then defined in different sites during graded muscle contraction, attention being directed not only to the shape and dimensions of the potentials but also to their initial firing rate and the rate at which they must fire before additional units are recruited. Finally, the interference pattern is compared to the strength of contraction during increasingly powerful contractions, until full voluntary power is being exerted.

ELECTRICAL ACTIVITY OF NORMAL MUSCLE

In clinical electromyography electrical activity is recorded extracellularly from muscle fibers that are embedded in tissue which is itself a conducting medium. The action potentials that are recorded in this way have a tri- or biphasic configuration, and the basis for this is illustrated schematically in Figure 6.1, where the active electrode is shown on the surface of a fiber and the reference electrode is placed at a remote point in the conducting medium. Since there is a flow of current into the fiber (that is, a current "sink") at the point of excitation and an outward flow of current in adjacent regions, the propagated impulse can be considered as a moving sink of current, preceded and followed by current sources. Accordingly, when an impulse travels toward the active electrode, this electrode becomes relatively more positive as it comes to overlie the current source preceding the action potential (Fig. 6.1A). A short time later, as the impulse itself arrives, the active electrode registers a negative potential in relation to the distance electrode (Fig. 6.1B), and then a relatively positive potential as the impulse passes on and is followed by the current source behind it (Fig. 6.1C). As this too passes on, the electrode comes again to be on a resting

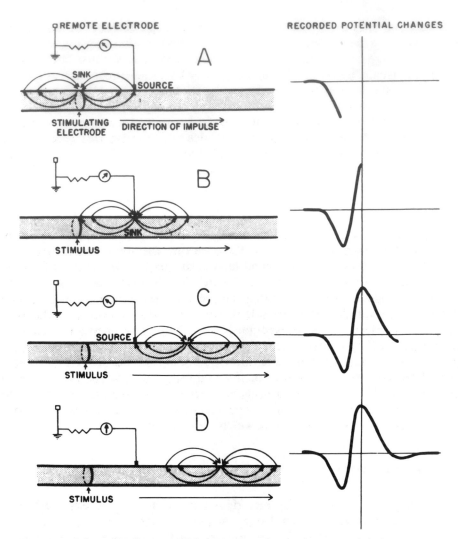

Fig. 6.1. *Schematic diagram of the passage of an action potential along a nerve or muscle fiber in a conducting medium. The active electrode is on the surface of the fiber, and the reference electrode is at a remote point in the conducting medium (from Brazier, M. A. B. 1977. Electrical activity of the nervous system, 4th edn. Pitman Medical, London).*

portion of the fiber and the potential between the two electrodes returns to the baseline (Fig. 6.1D). Clearly, the recorded action potential will be biphasic with a negative onset (rather than triphasic with a positive onset) if the active electrode is placed over the region of the fiber at which the impulse is initiated.

At Rest

Electrical activity cannot usually be recorded outside of the end-plate region of healthy muscle at rest, except immediately after insertion or movement

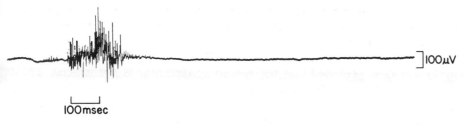

]100μV

└──┘
100msec

Fig. 6.2. *Insertion activity evoked in normal muscle. In accordance with convention, an upward deflection in this and subsequent figures indicates relative negativity of the active electrode.*

of the needle recording electrode. The activity related to electrode movement—*insertion activity*—is due to mechanical stimulation or injury of the muscle fibers, and usually stops within 2 or 3 seconds of the movement (Fig. 6.2). After cessation of this activity, spontaneous activity may be found in the end-plate region, but not elsewhere. This *end-plate noise,* as it is called, consists of monophasic negative potentials which have an irregular, high-frequency discharge pattern, a duration of between 0.5 and 2.0 msec, and an amplitude that is usually less than 100 μV. The potentials correspond to the miniature end-plate potentials that can be recorded with microelectrodes in experimental animals. Biphasic potentials with a negative onset are also a constituent of end-plate noise, and have a duration of 3 to 5 msec and an amplitude of 100 to 200 μV. They have been held to represent muscle fiber action potentials arising sporadically due to spontaneous activity at the neuromuscular junction (Buchthal and Rosenfalck, 1966), or activity in intramuscular nerve fibers (Jones, Lambert, and Sayre, 1955).

During Activity

Motor Unit Potentials. Excitation of a single lower motor neuron normally leads to the activation of all of the muscle fibers that it innervates, i.e. which comprise the motor unit. The motor unit potential is a compound potential representing the sum of the individual action potentials generated in the few muscle fibers of the unit which are within the pick-up range of the recording electrode. When recorded with a concentric needle electrode, motor unit potentials are usually bi- or triphasic (Fig. 6.3), but in the limb muscles about 12 percent may have 5 or more phases and are then described as polyphasic. The duration of the potentials, which is normally between 2 and 15 msec, relates to the anatomic scatter of end-plates of those muscle fibers, in the units under study, that are within the pick-up zone of the recording electrode. This is because of the different distances along which the muscle fiber action potentials will have to be conducted from the individual end-plates before they reach the recording zone of the electrode. The amplitude of the motor unit potentials is usually between 200 μV and 3 mV and is determined largely by the distance between the recording electrode and the active fibers that are closest to it; the number of active fibers lying close to the electrode and the temporal dispersion of their individual action potentials also affect the amplitude of the potentials, but to a lesser extent.

The configuration and dimensions of individual motor unit potentials are normally constant provided that the recording electrode is not moved. They are, however, influenced by the characteristics of the recording electrode and apparatus in the electromyograph system, and by physiologic factors, such as age, intramuscular temperature, the site of the recording electrode within the muscle, and the particular muscle under examination. Abnormalities in the parameters of motor unit potentials occur in patients with neuromuscular diseases, as is discussed below.

Motor Unit Recruitment Pattern. When a muscle is contracted weakly, a few of its motor units begin firing irregularly and at a low rate. As the force of contraction increases, the firing rate of these active units increases until it reaches a certain frequency when additional units are recruited. Eventually, so many units are active that the baseline is interrupted continuously by the potentials, and individual potentials cannot be distinguished from each other. The

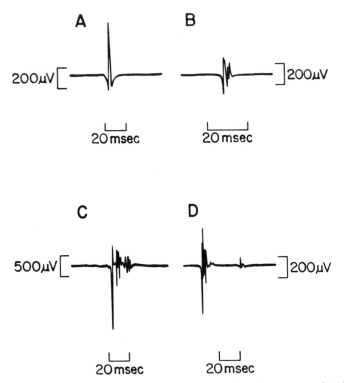

Fig. 6.3. Motor unit potentials. A, normal potential; B, low amplitude, short duration, polyphasic potential; C, long duration, polyphasic potential; D, polyphasic potential with a late component.

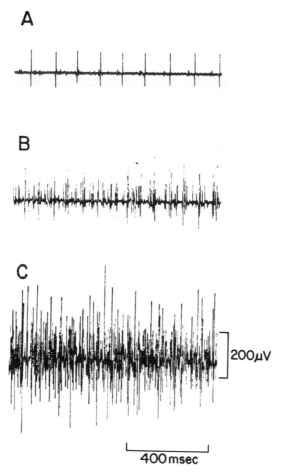

Fig. 6.4. Motor unit potentials recorded during slight (A), moderate (B), and maximal (C) voluntary contraction of muscle.

resulting appearance of the oscilloscope trace is referred to as the interference pattern (Fig. 6.4).

ELECTRICAL ACTIVITY FOUND IN PATHOLOGIC STATES

At Rest

Insertion Activity. Insertion activity is found only when some muscle tissue remains viable. It is prolonged in denervated muscle, and in polymyositis, the myotonic disorders, and some of the other myopathies.

After cessation of all insertion activity, various types of spontaneous activity may be recorded from fully relaxed muscle in patients with a neuromuscular disorder.

Fibrillation Potentials. Fibrillation potentials are action potentials that arise spontaneously from single muscle fibers. When they occur rhythmically their genesis may relate to oscillations of the resting membrane potential of denervated skeletal muscle fibers (Li, Shy, and Wells, 1957; Purves and Sakmann, 1974; Thesleff and Ward, 1975). In other instances they occur irregularly, and this has been attributed to the occurrence of random, discrete spontaneous depolarizations which originate in the transverse tubular system of the muscle fiber (Smith and Thesleff, 1976). The initiating events of both types of fibrillation are suppressed by tetrodotoxin or removal of external sodium ions, suggesting that they are related to changes in sodium conductance (Purves and Sakmann, 1974).

Fibrillation potentials usually have an amplitude of between 20 and 300 μV, a duration of less than 5 msec, and a firing rate of between 2 and 20 per second (Fig. 6.5). They have a bi- or triphasic shape, the first phase being positive except when the potentials are recorded in the end-plate region. This positive onset facilitates their distinction from end-plate noise. Over the loudspeaker they give rise to a high-pitched repetitive click, which aids their detection. They are found in denervated muscle, provided that some tissue remains viable and the muscle is warm when examined, but they may not appear for some two or three weeks after an acute neuropathic lesion. They are not in themselves diagnostic of denervation, however, for they are also seen in primary muscle diseases such as polymyositis and muscular dystrophy, and in patients with botulism, trichinosis, muscle trauma, or metabolic disorders such as acid maltase deficiency or hyperkalemic periodic paralysis. Indeed, scanty fibrillary potentials may occasionally be found in normal healthy muscle (Buchthal and Rosenfalck, 1966), and pathologic significance should therefore not be attributed to them unless they are detected in at least three separate sites within the muscle being examined.

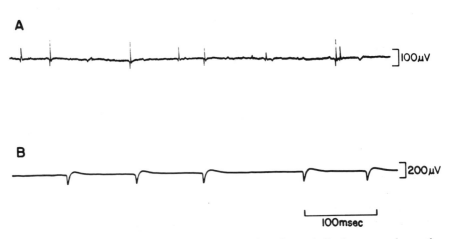

A

]100μV

B

]200μV

100msec

Fig. 6.5. Spontaneous activity recorded in relaxed, partially denervated muscle. A, fibrillation potentials; B, positive sharp waves.

Positive Sharp Waves. These are usually found in association with fibrillation potentials both in denervated muscle and in certain primary disorders of muscle, and are thought to arise from single muscle fibers which have been injured. As viewed on the oscilloscope, they consist of an initial positive deflection, following which there is a slow change of potential in a negative direction that may be extended into a small negative phase (Fig. 6.5). Their amplitude is usually about the same, or slightly greater, than that of fibrillation potentials, their duration is often 10 msec or more, and their discharge rate can be up to 100 per second.

Fasciculation Potentials. Fasciculation potentials are similar to motor unit potentials in their dimensions, and have been attributed to spontaneous activation of the muscle fibers of individual motor units (Denny-Brown and Pennybacker, 1938). Their detection is aided by the sudden dull thump that they produce over the loudspeaker. They may be found in normal muscle or in patients with chronic partial denervation, especially when this is due to spinal cord pathology. Forster, Borkowski, and Alpers (1946) considered that fasciculation potentials arose at the neuromuscular junctions and then spread antidromically by axonal reflex to the other nerve terminals of the motor unit. More recently, Wettstein (1977), using a collision technique, has studied the origin of these potentials in patients with anterior horn cell involvement due to various causes and found that they could originate at multiple sites along motor axons or the somas of diseased motor neurons.

Myotonic Discharges. These discharges consist of high-frequency trains of action potentials which are evoked by electrode movement or by percussion or contraction of the muscle, and are enhanced by cold. Some of the potentials resemble fibrillation potentials or positive sharp waves, while others resemble motor unit potentials. Their frequency and amplitude wax and wane (Fig. 6.6),

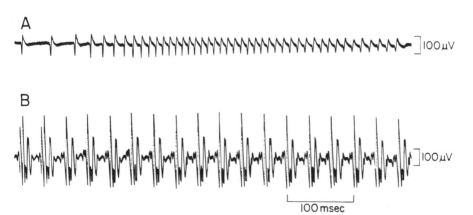

Fig. 6.6. *Spontaneous high-frequency activity. A, myotonic discharge recorded in a patient with myotonia congenita; B, bizarre high-frequency potentials recorded in a partially denervated muscle.*

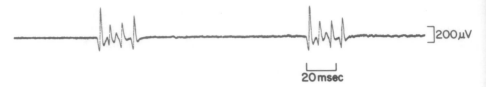

Fig. 6.7. Spontaneous repetitive motor unit activity, showing grouped discharges.

and in consequence the trains of potentials produce a sound like that of a dive bomber on the loudspeaker. Such discharges occur independently of any neural influence, and can thus be elicited even when neuromuscular blockage is induced by curare (Landau, 1952). Their pathogenesis is uncertain, but seems to relate to a disorder of the muscle fiber membrane. They are found in patients with one or other of the various myotonic disorders. They may also be found in hyperkalemic periodic paralysis, and occasionally in patients with neurogenic muscle weakness or the myopathy of acid maltase deficiency.

Bizarre High-Frequency Potentials. Trains of bizarre, high-frequency potentials are sometimes found in the muscles of patients with muscular dystrophy, polymyositis, or chronic partial denervation, and occasionally in patients with such metabolic disorders as hyperkalemic periodic paralysis, hypothyroidism, or certain of the glycogen storage diseases. The discharges occur spontaneously, and after electrode movement or voluntary contraction. They have an abrupt onset and termination, but unlike myotonic discharges their amplitude and frequency remain constant (Fig. 6.6). The individual potentials are often polyphasic, but their origin is uncertain.

Motor Unit Potentials. Motor unit activity may occur spontaneously and repetitively despite full voluntary relaxation of the muscle in patients with myokymia, muscle cramps, or tetany. Moreover, the individual potentials sometimes exhibit a rhythmic, grouped pattern of firing so that double, triple, or multiple discharges are seen, especially in patients with tetany or myokymia (Fig. 6.7).

During Activity

Motor Unit Potentials. Any change in the number of functional muscle fibers contained in motor units will affect the parameters of motor unit potentials. This is best exemplified by considering the character of the potentials that are recorded from a muscle when the number of muscle fibers per unit is reduced. The mean duration of the potentials is shortened due to loss of some of the distant fibers that previously contributed to their initial and terminal portions, while their mean amplitude is reduced due to loss of some of the fibers lying close to the electrode. If the spikes generated by the surviving muscle fibers of individual units are widely separated in time, there may also be an increased incidence of polyphasic potentials. As might be expected, therefore, the mean duration and amplitude of motor unit potentials are reduced in patients with myopathic disorders (Fig. 6.3), and there is an increased incidence of polyphasic potentials. Similar findings may also be encountered in patients with disorders of neuromuscular transmission such as myasthenia gravis or the myasthenic syndrome, and during the reinnervation of muscle following severe peripheral nerve injury, but the characteristic feature in such circumstances is the variability that the potentials exhibit in their parameters, and especially in their amplitude, during continued activity (Fig. 6.8).

In neuropathic disorders it is the number of functional motor units that is reduced, and the average number of muscle fibers per unit may actually be increased if denervated muscle fibers are reinnervated by collateral branches from the nerve fibers of surviving units. The motor unit potentials recorded in such circumstances are of longer duration than normal, and may be polyphasic (Fig. 6.3). This is because the activity recorded by the electrode is temporally more dispersed than normal, due primarily to the greater anatomic scatter of end-plates in the units, but also to the reduced conduction velocity at which immature collateral branches conduct impulses. The potentials may also have a greater amplitude than normal if the number of muscle fibers lying close to the electrode is increased, and such potentials are often particularly conspicuous in patients with spinal cord involvement.

Motor unit potentials are sometimes followed by smaller potentials after an interval of about 15 to 25 msec or more (Fig. 6.3). These late components of motor unit potentials have been reported both in progressive neurogenic disorders (Borenstein and Desmedt, 1973) and in such muscle diseases as polymyositis and muscular dystrophy (Desmedt and Borenstein, 1976). They have also been described in a patient with myoglobinuria attributed to a viral myositis (Pickett, 1978). They can be explained by the presence of an ectopic end-plate or by delayed conduction along unmyelinated collateral nerve sprouts innervating previously denervated muscle fibers, but in the latter case a change in the latency of the late component would be expected to occur with sprout myelination. In muscular dystrophy, the denervated fibers are thought to arise

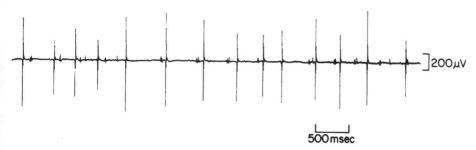

Fig. 6.8. Variation in amplitude of a motor unit potential during continued, weak voluntary activity of a reinnervated muscle.

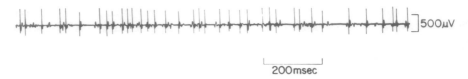

Fig. 6.9. *Activity recorded during maximal voluntary contraction of a partially denervated muscle.*

by segmentation of existing muscle fibers or by muscle regeneration (Desmedt and Borenstein, 1976).

Abnormalities of Recruitment Pattern. When the number of functional motor units is reduced, as in patients with neurogenic weakness, there may be a diminution in the density of electrical activity that can be recorded from affected muscles during a maximal voluntary contraction, and in severe cases it may be possible to recognize individual motor unit potentials (Fig. 6.9). In such circumstances there is an increase in the rate at which individual units begin to fire, and also in the rate at which they must fire before additional units are recruited (Petajan, 1974).

In patients with myopathic disorders the number of functional units remains unchanged until an advanced stage of the disorder, and the interference pattern therefore remains full. Indeed, it may be more complete than normal for a given degree of voluntary activity because there is an increase in the number of active units to compensate for the reduced tension that individual units—with their reduced fiber content—are able to generate. Motor unit firing rates tend toward normal unless the myopathy is severe, when the frequency of firing at onset and at recruitment of other units may be increased (Petajan, 1974).

ELECTROMYOGRAPHIC FINDINGS IN VARIOUS CLINICAL DISORDERS

Myopathic Disorders

The electromyographic findings in myopathic disorders do not, in themselves, indicate the etiology of the underlying muscle disease. Indeed, the findings do not even establish with certainty that the underlying pathology is a primary disorder of muscle. During the reinnervation of muscle after a severe peripheral nerve lesion, for example, the electromyographic appearance may be similar to that in a myopathy (Kugelberg, 1947). Again, several hypothetical neurogenic mechanisms could lead to motor unit potentials resembling those traditionally associated with myopathic disorders (Engel, 1975). Nevertheless, electromyography is of undoubted practical usefulness in the diagnosis of myopathies at the present time, provided that the clinical context of the examination is borne in mind and the findings are integrated wtih the results of other laboratory procedures.

An increased amount of insertion activity may be found in myopathic disorders, and abnormal spontaneous activity is sometimes present, particularly in patients with inflammatory diseases of muscle. Indeed, in the myotonic disorders the characteristic electromyographic finding consists of spontaneous high-frequency discharges of potentials that wax and wane in frequency and amplitude, thereby producing a sound like that of a dive bomber on the loudspeaker. The features that are most helpful in the electromyographic recognition of myopathic disorders, however, relate to the character and recruitment pattern of motor unit potentials. The number of short and/or small potentials is characteristically increased, and many of the potentials are polyphasic. Such potentials produce a characteristic crackle on the loudspeaker, and this aids their detection. Because there is a reduction in the tension that individual motor units can generate, an excessive number of units is activated in weak contractions. During strong voluntary contractions a full interference pattern is seen, but the potentials are lower in amplitude and more spiky than in normal muscle.

In assessing the electromyographic findings in patients with a suspected myopathic disorder, it must be appreciated that abnormalities may not be detected despite a meticulous search and quantitative analysis of the data so obtained. The findings in various myopathic disorders are discussed below, with attention being directed to the manner in which they may differ from the changes just described. Further details are given by Aminoff (1978).

Muscular Dystrophies. In the muscular dystrophies the usual electromyographic findings are as described above, although abnormalities are sometimes inconspicuous, particularly in the relatively benign forms of muscular dystrophy such as the limb-girdle or facioscapulohumeral varieties (Buchthal, 1962). Attempts to identify female carriers of the gene of the sex-linked variety of muscular dystrophy by studying the parameters of motor unit potentials (Van den Bosch, 1963; Gardner-Medwin, 1968), the refractory period of muscle fibers (Caruso and Buchthal, 1965), or the pattern of electrical activity of muscle (Willison, 1967) have met with only limited success and are of little practical significance at the present time.

Inflammatory Disorders of Muscle. In polymyositis the character and recruitment pattern of motor unit potentials are similar to those seen in other myopathic disorders, but insertion activity is frequently excessive and spontaneous fibrillation potentials, positive sharp waves, and bizarre high-frequency potentials are found more often and are usually much more conspicuous than in patients with muscular dystrophy. These findings are patchy in distribution, but are usually prominent when the disease is in an active phase. Similar findings may be encountered in other inflammatory disorders, such as trichinosis (Waylonis and Johnson, 1964) and toxoplasmosis (Rowland and Greer, 1961; Buchthal and Rosenfalck, 1963), but in patients with polymyalgia rheumatica the electromyographic findings are usually normal.

Endocrine and Metabolic Myopathies. In patients with an endocrine myopathy the electrophysiologic findings are again similar to those of other myopathies, and abnormal spontaneous activity is usually not seen. Abnormalities are often inconspicuous in patients with a steroid-induced myopathy, however, presumably because it is the type 2 muscle fibers that are affected predominantly in this condition.

In thyrotoxicosis, fasciculation potentials may be conspicuous. In hypothyroidism, insertion activity is sometimes increased (Ross et al, 1958; Waldstein et al, 1958; Ozker, Schumacher, and Nelson, 1960), and spontaneous fibrillation and fasciculation potentials, together with trains of bizarre repetitive discharges, may also be found (Ozker et al, 1960). In interpreting the findings in patients with endocrine disturbances, it must be remembered that a myopathy may coexist with other types of neuromuscular disorder, and these may complicate the electromyographic findings. For example, patients with hypothyroidism are liable to develop peripheral nerve entrapment syndromes, while myasthenia gravis sometimes occurs in association with thyrotoxicosis.

The electromyographic features of a myopathy may also be found in patients with osteomalacia, chronic renal failure, and a number of other less common metabolic disorders. In patients with hypokalemic periodic paralysis, the electromyographic findings between attacks may be normal, or less commonly are suggestive of a proximal myopathy. During the attacks, no abnormality of insertion or spontaneous activity is found, but motor unit potentials are reduced in duration and number; the interference pattern during attempted voluntary contraction is diminished, and in severe cases there may be complete electrical silence (Shy et al, 1961). During attacks of hyperkalemic or normokalemic periodic paralysis, insertion activity is increased, spontaneous fibrillation potentials, myotonic discharges, and bizarre high-frequency potentials may be found, and motor unit potentials are reduced in duration and number (Buchthal, Engbaek, and Gamstorp, 1958; Layzer, Lovelace, and Rowland, 1967).

In the glycogen storage diseases due to deficiency of phosphorylase (McArdle's disease) or phosphofructokinase the electromyogram of the resting muscle is usually normal but occasionally is suggestive of a myopathy. No electrical activity can be recorded during the contractures that may develop during continued exercise (McArdle, 1951; Layzer, Rowland, and Ranney, 1967). In patients with acid maltase deficiency (Pompe's disease), electromyography may reveal increased insertion activity and profuse, spontaneous fibrillation, positive sharp waves, myotonic discharges and bizarre high-frequency potentials, but the motor unit potentials are similar in character to those seen in other myopathies (Swaiman, Kennedy, and Sauls, 1968; Engel, 1970).

Myopathy due to drugs or alcohol. Changes suggestive of a myopathy may be found at electromyography in patients with chronic alcoholism, or those taking certain drugs such as bretylium tosylate (Campbell and Montuschi, 1960), colchicine (Kontos, 1962) and chloroquine (Whisnant et al, 1963). In the case of chloroquine, however, the number of functional motor units is sometimes reduced and conduction velocity may be slowed in peripheral nerves, suggesting that there is also a neurogenic component to the weakness that develops.

Congenital myopathies of uncertain etiology. A number of congenital myopathies have been described, and these may be associated with specific structural changes that enable distinct entities to be recognized. Appropriate EMG changes may be found in some cases, but in others the findings are normal. In nemaline and centronuclear myopathy, however, abnormal spontaneous activity may be a conspicuous feature.

Myotonic disorders. The characteristic electromyographic feature in dystrophia myotonica, the dominant and recessive forms of myotonia congenita, paramyotonia congenita, and chondrodystrophic myotonia (Aberfeld et al, 1970) is the occurrence of myotonic discharges that are evoked by electrode movement and by percussion or voluntary contraction of the muscle being examined. Motor unit potentials are normal in appearance except in dystrophia myotonica and the recessive type of myotonia congentia, when an excess of small, short duration and/or polyphasic potentials may be found as in other myopathic disorders. Dystrophia myotonica is a dominantly inherited disorder and electromyography has a definite place in the investigation of apparently unaffected relatives to determine whether they are at risk of developing the disease, since abnormalities may be present in asymptomatic subjects (Bundey, Carter, and Soothill, 1970; Polgar et al, 1972).

Neuropathic Disorders

Immediately after the development of an acute neuropathic lesion, electromyography reveals no abnormality other than a reduction in the number of motor unit potentials under voluntary control. A complete interference pattern is not seen during maximal effort despite an increase in the firing rate of individual units, and in severe cases there may be no surviving units. The subsequent changes depend on whether or not denervation has occurred. If it has, the amount of insertion activity increases after several days, and abnormal spontaneous activity may subsequently be found, although its appearance may be delayed for up to about three weeks depending upon the site of the lesion. In particular, fibrillation potentials are usually detected sooner when the lesion is close to the muscle than with a more distant lesion. As reinnervation occurs, spontaneous activity becomes less conspicuous and low amplitude motor unit potentials are seen. These potentials may exhibit a marked variability in their size and configuration, and some have a complex polyphasic configuration. With time, many of these potentials regain a normal appearance and the interference pattern becomes more complete, but the extent of any residual electromyographic abnormality depends on the completeness of recovery.

In patients with chronic partial denervation, insertion activity is increased and spontaneous fibrillations, positive sharp waves, and bizarre high-frequency potentials are found. Fasciculation potentials are often conspicuous in patients with diseases such as motor neuron disease or poliomyelitis, in which the lower motor neurons in the spinal cord are affected, but may also be found with more peripheral lesions. The mean duration of motor unit potentials is increased and—especially in patients with spinal cord involvement—there may be an increased incidence of large units. In addition an excessive number of polyphasic motor unit potentials is usually encountered. There is an increase in the rate at which individual units begin firing and at which they must fire before additional units are recruited, and the interference pattern during maximal contractions is reduced.

Spinal Cord Pathology. Signs of chronic partial denervation are found in the affected muscles of patients with chronic myelopathies if the anterior horn cells are involved. Insertional activity is increased, and spontaneous fasciculations, fibrillation, positive sharp waves, and bizarre high-frequency potentials may be found. The mean duration and amplitude of motor unit potentials—and the number of polyphasic potentials—are increased, giant potentials may be encountered, and the firing rate of individual potentials is increased while the interference pattern is reduced.

By making it possible to define the precise segmental distribution of a lesion involving lower motor neurons, the electromyographic examination can aid in the localization of spinal cord lesions. Electromyography, therefore, has an important role in distinguishing motor neuron diseases from discrete, surgically remediable conditions affecting the spinal cord. The examination should be continued until it is clear whether or not the pattern of involved muscles can be accounted for by a restricted cord lesion.

Spinal cord disorders can usually be distinguished from peripheral nerve or plexus lesions by the pattern of muscle involvement, and measurement of motor and sensory conduction velocity may also be helpful in this respect. It is harder to distinguish a discrete spinal cord lesion from a root lesion, because in both instances electromyographic abnormalities may have a segmental distribution and changes may be found in the paraspinous muscles. In the former, however, several segments may be involved and bilateral changes can usually be expected. Electromyography per se does not provide any direct information regarding the pathology of the underlying abnormality.

Root Lesions. Electromyographic signs of chronic partial denervation may be found in muscles supplied by the affected segment. The number of limb muscles examined must be sufficient to distinguish a root lesion from more peripheral (plexus or peripheral nerve) involvement by the distribution of electrical abnormalities. The importance of this is shown most clearly by means of a simple example. Thus, neurogenic weakness of the elbow, wrist, and finger extensors may result from a lesion in any one of several sites, and the examination of a patient with such a deficit must be planned with meticulous care if correct localization of the lesion is to be achieved. In this particular instance, electromyographic evidence that flexor carpi radialis (C6,7) is involved but brachioradialis (C5,6) is spared would favor a lesion of the C7 root or the middle trunk of the brachial plexus; conversely, involvement of brachioradialis but sparing of flexor carpi radialis would suggest a radial nerve lesion unless the deltoid (C5,6) muscle is also affected, in which case the posterior cord of the brachial plexus may well have been involved.

It is often helpful to examine the paraspinous muscles because these are supplied from the spinal roots by their posterior primary rami, while the limb plexuses and peripheral nerves are derived from the anterior primary rami. Abnormalities in the paraspinous muscles are, therefore, common in patients with a radiculopathy and may precede changes in the limb muscles, but would not be expected in patients with a plexus or peripheral nerve lesion. No conclusions should be reached about the level of the lesion from the findings in these muscles, however, because there is a marked overlap in the territory supplied by the posterior primary rami. Moreover, abnormalities may be found in patients who have previously undergone back surgery, and in such circumstances are of questionable significance.

Plexus Lesions. As is shown in Figure 6.10, the brachial plexus is formed from the anterior primary rami of the C5, C6, C7, C8, and T1 roots, with a variable contribution from C4 (pre-fixed) and T2 (postfixed plexus). The C5 and C6 roots combine to form the upper trunk, C7 continues as the middle trunk, and C8 and T1 join to form the lower trunk. The trunks traverse the supraclavicular fossa and at the upper border of the clavicle each divides into anterior and posterior divisions. The three posterior divisions then combine to form the posterior cord of the plexus, while the anterior divisions of the upper two trunks unite to form the lateral cord and the anterior division of the lower trunk continues as the medial cord. It is the cords which give rise to the main peripheral nerves of the arm.

The lumbar portion of the lumbosacral plexus is derived from the anterior primary rami of the first four lumbar roots, while the sacral portion is formed from the lumbosacral trunk (L4 and L5) and the anterior primary rami of the first four sacral roots.

Needle electromyography may be helpful in assessing the functional integrity of a nerve plexus, in attempting to localize a plexus lesion, and in distinguishing such a lesion from root or peripheral nerve pathology. The muscles examined should include those supplied by each of the main peripheral nerves and spinal roots in question, so that the site of the lesion can be determined by the pattern of involved muscles. The importance of examining the paraspinous muscles when attempting to distinguish between a root and plexus lesion has already been stressed. Such a distinction can sometimes also be made by stimulation techniques in which appropriate sensory action potentials are recorded in the extremities (Ch. 7). These potentials may be small or absent in patients with lesions that are distal to the dorsal root ganglia and have caused afferent fibers to degenerate, but are preserved in patients with radiculopathy because the lesion is more proximal and peripheral sensory fibers therefore remain intact.

These principles are well-exemplified by the findings in patients in whom the

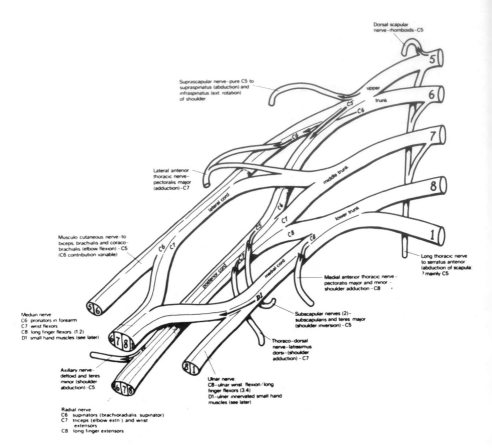

Fig. 6.10. *Anatomy of the brachial plexus (from Patten, J. P. 1977. Neurological Differential Diagnosis, Springer-Verlag, New York).*

lower trunk of the brachial plexus, or the anterior primary rami of the C8 and T1 nerve roots, are compressed or angulated by a cervical rib or band. The muscle wasting that results may be restricted to, or especially conspicuous in, the lateral part of the thenar pad, but careful clinical and electromyographic examination shows that motor involvement is more extensive than can be accounted for by a median nerve lesion alone, conforming instead to the distribution of muscles supplied by the C8 and T1 segments. Moreover, sensory action potentials may be small or absent when recordings are made from the ulnar nerve at the wrist after stimulation of its digital fibers in the little finger, indicating that the lesion is distal to the dorsal root ganglia (Gilliatt et al, 1970).

Peripheral Nerve Lesions. The electromyographic distinction of peripheral nerve from other neuropathic lesions has been discussed above. In addition to the detection of signs of denervation in muscle supplied by the individual peripheral nerves, motor and sensory conduction can be studied in these nerves, and this is discussed in the following chapter.

Needle electromyography has an important role in providing a guide to prognosis after peripheral nerve injuries, and in following the course of recovery. After injuries in which the function of a nerve is temporarily deranged but its structure remains intact, needle electromyography reveals only a reduction in the number of motor units under voluntary control. If the anatomic continuity of nerve fibers is interruped, however, the amount of insertion activity increases after a few days and abnormal spontaneous activity is eventually found, as described on p. 211 where the subsequent changes that occur with regeneration and reinnervation were also considered. In evaluating patients with peripheral nerve injuries, needle electromyography may provide evidence that some motor units remain under voluntary control after an apparently complete nerve lesion, and this implies a more favorable prognosis than otherwise, provided the possibility of these units being innervated anomalously has been excluded. Again, it is an important method of determining whether denervation has occurred, and this too has prognostic significance. Finally, needle electromyography may indicate at an early stage whether recovery is occurring after a complete palsy, since voluntary motor unit activity reappears long before any signs of clinical recovery.

Disorders of Neuromuscular Transmission

The electromyographic findings in patients with disorders of neuromuscular transmission are discussed in Chapter 8. The only point that need be made here is that individual motor unit potentials may show a marked variation in their dimensions and configuration due to blocking of impulse transmission to individual muscle fibers within the motor unit. Such variability is, therefore, a common finding in patients with myasthenia gravis, the Eaton-Lambert syndrome, or botulism, and is also encountered as reinnervation occurs after a neuropathic lesion, and following muscle trauma. There may also be an increased incidence of short duration and/or polyphasic motor unit potentials in patients with myasthenia gravis, due to a reduction in the number of functional muscle fibers per unit or to the development of a secondary myopathy, and similar findings may again be encountered in the Eaton-Lambert syndrome or botulism due to the defect in neuromuscular transmission.

Miscellaneous Disorders

Intermittent bursts of high-frequency, repetitive motor unit discharges are found in different parts of the muscle in patients with cramps, the bursts having an abrupt onset and termination (Denny-Brown and Foley, 1948). In patients with myokymia, electromyography may reveal prolonged bursts of repetitive motor unit potentials, or repetitive multiplets containing from 2 to over 200 potentials with intervals of about 20 msec between component spikes (Gardner-Medwin and Walton, 1969). Hjorth and Willison (1973) found that single or double discharges of individual motor units occurred spontaneously and regularly at intervals of 100 to 200 msec in patients with facial myokymia, while Lambert, Love, and Mulder (1961) found intermittent firing of motor units for up to 900 msec at intervals of 2 to 4 seconds at rates of 30 to 40 per second. The findings in patients with myotonia, cramps, or myokymia must be distinguished from the spontaneous, high-frequency (up to 300 per second) motor unit discharges that are seen in patients with "neuromyotonia." These discharges may be continuous in severe cases, but there is a marked variability in the configuration and dimensions of the potentials that are found, some being of particularly low amplitude and short duration (Isaacs, 1967). The spontaneous discharges are increased temporarily by voluntary activity, but a brief period of electrical silence may follow strenuous, continuous activity; they persist despite local nerve block, disappear after intravenous curare or succinylcholine, and are reduced by treatment with diphenylhydantoin.

Two types of abnormal movements have been described in patients with hemifacial spasm (Hjorth and Willison, 1973). The first consists of brief twitches which affect several different muscles simultaneously, and is accompanied electromyographically by isolated bursts of repetitive, high-frequency motor unit discharges, each burst consisting of discharges from the same unit. The second type of abnormal movement consists of a prolonged, irregular fluctuating contraction during which motor units fire irregularly at lower frequencies, although bursts of activity identical to those just described are also seen.

During the spasms of tetany, motor unit potentials may be seen to fire repetitively in doublets, triplets, and/or multiplets (Kugelberg, 1948).

QUANTITATIVE ASPECTS OF ELECTROMYOGRAPHY

In an endeavor to improve the accuracy, reliability, and speed with which the examination is performed and to gain further insight into the pathophysiology of neuromuscular disorders, a number of quantitative techniques have been developed by different workers over the years. In the following section a brief account is provided of some of the more important of these methods, but readers interested in the application of computers to electromyography are referred to the detailed review by Basmajian et al (1975).

Measurement of Motor Unit Parameters

The most commonly used quantitative technique consists of measuring the parameters of individual motor unit potentials. The technique is described in detail by Buchthal and Pinelli (1953 a,b). In brief, 20 or more potentials are each recorded photographically five times during slight voluntary activity of the muscle under examination, and their amplitude and duration are measured. The data are then compared to the values obtained from the corresponding muscle in age-matched normal subjects examined in the same laboratory under the same conditions and with the same recording electrode and arrangements. The method has been used in a number of clinical contexts by different workers, but it is time-consuming and provides information concerning primarily the motor unit potentials activated during slight effort.

Motor Unit Territory

The distribution of potentials containing spikes from a single motor unit can be measured by inserting two multielectrodes at right angles to each other across the muscle. Recordings are then made at intervals along the length of each electrode. The motor unit territory in limb muscles is roughly circular in area, and normally has a diameter of between 5 and 7 mm in the upper extremities, and 7 and 10 mm in the lower (Buchthal, Erminio, and Rosenfalck, 1959). The density of active muscle fibers is held to be reflected by the amplitude of the largest spikes recorded in this way. Motor unit territory is increased by up to about 40 percent in patients with neurogenic weakness, due presumably—at least in part—to reinnervation of denervated muscle fibers by collateral sprouting from surviving axons. In contrast, motor unit territory is often reduced in patients with such myopathic disorders as muscular dystrophy and polymyositis, due to loss of some of the muscle fibers from individual units (Erminio, Buchthal, and Rosenfalck, 1959; Buchthal, Rosenfalck, and Erminio, 1960).

Integration

A number of workers have been concerned with integration of the electromyogram. Basmajian et al (1975) have critically reviewed such studies and the often unwarranted conclusions that have been drawn from them, stressing some of their technical and other inadequacies. At the present time, such sophisticated approaches have little relevance to the clinician in a diagnostic situation, and will not be discussed further.

Frequency Analysis

Automatic methods of frequency analysis have been used in the diagnosis of muscle disease by several workers. Richardson (1951) described a method of analysis in which the amount of activity at or above 400 Hz in a full interference pattern was compared to that below 400 Hz, and showed a shift to the higher frequencies in myopathies. Walton (1952) used an audiofrequency spectrometer for more detailed frequency analysis of the full interference pattern. The apparatus consisted of 27 resonant circuits which were tuned to different frequencies throughout the range of 40 to 16,000 Hz. Upon contraction of the muscles, the storage condensors in the filter circuits for each of the frequencies were charged in proportion to the amount of activity of that frequency appearing in the wave forms being analyzed. These currents were then fed into a cathode ray oscilloscope for display. Walton found that in the electromyograms of normal control subjects activity was confined to the frequency bands below 800 Hz in the major limb muscles, the peak frequency being at 100 to 200 Hz, while in 98 of 100 patients with muscular dystrophy there was a shift of the dominant frequency to higher values. In a critical evaluation of this method, Fex and Krakau (1957) obtained similar results to those of Walton but concluded that the method was of limited diagnostic value in itself.

Estimation of Motor Unit Number

McComas and a number of other workers have attempted to estimate the number of motor units in the extensor digitorum brevis and other limb muscles on the basis of the amplitude of the compound muscle action potentials recorded by surface electrodes following nerve stimulation (McComas et al, 1971; Brown, 1972; Sica et al, 1974). Successive motor units are recruited singly by grading the intensity of the electrical stimulus to the nerve, as illustrated in Figure 6.11, so that the mean motor unit potential amplitude can be calculated. The response of all the motor units in the muscle is then evoked by a maximal nerve stimulus, and the number of units within the muscle is determined by division. The method depends on a number of questionable underlying assumptions

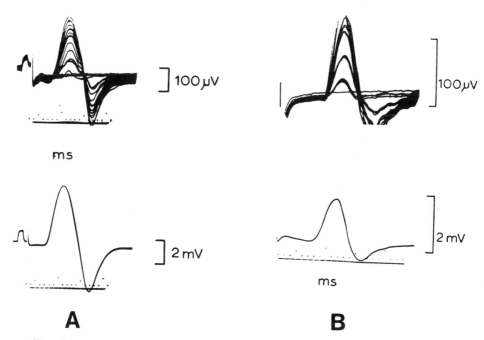

Fig. 6.11. *Action potentials in extensor digitorum brevis evoked by stimulation of the anterior tibial nerve in (A) control subject, and (B) a 16-year-old boy with Duchenne dystrophy. In both instances the upper records display superimposed traces of responses as stimulus intensity was gradually increased above threshold; the incremental nature of the potentials is clearly seen. The lower records show the responses to supramaximal stimuli (from McComas, A. J., Sica, R. E. P. and Currie, S. 1970. Nature, 226, 1263.)*

(Brown and Milner-Brown, 1976), and has been criticized on a number of other grounds (for example, by Panayiotopoulos, Scarpalezos, and Papapetropoulos, 1974) but in particular as to whether it is sensitive enough to distinguish the small motor units that can occur in myopathic disorders. Despite these objections, McComas and his colleagues have concluded that conditions such as the muscular dystrophies, previously regarded as primary degenerative disorders of muscle, are neurogenic in origin, because they found an apparent reduction in the number of motor units contained in muscle (McComas, Campbell, and Sica, 1971; McComas, Sica, and Currie, 1971; Sica and McComas, 1971).

More recently, Ballantyne and Hansen (1974a) have described a modification of the method, incorporating on-line computer analysis, which is said to be a more sensitive means of estimating the number of motor units in muscle, especially when the configuration of motor unit potentials is qualitatively altered from normal. They reported normal numbers of motor units in the muscles of patients with Duchenne, limb-girdle, and facioscapulohumeral muscular dystrophy, but significantly reduced numbers in patients with myotonic dystrophy (Ballantyne and Hansen, 1974b). The method of McComas and his colleagues has also been modified by Milner-Brown and Brown (1976) to correct for fluctuations in the response of motor units to electrical excitation, and for any overlap in the firing levels of motor axons. By this means, they found that previous estimates of the number of motor units in a muscle were generally too high, and concluded that a number of problems still remained to be solved before electrophysiologic methods could reliably be used to make such estimates.

Single Fiber Electromyography

Single fiber electromyography is a particularly exciting, new quantitative approach to the subject. The technical details of the procedure are discussed at length by Ekstedt and Stålberg (1973), to whose paper the interested reader is referred. In brief, muscle fiber action potentials are recorded from a needle electrode which has one or several electrode surfaces mounted in its side, and which is inserted into the muscle while the latter is under slight voluntary activation. The potentials have a constant shape for consecutive discharges, provided that the time resolution of the display is 10 μsec. They are essentially biphasic, and often are followed by a small, long-duration terminal phase. They are usually 5 to 10 mV in amplitude and have a total duration of less than 1 msec, and the rise time of the positive-negative deflection is less than 200 μsec. With the electrode appropriately positioned, activity is usually recorded from only one muscle fiber in an individual motor unit. In a certain number of cases, however, activity can be recorded from two or more muscle fibers belonging to the same motor unit. In such circumstances the time interval between the recorded action potentials depends on differences in conduction time along the nerve and muscle fibers, and on the anatomic localization of motor end-plates. A temporal variability, the jitter, is found between the two action potentials at consecutive discharges, and this is due mainly to variation in the neuromuscular transmission time in the two motor end-plates involved. The jitter can be expressed numerically as the mean value of consecutive differences (MCD) of 200 to 500 interpotential intervals, and is normally between 5 and 50 μsec depending on the muscle examined. Its value does not depend upon the recording site, suggesting that variability in the conduction velocity of muscle or nerve fibers contributes only a minor proportion of the jitter.

Measurement of jitter is a sensitive means of evaluating neuromuscular transmission. When there is uncertain transmission in the terminal nerve twigs or immature motor end-plates, such as occurs following reinnervation, jitter is increased and there may be a partial or total conduction block. In patients with myasthenia gravis, increased jitter and impulse blocking are the expected findings (Fig. 6.12), especially in muscles that clinically are affected. In patients

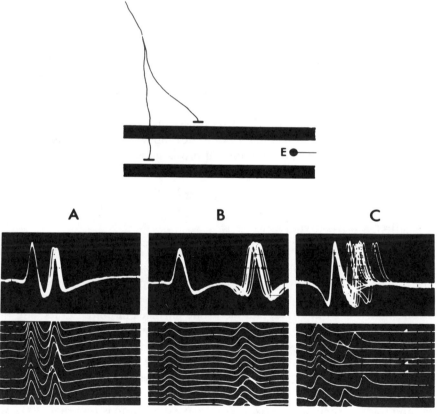

Fig. 6.12. *The Jitter. Electrode E is recording activity from two muscle fibers belonging to the same motor unit. A represents a recording from a normal muscle, B and C from a myasthenic. The oscilloscope sweep is triggered by the first action potential and interval variability between the potentials is seen as a variable position of the second potential. In the upper row 10–15 action potentials are superimposed. In the lower row the oscilloscope sweep is moved downwards. There is normal jitter in A, increased jitter but no impulse blockings in B, and increased jitter and occasional blockings (arrows) in C. Calibration 500 μsec (from Stålberg, E. 1974. Single fiber electromyography, Disa electronics).*

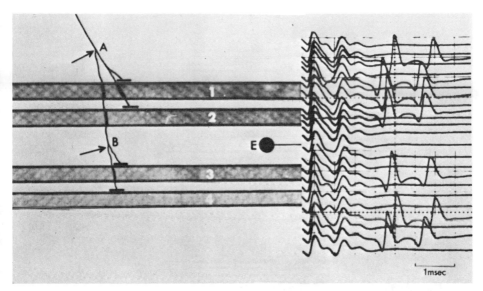

Fig. 6.13. *Schematic drawing of recording from four muscle fibers innervated by the same nerve axon—two of them (three and four) by a sprout branching off in A. To the right an original recording from the electrode E of mainly four potentials, two of them blocking together (three and four). They behave as a unit which also has a large jitter in relation to the rest of the action potential complex (from Stålberg, E. and Thiele, B. 1972. J. Neurol. Neurosurg. Psychiatry, 35, 52).*

with myopathy, a slight increase in jitter may be seen in 10 to 15 percent of the recordings and blockings may be found in 5 to 10 percent (Stålberg and Ekstedt, 1973). Jitter is normal in myotonia congenita but is increased in myotonic dystrophy. In neurogenic disorders, the jitter is markedly increased and frequent blocking is found. When recordings are made from three or more muscle fibers at the same time, it is sometimes apparent that two or more of the components will only block together, and they show a common large jitter in relation to the rest of the action potential complex as can be seen in Fig. 6.13. This is due to impaired or blocked transmission in the distal axonal branch supplying the muscle fibers whose action potentials are affected in this way (Stålberg and Ekstedt, 1973).

Single fiber electromyography can also provide an estimate of mean fiber density of motor units. The electrode is positioned so that a muscle fiber action potential is recorded at maximal amplitude. This action potential is then made to trigger the oscilloscope sweep, and the number of synchronous action potentials that are larger than 200 μV and have a rise time of less than 300 μsec is counted for this particular electrode position. In order to obtain a measure of fiber density in the motor units of the muscle under examination, the process is then repeated for at least 20 different positions of the recording electrode, and the mean number of responses is calculated. The number of fiber potentials

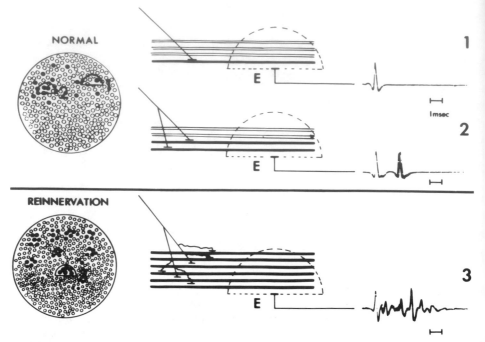

Fig. 6.14. *Single fiber EMG recordings in normal and reinnervated muscle. The diagram illustrates the number of muscle fibers of one motor unit (blackened). The uptake area of the recording electrode is represented as the half circle and E. In the normal (1 and 2) only action potentials from one or two fibers are recorded. In reinnervation (3) many fiber action potentials are recorded due to increased fiber density in the motor unit (right part of figure) (from Hakelius, L. and Stålberg, E. 1974. Scand. J. Plast. Reconstr. Surg., 8, 211).*

recorded with random electrode placements in this way normally averages 1.4 to 1.5, and seldom is it possible to record from three or more muscle fibers belonging to the same motor unit in any one electrode position. After reinnervation, however, fiber density is increased due to collateral sprouting and it may be possible to record potentials from up to about 10 fibers of the same motor unit with the electrode in one position, as shown in Figure 6.14.

Analysis of the Pattern of Electrical Activity of Muscle

Quantitative analysis of the pattern of electrical activity of muscle during contraction against a standard load (usually of 2 kg, as shown in Figure 6.15) has been used to distinguish between patients with myopathy and normal subjects. Fitch and Willison (1965) measured those features of an interference pattern which are usually evaluated subjectively by converting the EMG into two serial pulse trains. As can be seen in Figure 6.16, a turn pulse was generated each time the EMG signal changed its direction from positive to negative or vice versa, provided that the deflection exceeded a certain level of significance (usually 100 μV), and an amplitude pulse was generated whenever the potential between each turn in the signal reached 100 μV, irrespective of the direction of potential change. The two pulse trains were counted over specified intervals to determine the number of spikes (turns) for each 5-second period, the amplitude of the potential changes between spikes, and the distribution of time intervals between spikes. A small computer was used for more detailed analysis (Dowling, Fitch, and Willison, 1968).

The application of the method to the diagnosis of myopathic disorders has been described by Rose and Willison (1967). The characteristic finding is an increase in the mean turns count as might be expected from the shortened duration of motor unit potentials. In patients with chronic partial denervation, Hayward and Willison (1973, 1977) found that a change in mean amplitude between turns was characteristic, while there was no significant change in the mean spike count. This was attributed to an increase in the density of muscle fibers in individual motor units due to reinnervation.

Fuglsang-Frederiksen and Månsson (1975) have analyzed, by a similar technique, the electrical activity of muscle at different degrees of voluntary activity. They measured the activity during contractions against a load related to the subject's maximal voluntary effort, rather than against a fixed load, and

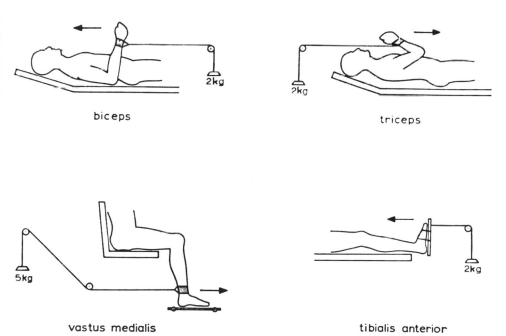

Fig. 6.15. Arrangement of the patient for quantitative analysis of the pattern of electrical activity of muscle as performed by Willison and his colleagues (from Hayward, M. and Willison, R. G. 1973. New Developments in Electromyography and Clinical Neurophysiology, Desmedt, J. E., Ed., vol. 2, p. 448, S. Karger, Basel).

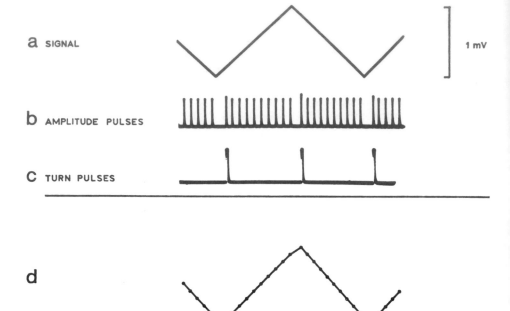

a SIGNAL   1 mV

b AMPLITUDE PULSES

c TURN PULSES

d

Fig. 6.16. Oscilloscope tracings of a, calibration signal; b, and c, outputs of pulse generators. A reconstruction of the signal, d, was obtained by plotting the information given by the pulse trains (from Hayward, M. and Willison, R. G. 1973. New Developments in Electromyography and Clinical Neurophysiology, Desmedt, J. E., Ed., vol. 2, p. 448, S. Karger, Basel).

found that a force of 2 kg resulted in a lower number of turns when subjects were capable of high maximum force than when the maximum force that they could generate was low. If subjects exerted the same relative force, however, the number of turns was independent of maximum force. They concluded, therefore, that a fixed relative force (e.g. 30 percent maximum) was less likely to give false positive data or to obscure abnormalities than a fixed absolute load.

When the pattern of electrical activity was analyzed during a force which was a fixed fraction (30 percent) of maximum in 41 patients with myopathy, the ratio of number of turns in 5 seconds to mean amplitude between turns gave a diagnostic yield of 70 percent. The yield was increased to 87 percent when abnormalities in the number of turns per 5 seconds, the incidence of short time intervals between turns, and mean amplitude were included. In the same muscles, measurement of the mean duration of motor unit potentials during weak effort enabled a diagnosis of myopathy to be made in 60 percent of the patients, while if attention was also directed at the number of polyphasic potentials the diagnosis was made in 89 percent of cases. The two methods supplemented each other, as in some instances the myopathy could only be identified by one or other of the two procedures (Fuglsang-Frederiksen, Scheel, and Buchthal, 1976).

Patients with neurogenic weakness were investigated in a later study by these same authors (Fuglsang-Frederiksen, Scheel, and Buchthal, 1977), who again found that the best diagnostic yield from the pattern of electrical activity was obtained when the force was 30 percent of maximum. The number of spikes (turns) per 5 seconds was diminished in 70 percent of their patients, and this was attributed mainly to a prolongation in the duration of motor unit potentials. They also found an increased incidence of long duration intervals between turns, and an increased amplitude between turns.

REFERENCES

Aberfeld, D. C., Namba, T., Vye, M. V., and Grob, D. (1970). Chondrodystrophic myotonia: a report of two cases. Arch. Neurol., *22:*455.

Adrian, E. D. and Bronk, D. W. (1929). The discharge of impulses in motor nerve fibres. Part II. J. Physiol., *67:*119.

Aminoff, M. J. (1978). Electromyography in Clinical Practice. Addison-Wesley, Menlo Park.

Ballantyne, J. P. and Hansen, S. (1974a). A new method for the estimation of the number of motor units in a muscle. 1. Control subjects and patients with myasthenia gravis. J. Neurol. Neurosurg. Psychiatry, *37:*907.

Ballantyne, J. P. and Hansen, S. (1974b). New method for the estimation of the number of motor units in a muscle. 2. Duchenne, limb-girdle and facioscapulohumeral, and myotonic muscular dystrophies. J. Neurol. Neurosurg. Psychiatry, *37:*1195.

Basmajian, J. V., Clifford, H. C., McLeod, W. D., and Nunnally, H. N. (1975). Computers in Electromyography. Butterworths, London.

Borenstein, S. and Desmedt, J. E. (1973). Electromyographical signs of collateral reinnervation. In: New Developments in Electromyography and Clinical Neurophysiology, Vol. 1, Desmedt, J. E., Ed., p. 130, Karger, Basel.

Brown, W. F. (1972). A method for estimating the number of motor units in thenar muscles and the changes in motor unit count with ageing. J. Neurol. Neurosurg. Psychiatry, *35:*845.

Brown, W. F. and Milner-Brown, H. S. (1976). Some electrical properties of motor units . . . . J. Neurol. Neurosurg. Psychiatry, *39:*249.

Buchthal, F. (1962). The electromyogram. Its value in the diagnosis of neuromuscular disorders. World Neurology, *3:*16.

Buchthal, F. and Pinelli, P. (1953a). Muscle action potentials in polymyositis. Neurology, *3:*424.

Buchthal, F. and Pinelli, P. (1953b). Action potentials in muscular atrophy of neurogenic origin. Neurology, *3:*591.

Buchthal, F. and Rosenfalck, P. (1963). Electrophysiological aspects of myopathy with particular reference to progressive muscular dystrophy. In: Muscular Dystrophy in Man and Animals, Bourne, G. W. and Golarz, M. N., Eds., p. 193. Karger, Basel.

Buchthal, F. and Rosenfalck, P. (1966). Spontaneous electrical activity of human muscle. Electroencephalogr. Clin. Neurophysiol., *20:*321.

Buchthal, F., Engbaek, L., and Gamstorp, I. (1958). Paresis and hyperexcitability in adynamia episodica hereditaria. Neurology, *8:*347.

Buchthal, F., Erminio, F., and Rosenfalck, P. (1959). Motor unit territory in different human muscles. Acta Physiol. Scand., *45:*72.

Buchthal, F., Rosenfalck, P., and Erminio, F. (1960). Motor unit territory and fiber density in myopathies. Neurology, *10:*398.

Bundey, S., Carter, C. O., and Soothill, J. F. (1970). Early recognition of heterozygotes for the gene for dystrophia myotonica. J. Neurol. Neurosurg. Psychiatry, *33:*279.

Campbell, E. D. R. and Montuschi, E. (1960). Muscle weakness caused by bretylium tosylate. Lancet, *2:*789.

Caruso, G. and Buchthal, F. (1965). Refractory period of muscle and electromyographic findings in relatives of patients with muscular dystrophy. Brain, *88:*29.

Denny-Brown, D. and Foley, J. M. (1948). Myokymia and the benign fasciculation of muscular cramps. Trans. Assoc. Am. Physicians, *61:*88.

Denny-Brown, D. and Pennybacker, J. B. (1938). Fibrillation and fasciculation in voluntary muscle. Brain, *61:*311.

Desmedt, J. E. and Borenstein, S. (1976). Regeneration in Duchenne muscular dystrophy. Electromyographic evidence. Arch. Neurol. *33:*642.

Dowling, M. H., Fitch, P., and Willison, R. G. (1968). A special purpose digital computer (Biomac 500) used in the analysis of the human electromyogram. Electroencephalogr. Clin. Neurophysiol., *25:*570.

Doyle, A. M. and Mayer, R. F. (1969). Studies of the motor unit in the cat. A preliminary report. Bull. School of Med., Univ. of Maryland, *54:*11.

Ekstedt, J. and Stålberg, E. (1973). Single fibre electromyography for the study of microphysiology of the human muscle. In: New Developments in Electromyography and Clinical Neurophysiology, Vol. 1, Desmedt, J. E., Ed., p. 89, Karger, Basel.

Engel, A. G. (1970). Acid maltase deficiency in adults: studies in four cases of a syndrome which may mimic muscular dystrophy or other myopathies. Brain, *93:*599.

Engel, W. K. (1975). Brief, small, abundant motor-unit action potentials: a further critique of electromyographic interpretation. Neurology, *25:*173.

Erminio, F., Buchthal, F., and Rosenfalck, P. (1959). Motor unit territory and muscle fiber concentration in paresis due to peripheral nerve injury and anterior horn cell involvement. Neurology, *9:*657.

Fex, J. and Krakau, C. E. T. (1957). Some experiences with Walton's frequency analysis of the electromyogram. J. Neurol. Neurosurg. Psychiatry, *20:*178.

Fitch, P. and Willison, R. G. (1965). Automatic measurement of the human electromyogram. J. Physiol., *178:*28P.

Forster, F. M., Borkowski, W. J., and Alpers, B. J. (1946). Effects of denervation on fasciculations in human muscle. Arch. Neurol. Psychiatry, *56:*276.

Fuglsang-Frederiksen, A. and Månsson, A. (1975). Analysis of electrical activity of normal muscle in man at different degrees of voluntary effort. J. Neurol. Neurosurg. Psychiatry, *38:*683.

Fuglsang-Frederiksen, A., Scheel, U., and Buchthal, F. (1976). Diagnostic yield of analysis of the pattern of electrical activity and of individual motor unit potentials in myopathy. J. Neurol. Neurosurg. Psychiatry, *39:*742.

Fuglsang-Frederiksen, A., Scheel, U., and Buchthal, F. (1977). Diagnostic yield of the analysis of the pattern of electrical activity of muscle and of individual motor unit potentials in neurogenic involvement. J. Neurol. Neurosurg. Psychiatry, *40:*544.

Gardner-Medwin, D. (1968). Studies of the carrier state in the Duchenne type of muscular dystrophy. 2. Quantitative electromyography as a method of carrier detection. J. Neurol. Neurosurg. Psychiatry, *31:*124.

Gardner-Medwin, D. and Walton, J. N. (1969). Myokymia with impaired muscular relaxation. Lancet, *1:*127.

Gilliatt, R. W., Le Quesne, P. M., Logue, V., and Sumner, A. J. (1970). Wasting of the hand associated with a cervical rib or band. J. Neurol. Neurosurg. Psychiatry, *33:*615.

Guld, C., Rosenfalck, A., and Willison, R. G. (1970). Report of the Committee on EMG instrumentation. Technical factors in recording electrical activity of muscle and nerve in man. Electroencephalogr. Clin. Neurophysiol., *28:*399.

Hayward, M. and Willison, R. G. (1973). The recognition of myogenic and neurogenic lesions by quantitative EMG. In: New Developments in Electromyography and Clinical Neurophysiology, Vol. 2, Desmedt, J. E., Ed., p. 448. Karger, Basel.

Hayward, M. and Willison, R. G. (1977). Automatic analysis of the electromyogram in patients with chronic partial denervation. J. Neurol. Sci., *33:*415.

Hjorth, R. J. and Willison, R. G. (1973). The electromyogram in facial myokymia and hemifacial spasm. J. Neurol. Sci., *20:*117.

Isaacs, H. (1967). Continuous muscle fibre activity in an Indian male with additional evidence of terminal motor fibre abnormality. J. Neurol. Neurosurg. Psychiatry, *30:*126.

Jones, R. V., Lambert, E. H., and Sayre, G. P. (1955). Source of a type of "insertion activity" in electromyography with evaluation of a histologic method of localization. Arch. Phys. Med. Rehabil., *36:*301.

Kontos, H. A. (1962). Myopathy associated with chronic colchicine toxicity. New Engl. J. Med., *266:*38.

Kugelberg, E. (1947). Electromyograms in muscular disorders. J. Neurol. Neurosurg. Psychiatry, *10:*123.

Kugelberg, E. (1948). Activation of human nerves by ischemia. Trousseau's phenomenon in tetany. Arch. Neurol. Psychiatry, *60:*140.

Lambert, E. H., Love, J. G., and Mulder, D. W. (1961). Facial myokymia and brain tumor: electromyographic studies. Newsletter. Am. Assoc. Electromyography and Electrodiagnosis, *8:*8.

Landau, W. H. (1952). The essential mechanism in myotonia. An electromyographic study. Neurology, *2:*369.

Layzer, R. B., Lovelace, R. E., and Rowland, L. P. (1967). Hyperkalemic periodic paralysis. Arch. Neurol., *16:*455.

Layzer, R. B., Rowland, L. P., and Ranney, H. M. (1967). Muscle phosphofructokinase deficiency. Arch. Neurol., *17:*512.

Li, C.-L., Shy, G. M., and Wells, J. (1957). Some properties of mammalian skeletal muscle fibres with particular reference to fibrillation potentials. J. Physiol., *135:*522.

McArdle, B. (1951). Myopathy due to a defect in muscle glycogen breakdown. Clin. Science, *10:*13.

McComas, A. J., Campbell, M. J., and Sica, R. E. P. (1971). Electrophysiological study of dystrophia myotonica. J. Neurol. Neurosurg. Psychiatry, *34:*132.

McComas, A. J., Sica, R. E. P., and Currie, S. (1971). An electrophysiological study of Duchenne dystrophy. J. Neurol. Neurosurg. Psychiatry, *34:*461.

McComas, A. J., Fawcett, P. R. W., Campbell, M. J., and Sica, R. E. P. (1971). Electrophysiological estimation of the number of motor units within a human muscle. J. Neurol. Neurosurg. Psychiatry, *34:*121.

Milner-Brown, H. S. and Brown, W. F. (1976). New methods of estimating the number of motor units in a muscle. J. Neurol. Neurosurg. Psychiatry, *39:*258.

Ozker, R. R., Schumacher, O. P., and Nelson, P. A. (1960). Electromyographic findings in adults with myxedema: report of 16 cases. Arch. Phys. Med. Rehabil., *41:*299.

Panayiotopoulos, C. P., Scarpalezos, S., and Papapetropoulos, Th. (1974). Electrophysiological estimation of motor units in Duchenne muscular dystrophy. J. Neurol. Sci., *23:*89.

Petajan, J. H. (1974). Clinical electromyographic studies of diseases of the motor unit. Electroencephalogr. Clin. Neurophysiol., *36:*395.

Pickett, J. B. (1978). Late components of motor unit potentials in a patient with myoglobinuria. Ann. Neurol., *3:*461.

Polgar, J. G., Bradley, W. G., Upton, A. R. M., Anderson, J., Howat, J. M. L., Petito, F., Roberts, D. F., and Scopa, J. (1972). The early detection of dystrophia myotonica. Brain, *95:*761.

Purves, D. and Sakmann, B. (1974). Membrane properties underlying spontaneous activity of denervated muscle fibres. J. Physiol., *239:*125.

Richardson, A. T. (1951). Newer concepts in electrodiagnosis. St. Thomas Hospital Reports, *7:*164.

Rose, A. L. and Willison, R. G. (1967). Quantitative electromyography using automatic analysis: studies in healthy subjects and patients with primary muscle disease. J. Neurol. Neurosurg. Psychiatry, *30:*403.

Ross, G. T., Scholz, D. A., Lambert, E. H., and Geraci, J. E. (1958). Severe uterine bleeding and degenerative skeletal-muscle changes in unrecognized myxedema. J. Clin. Endocrinol. Metab., *18:*492.

Rowland, L. P. and Greer, M. (1961). Toxoplasmic polymyositis. Neurology, *11:*367.

Shy, G. M., Wanko, T., Rowley, P. T., and Engel, A. G. 1961. Studies in familial periodic paralysis. Exp. Neurol., *3:*53.

Sica, R. E. P. and McComas, A. J. (1971). An electrophysiological investigation of limb-girdle and facioscapulohumeral dystrophy. J. Neurol. Neurosurg. Psychiatry, *34:*469.

Sica, R. E. P., McComas, A. J., Upton, A. R. M., and Longmire, D. (1974). Motor unit estimations in small muscles of the hand. J. Neurol. Neurosurg. Psychiatry, *37:*55.

Smith, J. W. and Thesleff, S. (1976). Spontaneous activity in denervated mouse diaphragm muscle. J. Physiol., *257:*171.

Stålberg, E. and Ekstedt, J. (1973). Single fibre EMG and microphysiology of the motor unit in normal and diseased human muscle. In: New Developments in Electromyography and Clinical Neurophysiology, Vol. 1, Desmedt, J. E., Ed., p. 113, S. Karger, Basel.

Swaiman, K. F., Kennedy, W. R., and Sauls, H. S. (1968). Late infantile acid maltase deficiency. Arch. Neurol., *18:*642.

Thesleff, S. and Ward, M. R. (1975). Studies on the mechanism of fibrillation potentials in denervated muscle. J. Physiol., *244:*313.

Van den Bosch, J. (1963). Investigations of the carrier state in the Duchenne type dystrophy. In: Research in Muscular Dystrophy. Proc. 2nd Symp. Current Research in Muscular Dystrophy, Ed. Members of the Research Committee of the Muscular Dystrophy Group, p. 23, Pitman Medical, London.

Waldstein, S. S., Bronsky, D., Shrifter, H. B., and Oester, Y. T. (1958). The electromyogram in myxedema. Arch. Intern. Med., *101:*97.

Walton, J. N. (1952). The electromyogram in myopathy: analysis with the audiofrequency spectrometer. J. Neurol. Neurosurg. Psychiatry, *15:*219.

Waylonis, G. W. and Johnson, E. W. (1964). The electromyogram in acute trichinosis: report of four cases. Arch. Phys. Med. Rehabil., *45:*177.

Wettstein, A. (1977). The origin of fasciculations in motoneuron disease. Neurology, *27:*357.

Willison, R. G. (1967). Quantitative electromyography. The detection of carriers of Duchenne dystrophy. In: Progress in Neuro-Genetics, Vol. 1, Proc. 2nd Int. Cong. Neuro-Genetics and Neuro-Ophthalmology of the World Federation of Neurology, Barbeau, A. and Brunette, J. R., Eds., Excerpta Medica International Congress Series, No. 175, p. 123, Excerpta Medica Foundation, Amsterdam.

Whisnant, J. P., Espinosa, R. E., Kierland, R. R., and Lambert, E. H. (1963). Chloroquine neuromyopathy. Proc. Staff Meetings of Mayo Clinic, *38:*501.

7
Nerve Conduction Studies

JASPER R. DAUBE

INTRODUCTION

Nerve conduction studies assess peripheral motor and sensory function by recording the evoked response to stimulation of peripheral nerves. Motor nerve conduction studies require stimulation of a peripheral nerve, while recording from a muscle innervated by that nerve. Sensory nerve conduction studies are performed by stimulating a mixed nerve and recording from a cutaneous nerve, or by stimulating a cutaneous nerve and recording from a mixed or cutaneous nerve. Both motor and sensory nerve conduction studies have been used clinically for many years to locate peripheral nerve disease within single nerves and along the length of nerves, and to differentiate these disorders from diseases of the muscle or neuromuscular junction. Nerve conduction studies also can help distinguish axonal degeneration, segmental demyelination, and abnormal nerve irritability.

Motor nerve conduction studies were first described for clinical use by Hodes, Larrabee, and German in 1948. Subsequent studies defined normal values (Magladery and McDougal, 1950; Wagman and Lesse, 1952; Wagner and Buchthal, 1972) and the abnormalities seen in clinical disorders (Lambert, 1960, 1962), and have expanded steadily in application since then. Sensory nerve conduction studies were initially demonstrated by Dawson and Scott in 1949, and were shown to be of clinical value in 1958 by Gilliatt and Sears. Adequate assessment of any neuromuscular disease requires the combined application of a careful clinical evaluation, the needle examination as described in the previous chapter, and the nerve conduction studies described in this chapter.

MOTOR NERVE CONDUCTION STUDIES

The function of motor axons in any peripheral nerve innervating somatic muscle can be evaluated by motor nerve conduction studies, if the nerve can be stimulated and the response by one or more of the muscles that it innervates can be recorded electrically. Standard studies of motor nerve conduction assess the most accessible nerves—the ulnar and median nerves in the upper extremities, and the tibial and peroneal nerves in the lower extremities. Reliable motor nerve conduction studies can also be performed on the musculocutaneous, radial, facial, femoral, and phrenic nerves, but with increasing technical difficulty. Electrical studies of the axillary, suprascapular, and intercostal nerves are even more difficult and are rarely used clinically.

Stimulation of any of these nerves evokes both an electrical and a mechanical response in those muscles innervated by the nerve distal to the site of stimulation. The mechanical response, or muscle twitch, is not recorded in standard clinical nerve conduction studies, but it may be measured for strength-duration curves or other special studies. The electrical response is called the *compound muscle action potential* (Fig. 7.1), and is the summated electrical activity of the muscle fibers in the region of the recording electrode that are innervated by the nerve. The general techniques of stimulating and recording are similar for each of the nerves.

Stimulation

Nerve stimulation is most readily achieved with surface electrodes placed over a nerve where it is relatively superficial, such as over the ulnar nerve at the wrist and elbow. If there is overlying edema or fatty tissue, or if the nerve is deep, a needle electrode will permit more precise stimulation of the nerve, although carrying the risk of trauma or infection.

The standard stimulus is a square-wave pulse of current passing between two poles, the cathode (−) and anode (+). In the usual studies, the cathode is closer to the recording electrodes than the anode, because the cathode activates by depolarizing, and the anode may block conduction in some axons by hyperpolarization. A gradually increasing stimulus voltage results in a progressive increase in size of the compound muscle action potential as more and more axons in the nerve are activated. While large, low-threshold axons should be stimulated initially, variations in location of fascicles, as well as in patterns of current flow, often result in initial activation of smaller axons with slower conduction. The threshold of activation is too variable to allow selective measurement of slow-conducting fibers, and standard nerve conduction studies using a supramaximal stimulus therefore assess only the fast-conducting fibers. The supramaximal stimulus is generally selected to be one-third greater than that required to obtain the maximal amplitude response, in order to ensure that all fibers are activated. A stimulus of 100 V and of 0.1 msec duration is usually adequate, but abnormal nerves may require a stimulus of as much as 300 V for 0.5 msec. Such large stimuli may produce an error by inadvertently stimulating other nearby nerves.

Recording

The compound muscle action potential is recorded using electrodes placed in or near a muscle or group of muscles innervated by the nerve. Recordings are often made from one muscle innervated by the nerve and, therefore, will assess only the axons innervating that muscle. For instance, motor conduction of the

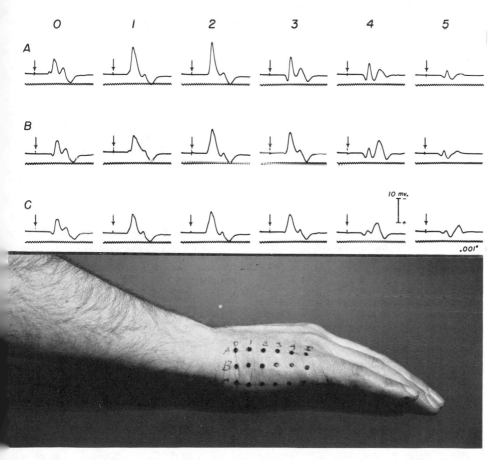

Fig. 7.1. *Compound muscle action potentials on ulnar nerve stimulation* (top tracings) *recorded at different locations of the G1 recording electrode* (bottom).

ulnar nerve is commonly tested by recordings from the hypothenar muscles, and selective damage to the axons innervating either the flexor carpi ulnaris muscle or the first dorsal interosseous muscle would, therefore, not be identified unless recordings were also made from those muscles.

Standard anatomic locations of recording electrodes provide reproducible potentials that can be compared with normal values. Measurements of an evoked response are most reliable when recordings are made over the end-plate region of the muscle, near the middle of the muscle belly. Recordings are made using a bipolar derivation, with an active (G1) electrode over the end-plate region and a reference (G2) electrode over the tendon. Because muscles vary widely in length, accurate amplitude recordings require different G1-to-G2 distances for muscles of different sizes.

Recordings may be made using surface or needle electrodes. Surface electrodes provide the advantage of nontraumatic recordings and less risk of infection, particularly in patients with hepatitis or Creutzfeldt-Jakob disease. Surface electrodes also can be more readily repositioned to obtain the maximal response. Needle electrodes have a somewhat higher impedance, but they can be fixed in a more stable position; and when placed in the subcutaneous tissue immediately adjacent to the muscle, they provide a more accurate reflection of the size of the compound muscle action potential than do surface electrodes, which may be a distance from the muscle. Needle electrodes within muscle are less reliable because of an unstable configuration and amplitude of the evoked response during muscle movement. However, intramuscular electrodes can record from a more limited area of the muscle and may be of value in assessing individual motor branches of a nerve or an anomalous pattern of innervation.

Measurements

The directly evoked compound muscle action potential recorded after stimulation of a peripheral nerve is called an *M wave*. With supramaximal stimulation, all the fibers in a muscle innervated by the nerve contribute to the potential. The earliest component is elicited by the fastest conducting motor axons. The M wave is described by its latency, amplitude, and configuration. The *latency* is the time in milliseconds from the application of a stimulus to the initial deflection from the baseline, and is the time required for the action potentials in the fastest conducting fibers to reach the nerve terminals and activate the muscle fibers (Fig. 7.2). The latency of the evoked response includes the time required for the stimulus to activate an action potential in the underlying nerve, and the time for neuromuscular transmission to activate the muscle fiber action potentials, as well as time for the action potential to travel from the site of stimulation to the nerve terminal. The latency varies directly with the distance of the stimulating electrode from the muscle.

The area of the negative phase of the action potential is directly proportional to the number of the muscle fibers depolarized, but it is also dependent on the distance of the muscle from the recording electrodes. Area is difficult to measure, and a measurement of amplitude can serve the same purpose if the dura-

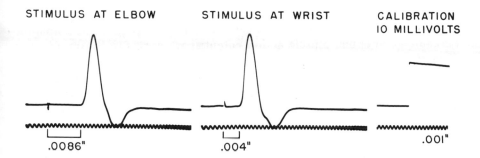

STIMULUS AT ELBOW   STIMULUS AT WRIST   CALIBRATION
10 MILLIVOLTS

.0086"   .004"   .001"

CONDUCTION TIME, elbow to wrist   .0086 — .004 =   .0046 SECONDS
CONDUCTION DISTANCE, elbow to wrist   .245   METERS
CONDUCTION VELOCITY   .245 ÷ .0046 = 53 METERS/SECOND

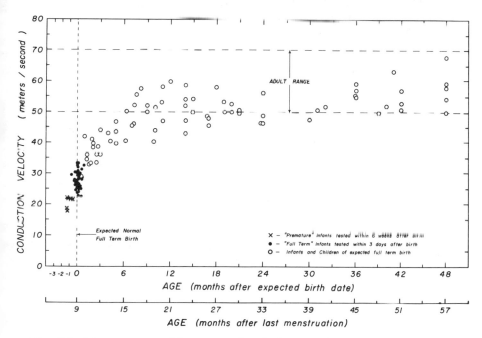

Fig. 7.2. *Measurement of latency and calculation of conduction velocity in ulnar nerve recording hypothenar muscle action potential* (top tracing) *and the change with age in children* (bottom) (*modified from Thomas, J. E., and Lambert, E. H. 1960. Ulnar nerve conduction velocity and H-reflex in infants and children. J. Appl. Physiol., 15, 1. By permission of the American Physiological Society*).

tion of the evoked response is normal. The *amplitude* of the compound muscle action potential is the height in millivolts from the baseline to the peak of the negative phase. The amplitude normally is somewhat lower with stimulation at more proximal sites, and generally ranges between 2 and 20 mV. The amplitude and area of a compound muscle action potential are normally constant in size on repeated stimulation. In the presence of disorders of neuromuscular transmission and in some disorders of nerve and muscle, consecutive evoked responses may show changes in their amplitude, configuration, or latency on repetitive stimulation, by either an increment or decrement in the evoked response. Such changes are dependent on the rate of stimulation and are discussed in Chapter 8.

The duration of the response is the time in milliseconds from the onset to the end of the initial negative phase of the potential. The duration reflects the synchrony of discharge of the individual muscle fibers; that is, when the muscle fibers are discharged in near synchrony, the action potential is of shorter duration. If the conduction velocities vary widely among different axons, some muscle fibers are activated earlier than others, and this results in a longer duration of the negative phase of the compound muscle action potential. The duration normally increases slightly at more proximal sites of stimulation.

The normal configuration of the compound muscle action potential recorded over the end-plate region of the muscle is biphasic, negative-positive. If the active electrode is not over the end-plate region, the potential is triphasic with an initial positivity, which makes latency measurements less accurate. Normally, only minimal changes in configuration occur at proximal sites of stimulation.

If the nerve is accessible, it is stimulated at more than one site along its course to obtain two or more evoked responses from the muscle. The latencies, amplitudes, and configurations of the evoked responses at each site are compared. The latency progressively increases at more proximal sites of stimulation, because the action potentials have to traverse longer segments of nerve. Typically, the amplitude of the response to proximal stimulation is slightly lower because the different rates of conduction within the motor axons increase the temporal dispersion of the potentials. There is usually little change in configuration of the evoked response. Measurements of the differences in distance and latency between sites of stimulation allow calculation of conduction velocity in meters per second in the intervening segment of nerve. Comparison of conduction between segments of the nerve and with normal values can localize lesions to selected areas along the length of a nerve. Normal conduction velocities in the legs range from 40 to 55 m per second, and in the arms from 50 to 70 m per second. Normal values for latency, amplitude, and conduction velocity vary with patient age and the measuring technique. Each laboratory, therefore, should determine its own normal values.

When a peripheral nerve is stimulated, in addition to the direct M response, other waveforms may be elicited. A nerve stimulus normally evokes action potentials that propagate proximally toward the anterior horn cell (antidromically), as well as peripherally to activate the muscle directly. The antidromic potentials are often blocked by hyperpolarization at the anode, but if the cathode is placed proximally, all of the motor axons can be activated antidromically. A small proportion of the anterior horn cells are activated antidromically, in either the cell body or the axon hillock, to discharge another action potential orthodromically along the axon. These recurrent discharges produce a small muscle potential after a delay of 20 to 50 msec, depending on the distance from the site of stimulation to the spinal cord. These late responses are referred to as *F waves* and were first described by Magladery and McDougal (1950) (Fig. 7.3). Individual F waves are the action potentials of a single or a few motor units. Although F waves represent only a small sampling of the axons in the nerve and have variable latencies as different axons are activated, they can provide an estimate of conduction in the central segments of motor fibers. F wave latencies are most readily performed by comparing the measured latency with normal values at the same distance. Because the major application of F waves has been the assessment of conduction in central segments, various methods of calculation have been devised to obtain estimates of conduction velocities in these segments. Each of these methods is associated with potential technical errors in measurement and calculation, and none has been shown to be of greater value than F wave latency measurements against distance (Ch. 9).

Other small electrical responses from various sources may occur after the M wave. For instance, if a few axons are conducting at a slower rate than the remainder, a small late potential may be seen after the action potential and may be time-locked to it (Fig. 7.4). Or, in some disease processes, the axon may branch in the peripheral nerve, so that stimulation distal to the site of branching produces a late response via the axon branches, as an axon reflex. This poten-

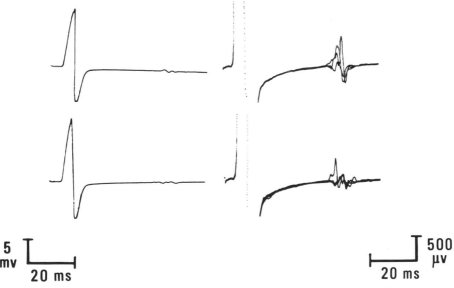

5 mv

20 ms

500 µV

20 ms

Fig. 7.3. F waves recorded from abductor hallucis brevis muscle on tibial nerve stimulation at standard (left) and high amplification (right).

STIMULATE

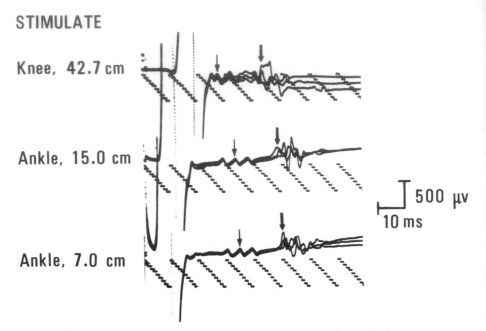

Knee, 42.7 cm

Ankle, 15.0 cm

Ankle, 7.0 cm

500 μv
10 ms

Fig. 7.4. *Late responses in abductor hallucis brevis muscle to tibial nerve stimulation.* Broad arrow *indicates F waves;* narrow arrow *indicates axon reflex.*

tial, like the F wave, becomes of shorter latency as the site of stimulation moves proximally. A third late response occurs in some diseases of peripheral nerve in which there is an unusual irritability, such as in hypocalcemia. In these diseases, the nerve and muscle discharge repetitively in response to a single stimulus.

SENSORY NERVE CONDUCTION STUDIES

Direct evaluation of sensory axons in peripheral nerves may be performed by stimulating and recording from a cutaneous nerve, recording from a cutaneous nerve while stimulating a mixed nerve, recording from a mixed nerve while stimulating a cutaneous nerve, or recording from the cerebral hemispheres while stimulating a cutaneous or mixed nerve. The potentials recorded by the latter technique are called somatosensory evoked potentials and are discussed in Chapter 13. The other methods can be readily applied to the ulnar, median, radial, plantar, and sural nerves. Sensory recordings from the musculocutaneous and peroneal nerves are more difficult, and recordings from the lateral femoral cutaneous, and saphenous nerves are not sufficiently reliable for routine clinical application. Sensory conduction studies of these nerves can add much to motor conduction studies, such as evidence of diffuse sensory fiber disorders, localized lesions involving a cutaneous nerve, or disorders that have preferentially damaged the sensory fibers in a mixed nerve. Sensory nerve conduction studies are more sensitive than motor conduction studies in detecting early or mild disorders so that they have become a necessary part of the electrophysiologic evaluation of peripheral neuromuscular disease.

Two other techniques, the blink reflex and the H reflex, indirectly assess sensory axons and are discussed in Chapter 9. In each, sensory fibers are stimulated while a reflex response mediated by the central nervous system is recorded.

Stimulation

Because the speed of conduction in axons is the same orthodromically and antidromically, action potentials may be evoked in either direction for testing sensory conduction (Fig. 7.5). Each has advantages and disadvantages that make it more appropriate for particlar clinical situations. Stimulation of a cutaneous nerve at a distal site, such as the digital nerves in a digit, produces an orthodromic nerve action potential that can be recorded over the proximal mixed nerve that it joins. Stimulation also can be applied over a mixed nerve to record an antidromic nerve action potential over the cutaneous nerve, but it is often associated with a motor response that may be difficult to distinguish from the sensory nerve action potential.

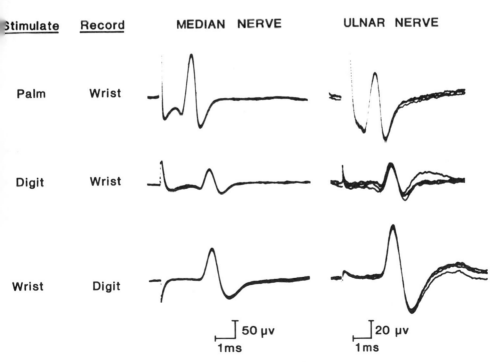

Fig. 7.5. Orthodromic and antidromic surface recordings of median sensory nerve action potentials.

Stimulation parameters for sensory nerve conduction studies are similar to those for motor studies and stimuli should again be supramaximal. The location and orientation of the stimulating electrodes are important in obtaining artifact-free recordings.

Recording

Because of their small size, compound nerve action potentials are technically more difficult to record than compound muscle action potentials. Recording electrodes placed on the surface over a mixed nerve or cutaneous nerve are most convenient, but needle recording electrodes placed near the nerve can enhance significantly the amplitude of the response. The potential typically has a positive onset and is triphasic, with a latency proportional to the distance from the stimulating electrodes and an amplitude proportional to the number of active axons, their synchrony of firing, and the distance from the nerve to the recording electrodes.

The high amplification in sensory recording makes a stimulus artifact more common and more of a problem. Greater attention, therefore, is required to the appropriate placement of ground electrodes and the elimination of conducting bridges between the ground and the stimulating electrodes, isolation of the stimulating electrodes, and proper orientation of the stimulating and recording electrodes. Another common problem in recording sensory potentials is the appearance of background muscle activity; this is reduced effectively by providing the patient with an auditory feedback of his muscle contractions. Sensory studies require particular attention to temperature, because the superficial location of the cutaneous nerves makes it more likely that mild slowing in conduction may be due to low temperature.

Technically, the easiest and more reliable sensory nerve action potential recordings are obtained by orthodromic activation of the axons during stimulation of cutaneous nerves, while recording either from the cutaneous nerve more proximally or from the mixed nerve it joins. This is true of both the ulnar and median digital nerves. Radial and sural nerves, however, are as readily tested with an antidromic volley, recording over a distal branch while stimulating the main trunk of the cutaneous nerve.

Measurements

Compound nerve action potentials are measured in the same manner as the compound muscle action potentials. The sensory nerve action potential is a moving wave recorded in a volume conductor and, therefore, typically has an initial positivity due to current flow ahead of the area of depolarization. The amplitude of the response measured from positive peak to negative peak provides an estimate of the total number of fibers activated, although it is heavily influenced by the distance of the recording electrode from the nerve. The latency of the response is directly related to the rate of conduction and the distance between the stimulating and the recording electrodes. Comparisons of

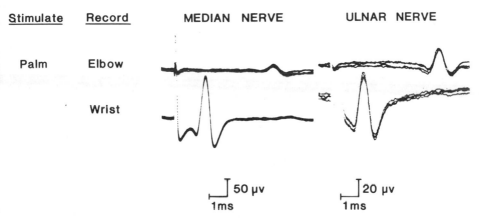

Fig. 7.6. Surface recordings of sensory nerve action potentials on palmar stimulation.

differences in latency and distance at different sites allow calculations of conduction velocity. Identifying the onset of the potential for measuring latency is more difficult than in motor conduction, but is most accurately made to the initial positive peak. Difficulty in identifying this point because of background noise makes measurement of the latency to the peak of the potential more common, particularly for distal measurements. However, peak latencies are less reliable for conduction velocities, because they provide estimates of conduction in slower fibers. With distal stimulation, potentials are small at proximal sites and, at times, this precludes their direct recording without averaging. Larger potentials can be obtained by stimulation of the mixed nerve or by stimulation of unbranched digital nerves, as can be obtained by stimulation of the median or ulnar nerves in the palm, distal to the main motor branches. With palmar stimulation, orthodromic sensory potentials can be recorded at proximal sites without averaging (Fig. 7.6).

Sensory compound nerve action potentials range from a few microvolts to 200 μV. Their conduction velocities are generally faster than motor conduction, but a greater dispersion of response and a greater reduction in amplitude occur with distant stimulation because of the larger range of conduction velocities among sensory fibers.

Less direct measures of sensory nerve conduction may be obtained by recording H wave latency (Ch. 9) or somatosensory cerebral or spinal evoked responses (Chs. 13 and 14).

ANOMALIES OF INNERVATION

In standard nerve conduction studies it is assumed that a patient's nerves follow the normal anatomic patterns. However, as many as 20 percent of persons may have anomalous innervation in the arm or leg, and this can result in

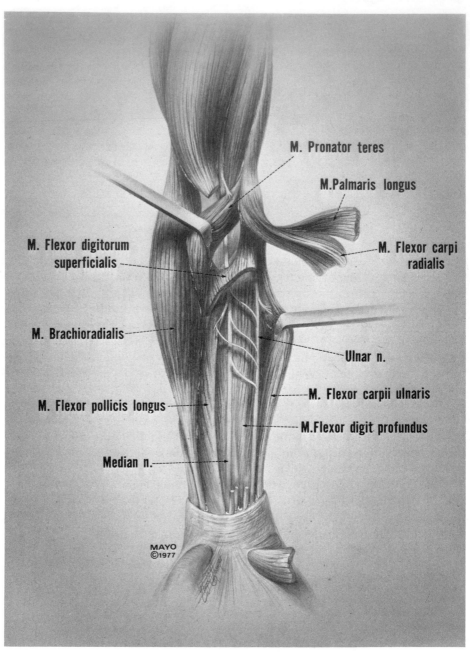

Fig. 7.7. *Schematic drawing of sites of anastomotic fibers crossing from median to ulnar nerve.*

unusual evoked responses. If not recognized, these unusual responses may be misinterpreted as indicative of disorders of the peripheral nerves. Two types of anomaly are of particular concern: median-to-ulnar nerve anastomosis in the forearm (Martin-Gruber), and the presence of a deep accessory branch of the superficial peroneal nerve in the leg.

Median-Ulnar Nerve Anastomosis

Fifteen to 20 percent of normal persons have anomalous axons passing from the median to the ulnar nerve in the proximal third of the forearm (Fig. 7.7). These axons may leave either the main trunk of the median nerve or the anterior interosseous nerve, and join the main trunk of the ulnar nerve. Axons leaving or joining a nerve between two sites of stimulation will cause an unanticipated change in the size or shape of the evoked response (Fig. 7.8). In ulnar nerve stimulation, the amplitude is lower at more proximal sites of stimulation, while in median nerve stimulation the amplitude is higher at more proximal sites of stimulation. The axons crossing from the median to the ulnar nerve may innervate any of a number of intrinsic hand muscles, most commonly the first dorsal interosseous. For standard nerve conduction studies, the most important sites of innervation are the thenar and hypothenar muscles (Fig. 7.9). This

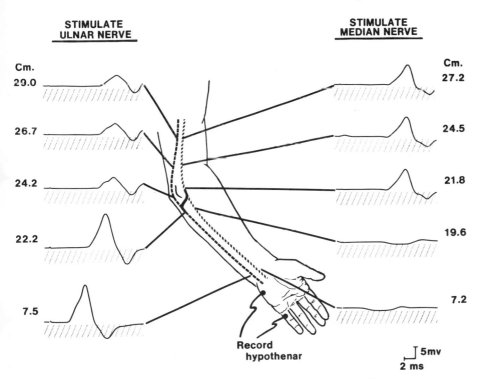

Fig. 7.8. Hypothenar muscle evoked responses to ulnar and median nerve stimulation with median-to-ulnar anastomosis in proximal forearm.

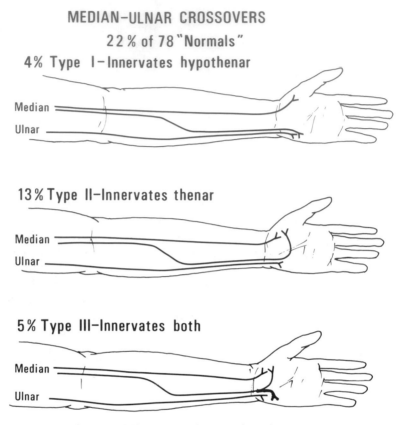

MEDIAN-ULNAR CROSSOVERS
22% of 78 "Normals"
4% Type I-Innervates hypothenar

Median

Ulnar

13% Type II-Innervates thenar

Median

Ulnar

5% Type III-Innervates both

Median

Ulnar

Fig. 7.9. Distribution of fibers in median-to-ulnar forearm anastomosis in normal subjects (data from Wilbourn, A. and Lambert, E. H. 1976. The forearm median-to-ulnar nerve communication; electrodiagnostic aspects [abstract]. Neurology, 26, 368).

anomaly can be particularly confusing in the presence of a carpal tunnel syndrome (Gutmann, 1977).

Deep Accessory Branch of Superficial Peroneal Nerve

The other potentially confusing anomaly concerns the innervation of the extensor digitorum brevis muscle on the foot, via the superficial rather than the deep peroneal nerve. The axons pass posterior to the lateral malleolus rather than anterior to the ankle. The detour of fibers away from the deep peroneal nerve results in a lower amplitude response with distal than with proximal stimulation, and can be seen in 15 to 20 percent of normal persons (Lambert, 1969b). This can be especially confusing in the presence of a peroneal neuropathy with a partial conduction block (Fig. 7.10).

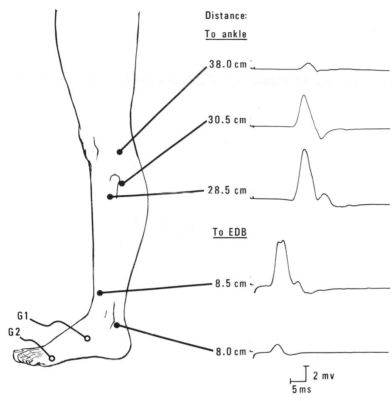

Fig. 7.10. *Changes in evoked response amplitude from extensor digitorum brevis muscle (EDB) on peroneal nerve stimulation in presence of a localized peroneal neuropathy at the head of the fibula and an anomalous deep accessory peroneal nerve.*

PATHOPHYSIOLOGY

Disorders of peripheral nerve produce only a limited number of electrophysiologic alterations, and these can be classified into disorders with *conduction slowing,* disorders with *conduction block,* and disorders with a reduced or absent electrical response. Each of these may be focal or diffuse in distribution. A block of conduction occurs with a metabolic alteration in the membrane, as with a local anesthetic block, or with a structural alteration in the myelin, such as telescoping or segmental demyelination. Slowing of conduction also can occur with segmental demyelination or with narrowing of the axons. Reduced or absent responses are the result of wallerian degeneration after axonal disruption, or of axonal degeneration as in "dying-back" neuropathies.

The hallmark of a conduction block is a reduction in evoked response amplitude proximal to the site of block, while conduction slowing is seen as prolonged latency. These may be seen in combination, but they often occur independently. A block is more common in rapidly developing disorders and slowing is more common in chronic disorders. Lack of function is best identified by an absent or reduced response to stimulation at any site, in combination with fibrillation potentials. These parameters can help categorize nerve damage into broad groups. For instance, in traumatic injuries of a nerve, there is usually a conduction block with an amplitude change or axonal disruption with fibrillation potentials (or some combination of both). The clinical defect in either instance may have a variable duration (Table 7.1).

Thus, no single finding in nerve conduction studies is typical of the clinical phenomenon of neurapraxia, in which there is a transient loss of function without atrophy. Neurapraxia may be of relatively short duration, lasting only a few minutes, or of very long duration, lasting up to weeks or months, depending on the underlying pathology. The findings obtained by nerve conduction studies will be a function of the underlying pathology of the disorder rather than its duration. Table 7.2 summarizes some patterns of abnormality.

Localized Peripheral Nerve Damage

This damage is characterized by low-amplitude responses, slow conduction, or a change in evoked response amplitude. The amplitude of the evoked responses may be low at all sites of stimulation if there is muscle atrophy, or if portions of the muscle are not innervated by the nerve. A lower amplitude response at proximal sites than at distal sites of stimulation is evidence of a block of conduction, in which some of the axons are unable to transmit an action potential through the damaged segment but are functioning distal to it (Trojaborg, 1977). If all axons are blocked in a segment, no response will be obtained by stimulation proximal to the site of the lesion. A block in conduction must be distinguished from slowing in conduction, which may occur with or without a conduction block (Fig. 7.11). Slowing of nerve conduction in some of the axons in the nerve also is associated with a reduction in amplitude on proximal stimulation, because of dispersion and increased duration of the response; however, the area of the evoked response remains constant.

Table 7.1. DURATION OF DEFICIT AFTER PERIPHERAL NERVE INJURY

Conduction block (amplitude change)
    Metabolic—seconds to minutes
    Myelin loss—days to weeks
    Axonal distortion—weeks to months
Axonal disruption (fibrillation potentials)
    Scattered axons—no deficit
    Many axons—weeks to months
    Total—months to years

Table 7.2. PATTERNS OF ABNORMALITY IN NERVE CONDUCTION STUDIES OF PERIPHERAL NEUROMUSCULAR DISORDERS

Disorder	Motor nerve conduction			Sensory nerve conduction			F & H Latency
	Amplitude	Conduction Velocity	Duration	Amplitude	Conduction Velocity	Duration	
Axonal neuropathy	→	>70%	Normal	↓↓	>70%	Normal	Mild ↑
Demyelinating neuropathy	↓ Proximal	<50%	↑ Proximal	→	<50%	↑ Proximal	↑
Mononeuropathy	→	→	→	↓↓	→	→	↑
Regenerated nerve	→	→	→	→	→	→	↑
Motor neuron disease	↓↓	>70%	Normal	Normal	Normal	Normal	Mild ↑
Neuromuscular transmission defect	(↓)*	Normal	Normal	Normal	Normal	Normal	Normal
Myopathy	(↓)*	Normal	Normal	Normal	Normal	Normal	Normal

* Sometimes present.

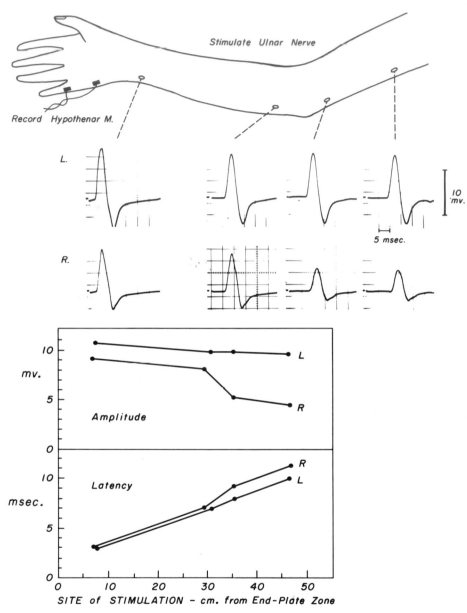

Fig. 7.11. Changes in amplitude and latency of hypothenar muscle evoked re-sponses to ulnar nerve stimulation in presence of a localized right ulnar neuropathy at the elbow. Normal responses are present on left side (by permission of E. H. Lambert, Mayo Clinic, Rochester, Minnesota).

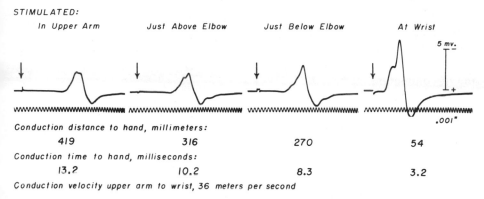

STIMULATED:

In Upper Arm   Just Above Elbow   Just Below Elbow   At Wrist

5 mv.

.001"

Conduction distance to hand, millimeters:

419   316   270   54

Conduction time to hand, milliseconds:

13.2   10.2   8.3   3.2

Conduction velocity upper arm to wrist, 36 meters per second

Fig. 7.12. Dispersion of evoked potentials and reduction of evoked response amplitude from hypothenar muscles in severe neuropathy (by permission of E. H. Lambert, Mayo Clinic, Rochester, Minnesota).

Diffuse Peripheral Nerve Damage

Nerve conduction studies, at times, can distinguish among general categories of nerve disorders (Gilliatt, 1966; Thomas, 1971; McLeod, Prineas, and Walsh, 1973). A disorder associated with axonal destruction, as in the axonal dystrophies and dying-back neuropathies, is associated predominantly with a reduction in amplitude of the evoked response at all sites of stimulation with relatively little (or at the most up to 30 percent) slowing in conduction velocity. In contrast, segmental demyelination is associated with pronounced slowing of conduction, usually to less than 50 percent of normal, and with a progressive reduction in amplitude in the evoked reponse due to dispersion of the response (Fig. 7.12). Other disorders also have been associated with nerve conduction abnormalities, but less specifically.

PERIPHERAL NEUROPATHIES

Variations in the type and distribution of pathologic changes in peripheral neuropathies result in different patterns of electrophysiologic abnormality. Although the location and severity of nerve disease are readily defined by nerve conduction studies, the presence of mixed patterns or mild changes in nerve conduction studies precludes characterization of the histologic changes in most peripheral neuropathies. For example, in diabetes, a wide variety of patterns of abnormality may be seen on nerve conduction studies (Mulder et al, 1961; Williams and Mayer, 1976; Behse, Buchthal, and Carlsen, 1977). Among the most common is a mononeuropathy of the median nerve at the wrist, ulnar nerve at the elbow, or peroneal nerve at the knee, with localized slowing of conduction or conduction block. Often, these focal mononeuropathies are superimposed on mild, diffuse change, with generalized reduction in amplitudes of the evoked responses and mild slowing of conduction. The needle examination often shows only mild changes, usually distally. However, some patients with diabetes have a lumbosacral polyradiculopathy manifested primarily by diffuse fibrillation potentials in paraspinal and L-2 to L-4 muscles. This pattern may be associated with prolongation of F wave latencies due to proximal slowing of conduction.

The Guillain-Barré syndrome, or inflammatory polyradiculoneuropathy, also has a range of electrophysiologic changes (McLeod et al, 1976; Raman and Taori, 1976; Miyoshi and Oh, 1977; Kimura, 1978). There may be no abnormalities on nerve conduction studies, or the abnormalities may be limited to proximal slowing with prolongation of the F wave or H reflex latency. Distal recording with stimulation at proximal sites, such as a spinal nerve or the brachial plexus, also may be abnormal. More commonly, however, the Guillain-Barré syndrome is associated with prolonged distal latencies of a mild-to-moderate degree and variable slowing of conduction velocities, which may be symmetric or asymmetric. The facial nerves or other cranial nerves may be involved with abnormalities on blink reflex testing, or on facial nerve stimulation (Fig. 7.13). While these patients with Guillain-Barré syndrome usually have only mild changes on needle examination, some patients have prominent fibrillation potentials, indicating severe axonal destruction and a poorer prognosis.

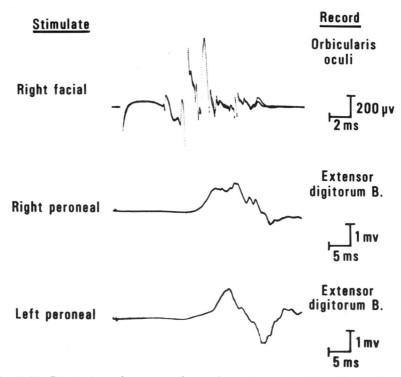

Fig. 7.13. Dispersion of compound muscle action potentials with needle and surface electrode recordings in Guillain-Barré syndrome.

Table 7.3. PATTERNS OF ELEC-
TROPHYSIOLOGIC ABNORMALITY IN
PERIPHERAL NEUROPATHY

Predominantly "axonal degeneration"
  Diabetes (some patients)
  Guillain-Barré syndrome (some patients)
  Toxic—vincristine, acrylamide, others
  Alcohol
  Uremia
  Acute intermittent porphyria
  Collagen-vascular diseases
  Carcinoma
  Amyloid
Predominantly "segmental demyelination"
  Diabetes (some patients)
  Guillain-Barré syndrome (some patients)
  Déjérine-Sottas disease
  Diphtheria
  Chronic inflammatory
  Refsum's disease
  Leukodystrophies

Although many patients with neuropathies show mixed findings on nerve conduction studies, some patients may have a predominantly axonal degeneration or segmental demyelination (Table 7.3).

Axonal Neuropathies

Axonal neuropathies primarily affect the axon, with either diffuse degeneration or dying-back of its distal portion, and are particularly common in toxic and metabolic disorders. The major change found by nerve conduction studies is a reduction in the amplitude of the compound muscle action potential or the compound nerve action potential (or both) which is proportional to the severity of the disease. Some axonal neuropathies predominantly affect sensory fibers, such as vitamin B_{12} deficiency, carcinomatous neuropathy, and Friedreich's ataxia, while others, such as the lead neuropathies, have a greater effect on motor fibers. The sensory axons are commonly involved earlier and more severely than motor axons. Sensory potentials can be of very low amplitude and be associated with only mild sensory symptoms. In contrast to the change in amplitude, the latencies or conduction velocity usually are altered very little, because conduction in individual axons generally remains normal until the axon has degenerated. Normal conduction velocities, therefore, should not be considered evidence against the presence of a neuropathy. Often the only finding will be fibrillation potentials on needle examination of distal muscles, especially intrinsic foot muscles, with or without low-amplitude evoked responses.

If many of the large axons are lost there may be a mild reduction in the conduction velocity, but not to less than 70 percent of normal. Axonal neuropathies typically affect the longer axons earlier and, therefore, are first manifested in the lower extremities. Those nerves that are more susceptible to local trauma because of a superficial location also are more sensitive, and so these disorders are commonly manifested initially as peroneal neuropathies with low-amplitude or absent responses, while other motor nerves remain intact. Axonal neuropathies may be associated with a change of the refractory period of the nerve and with a relative resistance to ischemia.

Segmental Demyelinating Neuropathies

Segmental demyelinating neuropathies are usually subacute inflammatory disorders, such as Guillain-Barré syndrome or diphtheritic neuropathies, but similar patterns may be seen in hypertrophic neuropathies such as Déjérine-Sottas disease and hereditary motor sensory neuropathy. Demyelinating neuropathies are typically associated with prolonged latencies and a pronounced slowing of conduction, often in the range of 10 to 20 m per second. In some hereditary disorders, such as Déjérine-Sottas disease, the velocity may be only a few meters per second. Commonly, there is a relative preservation of the amplitude on distal stimulation, but a progressive reduction in the amplitude and dispersion of the evoked response on proximal stimulation (Fig. 7.12). Demyelinating neuropathies commonly affect sites of nerve compression early, producing symmetric neuropathies of the peroneal, ulnar, or median nerves at the knee, elbow, or wrist, respectively. The refractory period in demyelinating neuropathies is reduced, often to the extent that repetitive stimulation at rates as low as 5 Hz will result in a decrement, although the decrement more commonly does not appear until rates of 10 or 20 Hz are used (Simpson, 1966).

FOCAL NEUROPATHIES

In mononeuropathies the electrophysiologic changes found by nerve conduction studies vary with the rapidity with which the neuropathy developed, the duration of damage, and the severity of damage, as well as with the underlying disorder (Fowler, Danta, and Gilliatt, 1972; Nakano, 1978). Localized narrowing, or paranodal or internodal demyelination with a chronic compressive lesion, produces localized slowing of conduction. Narrowing of axons distal to a chronic compression results in slowing of conduction along the entire length of the nerve. Telescoping of axons with intussusception of one internode into another distorts and obliterates the nodes of Ranvier and blocks conduction. Moderate segmental demyelination and local metabolic alterations often are associated with a conduction block. Such conduction blocks are manifested as a lower-amplitude evoked response with stimulation proximal to the site of damage than distal to it. The segment of nerve distal to an acute lesion in which

Table 7.4. COMPOUND ACTION POTENTIAL AMPLITUDE AFTER PERIPHERAL NERVE INJURY *

	0–5 Days	After 5 Days	Recovery
Conduction block			
Proximal stimulation	Low	Low	Increases
Distal stimulation	Normal	Normal	Normal
Axonal disruption			
Proximal stimulation	Low	Low	Increases
Distal stimulation	Normal	Low	Increases

* Supramaximal stimulation.

there has been disruption of axons may continue to function normally for as long as 5 days. Then, as the axons undergo wallerian degeneration, their conduction ceases and the evoked response diminishes in amplitude and finally disappears. One week after an acute injury, the amplitude of the evoked response can be used as an approximation of the number of intact, viable axons (Table 7.4).

The findings on needle examination may also aid the electrophysiologic evaluation of peripheral nerve injury and in characterizing mononeuropathies (Table 7.5).

Adequate assessment of a peripheral nerve injury, therefore, should include both the needle examination and the nerve conduction studies. The significance of changes with time after injury is outlined in Table 7.6.

Median Neuropathies

One of the most common focal mononeuropathies is the carpal tunnel syndrome, in which the median nerve is compressed in the space formed by the wrist bones and the carpal ligament. Early or mild compression of the median nerve in the carpal tunnel may not be associated with electrophysiologic abnormalities. However, more than 90 percent of symptomatic patients have localized slowing of conduction in sensory fibers (Thomas, Lambert, and

Table 7.5. NEEDLE EXAMINATION AFTER PERIPHERAL NERVE INJURY

	0–15 Days	After 15 Days	Recovery
Conduction block			
Fibrillation potentials	None	None	None
Motor unit potentials	↓ Recruitment	↓ Recruitment	↑ Recruitment
Axonal disruption			
Fibrillation potentials	None	Present	Reduced
Motor unit potentials	↓ Recruitment	↓ Recruitment	"Nascent"

Table 7.6. INTERPRETATION OF ELECTROPHYSIOLOGIC FINDINGS AFTER PERIPHERAL NERVE INJURY

Finding	Interpretation
0–5 Days	
Motor unit potentials present	Nerve intact, functioning axons
Fibrillations present	Old lesion
Low compound action potential	Old lesion
5–15 Days	
Compound action potential distal only	Conduction block
Low compound action potential	Amount of axonal disruption
Motor unit potentials present	Nerve intact
After 15 Days	
Compound action potential distal only	Conduction block
Motor unit potentials present	Nerve intact
Fibrillation potentials	Amount of axonal disruption
	Distribution of damage
Recovery	
Increasing compound action potential	Block clearing
Increasing number of motor unit potentials	Block clearing
Decreasing number of fibrillations	Reinnervation
"Nascent" motor unit potentials	Reinnervation

Cseuz, 1967; Buchthal and Rosenfalck, 1971). The sensory latency through the carpal tunnel (i.e. stimulating the digital nerves in the palm while recording at the wrist) is the most sensitive measurement in identifying the earliest abnormality (Fig. 7.14). This so-called "palmar latency" may be compared with normal values, but it is more reliable if compared with the latency in ulnar sensory fibers over the same distance. More severe nerve compression reduces the amplitude of the sensory nerve action potential and prolongs the latency to a greater extent and over a longer distance. Severe median neuropathy at the wrist also increases the distal motor latency to the thenar muscles and reduces the thenar compound muscle action potential (Fig. 7.15). Reduction of the compound muscle action potential is often associated with mild slowing of the motor conduction velocity in the forearm and with the presence of fibrillation potentials in the abductor pollicis brevis muscle. Patients with carpal tunnel syndromes of moderate severity may have anomalous innervation of the thenar muscles, with the amplitude of the response being higher on elbow stimulation than on wrist stimulation (Fig. 7.16).

A median neuropathy may be an early finding in patients with more diffuse neuropathies, and assessment of other nerves to exclude this possibility is a necessity. Many patients with carpal tunnel syndrome have bilateral abnormalities on nerve conduction studies, even though the symptoms may be unilateral, and conduction in the opposite extremity should, therefore, be measured as well, if a median neuropathy at the wrist is identified. A few patients

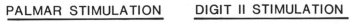

PALMAR STIMULATION DIGIT II STIMULATION

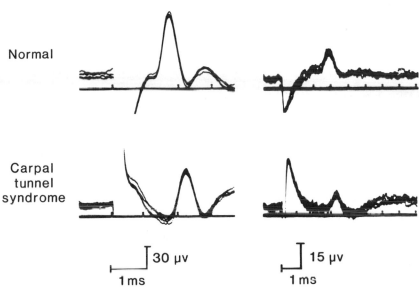

Normal

Carpal
tunnel
syndrome

30 μv

1 ms

15 μv

1 ms

Fig. 7.14. *Sensory nerve action potentials in carpal tunnel syndrome. Palmar latency is prolonged (2.4 msec), while digital latency is still in the normal range (3.3 msec).*

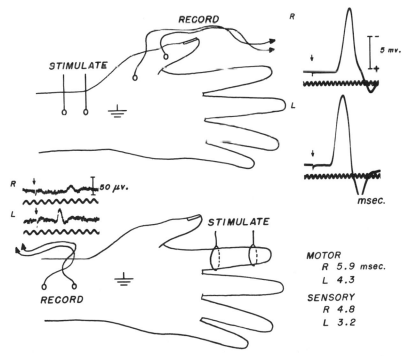

RECORD   R

STIMULATE

5 mv.

L

msec.

R   50 μv.

L

STIMULATE

RECORD

MOTOR
R 5.9 msec.
L 4.3

SENSORY
R 4.8
L 3.2

Fig. 7.15. *Prolonged motor and sensory latencies with carpal tunnel syndrome in right hand (from Mayo Clinic Department of Neurology and the Department of Physiology and Biophysics. 1971. Clinical Examinations in Neurology, 3rd edn. W. B. Saunders Company, Philadelphia).*

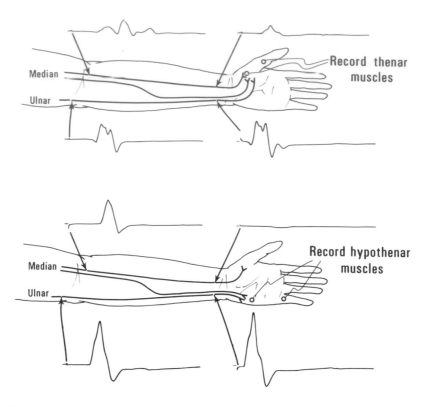

Fig. 7.16. Carpal tunnel syndrome with anomalous median-to-ulnar nerve anastomosis. Thenar response with median nerve stimulation at elbow is larger and more complex and has too short a latency.

have a normal sensory response and a prolonged distal motor latency, and this may have a number of causes. For instance, there may be slowing with a chronic neurogenic atrophy because of a more proximal lesion, such as damage to a spinal nerve or anterior horn cells. Or a radial sensory response may be evoked inadvertently by high-voltage stimulation of the median nerve and recorded as an apparent median sensory potential. Occasionally, patients have sensory branches to one or more fingers which are anatomically separated from the motor fibers and are relatively spared. The compression also may vary in its severity on the fascicles of the median nerve, resulting in greater slowing in the axons to some digital nerves than others.

Median neuropathies in the forearm are much less common and only rarely show any abnormality on nerve conduction studies other than low-amplitude sensory and motor responses (Buchthal, Rosenfalck, and Trojaborg, 1974). Both the anterior interosseous neuropathy and the pronator syndrome are usually manifested electrophysiologically by fibrillation potentials in the appropriate muscles. Only infrequent patients have localized slowing of conduction in the damaged segment of nerve.

Ulnar Neuropathies

The electrophysiologic alteration in ulnar neuropathies varies with the severity and location of the lesion (Payan, 1969). The rare patient with compression of the ulnar nerve in the hand will have a prolonged latency only to the first dorsal interosseous muscle. In such a patient, the hypothenar muscles should not be the only recording site for ulnar nerve conduction studies. In most patients with ulnar neuropathy, the abnormality is at the elbow and can be identified with recordings from the hypothenar muscle (Figs. 7.11 and 7.17). As in the carpal tunnel syndrome, sensory fibers are more likely than motor fibers to be damaged, so that the compound sensory action potential is commonly lost early. In some patients, focal slowing in ulnar sensory fibers across the elbow can be demonstrated. The most common localizing finding in ulnar neuropathy of recent onset is a block of conduction at the elbow (Fig. 7.15). Amplitudes are normal with stimulation at the wrist and below the elbow, but are lower by 30 percent or more with stimulation just above the elbow and more proximally. The block of conduction may be associated with local slowing. Long-standing or chronic ulnar neuropathy usually results in slowing of conduction which may not be localized to the elbow. Although an occasional patient may have slowing of conduction to the flexor carpi ulnaris, this muscle usually shows little or no change on nerve conduction studies and needle examination. In both the ulnar and median neuropathies, the F-wave latency is prolonged in proportion to the

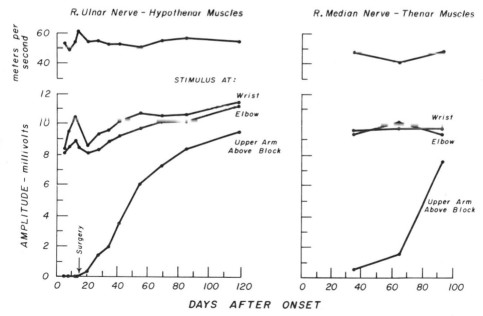

Fig. 7.17. Evolution of latency and amplitude changes of hypothenar muscle and thenar muscle evoked responses in ulnar and median neuropathy due to compression in upper arm (by permission of E. H. Lambert, Mayo Clinic, Rochester, Minnesota).

slowing in the peripheral segments. Because ulnar neuropathies also are commonly bilateral, the opposite extremity must be tested if an ulnar neuropathy is evident on one side.

Peroneal Neuropathies

Neuropathies of the peroneal nerve at the head of the fibula are another common focal lesion. Peroneal neuropathy of recent onset due to compression is associated most frequently with a block of conduction at the head of the fibula and can be localized precisely by stimulation at short intervals along the nerve to identify the area at which the evoked response decreases (Fig. 7.18). Conduction across this segment is generally not slowed, although in lesions of longer duration slowing does become much more prominent (Singh, Behse, and Buchthal, 1974). Nerve conduction studies of the superficial peroneal nerve may be of value, but they are technically more difficult. Some patients with a moderately severe peroneal neuropathy may show no evoked response from the extensor digitorum brevis, the most common site of recording. In these circumstances, recordings from the anterior tibial and other anterior compartment muscles with stimulation at the head of the fibula and the knee may still demonstrate a block or slowing of conduction in the nerve. F wave latencies

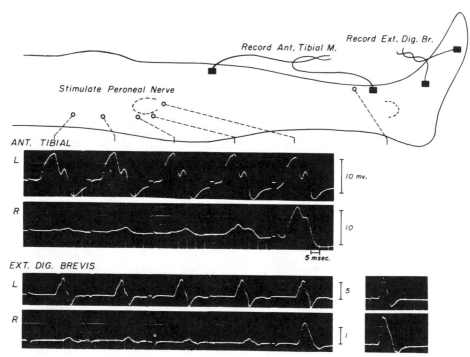

Fig. 7.18. *Localized conduction block at head of fibula in "crossed-leg" peroneal neuropathy (by permission of E. H. Lambert, Mayo Clinic, Rochester, Minnesota).*

may aid in distinguishing peroneal neuropathies from L-5 root lesions by providing evidence of proximal slowing. Anomalous innervation of the extensor digitorum brevis muscle, via a deep accessory branch of the superficial peroneal nerve, may complicate the recognition of a peroneal neuropathy. In apparent peroneal neuropathies without localized slowing of conduction, the short head of the biceps femoris muscle must be tested for fibrillation potentials. Sciatic nerve lesions may present with only peroneal deficit, and sciatic nerve conduction studies are technically more difficult to perform.

Other Neuropathies

A few other neuropathies, such as those of the radial and tibial nerves, may similarly be localized by nerve conduction studies (Johnson and Ortiz, 1966; Trojaborg, 1970), but evaluation of many others is not aided by nerve conduction studies because they do not show localized slowing. In facial neuropathies like Bell's palsy, the examination provides only limited information because stimulation cannot be applied just proximal and distal to the site of the lesion. The usual findings in Bell's palsy with neurapraxia are normal amplitudes and latencies of the evoked responses; in axonal degeneration, the amplitude of the evoked response is decreased in proportion to the axonal destruction (Olsen, 1975). Blink reflexes can measure conduction across the involved segment, but they are commonly absent in Bell's palsy (Kimura, Giron, and Young, 1976). Conduction studies can help differentiate hemifacial spasm from other facial movements by demonstrating aberrant reinnervation. The normal early response blink reflex occurs only in the ocular muscles on the side stimulated. After aberrant reinnervation in Bell's palsy, and in patients with hemifacial spasm, an early response can be recorded over the perioral muscles on stimulation of the first division of the trigeminal nerve (Stöhr, 1976).

Most brachial plexus lesions are traumatic, and nerve conduction studies are of limited value. Most commonly, the amplitude of compound muscle action potential is reduced, and sensory responses are absent in the distribution of the damaged fibers. With lower trunk lesions, the ulnar sensory response is absent; with upper trunk lesions, the median sensory response of the index finger is reduced or absent. In patients with slow, compressive lesions of the plexus, such as tumors, a localized slowing of conduction of motor or sensory fibers, and occasionally a conduction block, may be identified on stimulation at the supraclavicular or nerve root level. The clinical entity of a thoracic-outlet syndrome, which has been reported to show abnormalities on nerve conduction studies, is usually a vascular syndrome with a change, if any, only in sensory potential amplitudes, and no slowing of nerve conduction (Gilliatt et al, 1978).

Radiculopathies

Cervical and lumbosacral radiculopathies are usually not associated with changes in the findings obtained by nerve conduction studies; however, if there is sufficient destruction of axons and wallerian degeneration in the distribution of the nerve being tested, the amplitude of the evoked motor response may be reduced. For instance, in an L-5 radiculopathy, the response of the extensor digitorum brevis muscle to peroneal nerve stimulation is often of low amplitude or absent. In the presence of atrophy and a low compound muscle action potential, there may be mild slowing of conduction in the motor axons innervating the atrophic muscle. In a few patients with a mild lumbosacral radiculopathy, measurements of F wave or H reflex latencies have been of value in identifying proximal slowing of conduction (Braddom and Johnson, 1974). Because most lesions of the spinal nerve and nerve root occur proximal to the dorsal root ganglion, the sensory potentials usually are normal, even in the distribution of a sensory deficit. This phenomenon is valuable in identifying avulsion of a nerve root, in which there is total anesthesia and loss of motor function with normal sensory potentials.

SYSTEM DEGENERATIONS

Among the system degenerations of the central nervous system are some that involve either dorsal root ganglia or anterior horn cells. Because the peripheral axons of the anterior horn cells and dorsal root ganglia are assessed in nerve conduction studies, both groups will show abnormalities on electrophysiologic testing.

Motor System

System degenerations include motor neuron disease, such as amyotrophic lateral sclerosis, spinal muscular atrophy, the neuronal form of Charcot-Marie-Tooth disease, Kugelberg-Welander disease, and Werdnig-Hoffmann disease (Lambert, 1969a; Ryniewicz, 1977). Each of these disorders is characterized by degeneration of the anterior horn cells and, consequently, loss of peripheral motor axons. In these disorders, the individual axons conduct normally until their function ceases. Therefore, nerve conduction does not become slow unless the loss of large axons is significant. The conduction velocity, as measured from the whole nerve when large, fast conducting axons are lost, is never less than 70 percent of normal.

The most striking change found by the nerve conduction studies in patients with motor neuron diseases is a reduction in amplitude of the compound muscle action potential, and this is proportional to the loss of innervation of the muscle. However, the reduction in amplitude may not reflect the duration or severity of disease. In slowly progressive disorders, if collateral sprouting and reinnervation can compensate for the loss of anterior horn cells, the evoked response amplitude may remain normal. A mild slowing of conduction may be seen in these circumstances, but is usually not found until the action potential amplitude has decreased below normal. Occasional patients with motor neuron diseases have a decrement on repetitive stimulation.

In motor neuron diseases, sensory fibers are not involved and sensory conduction studies are usually normal. Some afferent axons may, however, show mild histopathologic changes, and this is reflected in the occasional patient with a clinical motor neuron disease who has either a mild reduction in amplitude in the sensory nerve action potential or a slight slowing of sensory conduction.

Sensory System

System degenerations manifested in peripheral sensory fibers are the spinocerebellar degenerations, particularly Friedreich's ataxia, and vitamin B_{12} deficiency. Carcinomatous sensory neuropathy may have a similar basis (Dunn, 1973; Roos, 1977). The degeneration seen in the posterior and lateral columns of the spinal cord in these disorders is due to degeneration of their cells of origin in the dorsal root ganglia. These cells also give rise to the large sensory fibers in the peripheral nerves which are the source of the largest proportion of the compound nerve action potential recorded in sensory nerve conduction studies. In this group of disorders, the amplitude of the compound sensory action potential is typically reduced, and often sensory nerve action potentials are not recordable with surface techniques. These patients also may show mild changes in motor nerve conduction studies, but the changes are much less than those found in sensory studies.

DISORDERS OF THE NEUROMUSCULAR JUNCTION

Of the disorders of neuromuscular transmission, the myasthenic syndrome and *Clostridia botulinum* intoxication are most likely to show changes on nerve conduction studies. Both of these conditions have very low rates of release of acetylcholine from the nerve terminals and both have a block of neuromuscular transmission to a large proportion of the muscle fibers. The compound muscle action potentials are, therefore, usually low with single stimuli (Fig. 7.19). A patient with a clinical history of weakness, who has low amplitude compound muscle action potentials, should always be further tested with slow repetitive stimulation and exercise in search of evidence of a decrement or facilitation, the usual sign of a defect of neuromuscular transmission (Ch. 8). In myasthenia gravis the average evoked response amplitude may be lower than normal, but most patients have amplitudes that are within the normal range. Motor nerve conduction velocities and sensory nerve conduction are normal.

PRIMARY MUSCLE DISEASES

Most myopathies predominantly affect the proximal muscles that are not tested by routine nerve conduction studies. There is, therefore, little change on these studies. However, with proximal nerve conduction studies, or with a myopathy involving distal muscles, the compound muscle action potential amplitude is often reduced proportionately to the amount of muscle atrophy

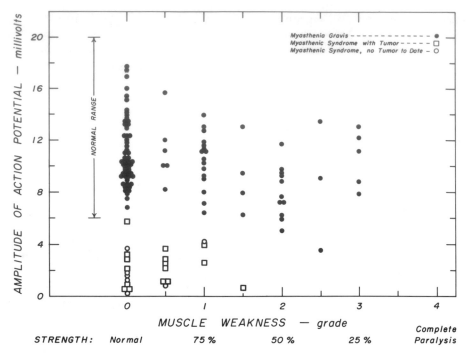

Fig. 7.19. *Amplitudes of hypothenar compound muscle action potentials in myasthenia gravis and the myasthenic syndrome at different grades of muscle weakness (by permission of E. H. Lambert, Mayo Clinic, Rochester, Minnesota).*

(Buchthal, 1970) (Fig. 7.20). Motor and sensory conduction velocity and latency are normal. In some myopathies, particularly those associated with myotonia, such as periodic paralysis and myotonic dystrophy, the excitability of the muscle fiber membrane varies. The compound muscle action potential during nerve conduction studies may change with repetitive stimulation or slowly during a period of 30 to 60 minutes (Brown, 1974; Aminoff et al, 1977). After prolonged exercise, the amplitude may decrease to half normal before it slowly returns to normal (Fig. 7.21). If a patient with a myotonic disorder has been active just before nerve conduction studies are performed, the compound muscle action potentials may be of low amplitude initially and then return graduálly to normal levels. Some patients with myotonic dystrophy have mild slowing of motor conduction in the lower extremities.

DISORDERS ASSOCIATED WITH INVOLUNTARY ACTIVITY OF PERIPHERAL NERVE ORIGIN

A small group of disorders are manifested as stiffness of muscles, myokymia, and cramping, due to excessive discharges in peripheral axons (Wallis, Van Poznak, and Plum, 1970). In this group, there are many different clinical patterns and an even wider variation in electrical manifestations. Their categorization has not been fully accepted, but they can be subdivided into (1) those associated with clinical and pathologic evidence of peripheral nerve disease; (2) those associated with disorders of calcium, such as tetany and hypocalcemia; (3) those of unknown origin, which have been called continuous muscle fiber activity, neuromyotonia, or Isaac's syndrome; and (4) those that are hereditary. Each has different findings on clinical needle electromyography which can provide identification and distinction of the groups, but abnormalities also are seen on nerve conduction studies. Except for the first group, conduction velocities and amplitudes of evoked responses are normal in both

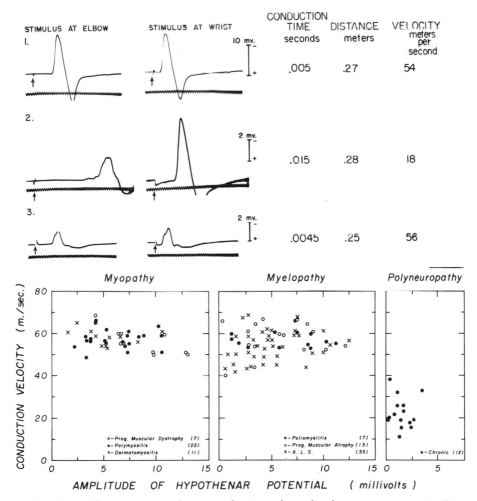

Fig. 7.20. *Ulnar nerve conduction velocity and amplitude measurements in (1) normal person, (2) peripheral neuropathy, and (3) myositis and myelopathy (from Mayo Clinic Department of Neurology and the Department of Physiology and Biophysics. 1971. Clinical Examinations in Neurology. 3rd edn. W. B. Saunders Company, Philadelphia).*

DURING EXERCISE (After 40 Minutes Rest)

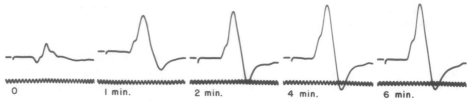

| 0 | I min. | 2 min. | 4 min. | 6 min. |

DURING REST (After 6 Minutes Exercise)

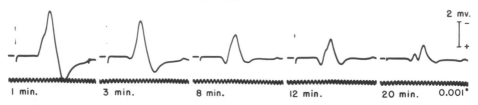

| I min. | 3 min. | 8 min. | 12 min. | 20 min. | 0.001" |

Fig. 7.21. Hypothenar muscle evoked response amplitude on supramaximal ulnar nerve stimulation in a patient with hypokalemic periodic paralysis (by permission of E. H. Lambert, Mayo Clinic, Rochester, Minnesota).

motor and sensory nerves. In each disorder, though, motor nerve stimulation produces a repetitive discharge of the muscle. Instead of a single compound muscle action potential after a single stimulus, a group of two to six potentials occur at regular intervals, with decreasing amplitudes.

REFERENCES

Aminoff, M. J., Layzer, R. B., Satya-Murti, S., and Faden, A. I. (1977). The declining electrical response of muscle to repetitive nerve stimulation in myotonia. Neurology, *27*:812.

Behse, F., Buchthal, F., and Carlsen, F. (1977). Nerve biopsy and conduction studies in diabetic neuropathy. J. Neurol. Neurosurg. Psychiatry, *40*:1072.

Braddom, R. I. and Johnson, E. W. (1974). Standardization of H reflex and diagnostic use in S1 radiculopathy. Arch. Phys. Med. Rehabil., *55*:161.

Brown, J. C. (1974). Muscle weakness after rest in myotonic disorders: an electrophysiological study. J. Neurol. Neurosurg. Psychiatry, *37*:1336.

Buchthal, F. (1970). Electrophysiological abnormalities in metabolic myopathies and neuropathies. Acta Neurol. Scand., Suppl. *43*:129.

Buchthal, F. and Rosenfalck, A. (1971). Sensory conduction from digit to palm and from palm to wrist in the carpal tunnel syndrome. J. Neurol. Neurosurg. Psychiatry, *34*:243.

Buchthal, F., Rosenfalck, A., and Trojaborg, W. (1974). Electrophysiological findings in entrapment of the median nerve at wrist and elbow. J. Neurol. Neurosurg. Psychiatry, *37*:340.

Dawson, G. D. and Scott, J. W. (1949). The recording of nerve action potentials through skin in man. J. Neurol. Neurosurg. Psychiatry, *12*:259.

Dunn, H. G. (1973). Nerve conduction studies in children with Friedreich's ataxia and ataxia-telangiectasia. Dev. Med. Child Neurol., *15*:324.

Fowler, T. J., Danta, G., and Gilliatt, R. W. (1972). Recovery of nerve conduction after a pneumatic tourniquet: observations on the hind-limb of the baboon. J. Neurol. Neurosurg. Psychiatry, *35:*638.

Gilliatt, R. W. (1966). Nerve conduction in human and experimental neuropathies. Proc. R. Soc. Med., *59:*989.

Gilliatt, R. W. and Sears, T. A. (1958). Sensory nerve action potentials in patients with peripheral nerve lesions. J. Neurol. Neurosurg. Psychiatry, *21:*109.

Gilliatt, R. W., Willison, R. G., Dietz, V., and Williams, I. R. (1978). Peripheral nerve conduction in patients with a cervical rib and band. Ann. Neurol., *4:*124.

Gutmann, L. (1977). Median-ulnar nerve communications and carpal tunnel syndrome. J. Neurol. Neurosurg. Psychiatry, *40:*982.

Hodes, R., Larrabee, M. G., and German, W. (1948). The human electromyogram in response to nerve stimulation and the conduction velocity of motor axons. Studies on normal and on injured peripheral nerves. Arch. Neurol. Psychiatry, *60:*340.

Johnson, E. W. and Ortiz, P. R. (1966). Electrodiagnosis of tarsal tunnel syndrome. Arch. Phys. Med. Rehabil., *47:*776.

Kimura, J. (1978). Proximal versus distal slowing of motor nerve conduction velocity in the Guillain-Barré syndrome. Ann. Neurol., *3:*344.

Kimura, J., Giron, L. T., Jr., and Young, S. M. (1976). Electrophysiological study of Bell palsy. Electrically elicited blink reflex in assessment of prognosis. Arch. Otolaryngol., *102:*140.

Lambert, E. H. (1960). Neurophysiological techniques useful in the study of neuromuscular disorders. Res. Publ. Assoc. Res. Nerv. Ment. Dis., *38:*247.

Lambert, E. H. (1962). Diagnostic value of electrical stimulation of motor nerves. Electroencephalogr. Clin. Neurophysiol., Suppl. *22:*9.

Lambert, E. H. (1969a). Electromyography in amyotrophic lateral sclerosis. In: Norris, F. H., Jr., and Kurland, L. T., Eds. Motor Neuron Diseases: Research on Amyotrophic Lateral Sclerosis and Related Disorders. Vol. 2, p. 135. Grune and Stratton, New York.

Lambert, E. H. (1969b). The accessory deep peroneal nerve. A common variation in innervation of extensor digitorum brevis. Neurology, *19:*1169.

Magladery, J. W. and McDougal, D. B., Jr. (1950). Electrophysiological studies of nerve and reflex activity in normal man. I. Identification of certain reflexes in the electromyogram and the conduction velocity of peripheral nerve fibres. Bull. Johns Hopkins Hosp., *86:*265.

McLeod, J. G., Prineas, J. W., and Walsh, J. C. (1973). The relationship of conduction velocity to pathology in peripheral nerves: a study of the sural nerve in 90 patients. In: New Developments in Electromyography and Clinical Neurophysiology, Desmedt, J. E., Ed. Vol. 2, p. 248. Karger, Basel.

McLeod, J. G., Walsh, J. C., Prineas, J. W., and Pollard, J. D. (1976). Acute idiopathic polyneuritis. A clinical and electrophysiological follow-up study. J. Neurol. Sci., *27:*145.

Miyoshi, T., and Oh, S. J. (1977). Proximal slowing of nerve conduction in the Guillain-Barre syndrome. Electromyogr. Clin. Neurophysiol., *17:*287.

Mulder, D. W., Lambert, E. H., Bastron, J. A., and Sprague, R. G. (1961). The neuropathies associated with diabetes mellitus. A clinical and electromyographic study of 103 unselected diabetic patients. Neurology, *11:*275.

Nakano, K. (1978). The entrapment neuropathies. Muscle Nerve, *1:*264.

Olsen, P. Z. (1975). Prediction of recovery in Bell's palsy. Acta Neurol. Scand., Suppl. *61:*1.

Payan, J. (1969). Electrophysiological localization of ulnar nerve lesions. J. Neurol. Neurosurg. Psychiatry, *32:*208.

Raman, P. T. and Taori, G. M. (1976). Prognostic significance of electrodiagnostic studies in the Guillain-Barré syndrome. J. Neurol. Neurosurg. Psychiatry, *39:*163.

Roos, D. (1977). Electrophysiological findings in gastrectomized patients with low serum B_{12}. Acta Neurol. Scand., *56:*247.

Ryniewicz, B. (1977). Motor and sensory conduction velocity in spinal muscular atrophy. Follow-up study. Electromyogr. Clin. Neurophysiol., *17:*385.

Simpson, J. A. (1966). Disorders of neuromuscular transmission. Proc. R. Soc. Med., *59:*993.

Singh, N., Behse, F., and Buchthal, F. (1974). Electrophysiological study of peroneal palsy. J. Neurol. Neurosurg. Psychiatry, *37:*1202.

Stöhr, M. (1976). Der Orbicularis oculi-Reflex bei der Beurteilung defektgeheilter peripherer Facialisparsen. J. Neurol., *212:*85.

Thomas, J. E., Lambert, E. H., and Cseuz, K. A. (1967). Electrodiagnostic aspects of the carpal tunnel syndrome. Arch. Neurol., *16:*635.

Thomas, P. K. (1971). The morphological basis for alterations in nerve conduction in peripheral neuropathy. Proc. R. Soc. Med., *64:*295.

Trojaborg, W. (1970). Rate of recovery in motor and sensory fibres of the radial nerve: clinical and electrophysiological aspects. J. Neurol. Neurosurg. Psychiatry, *33:*625.

Trojaborg, W. (1977). Prolonged conduction block with axonal degeneration. An electrophysiological study. J. Neurol. Neurosurg. Psychiatry, *40:*50.

Wagman, I. H. and Lesse, H. (1952). Maximum conduction velocities of motor fibers of ulnar nerve in human subjects of various ages and sizes. J. Neurophysiol., *15:*235.

Wagner, A. L. and Buchthal, F. (1972). Motor and sensory conduction in infancy and childhood. Reappraisal. Dev. Med. Child Neurol., *14:*189.

Wallis, W. E., Van Poznak, A., and Plum, F. (1970). Generalized muscular stiffness, fasciculations, and myokymia of peripheral nerve origin. Arch. Neurol., *22:*430.

Williams, I. R. and Mayer, R. F. (1976). Subacute proximal diabetic neuropathy. Neurology, *26:*108.

8

The Electrophysiologic Study of Disorders of Neuromuscular Transmission

J. A. R. LENMAN

INTRODUCTION

Failure of neuromuscular conduction in man can readily be brought about by drugs such as curare, and preparations which produce paralysis by interfering with neuromuscular transmission have found a place as relaxant drugs in connection with surgical anesthesia. Many toxins occurring in nature, such as botulinus toxin and certain varieties of snake venom, also act by producing neuromuscular block. Again, an interference with neuromuscular transmission is a side effect of a number of drugs, including certain antibiotics. However, the most important clinical disorder in which neuromuscular block occurs is myasthenia gravis. Neuromuscular block is also a feature of the myasthenic syndrome seen in association with bronchial carcinoma, and neuromuscular conduction may be impaired in several forms of myopathic disorder and in patients with peripheral neuropathy or amyotrophic lateral sclerosis.

Although the mechanism for conduction of the impulse from nerve to muscle is complex, it has been clarified both by clinical observation and by experimental work involving histologic, pharmacologic and electrophysiologic methods. It is evident that the process of neuromuscular transmission can be interfered with at several sites and by differing mechanisms, and these are exemplified in varying degree by the different disorders of neuromuscular function which occur clinically. The application of electrophysiologic methods to the study of these disorders has been helpful both in providing a means of establishing the clinical diagnosis and in clarifying the nature of the underlying defect. In this chapter consideration will be given first to the anatomy of the neuromuscular junction and the physiology of transmission across it. This will be followed by a discussion of the mechanisms underlying neuromuscular block, and finally by an account of the clinical conditions in which neuromuscular block occurs and the electrophysiologic methods which have been found helpful in its study.

NEUROMUSCULAR TRANSMISSION

Structure of Neuromuscular Junction

The neuromuscular junction is a specialized form of synapse, a synapse consisting of the site of connection between one nerve cell and another or between a nerve and an effector organ. Although synapses show considerable variation in structure, mammalian synapses always include a presynaptic portion, the terminal membrane of which is separated from the postsynaptic membrane by a cleft or space of approximately 25 nanometers in width. Under the electron microscope the presynaptic portion is seen to be rich in mitochondria and to contain vesicular structures of approximately 50 nanometers in diameter. The vesicles contain a transmitter substance liberated by the nerve impulse, and at the neuromuscular junction this transmitter is acetylcholine.

In the neuromuscular junction the presynaptic membrane is part of the fine terminal of the nerve fiber, and the postsynaptic membrane is the part of the muscle fiber membrane which lies underneath the nerve ending. The fine terminal of the nerve fiber has no myelin sheath, being enveloped by Schwann cells which separate it from the surrounding tissues. The postsynaptic membrane lies under the nerve ending and is sometimes referred to as the motor end-plate. It forms a depression, known as the synaptic gutter, on the surface of the muscle fiber, and the nerve terminal lies in this. The space which separates the nerve terminal from the surface of the muscle end-plate is known as the primary synaptic cleft. The zone which lies under the end-plate membrane is known as the subneural apparatus, and into this are invaginated folds of surface membrane which are called junctional folds or secondary synaptic clefts. Under the electron microscope the subneural apparatus is seen to contain large numbers of mitochondria, and histochemical staining has shown that the enzyme acetylcholinesterase is present in high concentration. The use of alpha-bungarotoxin, which is derived from the venom of the banded krait and reacts specifically with acetylcholine receptors, has made it possible to identify these receptors. They are distributed along the postsynaptic membrane, particularly in

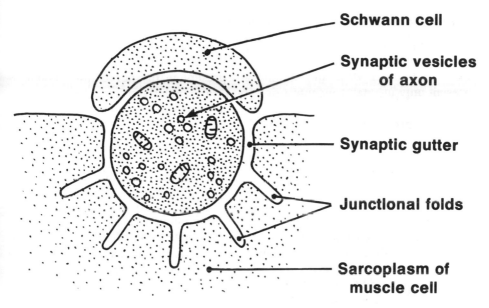

Fig. 8.1. Structure of the neuromuscular junction.

those portions of the junctional fold which face the motor nerve terminal. The nerve terminals also contain many mitochondria, and the synaptic vesicles observed under the electron microscope (Robertson, 1956) are considered to contain stores of acetylcholine (Fig. 8.1).

Transmission Across the Synapse

It is now generally recognized that transmission of an impulse from nerve to muscle is mediated by acetylcholine, which is liberated from the nerve ending to diffuse across the synaptic cleft. By reacting with the receptors on the postsynaptic membrane it depolarizes the membrane to set up a propagated action potential. The effect of acetylcholine on the end-plate can be reproduced experimentally by applying acetylcholine iontophoretically from a pipette close to the postsynaptic membrane. It is only effective if applied to the outer surface of the membrane (del Castillo and Katz, 1956) in the end-plate zone (Miledi, 1960). In fetal muscle, however, sensitivity extends over the entire surface of the muscle fiber (Diamond and Miledi, 1962), and in denervated muscle also the sensitivity of the muscle membrane extends beyond the end-plate region (Axelsson and Thesleff, 1959). The effect of acetylcholine on the receptor is to allow the passage of ions across the membrane, and this sets off the process of depolarization. The action of acetylcholine is rapidly terminated since it is inactivated by the acetylcholinesterase which is present in the subneural apparatus. Following the action potential there is a rapid process of recovery and repolarization so that the muscle can again respond to a further nerve impulse.

Formation and Release of Acetylcholine

The enzyme choline acetylase brings about the synthesis of acetylcholine by catalyzing the transfer of acetyl groups from acetyl coenzyme A to choline. Both choline acetylase and choline are present in the nerve, but choline is present only in small concentrations and is largely derived from the extracellular fluid. Acetylcholine is synthesized in the axoplasm and most of it is taken up and concentrated in the synaptic vesicles.

The release of acetylcholine occurs continuously in small amounts even in the absence of a nerve impulse. There is evidence that this acetylcholine is liberated in the form of discrete packets or quanta. Each quantum probably contains approximately 10,000 molecules of acetylcholine. The arrival of spontaneously released quanta of acetylcholine at the postsynaptic membrane gives rise to small potentials of about 0.50 mV in amplitude which can be recorded from a micro-electrode inserted into the end-plate zone of a resting muscle. These potentials are known as miniature end-plate potentials. In response to a nerve impulse a more substantial amount of acetylcholine, perhaps 200 to 300 quanta, is released (Hubbard and Wilson, 1973). This gives rise to a very much larger potential which is known as the end-plate potential. The end-plate potential can best be studied if a muscle is curarized, as this will prevent depolarization proceeding to the extent of giving rise to a propagated action potential. The effect of the reaction of acetylcholine with its receptor on the postsynaptic membrane is to increase the permeability of the membrane to ions, in particular those of sodium, potassium, and ammonium, so that the membrane becomes partially depolarized. In the presence of curare only a localized end-plate potential is recorded; normally, however, a progressive fall in membrane potential occurs till the depolarization threshold is reached and a propagated action potential spreads along the muscle fiber membrane. The mechanism whereby the propagated action potential leads to muscle contraction is not fully understood. There is evidence that excitation passes along the membrane of the transverse tubules of the muscle fibers, which are in continuity with the muscle fiber membrane (Huxley and Taylor, 1958). In this way excitation is transmitted to the sarcoplasmic reticulum where calcium is released from terminal cisternae to diffuse to the region in the myofibrils where the thick and thin filaments overlap. By reacting with the inhibitory protein troponin, calcium ions release the tension-generating mechanism.

Calcium is also necessary for the release of acetylcholine from the nerve. Calcium ions enter the nerve terminal from the extracellular fluid as the terminal becomes depolarized with the entry of the nerve impulse, and may bring about the release of acetylcholine by disrupting the acetylcholine-containing vesicles (MacIntosh, 1958). The process whereby calcium brings about the release of transmitter accounts for most of the synaptic delay between the time that the nerve terminal is excited and the development of the muscle action potential, which in the mammalian neuromuscular junction is of the order of 0.2msec. Magnesium has the opposite effect to calcium and can produce block of neuromuscular transmission by preventing the release of acetylcholine.

Botulinus toxin may also produce neuromuscular block by interfering with the output of transmitter (Burgen, Dickens, and Zatman, 1949). Hemicholinium (HC_3) is a quaternary base which interferes with the manufacture of acetylcholine by inhibiting the carrier mechanism for transporting choline into the nerve.

The size of the end-plate potentials evoked by a stimulus may be altered if the test shock is preceded by a conditioning stimulus. At short intervals between the two stimuli, there is increased release of acetylcholine—and thus a larger end-plate potential—following the second shock, due to the presence within the nerve terminal of the calcium that accumulated after the initial stimulus. With longer intervals between the two shocks, the end-plate potentials evoked by the second stimulus are reduced in amplitude because the acetylcholine immediately available for release and the probability of release of individual quanta are reduced. A conditioning period of tetanic stimulation also influences the size of the end-plate potentials elicited by a test stimulus, enhancing them when the interval between conditioning and test stimuli is short, and reducing them at longer intervals. This does not affect neuromuscular transmission in normal subjects because the amount of acetylcholine released—and the size of the end-plate potentials produced—by a nerve impulse are anyway much greater than is needed to generate propagated action potentials in the muscle fibers. If this safety factor is reduced, however, previous junctional activity may reduce the number of muscle fibers activated, by reducing the number of end-plate potentials which reach threshold values in response to a test stimulus.

NEUROMUSCULAR BLOCK

Failure of neuromuscular transmission may occur through a disturbance affecting either the presynaptic or the postsynaptic part of the neuromuscular junction.

Presynaptic block may come about through failure of the nerve impulse to invade the fine terminals of the axon. This is a probable explanation for the paralysis which occurs in mice with motor end-plate disease (Duchen and Stefani, 1971) and for the neuromuscular block which may be seen in neuropathies where the terminal axons are abnormally attenuated. Small nerve terminals may also contain an inadequate number of synaptic vesicles. Failure to synthesize acetylcholine may be brought about by hemicholinium, and magnesium will prevent the liberation of acetylcholine from the synaptic vesicles.

Postsynaptic block can be of the competitive variety, in which another substance is present which competes with acetylcholine for the acetylcholine receptor site. Depolarization block, on the other hand, is due to an agent producing prolonged depolarization of the end-plate. Curare acts by giving rise to a competitive block and its effect is to reduce the size of the end-plate potential so that it fails to initiate the propagated action potential. A competitive block is antagonized by acetylcholine or by an anticholinesterase. If a muscle is partially blocked by curare and tetanic stimulation is applied to it through its nerve, the tetanus will not be well sustained; if stimuli are applied at a low frequency at the end of a tetanus, however, there is a rapid and prolonged restoration of the size of the action potentials. A postsynaptic block will also occur in the absence of any competitive blocking agent if there is a marked reduction in number of acetylcholine receptors. Depolarization block can be produced by an anticholinesterase such as neostigmine, or by either acetylcholine itself or substances which have a similar action to it in that they combine with the receptors to depolarize the postsynaptic membrane.

In myasthenia gravis the essential defect is a lack of postsynaptic acetylcholine receptor sites (Fambrough, Drachman, and Satyamurti, 1973) which comes about through an autoimmune reaction against the acetylcholine receptor protein (Patrick and Lindstrom, 1973). Other clinical disorders of neuromuscular transmission may be the result of presynaptic deficiency. In the Eaton-Lambert myasthenic syndrome which may be associated with bronchial carcinoma there is a defect in the release of acetylcholine from the synaptic vesicles similar to that occurring in magnesium poisoning. Recently Engel, Lambert, and Gomez (1977) have described a patient with a conduction defect associated with very small nerve endings in which the limited number of synaptic vesicles gives rise to inadequate acetylcholine release. In this patient also, acetylcholinesterase was found to be absent from the motor end-plates. Antibiotics such as neomycin which interfere with neuromuscular transmission may do so by preventing the release of acetylcholine from the synaptic vesicles.

MYASTHENIA GRAVIS

Myasthenia gravis is a specific disorder of muscle which is characterized by an abnormal degree of fatigability so that muscular weakness characteristically develops after a period of activity. The earliest recorded description was the case described by Thomas Willis in 1672. Fuller accounts came at the end of the 19th century with the case reports of Wilkes, Erb, and Goldflam. Jolly in 1895 was able to show that the defect was peripheral in situation—if a muscle was stimulated through its motor nerve by applying a faradic current the initial brisk contraction was followed by a falling-off in tension. He described this effect as the myasthenic reaction. Later it was shown that the tension could be restored by direct stimulation of the muscle by a galvanic current. These observations suggested that the site of the lesion is in the neuromuscular junction and this was supported by Mary Walker's discovery in 1934 that physostigmine was effective in restoring the strength of myasthenic muscle. The historical development of electrophysiologic techniques for the study of neuromuscular block in myasthenia gravis has been reviewed by Slomić, Rosenfalck, and Buchthal (1968).

Although it has been clear for a long time that the site of the disturbance is at the neuromuscular junction, evidence as to whether the block is presynaptic or postsynaptic has been conflicting. Thus the similarity of the dysfunction in myasthenia to that produced by curare is consistent with myasthenic block being of a competitive postsynaptic variety, and the differing action of decamethonium on myasthenic patients compared with healthy subjects is also consistent with an abnormality affecting the end-plate (Churchill-Davidson and Richardson, 1952). On the other hand, the progressive fall in the size of the evoked responses in muscles following tetanization, which is similar to the effect of hemicholinium, is consistent with a presynaptic defect (Desmedt, 1958). Furthermore there are morphologic changes in the nerve endings and several groups of workers have found a prolongation of the distal latency following a nerve stimulus. An important landmark in understanding the nature of the defect in myasthenia was Simpson's suggestion in 1960 that myasthenia was essentially an autoimmune disorder in which an abnormal thymus gave rise to an antibody reacting against the acetylcholine receptors. This hypothesis was based on the recognition of the clinical association between myasthenia gravis and autoimmune disorders such as thyrotoxicosis and pernicious anaemia, and also on the effects of thymectomy on patients with myasthenia gravis. Evidence in support of this hypothesis includes the observation that in myasthenia gravis there is a decreased number of acetylcholine receptors (Fambrough, Drachman, and Satyamurti, 1973) and that serum from myasthenic patients can block the binding of alpha-bungaro-toxin to end-plate receptors (Almon, Andrew, and Appel, 1974).

Clinical Characteristics

Myasthenia gravis has a prevalence somewhere between 2 and 10 per 100,000, occurs approximately twice as frequently in women as in men, and has been seen at all ages. Clinically it presents with muscular weakness which may be generalized or affect selected muscle groups. In some patients it is virtually confined to the extra-ocular muscles. In others the bulbar muscles may be affected or the muscles of the neck, shoulder, and pelvic girdles are involved. The characteristic feature of the weakness is an undue fatigability so that sometimes the weakness may not be evident until the end of the day. In others it may be brought on by continued use of a muscle.

The simplest and the single most useful procedure for confirming the diagnosis is to test the response to an anticholinesterase, such as edrophonium chloride (Tensilon). This is made up as 10mg in a 1ml solution which is injected intravenously after the intravenous injection of a 0.2ml (2mg) test dose. In the myasthenic patient this can be expected to give rise to an improvement in muscle strength within about 1 minute, the effect lasting for up to 4 or 5 minutes. Healthy subjects may complain of a tight sensation round the eyes, and fasciculation of the facial muscles may be observed. This effect may also be seen in a myasthenic patient under treatment, and if the patient is weak due to an excess of cholinergic medication the injection of Tensilon may aggravate the weakness. This test may be combined with electrophysiologic studies. Other pharmacologic tests include testing the response to neostigmine or decamethonium, or assessing the sensitivity to curare or quinine. The use of these tests has been reviewed by Simpson (1974).

Electromyography

Electromyography using a concentric needle electrode may confirm the fatigability observed clinically, but in this respect the voluntary electromyogram is less helpful than recording the responses evoked by stimulation of a muscle through its nerve. Insertion of a needle electrode in myasthenic muscle rarely gives rise to an abnormal degree of insertion activity. Abnormal spontaneous activity—in the form of fibrillation potentials—is sometimes found in myasthenia gravis, but this is rare. During a voluntary contraction, although many of the motor unit potentials do not differ in amplitude, configuration, or duration from those seen in healthy muscle, they may exhibit a marked and abnormal variability in these parameters because defective neuromuscular transmission prevents activation of some of the fibers in the unit. Moreover, it is not uncommon to find motor units which are abnormally polyphasic, similar to the potentials which can be seen in muscular dystrophy or polymyositis. This could be due to a degree of neuromuscular block causing some of the fibers in a unit to drop out. In other instances it may be due to a myopathic change taking place in myasthenic muscle, and such a phenomenon may also explain the occasional development of neostigmine resistance in long-standing cases of myasthenia gravis. Since symptomatic myasthenia may be a feature of myopathic disorders such as polymyositis, it is important to exclude this possibility. In polymyositis, however, fibrillation and positive sharp waves are usually present in abundance.

During a sustained voluntary contraction of affected muscles in patients with myasthenia gravis, a gradual reduction in the amplitude of the interference pattern will be seen to occur, and this will continue until exhaustion is reached. At this point it may only be possible to observe single units, and these may suddenly appear to drop out. If edrophonium is given at the end of a sustained contraction the electrical response may be rapidly restored.

Neuromuscular Stimulation

A more precise measurement of fatigue is obtained by stimulating a muscle through its motor nerve and recording evoked potentials from the contracting muscle. This is most readily carried out on a peripheral nerve such as the ulnar nerve which can be stimulated at the wrist or elbow while evoked potentials are recorded from abductor digiti minimi.

As discussed in Chapter 7, such an evoked potential represents the summated electrical activity of the muscle fibers activated by the stimulus, and its amplitude provides an indication of the number of fibers so activated. Following supramaximal stimuli a decline in amplitude of the evoked potentials provides a measure of the degree of neuromuscular block. Although clinically useful, this technique has a number of disadvantages which may limit its value.

Firstly, the application of supramaximal stimuli, particularly at high rates, may be uncomfortable for the patient. Secondly, movement artifact may be a major difficulty and this cannot always be avoided even by careful splinting of the limb. Lastly, unless myasthenia gravis is generalized an abnormal response is not invariably recorded from the small muscles of the hand, even with high rates of stimulation.

In carrying out the test, careful preparation of the skin is essential and it is also important that the point at which the nerve is stimulated is located at the site where the smallest pulse will produce a supramaximal stimulus. The stimulus may be applied either through surface electrodes, which may be silver discs covered with gauze soaked in saline and strapped to the wrist, or through needle electrodes, which may be stainless steel electrodes coated with teflon except for 3mm at the tip. For recording, silver disc stick-on surface electrodes of the type used for EEG recording are satisfactory, one being placed over the muscle belly and the other over the muscle tendon. However, Slomić, Rosenfalck, and Buchthal (1968) recommend subcutaneous electrodes as less liable to give rise to artifact.

Healthy Subjects. In a healthy subject, repetitive stimulation at low rates may be carried out for extended periods of time without any decline in the size of the evoked potential. With tetanic frequencies, on the other hand, there may be a decline in the amplitude of the evoked potential depending on the rate of stimulation, and there is some variation between individuals. At rates greater than 10Hz the potentials which follow the first three to five stimuli show a progressive increase in amplitude and become shorter in duration. Between 100 and 200msec from the start of stimulation there may be a transient reduction in amplitude, possibly due to an artifact of movement. At stimulation frequencies up to 40Hz there will otherwise be no change in amplitude during the first 3 seconds of stimulation, but at rates above 65Hz the amplitude of the evoked response may fall to 50 percent of its initial value in 5 to 10 seconds. With stimulation at 50Hz a fall in amplitude of this magnitude may take 30 seconds or longer. After a period of tetanic stimulation, the potentials evoked by single stimuli are usually of the same size as those elicited before the tetanus (Harvey and Masland, 1941; Simpson, 1966; Brown, 1974; Lenman and Ritchie, 1977).

Myasthenic Subjects. In myasthenia gravis there is considerable variation in the response to repetitive stimulation. Thus in some patients an abnormal response will only be recorded at high rates of stimulation, though many severe or moderately affected patients will show a significant fall in amplitude of the evoked responses when short trains of stimuli at 3Hz are used (Slomić, Rosenfalck, and Buchthal, 1968). Some patients with myasthenia gravis show no pathologic response at all if the examination is confined to the small muscles of the hand.

In some patients a decrement may be recorded following a single pair of stimuli separated by anything from 20msec to 2 seconds, in which case the amplitude of the second potential may be significantly less than that of the first.

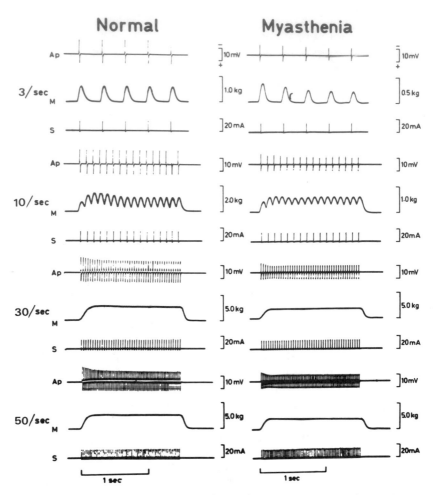

Fig. 8.2. *Action potentials (Ap), mechanical responses (M), and stimulus current (S) in trains, 1.5 sec in duration, evoked by stimuli given at a rate of 3, 10, 30, and 50 Hz. Normal subject U.S., male, 19 years old. Patient II, severe myasthenia gravis, female, 19 years old. The intramuscular temperature was 34–35°C (from Slomić, Rosenfalck, A., and Buchthal, F. 1968. Brain Res., 10, 1).*

These patients may show a progressive decline in the size of evoked responses to continued stimulation at rates as low as 3Hz, and Slomić, Rosenfalck, and Buchthal (1968) have found that trains of stimuli at 3Hz and lasting 1.5 seconds will give rise to a fall in amplitude of at least 10 percent in many severely or moderately severely affected patients with myasthenia gravis (Figs. 8.2 and 8.3). If the muscle is stimulated at 50Hz the most characteristic response is for a decrement to occur immediately or very early after the onset of the tetanus (Fig. 8.4); after stimulation for 1 or 2 seconds the amplitude of the potential may be maintained at a reduced but relatively constant level. In some subjects there may be little decrement with the first tetanus, but after several bursts of tetanus a decremental response is obtained. In other subjects, after repeated bursts of tetanus, a decremental response is seen even at rates of stimulation as low as 3Hz. Tetanic stimulation may also result in a progressive increment in action potential amplitude, similiar to that seen in the myasthenic syndrome.

Immediately after tetanic stimulation the action potentials evoked by single shocks are often of greater amplitude than those evoked before the tetanus in patients with myasthenia gravis. This is known as post-tetanic facilitation, and is similar to the phenomenon which can be seen in neuromuscular block induced by curare. It is due to an increased output of acetylcholine from the nerve endings following the tetanus (Johns, Grob, and Harvey,1956), and since it is not seen in normal subjects it is sometimes helpful in confirming the diagnosis of myasthenia gravis.

Repetitive Stimulation at Different Sites. Although the abductor digiti minimi is a satisfactory muscle to record from following stimulation of the ulnar nerve, only a proportion of patients with myasthenia gravis show an abnormal decremental response following stimulation in this situation. Other sites which have been studied include the deltoid muscle following stimulation at Erb's point on

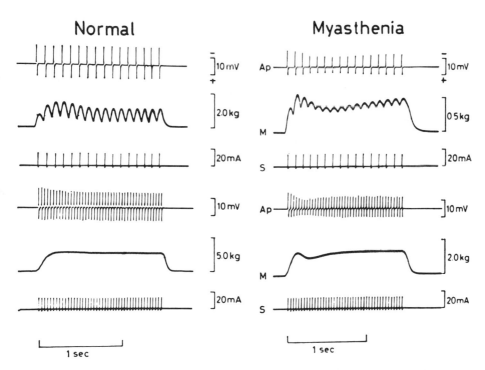

Fig. 8.3. *'Dip' in the action potential and the force in trains, at 10 Hz and 30 Hz for 1.5 sec in a patient with myasthenia gravis. Patient VI, severe myasthenia gravis, female, 19 years old; intramuscular temperature was 35°C (from Slomić, A., Rosenfalck, A., and Buchthal, F. 1968. Brain Res., 10, 1).*

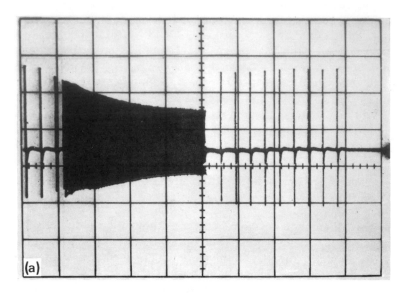

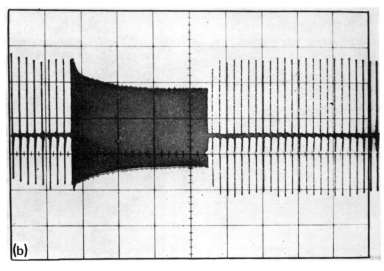

Fig. 8.4. *Evoked potentials in patient with myasthenia gravis obtained from abductor digiti minimi following repetitive stimulation of the ulnar nerve. In each record stimulation is at 5 and 50Hz. Height of squares in graticule represents 2.0mV. In record (a) amplitude of potentials decreases both at 5 Hz and at 50 Hz. In record (b) amplitude of potentials only decreases at 50 Hz, but the amplitude is increased following tetanic stimulation (from Lenman, J. A. R. and Ritchie, A. E. 1977. Clinical Electromyography. Pitman, London).*

the neck (Özdemir and Young, 1971) and the facial muscles (Kaeser, 1975). Özdemir and Young (1971), in a study of 30 patients with generalized myasthenia gravis, obtained significant changes in only 13 patients when they stimulated abductor digiti minimi, as compared with 23 patients when stimulating the deltoid. Twenty-six of the 30 patients showed a myasthenic response in one of three limb muscles studied, but in 6 this was only evident after vigorous exercise. Six out of 7 patients showed a decremental response when the orbicularis oculi was stimulated at rates of 3 to 8 Hz. Krarup (1977a and b) has carried out a detailed study of the responses evoked in the platysma muscle both in healthy subjects and in patients with myasthenia gravis, recording both the amplitude of the evoked action potential and the tension of the evoked isometric twitch. By this means it was possible to study the presence or absence of both a decremental response in action potential size, and of a staircase phenomenon (see below). Twenty-four patients were studied and it was found that the decrement in electrical and mechanical responses to repetitive stimuli was several times greater in the platysma than in the adductor pollicis, and the amplitude of post-tetanic facilitation was also several times greater in the platysma muscle. Edrophonium had a more pronounced effect in relieving the decrement in the platysma muscle than in the adductor pollicis. Although all 24 patients showed abnormalities in one or other of the muscles studied, abnormalities were either confined to, or more conspicuous in, the platysma in 16 (Fig. 8.5).

Post-tetanic Exhaustion. If stimulation is continued at a slow rate after a tetanus, there will be a progressive fall in size of the evoked potentials over about 20 minutes in myasthenia. A similar effect occurs in animals after

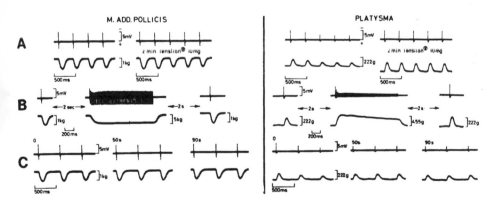

Fig. 8.5. Greater decrement in the electrical (upper traces) and the mechanical responses (lower traces) in the platysma than in the ADP in a patient with myasthenia gravis. A: 3 Hz trains (1.5 seconds in duration) before and after edrophonium, 10mg. B: tetanic stimuli (50 stimuli per second for 1.5 seconds) and single stimuli delivered before and after tetanus to show the greater post-tetanic facilitation of the action potential in the platysma than in the ADP. C: 2 Hz trains for 90 seconds; a staircase was absent in the platysma and in the ADP (from Krarup, C. 1977. J. Neurol. Neurosurg. Psychiatry, 40, 241).

hemicholinium, and this led Desmedt (1958) to postulate a failure of release of acetylcholine in myasthenia gravis. If short trains of stimuli are applied at 3Hz and at 1-minute intervals before and after maximum voluntary contraction lasting for half a minute, post-tetanic exhaustion can readily be demonstrated. Kaeser (1975) has shown that the procedure can also be carried out after prolonged trains of stimuli at 5Hz for 80 seconds or shorter trains of tetanus. Postactivation exhaustion may be aggravated by ischemia and this forms the basis of the double step test (Desmedt and Borenstein, 1977). In this test, muscles supplied by the ulnar nerve are activated through the nerve by supramaximal stimuli at 3 per second over a period of 4 minutes. This may be followed by a decrement which persists for as long as 20 minutes. Thirty minutes after the procedure a similar series of stimuli at 3 per second for 4 minutes is delivered after ischemia induced by a cuff placed around the arm proximal to the site of stimulation and inflated to 25 cm Hg. This is followed by a more profound decrement which gradually recovers after release of the cuff around the arm, and has proved useful in the recognition of subclinically involved muscles that reacted normally to the first step (Fig. 8.6).

Single Unit Stimulation. If graded threshold stimuli are applied to the ulnar or median nerve it is possible to isolate single motor unit responses from the thenar or hypothenar muscles (Kadrie and Brown, 1978a). The method is technically difficult, considerable experience being necessary to hold the stimulating electrode in position while the motor unit is studied in isolation, but it avoids the necessity to apply trains of stimuli of uncomfortable intensity to the patient. In a study of 8 patients with myasthenia gravis, 7 were found to show a decremental response in some of the motor units tested following stimulation. The proportion of motor units which showed abnormalities in neuromuscular transmission varied from 0 to 90 percent in different patients. When decrements were recorded, they tended to be greater for small than for large motor units, possibly indicating that small motor units have a lower margin for safe neuromuscular transmission (Kadrie and Brown, 1978b).

The Staircase Effect. The value of repetitive stimulation tests is enhanced if, in addition to recording the amplitude of evoked action potentials, the muscle tension is also recorded. The original myasthenic reaction described by Jolly was in fact a fall in tension following a stimulus, and if a fall in tension can be demonstrated by a transducer system which will record muscular tension, this aspect of the myasthenic response can be studied. A particularly interesting phenomenon which can only be studied by such means is the staircase phenomenon, which was originally described in cardiac muscle of the frog by Bowditch in 1870. If a muscle is stimulated repeatedly by electrical stimuli recurring slowly there is a progressive rise in twitch tension. This phenomenon was studied in man by Slomić, Buchthal, and Rosenfalck in 1968. They found that if contractions were evoked by trains of stimuli at 2Hz over a period of 1.5 minutes, there might be as much as a 40 percent increase in twitch tension without any comparable alteration in the amplitude of the evoked action potentials. In nearly all the cases of myasthenia gravis which they studied, however,

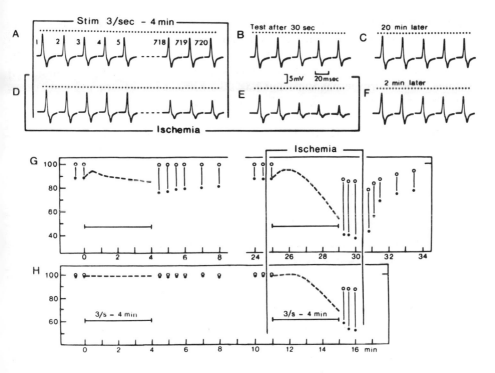

Fig. 8.6. *Female patient of 35 years with a moderately severe generalized myasthenia for about three months. Deprived of pyridostigmine for 5 hours. The double-step test is illustrated for the abductor muscle of the fifth finger on the left, which presents a significant (−12%) decrement of fifth muscle response in the rested state. Intramuscular temperature 36°C throughout. (A) First and last muscle responses (rank indicated) to ulnar nerve stimulation at 3 Hz for 4 minutes (first step). (B) Increased decrement (exhaustion) in the 3 Hz test 30 seconds after the series. (C) Fair recovery from exhaustion 20 minutes later. (D) Second step, under ischemia. (E) Thirty seconds later the first muscle response has increased in size with respect to the last response in the series, while the decrement of the fifth response is quite marked. (F) Partial recovery 2 minutes after release of the cuff. (G) Graph of the same experiment with the relative sizes of the first (circle) and fifth (dot) muscle response of each 3 Hz test (connected by a vertical line). This display indicates both the decrement and the changes in absolute size. The interrupted line represents changes in response size during the four-minute series. The period of ischemia is indicated. Abscissa, time in minutes. Ordinate, size of response as percent of the control response to a single stimulus before the tests. (H) Graph of a similar double-step test carried out after the patient had received 2.5 mg of neostigmine intramuscularly (from Desmedt, J. E. and Borenstein, S. 1977. Ann Neurol., 1, 55, with permission of Little, Brown).*

the staircase effect was absent. Absence of the staircase effect in particular was a sensitive indicator in mildly affected patients even when the muscle studied was clinically uninvolved, and monitoring the presence or absence of the staircase effect usefully increased the diagnostic yield of repetitive stimulation studies. The staircase phenomenon has also proved useful when the platysma muscle is examined (Krarup, 1977) (Figs. 8.5 and 8.7).

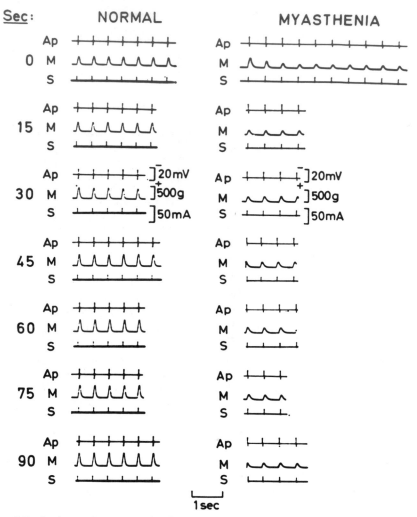

Fig. 8.7. *Staircase in a normal subject and absence of the staircase in a patient with severe myasthenia gravis. Action potential (Ap), force of the twitch (M), and stimulus current (S, 14 × threshold of the muscle action potential) at different times during the 1.5 min of supramaximal stimuli, given at a rate of 2 Hz to the ulnar nerve at the wrist. Left: Normal subject F. M. J., male, 22 years old; the intramuscular temperature was 34°C. Right: Patient No. VI with severe myasthenia gravis, female, 19 years old; the intramuscular temperature was 33°C (from Slomić, A., Rosenfalck, A., and Buchthal, F. 1968. Brain Res., 10, 1).*

Single Fiber Electromyography

If needle electrodes have a small enough recording surface it is possible to record action potentials from single muscle fibers, or from very small groups of muscle fibers, within a contracting muscle. If the muscle is activated electrically through stimulation of its motor nerve, repetitive stimulation will show that the latency of activated muscle fibers is not absolutely constant, but is subject to a small variation. This variation is known as jitter and is due to the variation which occurs in the time for conduction of the nerve impulse across the neuromuscular junction. The jitter phenomenon may be recorded by the multielectrode described by Ekstedt in 1964. This consists of a cannula containing 14 platinum wires which reach the surface through the side of the electrode to form a row of adjacent leading-off areas. For the purpose of recording variation in neuromuscular transmission time it is sufficient to have a simple electrode with 2 leading-off surfaces which should be designed to have an uptake radius of about 200 microns. With such an electrode it is possible to study jitter in voluntarily contracting muscle. To do this the electrode must be inserted so that it is able to record action potentials from two muscle fibers of the same unit, and one of these is made to trigger the oscilloscope sweep. The variation in the interval between these two potentials is the jitter (Fig. 8.8.). In healthy muscle the duration of jitter may be of the order of 20 μsec, but in neuromuscular block produced, for example, by curare this time may be considerably extended (Ekstedt and Stålberg, 1969). If jitter is to be expressed quantitatively it may be expressed in terms of MCD, which refers to the mean of the absolute consecutive differences of the interpotential intervals. To determine this precisely the time intervals can be recorded on digital tape and the mean consecutive differences extracted by means of a computer. In practice visual inspection of the oscilloscope screen will show whether there is an abnormal degree of jitter or not, but the degree of jitter can be measured manually by inspecting photographed recordings of a series of consecutive discharges. If 5 superimposed recordings, each of 10 consecutive discharges, are made and the range of interpotential interval for each recording is measured, the approximate MCD can be calculated according to the formula: MCD = mean range $_{(10)}$ × 0.37.

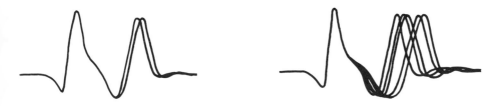

Fig. 8.8. Illustration to show variation in latency of second single fiber potential (jitter) when potentials from two fibers of same motor unit are recorded and potential from first triggers oscilloscope sweep. Degree of jitter in figure on the right is characteristic of neuromuscular block, and it is normal in figure on left.

(Ekstedt, Nilsson, and Stålberg, 1974). When myasthenic patients are studied one can expect to find an increase in jitter. The method is extremely sensitive as it is possible to study several potential pairs in a single muscle, and a variety of muscles can be examined. If no increase in jitter is found in any of the potential pairs examined, the diagnosis of myasthenia gravis becomes extremely unlikely. An increase in jitter, however, is not pathognomonic of myasthenia gravis since it may also be seen in other conditions, such as peripheral neuropathies, where reinnervation has taken place (Stålberg, Ekstedt, and Broman, 1974).

Jitter may also be recorded if the muscle is stimulated through its nerve. If myasthenic muscle is stimulated using submaximal pulses at a frequency of 2Hz, some potentials will be seen to drop out with continued stimulation. This procedure is again a very sensitive one, as blockings of single potentials may occur even in clinically unaffected muscles, and in patients with clinical manifestations of myasthenia that appear to be confined to the extraocular muscles (Schwartz and Stålberg, 1975). Single fiber electrode studies are on the whole well-tolerated by the patient and they do not require uncomfortable runs of supramaximal stimuli at tetanic frequency.

Terminal Latency and Numbers of Motor Units

A number of workers have shown that the terminal latency of motor unit potentials evoked by nerve stimulation is prolonged in patients with myasthenia gravis. This is so particularly with rapid rates of stimulation, but it has been found in severely affected patients even after a single stimulus. It has been shown that this increase in terminal latency applies also to single motor unit potentials which may be of short duration although of normal amplitude (Slomić, Buchthal, and Rosenfalck, 1968; Ballantyne and Hansen, 1974; Preswick, 1975). This observation adds little to the diagnostic information obtained by other methods, but it does provide evidence that there may be a terminal neuropathy in myasthenia gravis. It is consistent with morphologic evidence that the motor nerve terminals in myasthenia are abnormally fine and hence may conduct the impulses slowly

McComas, Sica, and Brown (1971) studied the extensor digitorum brevis muscle in 10 patients with myasthenia gravis and used an incremental stimulus technique (McComas, Sica, and Currie, 1970) to estimate the number of functioning motor units in the muscle. They found reduced populations of motor units in half the patients studied. Ballantyne and Hansen (1974), however, using a modified technique, were unable to find reduced numbers of motor units in the extensor digitorum brevis in the 20 myasthenic patients whom they studied.

The Response of Myasthenic Muscle to Relaxants

The use of edrophonium chloride (Tensilon) in the diagnosis of myasthenia gravis has been referred to above. It has a brief anticholinesterase action and it is effective, therefore, in distinguishing between myasthenic neuromuscular block and the cholinergic block which may occur in patients who are receiving more neostigmine than they are able to tolerate. Neostigmine is also effective in demonstrating the presence of a myasthenic block, but because of its prolonged latency and duration of action, it is a less satisfactory drug than edrophonium for this purpose. Edrophonium will counteract the decremental response of myasthenic muscle to repetitive stimulation, but it does not have this action on the staircase effect (Slomić, Buchthal, and Rosenfalck, 1968) and has no consistent effect on jitter. The action of decamethonium has been found to differ in myasthenic muscle as compared with healthy muscle (Churchill-Davidson and Richardson, 1952). In mildly affected patients its depolarizing action is less effective than it is in healthy muscle; in more severely affected patients it will produce neuromuscular block of the depolarization type, but this is succeeded by a competitive-type block which is reversible by Tensilon. Myasthenic muscle, on the other hand, is abnormally sensitive to curare, which will give rise to an increase in weakness in a much lower dose than is effective in a healthy subject. Both curare and quinine bisulphate, which also has a curare-like action, have been used in the diagnosis of myasthenia, but this application is not entirely free of hazard in view of the severe weakness which may develop.

THE MYASTHENIC SYNDROME

The association between bronchial carcinoma and a myasthenia-like syndrome was reported in 1953 by Anderson, Churchill-Davidson, and Richardson, and this condition was investigated electrophysiologically and fully described by Eaton and Lambert in 1957. Although the prominent symptoms of this condition are weakness and fatigability affecting particularly the proximal muscles, and there is undue sensitivity to muscle relaxants such as curare, the response to neostigmine and edrophonium is variable. On examination, tendon reflexes may be diminished or lost, sometimes to be temporarily restored following brief exercise. Although many cases have occurred in association with bronchial carcinoma and a smaller number in association with tumors from other sites such as the breast, stomach, or rectum, a number of cases have occurred in which no evidence of tumor has been found despite prolonged followup. It is not exceptional for the condition to present before the tumor is evident, and it has been reported following removal of a bronchial carcinoma. The therapeutic response to neostigmine is disappointing, but clinical improvement may follow the administration of guanidine which promotes the release of acetylcholine from the nerve endings.

Electron microscopy has shown that there is a normal content of synaptic vesicles in the nerve terminal and no deficiency of acetylcholine receptor in the postsynaptic membrane. Microelectrode studies of intercostal muscle biopsies have shown no alteration in the amplitude or discharge frequency of miniature end-plate potentials. During nerve stimulation, however, it has been found that the number of quanta of acetylcholine which are released may be insufficient to produce an adequate end-plate response. This is similar to the effect that might be expected if the nerve endings were exposed to an excess of magnesium. Addition of either calcium or guanidine to the bathing solution in the microelectrode recording chamber leads to an increase in size of the end-plate potentials (Lambert and Elmqvist, 1971).

The study of the effects of repetitive stimulation of a muscle through its peripheral nerve is of great assistance in establishing the diagnosis. The response to a single stimulus is abnormally small, and if the nerve is stimulated at a slow rate (1 to 2Hz) there is a progressive reduction in size of the evoked muscle potentials. On the other hand, with rapid rates of stimulation there is a progressive increase in the size of the potentials (Fig. 8.9). After tetanic stimulation has ceased there may be a short period of facilitation, and this is followed by a period of post-tetanic exhaustion similar to that seen in myasthenia gravis.

Recently Engel, Lambert, and Gomez (1977) have described a single patient who developed generalized weakness and fatigability, with diminished reflexes, soon after birth. On repetitive stimulation of the thenar muscles through the median nerve, there was a decremental response at both high and low frequencies of nerve stimulation. Neither anticholinesterase drugs nor guanidine had any effect on the condition. On electron microscopy the nerve terminals were found to be very small. Acetylcholine receptor was present in normal amounts in the postsynaptic region but acetylcholinesterase was found to be absent from the end-plates. When intercostal muscle was studied with microelectrodes,

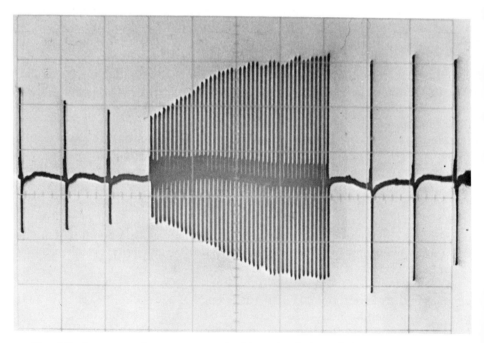

Fig. 8.9. Incremental response to repetitive stimulation of ulnar nerve recorded from patient with myasthenic syndrome.

miniature end-plate potentials of normal amplitude but decreased frequency were recorded. This syndrome, therefore, is characterized by two distinct features. First, the nerve terminals are very small and the release of acetylcholine from them is decreased, and second, the acetylcholine released is not inactivated by acetylcholinesterase.

MYOPATHIES AND NEUROPATHIES

Although they do not show the fatigability on clinical testing which is characteristic of myasthenia gravis, abnormal responses to repetitive stimulation are found in many patients with disorders of muscle. Thus patients with Duchenne, limb-girdle, or facioscapulohumeral muscular dystrophy may be found to show a decremental response in extensor digitorum brevis following repetitive stimulation of the muscle through its nerve (McComas, Sica, and Currie, 1970; Sica and McComas, 1971). In myotonia there may be a decremental response to rates of stimulation as low as 5Hz, but this is only present in rested muscle and is not evident if the muscle has already been conditioned by a train of stimuli (Brown, 1974). In polymyositis tetanic stimulation of the nerve may be followed either by a decrement or by a progressive increment in the amplitude of the evoked potentials. Decremental responses have also been reported in association with McArdle's syndrome when stimulation is continued for periods exceeding 4 seconds (Dyken, Smith, and Peak, 1967; Delwaide, Lemaire, and Reznik, 1968). A decremental response to stimulation was reported in 1948 by Hodes in patients with poliomyelitis, and has also been seen in motor neuron disease (Fig. 8.10) and in peripheral neuropathy (Mulder, Lambert, and Eaton, 1959; Simpson and Lenman, 1959). Changes tend to occur irregularly and the response to neostigmine is seldom striking.

ANTIBIOTICS

In addition to the neuromuscular blocking agents which have been described above, a number of antibiotics have been found to give rise to neuromuscular block. These include neomycin, streptomycin, tetracycline, and polymixin. It is not certain if all these drugs act in the same manner, but some would appear to prevent the release of acetylcholine from the nerve terminals.

BOTULISM

Botulinus toxin will produce neuromuscular block. On repetitive stimulation at low rates, there is a decrement in evoked muscle responses, but at rapid rates of stimulation there is an incremental response. These changes are similar

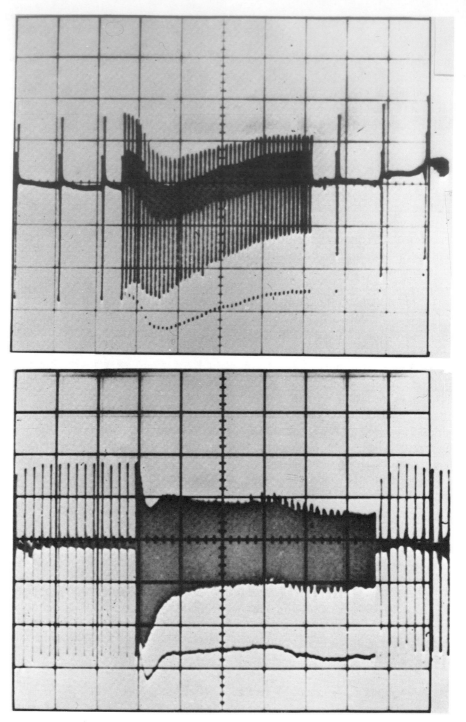

Fig. 8.10. *Fall in amplitude of potentials evoked in abductor digiti minimi during tetanic stimulation of the ulnar nerve in patient with motor neuron disease. In each record stimulation is at 5 and 50Hz. Height of squares on graticule represents 500 µV (from Lenman, J. A. R. and Ritchie, A. E. 1977. Clinical Electromyography, Pitman, London).*

to those seen in the Eaton-Lambert syndrome, and experimental evidence is consistent with the belief that there is a presynaptic block with impaired release of acetylcholine (Mayer, 1968; Harris and Miledi, 1971; Cherington, 1973).

ACKNOWLEDGMENTS

We are grateful to Miss M. Benstead, medical artist, Dundee University, who has provided a number of line drawings.

REFERENCES

Almon, R. R., Andrew, C. G., and Appel, S. H. (1974). Serum globulin in myasthenia gravis: inhibition of α-bungaro-toxin binding to acetylcholine receptors. Science, *186:*55.

Anderson, H. J., Churchill-Davidson, H. C., and Richardson, A. T. (1953). Bronchial neoplasm with myasthenia. Prolonged apnoea after administration of succinylcholine. Lancet, *II:*1291.

Axelsson, J. and Thesleff, S. (1959). A study of supersensitivity in denervated mammalian skeletal muscle. J. Physiol. (Lond.), *147:*178.

Ballantyne, J. P. and Hansen, S. (1974). Computer method for the analysis of evoked motor unit potentials. 1. Control subjects and patients with myasthenia gravis. J. Neurol. Neurosurg. Psychiatry, *37:*1187.

Brown, J. C. (1974). Repetitive stimulation and neuromuscular transmission studies. In: Disorders of Voluntary Muscle. 3rd Edn. J. N. Walton. Ed., Churchill Livingstone, Edinburgh.

Burgen, A. S. V., Dickens, F., and Zatman, L. J. (1949).The action of botulinum toxin on the neuromuscular junction. J. Physiol. (Lond.), *109:*10.

Castillo, J. del and Katz, B. (1956). Biophysical aspects of neuromuscular transmission. Progr. Biophys. Mol. Biol., *6:*122.

Cherington, M. (1973). Botulism: electrophysiologic and therapeutic observations. In: New Developments in Electromyography and Clinical Neurophysiology. Desmedt, J. E., Ed., Vol. 1. p. 375. S. Karger, Basel.

Churchill-Davidson, H. C. and Richardson, A. T. (1952). The action of decamethonium iodide (C10) in myasthenia gravis. J. Neurol. Neurosurg. Psychiatry, *15:*129.

Delwaide, P. J., Lemaire, R. and Reznik, M. (1968). EMG findings in a case of McArdle's myopathy. Electroencephalogr. Clin. Neurophysiol., *25:*414.

Desmedt, J. E. (1958). Myasthenic-like features of neuromuscular transmission after administration of an inhibitor of acetylcholine synthesis. Nature, *182:*1673.

Desmedt, J. E. and Borenstein, S. (1977). Double-step nerve stimulation test for myasthenic block: sensitization of postactivation exhaustion by ischemia. Ann. Neurol., *1:*55.

Diamond, J. and Miledi, R. (1962). A study of foetal and new-born rat muscle fibres. J. Physiol. (Lond.), *162:*393.

Duchen, L. W. and Stefani, E. (1971). Electrophysiological studies of neuromuscular transmission in hereditary 'motor end-plate disease' of the mouse. J. Physiol. (Lond.), *212:*535.

Dyken, M. L., Smith, D. M. and Peak, R. L. (1967). An electromyographic diagnostic screening test in McArdle's disease and a case report. Neurology, *17:*45.

Eaton, L. M. and Lambert, E. H. (1956). Electromyography and electric stimulation of nerves in diseases of motor unit. Observations on myasthenic syndrome associated with malignant tumors. J.A.M.A., *163:*1117.

Ekstedt, J. (1964). Human single-muscle fiber action potentials. Acta Physiol. Scand., *61:*suppl. 226, 1.

Ekstedt, J. and Stålberg, E. (1969). The effect of non-paralytic doses of D-tubocurarine on individual motor end-plates in man studied with a new electrophysiological method. Electroencephalogr. Clin. Neurophysiol., *27:*557.

Ekstedt, J., Nilsson, G, and Stålberg, E. (1974). Calculation of the electromyographic jitter. J. Neurol. Neurosurg. Psychiatry, *37:*526.

Engel, A. G., Lambert, E. H., and Gomez, M. R. (1977). A new myasthenic syndrome with end-plate acetylcholinesterase deficiency, small nerve terminals, and reduced acetylcholine release. Ann. Neurol., *1:*315.

Fambrough, D. M., Drachman, D. B., and Satyamurti, S. (1973). Neuromuscular junction in myasthenia gravis: decreased acetylcholine receptors. Science, *182:*293.

Harris, A. J. and Miledi, R. (1971). The effect of type D botulinum toxin on frog neuromuscular junctions. J. Physiol. (Lond.), *217:*497.

Harvey, A. M. and Masland, R. L. (1941). A method for the study of neuromuscular transmission in human subjects. Bull. Johns Hopkins Hosp., *68:*81.

Hubbard, J. I. and Wilson, D. F. (1973). Neuromuscular transmission in a mammalian preparation in the absence of blocking drugs and the effect of D-tubocurarine. J. Physiol. (Lond.), *228:*307.

Huxley, A. F. and Taylor, R. E. (1958). Local activation of striated muscle fibres. J. Physiol. (Lond.), *144:*426.

Johns, R. J., Grob, D. and Harvey, A. M. (1956). Studies in neuromuscular function. II. Effects of nerve stimulation in normal subjects and in patients with myasthenia gravis. Bull. Johns Hopkins Hosp., *99:*125.

Jolly, F. (1895). Uber myasthenia gravis pseudoparalytica. Berl. Klin. Wschr., *32:*33.

Kadrie, H. A. and Brown, W. F. (1978a). Neuromuscular transmission in human single units. J. Neurol. Neurosurg. Psychiatry, *41:*193.

Kadrie, H. A. and Brown, W. F. (1978b). Neuromuscular transmission in myasthenic single motor units. J. Neurol. Neurosurg. Psychiatry, *41:*205.

Kaeser, H. E., Ed. (1975). Nervous and muscular evoked potentials. In: Handbook of Electroencephalography and Clinical Neurophysiology. Vol. 16, A, Elsevier, Amsterdam.

Krarup, C. (1977a). Electrical and mechanical responses in the platysma and in the adductor pollicis muscle: in normal subjects. J. Neurol. Neurosurg. Psychiatry, *40:*234.

Krarup, C. (1977b). Electrical and mechanical responses in the platysma and in the adductor pollicis muscle: in patients with myasthenia gravis. J. Neurol. Neurosurg. Psychiatry, *40:*241.

Lambert, E. H. and Elmqvist, D. (1971). Quantal components of end-plate potentials in the myasthenic syndrome. Ann. N.Y. Acad. Sci., *183:*183.

Lenman, J. A. R. and Ritchie, A. E. (1977). Clinical Electromyography. Pitman, London.

MacIntosh, F. C. (1958). Formation, storage and release of acetylcholine at nerve endings. Canad. J. Biochem. Physiol., *37:*343.

Mayer, R. F. (1968). The neuromuscular defect in human botulism. Electroencephalogr. Clin. Neurophysiol., *25:*397.

McComas, A. J., Sica, R. E. P., and Brown, J. C. (1971). Myasthenia gravis: evidence for a "central" defect. J. Neurol. Sci., *13:*107.

McComas, A. J., Sica, R. E. P., and Currie, S. (1970). Muscular dystrophy: evidence for a neural factor. Nature, *226:*1263.

Miledi, R. (1960). Junctional and extra-junctional acetylcholine receptors in skeletal muscle fibres. J. Physiol. (Lond.), *151:*24.

Mulder, D. W., Lambert, E. H. and Eaton, L. M. (1959). Myasthenic syndrome in patients with amyotrophic lateral sclerosis. Neurology, *9:*627.

Özdemir, C. and Young, R. R. (1971). Electrical testing in myasthenia gravis. Ann. N.Y. Acad. Sci., *183:*287.

Patrick, J. and Lindstrom. J. (1973). Autoimmune response to acetylcholine receptor. Science, *180:*871.

Preswick, G. (1965). The myasthenic reaction. In: Neuromuscular Diseases. Proc. 8th Congress Neurologie, Vienna (1965), Vol. II, p. 525.

Robertson, J. D. (1956). The ultrastructure of a reptilian myoneural junction. J. Biophys. Biochem. Cytol., *2:*381.

Schwartz, M. S. and Stålberg, E. (1975). Single fibre electromyographic studies in myasthenia gravis with repetitive nerve stimulation. J. Neurol. Neurosurg. Psychiatry, *38:*678.

Sica, R. E. P. and McComas, A. J. (1971). Fast and slow twitch units in a human muscle. J. Neurol. Neurosurg. Psychiatry, *34:*113.

Simpson, J. A. (1960). Myasthenia gravis: a new hypothesis. Scott. Med. J., *5:*419.

Simpson, J. A. (1966). Disorders of neuromuscular transmission. Proc. R. Soc. Med., *59:*993.

Simpson, J. A. (1974). Myasthenia gravis and myasthenic syndromes. In: Disorders of Voluntary Muscle. 3rd Edn., J. N. Walton, Ed. Churchill Livingstone, Edinburgh.

Simpson, J. A. and Lenman, J. A. R. (1959). The effect of frequency of stimulation in neuromuscular disease. Electroencephalogr. Clin. Neurophysiol., *11:*604.

Slomić, A., Rosenfalck, A., and Buchthal, F. (1968). Electrical and mechanical responses of normal and myasthenic muscle. Brain Res., *10:*1.

Stålberg, E., Ekstedt, J., and Broman, A. (1974). Neuromuscular transmission in myasthenia gravis studied with single fibre electromyography. J. Neurol. Neurosurg. Psychiatry, *37:*540.

Walker, M. B. (1934). Treatment of myasthenia gravis with physostigmine. Lancet, *1:*1200.

9

Studies of Reflex Activity from a Clinical Viewpoint

BHAGWAN T. SHAHANI and ROBERT R. YOUNG

Introduction
The H reflex and F response
 Clinical applications
  Peripheral neuropathies

Entrapment neuropathies and root
 compression syndrome
Blink Reflexes
Concluding Comment

  Since the original description of the law concerning spinal nerve roots by Sir Charles Bell (1811) and Magendie (1822), there has been much interest in the reflex activity produced by a variety of peripheral stimuli. In the early part of this century, the epoch-making work of Sir Charles Sherrington, summarized in his Silliman lectures, "The integrative action of the Nervous System" (1906), marked a new era in the understanding of the fundamental principles of reflex physiology which form a basis for modern concepts of nervous integration. Although significant advances in electronic and computer technology have made it possible to study reflex activity quantitatively in intact human subjects, most neurologists still rely on gross clinical observations of altered responses to tonic or phasic stretches of muscles, or to skin irritation, in order to arrive at some understanding of altered physiology and thereby derive a neurologic diagnosis. However, in the past three decades, detailed electrophysiologic studies have shown that it is possible, using electromyographic techniques, to record most of the reflexes (both proprioceptive and exteroceptive) commonly studied in a clinical setting. These studies, in addition to providing better insight into the underlying physiologic mechanisms, provide an objective and quantitative measure of function of the central and peripheral nervous system in man. This chapter will review briefly the clinical reasons for studying three useful physiologic parameters: the monosynaptic H reflex, the F response (which is not a reflex), and the blink reflex which is an example of an exteroceptive reflex. We believe that studies of the H reflex, F response, and blink reflex have resulted in a substantial diagnostic yield and, therefore, that they should be performed, with certain limitations, in every clinical EMG laboratory.

THE H REFLEX AND F RESPONSE

  In 1918, Paul Hoffmann demonstrated that the compound muscle action potentials (CMAP) associated with the ankle and knee jerks were comparable in latency and configuration to those evoked by submaximal electrical shocks delivered percutaneously to the tibial and femoral nerves, respectively. He concluded that both the tendon jerks and the electrically induced "late responses" must represent activity in the same kind of stretch reflex. On the basis of his observations, which included a) abolition of the late response with supramaximal stimulation to the mixed nerve, and b) the relatively brief latency of the late response (e.g. 30 msec in the calf muscles), he reasoned that the afferent pathway of this reflex must consist of very fast conducting fibers and that the central delay must be extremely short. The conclusions from Hoffmann's remarkable experiments, which antedated the study of monosynaptic reflexes in animals by more than two decades (Lloyd, 1943), were subsequently confirmed by Magladery and McDougal (1950) who designated the electrically induced late response the H reflex after its discoverer. The even shorter latency CMAP evoked by direct electrical stimulation of motor axons was called the M response. In contrast to the large amplitude H reflex which could easily be recorded in the calf muscles following submaximal stimulation (Fig. 9.1), another type of late response was seen in intrinsic muscles of the hands and feet. This response (Fig. 9.2), which had a rather similar latency to that of the H reflex but required stronger stimulation, was named the F wave (or F response). Although Magladery and McDougal thought it was a polysynaptic reflex, it is now generally agreed that, to a large degree, F responses as recorded in the EMG laboratory are due to centrifugal discharges from individual motor neurons, each of which is initiated by an antidromic axonal volley (Dawson and Merton, 1956; Thorne, 1965; McLeod and Wray, 1966; Mayer and Feldman, 1967). Since their latencies are rather similar (the F response latency being a few milliseconds longer in the same muscle), it is not possible to ascertain exactly what percentage of a late response recorded with surface electrodes is made up of motor units active in the F response or in the H reflex. It is important to make a clear distinction between these two responses, because they provide a different type of information regarding the central and peripheral nervous system (Shahani and Young, 1976; Lachman, Shahani, and Young, 1979). Some of the distinguishing features of the H reflex and the F response are described in Table 9.1.

For many years, H reflexes have been used to study the excitability of the motor neuron pool; a submaximal reflex response is elicited before, during, and after a "conditioning" stimulus in normal subjects and in patients with lesions of the CNS (Magladery et al, 1952; Paillard, 1955; Angel and Hoffman, 1963; Ioku et al, 1965; Takamori, 1967; Yap, 1967; Zander Olsen and Diamantopoulos, 1967; Táboříková and Sax, 1969; Shahani, 1970a). It should be pointed out, however, that H reflex excitability curves are markedly affected by such independent variables as the position of the patient; the angle of the hip, knee, and ankle; and the amount of background voluntary or reflex muscular contraction in the leg muscles, as well as "remote" muscular contraction. In order to obtain reproducible responses, the subject must lie (or sit) still and relax in a comfortable position, and the limb must be rigidly fixed at various joints at appropriate angles to avoid changes in proprioceptive input. Even a slight

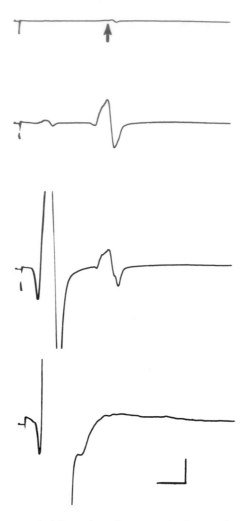

Fig. 9.1. *H reflex recorded from the soleus muscle. Increasing stimulus strength from the top to the bottom trace. Note the appearance of H reflex* (arrow) *before that of the direct M response. Details in the text. Calibration: 10 msec and 1 mV upper two traces, 500 µV lower two traces.*

change in the position of the head or neck, or in other sensory inputs (e.g. visual or auditory) can produce significant changes in motor neuron excitability, and this makes it very difficult to interpret the results of various studies. In all studies of H reflex excitability curves, it is important to demonstrate a small preceding M response of unchanging amplitude and configuration from one stimulus to the next, as a proof of the stability of the relationship between the nerve and the stimulating electrode. Although various methods have been tried in recent years (Johnson, Sax, and Feldman, 1974; Hays et al, 1979), in an attempt to represent adequately the characteristic fluctuations in the excitability of the motor neuron pool without incorporating variability due to randomly occurring supraspinal and segmental influences, we feel that plotting H reflex excitability curves in these ways is too tedious and time-consuming; therefore, they are not recommended for routine evaluation of the excitability of the motor neuron pool in the clinical EMG laboratory. Similarly, although we have demonstrated (Fisher, Shahani, and Young, 1978a) that certain CNS lesions produce changes in persistence and amplitude of the F response which may eventually provide a quantitative assessment of CNS function, we do not feel that such studies should be performed routinely in all EMG laboratories.

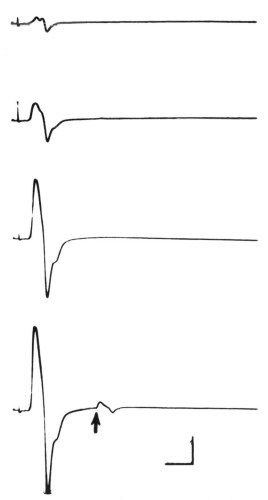

Fig. 9.2. *F response recorded from the abductor pollicis brevis muscle. Increasing stimulus strength from the top to the bottom trace. Note the appearance of the F response* (arrow) *with the supramaximal shock. Calibration: 10 msec and 1 mV.*

Table 9.1. FEATURES DISTINGUISHING BETWEEN THE
H REFLEX AND F RESPONSE

H Reflex	F Response
1. A monosynaptic reflex in which the afferent arc consists of group Ia afferent fibers from muscle spindles, and the efferent arc consists of alpha motor axons.	Not a reflex. Centrifugal discharge of a small percentage of motor neurons initiated by antidromic volleys in their axons. Both afferent and efferent arc consists of alpha motor axons.
2. Stimulus threshold lower than that required to evoke a direct M response. Supramaximal stimulation for the M response blocks the H reflex.	Stimulus threshold usually higher than that required for the H reflex and the M response.
3. Mean amplitude (5–10 responses) can be up to 50%–100% of the maximal M response.	Mean amplitude small, usually less than 5% of the maximal M response.
4. Appearance and persistence rather constant at low rates of stimulation (1 every 10–30 seconds).	Appearance and persistence rather variable, even at low rates of stimulation.
5. Easily recorded from the soleus muscle and some proximal "postural" muscles in adults. Present in intrinsic hand and foot muscles in newborn infants.	Can be recorded easily from almost every skeletal muscle.
6. Single motor units activated in the H reflex are different from those in the preceding M response.	Single motor units activated in the F response are same as those in the M response.
7. Fluctuation of latency of the single motor units activated in the H reflex is greater than for those in the F or the M response.	Fluctuation of single motor unit latency in the F response is less than that in the H reflex, but greater than that in the M response.

In recent years, these two late responses have been widely used to evaluate function in the peripheral nervous system (Ackil, Shahani, and Young, 1978a, b; Adams, Shahani, and Young, 1973; Albizzati et al, 1976; Braddom and Johnson, 1974; Conrad, Aschoff, and Fischler, 1975; Eisen, Schomer, and Melmed, 1977; Kimura, 1974; Kimura and Butzer, 1975; King and Ashby, 1976; Lachman, Shahani, and Young, 1977; Lefebvre-D'Amour et al, 1976; Mayer and Mawdsley, 1965; Panayiotopoulos, Scarpalezos, and Nastas, 1977, 1978; Shahani, Young, and Lachman, 1975; Wager and Buerger, 1974a, b; Young and Shahani, 1978). However, some of the techniques used are rather controversial. Some involve methods and formulae to convert minimal latencies of these two late responses into a conduction velocity in different segments (including proximal portions) of the peripheral nerve and nerve roots. Since these techniques are based on several unproven assumptions (previously discussed by Young and Shahani, 1978), we recommend that the clinical electromyographer restrict his studies to the measurement of *minimal latencies* of the F response and the H reflex. Conversion, using different formulae, of primary data (latencies) into conduction velocity may appear "scientific" to some, but in fact these methods introduce several errors and the results, therefore, can be rather misleading. The methodology for recording H reflexes and F responses has been well described previously (Hugon, 1973; Shahani and Young, 1976). As far as the use of late responses for evaluation of the peripheral nervous system is concerned, the rigid protocol (e.g. isometric recording and long interstimulus intervals) required to study CNS function may not be necessary. However, proper understanding of these two late responses and methods for differentiating between the two, as outlined in Table 9 1, is mandatory because they provide one with different types of information. Essentially, for recording H reflexes, the active surface electrode is placed over the middle part or on the medial bulge of the soleus muscle, below the level of the lower margin of the two heads of the gastrocnemius muscle, and the indifferent electrode is placed distally over the Achilles tendon. The tibial nerve is stimulated in the popliteal fossa using surface, bipolar stimulating electrodes, with the cathode being proximal. Stimuli, which usually are square wave pulses (duration 0.1 to 1 msec), are delivered at 0.5 Hz. The voltage is gradually increased (the H reflex usually appearing before the M response) until a maximal amplitude reflex response is recorded. After multiple recordings, the response with minimal latency is used for measurement. It may be noted that, although they are present in intrinsic hand muscles of newborn infants (Thomas and Lambert, 1960), H reflexes in normal adult subjects can be recorded easily *only* in the soleus muscle. This does not mean that the reflex pathway for the H reflex does not exist for various other muscles; in fact, H reflexes can be demonstrated in a variety of muscles in patients with certain CNS lesions, and in normal subjects under certain unusual physiologic conditions, such as by post-tetanic potentiation or by voluntary background contraction of the muscle (Hagbarth, 1962).

In contrast with the H reflex, the F response can be recorded easily from almost every skeletal muscle, making it more versatile for the evaluation of conduction in alpha motor axons. The method of recording and stimulation is similar to that used for measuring maximal motor conduction velocity (Ch. 7) in different nerves. In fact, F responses are evoked every time that tests for the measurement of motor conduction velocity are performed. In order to see them, however, the sweep speed of the oscilloscope must be changed to permit visualization of the trace for 100 msec after the stimulus. Ten responses are recorded and the minimal latency (measured to the first deflection from the baseline) provides information regarding the fastest conducting motor nerve fibers mediating the F response.

As expected, there is a direct relationship between the minimal latency of these two late responses and the height of the subject (Figs. 9.3 and 9.4) and/or length of the appropriate extremity (Conrad et al, 1975; Lefebvre-D'Amour et al, 1976; Young and Shahani, 1978; Lachman et al, 1979). On the whole it is easier, simpler, and more accurate to record heights and thus avoid unnecessary errors which are inherent in the measurement of distance between various

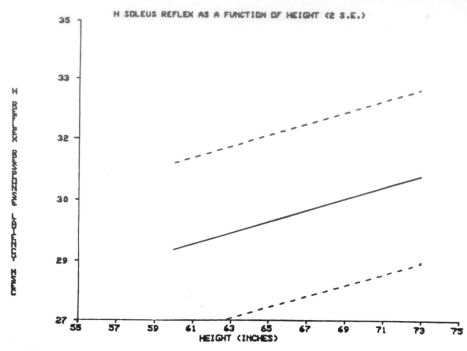

Fig. 9.3. *Relationship of minimal latency of the H reflex to the height in normal subjects.*

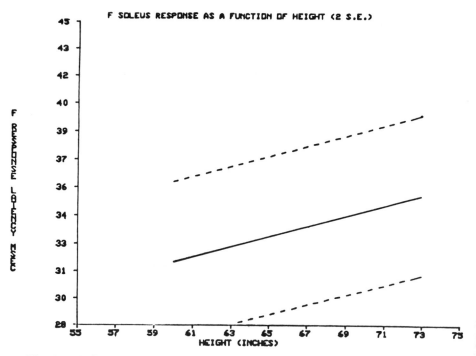

Fig. 9.4. *Relationship of minimal latency of the F response to the height in normal subjects.*

anatomic landmarks. Nomograms with minimal latency plotted for different heights provide accurate normative information regarding conduction in motor and/or group Ia afferent (in case of H reflex) nerve fibers. When one considers the adult population as a whole, maximal latencies for the H reflex in the soleus should be 34 msec or less, F response in soleus 38 msec or less, and F responses in the intrinsic hand muscles 30 msec or less. The interlimb difference in minimal latency of the H reflex in soleus muscle, or F responses in intrinsic hand muscles on the two sides, is normally less than 2 msec.

Clinical Applications

The usefulness of performing late response studies has been demonstrated in patients with a variety of disorders affecting the peripheral nervous system. Significant prolongation of minimal latency of H reflexes and F responses can be demonstrated at a time when conventional methods for studying motor and sensory conduction may not show an abnormality in an individual patient.

Peripheral Neuropathies. Abnormalities of late responses are seen in patients with a variety of peripheral neuropathies, including both the so-called "axonal" and the "segmental demyelinating" types (Lachman et al, 1979). In neuropathies in which there is a specific disorder of sensory fibers (e.g. Friedreich's ataxia) with preservation of the alpha motor axons, it can be shown that the H reflex is absent (Shahani, 1970b; Adams et al, 1973; Lachman et al, 1979), whereas F responses can be recorded with normal latency. In a variety of other neuropathies we have seen a gradual transition from the H reflex to the F response in the soleus muscle as the neuropathy has progressed with diminution and finally disappearance of the ankle jerk. F responses, in this instance, will have a prolonged latency if there is involvement of motor axons in addition to that of large afferent fibers which resulted in abolition of the H reflex. The minimal latency of the H reflex is usually (not always) relatively prolonged when the ankle jerk is diminished.

Because F responses can be recorded from a variety of skeletal muscles, they are valuable in providing information regarding motor conduction in the entire segment (proximal as well as distal) of peripheral nerves in different parts of the body. Moreover, since F responses are evoked whenever supramaximal stimulation is delivered to various nerves for determination of maximal motor conduction velocity, they provide additional information regarding the function of alpha motor axons, without extra effort on the part of the electromyographer or the need for an electronic averaging device.

In many neuropathies of the metabolic-nutritional type, such as alcoholic neuropathy, uremic neuropathy, and diabetic neuropathy (Lefebvre-D'Amour et al, 1976; Lachman et al, 1977; Ackil et al, 1978a, b), abnormalities of late responses can be demonstrated in individual patients in the distribution of the same nerve as that in which conventional methods of motor and sensory conduction do not show any abnormality. There are several possible explanations for this sensitivity of late response studies. In the first place, late responses studies evaluate function along the entire course of the motor axon so that abnormality in any particular segment can be detected. Secondly, the ranges of normal values for late responses are narrower compared to those for motor conduction velocity in different nerves, making it easier to detect mild abnormalities in individual patients.

In patients with neuropathies in which the primary pathologic process appears to be segmental demyelination (e.g. Guillain-Barré syndrome), prolongation of late response latencies may be the first objective recordable sign at an early stage in the disease, when diagnosis is difficult and when CSF protein and conventional motor and sensory conduction in the peripheral nerve segments are normal (Shahani et al, 1975; Lachman et al, 1977, 1979). Significant prolongation of late response latencies, with minor changes in conduction measured with conventional methods, also helps one localize a lesion to proximal segments, a finding which is sometimes seen in patients with Guillain-Barré idiopathic polyneuritis.

Entrapment Neuropathies and Root Compression Syndrome. In recent years we have demonstrated that, in addition to being useful in the diagnosis of mild or even subclinical peripheral neuropathies, measurements of late response latency can be an important adjunct to routine motor and sensory nerve conduction studies in establishing the diagnosis of entrapment neuropathies (Egloff-Baer, Shahani, and Young, 1978; Maccabee, Shahani, and Young, 1978; Shahani et al, 1979). In patients with carpal tunnel syndrome, the minimal latency of the F response in the median nerve innervated abductor pollicis brevis muscle may be significantly prolonged (>2 msec), when compared with the F response minimal latency in the ulnar innervated abductor digiti minimi in the same hand. Similarly, in patients with an ulnar entrapment syndrome at the elbow, the minimal latency for F responses in the abductor digiti minimi becomes relatively prolonged (>2 msec).

Since the soleus muscle is innervated primarily by S1 and S2 nerve roots, studies of the H reflex and F response in soleus can provide information regarding abnormalities of conduction in root compression syndromes affecting these nerve roots (Drechsler, Lastouka, and Kalvodova, 1966; Notermans and Vingerhoets, 1974; Braddom and Johnson, 1974; Fisher et al, 1978b; Tonzola et al, 1978). Minimal latency measurements in other muscles in the lower extremity such as extensor digitorum brevis (L5-S1) and abductor hallucis (S1-S2) provide further information regarding lesions of appropriate roots (Tonzola et al, 1978). In our experience, the minimal latency of the H reflex in the affected extremity is relatively prolonged only when there is reduction in the clinically elicited ankle jerk on the appropriate side. When the tendon jerk cannot be elicited, there is usually no H reflex, or if it is present, it is so small in amplitude that one cannot be certain, using surface electrodes, what percentage of the late response is an H reflex or an F response. In this instance, it is better to deliver supramaximal stimulation and record the F response which may or may not have a prolonged latency, depending upon the degree of compression of the alpha motor axons in a particular spinal root. It must be emphasized that there are a number of patients who have well-proven evidence of nerve root compression, although values for minimal latency of late responses are within normal limits. This is due to the fact that, as long as there are a few functional large diameter axons with normal conduction velocity that can mediate the late response, the minimal latency for that particular response will remain normal. However, whenever abnormal, studies of the H reflex and F responses can be extremely useful in localizing a lesion in patients with cervical or lumbosacral root disease. A number of patients are referred to EMG laboratories with a clinical diagnosis of thoracic outlet syndrome. In the majority of these patients, conventional motor and sensory conduction studies reveal no abnormality, and the results of late response studies are also normal. However, in well-documented cases of cervical rib and/or band compressing the lower cervical roots (C8, T1), we have often seen prolongation of minimal latencies of F responses in both median and ulnar innervated intrinsic hand muscles.

BLINK REFLEXES

The blink reflex, like many other cutaneous reflexes in man, is a double component polysynaptic reflex, the afferent arc of which is provided by sensory divisions (first and second) of the trigeminal nerve, whereas motor axons in the facial nerve form its efferent arc. There is no physiologic or anatomic evidence to suggest that the first component of the blink reflex is a monosynaptic proprioceptive reflex akin to the H reflex recorded from the soleus muscle (Shahani and Young, 1968; 1972a and b; 1973; 1977; Shahani, 1968; 1970b).

In most clinical studies, blink reflexes have been evoked either by a gentle mechanical tap on the glabella or by electrical stimulation of the supraorbital nerve near the supraorbital groove. Surface EMG recordings are made by placing electrodes over the outer two-thirds of the inferior orbicularis oculi muscle. When evoked by a mechanical tap on the glabella, two EMG components are seen on both sides (Fig. 9.5): the first shorter latency component (R_1) is more synchronized than the second longer latency, rather asynchronous component (R_2). On the other hand, electrical stimulation of the supraorbital nerve evokes both components on the side ipsilateral to the stimulation, whereas only a second component is seen on the contralateral side. Minimal latency for the first component in normal subjects ranges from 8 to 14 msec, and that for the second component 23 to 44 msec. The latency of mechanically evoked reflexes is 1 to 3 msec longer than those produced by electrical stimulation. The minimal latency difference for the first component on the two sides in the same individual is usually less than 1.0 msec.

Determination of minimal latencies of the two ipsilateral components (R_1 and R_2) and the second contralateral component (R_2) following electrical stimulation of the supraorbital nerve often helps in localizing a lesion to the trigeminal and/or facial nerves. If there is a lesion of the ipsilateral trigeminal nerve, both ipsilateral components of the blink reflex (R_1 and R_2) and the contralateral second component (R_2) will have a prolonged latency. On the other hand, if the

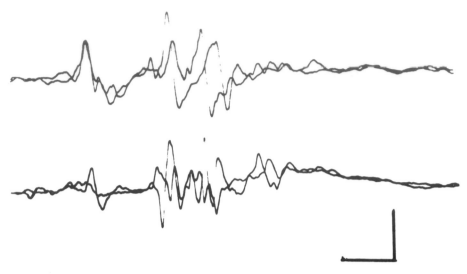

Fig. 9.5. *Two components of the blink reflex evoked by a mechanical tap on glabella in the normal subject. Calibration: 10 msec and 200 μV.*

lesion is confined to the facial nerve, there will be a delay in the latency of reflex components only on the affected side, regardless of the side of stimulation. Thus, blink reflex studies have proven useful in early detection of abnormalities of conduction in disorders affecting cranial nerves (Fig. 9.6), such as Bell's palsy or the Guillain-Barré syndrome (Shahani and Young, 1977). In patients with cerebellopontine angle tumors, abnormalities of blink reflex studies can be documented at a time when there is no evidence of clinical weakness of the facial muscles (Shahani and Parker, 1979). Alterations in the behavior of both components have also been noted in a variety of disorders of the CNS (Kimura and Lyon, 1972; Kimura, 1975; Fisher, Shahani, and Young, 1979).

CONCLUDING COMMENT

There is no longer any doubt that H reflex, F response, and blink reflex studies are useful in the early detection and documentation of various disorders of the peripheral nervous system in individual patients. However, it must be recognized that changes in these physiologic parameters can also be seen under different physiologic conditions as well as with various disorders of the CNS. Accordingly, proper interpretation of the results of these studies requires an understanding of the underlying neural mechanisms which, if affected, may alter these responses. Many of these studies, which may appear simple to a novice, therefore, require the expertise of a fully trained clinical neurophysiologist who has spent several years in the field of human reflexology.

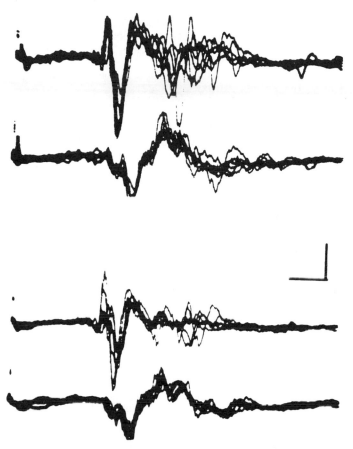

Fig. 9.6. *Two components of the blink reflex in a patient with Guillian-Barré syndrome. Note significantly prolonged latency for both components. Calibration: 10 msec and 200 μV.*

REFERENCES

Ackil, A. A., Shahani, B. T., and Young, R. R. (1978a). Usefulness of late response and sural conduction studies in patients with chronic renal failure. Amer. Assoc. EMG and Electrodiag. Program of 25th Annual Meeting, p. 28.

Ackil, A. A., Shahani, B. T., and Young, R. R. (1978b). Sural conduction studies and late responses in children undergoing hemodialysis. Arch. Phys. Med. Rehabil., *59*:562.

Adams, R. D., Shahani, B. T., and Young, R. R. (1973). A severe pansensory familial neuropathy. Trans. Am. Neurol. Assoc., *98*:67.

Albizzati, M. G.., Bassi, S., Passerini, D., and Crespi, V. (1976). F-wave velocity in motor neurone disease. Acta Neurol. Scand., *54*:269.

Angel, R. W., and Hoffman, W. W. (1963). The H reflex in normal, spastic and rigid subjects. Arch. Neurol., *8*:591.

Bell, C. (1811). Idea of a new anatomy of the brain submitted for the observations of his friends. Strahan and Preston, London.

Braddom, R. I., and Johnson, E. W. (1974). Standardization of H-reflex and diagnostic use in S-1 radiculopathy. Arch. Phys. Med. Rehabil., *55:*161.

Conrad, B., Aschoff, J. C., and Fischler, M. D. (1975). Der diagnostische wert der F-wellen-latenz. J. Neurol., *210:*151.

Dawson, G. D., and Merton, P. A. (1956). Recurrent discharges from motoneurones. Proc. 2e Congr. Int. Physiol., Bruxelles. p. 221.

Drechsler, B., Lastouka, M., and Kalvodova, E. (1966). Electrophysiological study of patients with herniated intervertebral disc. Electromyography, *6:*187.

Egloff-Baer, S., Shahani, B. T., and Young, R. R. (1978). Usefulness of late response studies in diagnosis of entrapment neuropathies. Electroencephalogr. Clin. Neurophysiol., *45:*16P.

Eisen, A., Schomer, D., and Melmed, C. (1977). The application of F-wave measurements in the differentiation of proximal and distal upper limb entrapments. Neurology, *27:*662.

Fisher, M. A., Shahani, B. T., and Young, R. R. (1978a). Assessing segmental excitability after acute rostral lesions. I. The F response. Neurology, *28:*1265.

Fisher, M. A., Shahani, B. T., and Young, R. R. (1979). Assessing segmental excitability after acute rostral lesions. II. The blink reflex. Neurology, *29:*45.

Fisher, M. A., Shivde, A. J., Teixera, C., and Grainer, L. S. (1978b). Clinical and electrophysiological appraisal of the significance of radicular injury in back pain. J. Neurol. Neurosurg. Psychiatry, *41:*303.

Hagbarth, K.-E. (1962). Post-tetanic potentiation of myotatic reflexes in man. J. Neurol. Neurosurg. Psychiatry, *25:*1.

Hays, K. C., Robinson, K. L., Wood, G. A., and Jennings, L. S. (1979). Assessment of the H reflex excitability curve using a cubic spline function. Electroencephalogr. Clin. Neurophysiol., *46:*114.

Hoffmann, P. (1918). Über die Beziehungen der Sehnenreflexe zur Willkurlichen Bewegung und zum tonus. Z. Biol., *68:*351.

Hugon, M. (1973). Methodology of the Hoffmann reflex in man. In: New Developments in Electromyography and Clinical Neurophysiology. J. E. Desmedt, Ed., Vol. 3, p. 277. Karger, Basel.

Ioku, M., Ribera, V. A., Cooper, I. S., and Matsuoka, S. (1965). Parkinsonism: electromyographic studies of monosynaptic reflex. Science, *150:*1472.

Johnson, T. L., Sax, D. S., and Feldman, R. G. (1974). A technique for feature extraction and interpatient comparison of H reflex conditioning curves. Electroencephalogr. Clin. Neurophysiol., *37:*188.

Kimura, Jun (1974). F-wave velocity in the central segment of the median and ulnar nerves. A study in normal subjects and in patients with Charcot-Marie-Tooth Disease. Neurology, *24:*539.

Kimura, Jun (1975). Electrically elicited blink reflex in diagnosis of multiple sclerosis— review of 260 patients over a seven year period. Brain, *98:*413.

Kimura, Jun and Butzer, J. F. (1975). F-wave conduction velocity in Guillain-Barré syndrome. Arch. Neurol., *32:*524.

Kimura, Jun and Lyon, L. W. (1972). Orbicularis oculi reflex in the Wallenberg syndrome: alteration of the late reflex by lesions of the spinal tract and nucleus of the trigeminal nerve. J. Neurol. Neurosurg. Psychiatry, *35:*228.

King, D. and Ashby, P. (1976). Conduction velocity in the proximal segments of a motor nerve in the Guillain-Barré syndrome. J. Neurol. Neurosurg. Psychiatry, *39:*538.

Lachman, T., Shahani, B. T., and Young, R. R. (1977). Late responses as diagnostic aids in Landry-Guillain-Barré syndrome. Electroencephalogr. Clin. Neurophysiol., *43:*147.

Lachman, T., Shahani, B. T., and Young, R. R. (1979). Late responses as aids to diagnosis in peripheral neuropathy. In press.

Lefebvre-D'Amour, M., Shahani, B. T., Young, R. R., and Bird, K. T. (1976). Importance of studying sural conduction and late responses in the evaluation of alcoholic subjects. Neurology, *26:*368.

Lloyd, D. P. C. (1943). Conduction and synaptic transmission of the reflex response to stretch in spinal cats. J. Neurophysiol., 6:317.

Maccabee, P. J., Shahani, B. T., and Young, R. R. (1978). Usefulness of double simultaneous recording (DSR) and F response studies in the diagnosis of carpal tunnel syndrome (CTS). Amer. Assoc. EMG and Electrodiag. Program of 25th Annual Meeting, p. 21.

Magendie, F. (1822). Experiences sur les fonctions des racines des nerfs rachidiens. J. Physiol. Exp., 2:276.

Magladery, J. W., and McDougal, D. B. (1950). Electrophysiological studies of nerve and reflex activity in normal man. I. Identification of certain reflexes in the electromyogram and the conduction velocity of peripheral nerves. Bull Johns Hopkins Hosp., 86:265.

Magladery, J. W., Teasdale, R. D., Park, A. M., and Languth, H. W. (1952). Electrophysiological studies of reflex activity in patients with lesions of the nervous system. I. A comparison of spinal motoneurone excitability following afferent nerve volleys in normal persons and patients with upper motor neurone lesions. Bull Johns Hopkins Hosp., 91:219.

Mayer, R. F. and Feldman, R. G. (1967). Observations on the nature of the F-wave in man. Neurology, 17:147.

Mayer, R. F. and Mawdsley, C. (1965). Studies in man and cat of the significance of the H-reflex. J. Neurol. Neurosurg. Psychiatry, 28:201.

McLeod, J. G. and Wray, S. H. (1966). An experimental study of the F-wave in the baboon. J. Neurol. Neurosurg. Psychiatry, 29:196.

Notermans, S. L. H. and Vingerhoets, H. M. (1974). The importance of the Hoffmann reflex in the diagnosis of lumbar root lesions. Clin. Neurol. Neurosurg., 1:54.

Paillard, J. (1955). Reflexes et regulations d'origine proprioceptive chez l'homme. Arnette, Paris.

Panayiotopoulos, C. P., Scarpalezos, S., and Nastas, P. E. (1977). F-wave studies in the deep peroneal nerve. Part 1. Control subjects. J. Neurol. Sci., 31:319.

Panayiotopoulos, C. P., Scarpalezos, S., and Nastas, P. E. (1978). Sensory (Ia) and F-wave conduction velocity in the proximal segment of the tibial nerve. Muscle and Nerve, 1:181.

Shahani, B. T. (1968). Effects of sleep on human reflexes with a double component. J. Neurol. Neurosurg. Psychiatry, 31:574.

Shahani, B. T. (1970a). Flexor reflex afferent nerve fibres in man. J. Neurol. Neurosurg. Psychiatry, 33:786–791.

Shahani, B. T. (1970b). The human blink reflex. J. Neurol. Neurosurg. Psychiatry, 33:792.

Shahani, B. T. and Parker, S. (1979). Electrophysiological studies in patients with cerebellar-pontine angle lesions. Neurology, 29:582.

Shahani, B. T. and Young, R. R. (1968). A note on blink reflexes. J. Physiol. (Lond.), 198:103.

Shahani, B. T. and Young, R. R. (1972a). Human orbicularis oculi reflexes. Neurology, 22:149.

Shahani, B. T. and Young, R. R. (1972b). The cutaneous nature of the first component of the monkey's blink reflex. Neurology, 22:438.

Shahani, B. T. and Young, R. R. (1973). Blink reflexes in orbicularis oculi. In: New Developments in Electromyography and Clinical Neurophysiology. Desmedt, J. E., Ed., Vol. 3, p. 641. S. Karger, Basel.

Shahani, B. T. and Young, R. R. (1976). Effect of vibration on the F response. In: The Motor System. Neurophysiology and Muscle Mechanisms. Shahani, M., Ed., p. 189. Elsevier, Amsterdam.

Shahani, B. T. and Young, R. R. (1977). The blink reflex. In: Electrodiagnosis of Neuromuscular Diseases. Goodgold, J. and Eberstein, A. pp. 245–250.

Shahani, B. T., Young, R. R., and Lachman, T. (1975). Late responses as aids to diagnosis in peripheral neuropathy. J. Postgrad. Med., 21:7.

Shahani, B. T., Young, R. R., Potts, F., and Maccabee, P. (1979). Terminal latency index (TLI) and late response studies in motor neuron disease (MND), peripheral neuropathies and entrapment syndromes. Acta Neurol. Scand., Supp. 73. Vol. 60:118.

Sherrington, C. S. (1906). The integrative action of the nervous system. Yale University Press, New Haven.

Táboříková, H. and Sax, D. S. (1969). Conditioning of H-reflexes by a preceding subthreshold H-reflex stimulus. Brain, *92:*203.

Takamori, M. (1967). H reflex study in upper motoneuron diseases. Neurology, *17:*32.

Thomas, J. E. and Lambert, E. H. (1960). Ulnar nerve conduction velocity and H-reflex in infants and children. J. Applied Physiol., *15:*1.

Thorne, J. (1965). Central responses to electrical activation of the peripheral nerves supplying the intrinsic hand muscles. J. Neurol. Neurosurg. Psychiatry, *28:*482.

Tonzola, R., Ackil, A. A., Shahani, B. T., and Young, R. R. (1978). Usefulness of electrophysiological studies in the diagnosis of lumbosacral root disease. Amer. Assoc. EMG and Electrodiag. Program of 25th Annual Meeting, p. 18.

Wager, E. E., Jr. and Buerger, A. A. (1974a). H-reflex latency and sensory conduction in normal and diabetic subjects. Arch. Phys. Med. Rehabil., *55:*126.

Wager, E. E., Jr. and Buerger, A. A. (1974b). A linear relationship between the H-reflex latency and sensory conduction velocity in neuropathy. Neurology, *24:*711.

Yap, C. B. (1967). Spinal segmental and long-loop reflexes on spinal motoneuron excitability in spasticity and rigidity. Brain, *90:*887.

Young, R. R. and Shahani, B. T. (1978). Clinical value and limitations of F-wave determination. Muscle and Nerve, *1:*248.

Zander Olsen, P. and Diamontopoulos, E. (1967). Excitability of spinal motor neurones in normal subjects and patients with spasticity, Parkinsonian rigidity and cerebellar hypotonia. J. Neurol. Neurosurg. Psychiatry, *30:*325.

10

Electroretinography

JOHN C. ARMINGTON

INTRODUCTION

The electroretinogram, an intricate potential produced by the light-sensitive tissues of the retina, has significant value in the diagnosis of visual disorders as well as broad applications in clinical and basic research. It is conveniently obtained from the human eye in comfort and safety under well-defined stimulus conditions. It is a unique indicator of receptor and early central nervous system action. Although much remains to be learned of its physiology, it is better understood than most mass action potentials, particularly those that are obtained with remote recording electrodes. The data that it provides, when joined with those of evoked potential recording and psychophysics, already make it possible to trace the transmission of visual information through several levels of processing with some success, and its usefulness in this regard undoubtedly will increase in the future. There is, therefore, every reason that it should be part of the battery of electrophysiologic techniques available to the neurologist. This chapter is concerned with human electroretinography at its current state of development and emphasizes those aspects that have an application for clinical diagnosis.

The first human electroretinogram (ERG) was recorded more than a century ago when Dewar (1877) placed an electrode against the eye and observed a response to light with a simple galvanometer. A substantial mass of information has accumulated since his time (Armington, 1974). The present discussion begins with an examination of the physiologic and anatomic basis upon which electroretinography rests. Then attention is given to the stimulus conditions that influence the waveforms and amplitudes of the recordings. The third section examines the recording techniques and methods of analysis that are unique for electroretinography. The chapter concludes with a review of some clinical findings.

Nature of the Electroretinogram

Identification of Components. The ERG can be regarded as having two parts: a steady resting potential, and a multiphasic transient potential that is released by a flash of light. It is the latter which has received the most experimental and clinical attention. Despite the fact that the ERG is produced deep within the eye, its main features are readily seen with external electrodes. Various of these may or may not be conspicuous in any individual recording, however, depending upon the specific testing conditions that are employed. Figure 10.1 is a sketch of the principal transient features and illustrates the waves that make up the ERG. Examples of actual recordings, which differ markedly with respect to the appearance and relative prominence of the several features, are shown in later figures. It can be seen that the recording first moves downward to reach a minimum within a few (~15) milliseconds of stimulus onset. Since it is customary to plot positivity upwards and negativity downwards, this deflection charts a negativity of the anterior surface of the retina with respect to the back. After the negativity subsides there is a shift in the position direction so that a positive maximum occurs some 60 to 70 msec after stimulus onset. This potential then drops, to be followed by a second shift again in the positive direction after some considerable delay. Einthoven and Jolly (1908) who were among the first to obtain accurate representations of the electroretinal waveform, named these peaks the *a* wave, the *b* wave, and the *c* wave respectively, names that are still in use today. Although not usually prominent in the human ERG, a potential called the *off* effect may appear when a steady stimulus is shut off. The positive aspect of this wave is termed the *d* wave.

With the main features of the ERG in mind, attention may now be directed to those that are less conspicuous. Frequently, these components have been given names which draw attention to their presumed anatomical origin, or in other cases to their role in retinal function. These implications will be discussed after the components have been identified. Proceeding from the left to right, the first activity is a biphasic potential that occurs immediately upon stimulus onset. It is the early receptor potential, often referred to by its initials, ERP. It gives way to the *a* wave which, because of a discontinuity that appears in its waveform, has been regarded as having two parts, A_p and A_s (Armington,

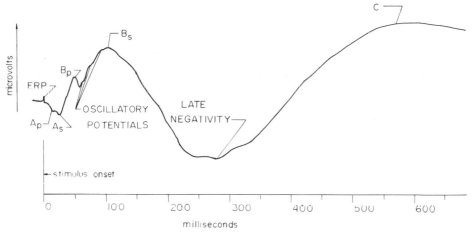

Fig. 10.1. *Features of the electroretinogram. Positivity of the front of the eye is indicated by an upward deflection. Note that this is a diagram illustrating the principal waves that can appear in the human electroretinogram. No one testing condition brings them all forth at the same time. ERP marks the early receptor potential. It is seen only with very strong stimuli. The two sections of the a wave (A_p, A_s) and of the b wave (B_p, B_s) are described in the text.*

Johnson, and Riggs, 1952). The *b* wave which follows can be similarly divided into sections, B_p and B_s (Adrian, 1945; Johnson, 1958). In some circumstances, the B_p component is termed the *x* wave. Frequently, a number of small peaks or ripples give the *b* wave an irregular contour. The first of these may appear during the *a* wave, dividing it into the two sections identified above (Bornschein and Goodman, 1957; Brunette, 1972). The remaining ones are superimposed on the broader *b* wave. Their spacing suggests a periodic activity, and hence, collectively they are known as the oscillatory potential (Yonemura, Masuda, and Hatta, 1963). Nevertheless, a body of evidence indicates that they are independent events and not true oscillations. The *b* wave is followed by additional potentials. A negative potential that is termed the afterpotential, or alternately the late negative potential, follows the *b* wave (Armington, Corwin, and Marsetta, 1971). Several smaller potentials may be superimposed upon this section of the ERG, but they have not been named. The *c* wave is frequently not prominent in the human eye under typical recording conditions (Bornschein, 1966).

The existence of many peaks or waves whose prominence can be changed experimentally indicates the ERG is a combination of several more or less independent components. Each of these is a waveform that extends over a period of time. Many efforts have been made to resolve the ERG into its components. After the early work of Piper (1911), Granit (1933) made the analysis shown in Figure 10.2. Three processes, PI, PII, and PIII, add together to produce the ERG. Although this analysis, which only accounts for the gross features of the ERG, is chiefly of historic interest today, the concept of compo-

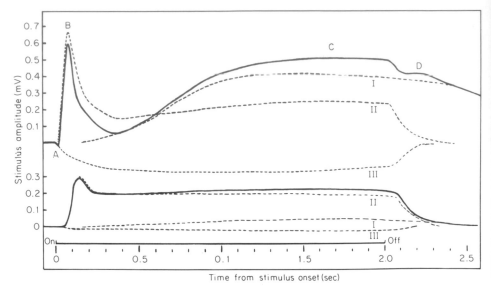

Fig. 10.2. *An analysis of the electroretinogram. Using a variety of physiologic techniques, Granit separated the electroretinogram into three processes: PI, PII, and PIII. They add together to produce an electroretinogram with* a, b, *and* c *waves and an off-effect, the* d *wave. A stronger stimulus was used to obtain the upper recording than the lower one (from Granit, R. 1933. J. Physiol., 77, 207).*

nents adding together is still fundamental. Furthermore, reference is occasionally made to one or another of Granit's processes in physiologic work and in clinical work where the response has been altered because of retinal disease.

Anatomic and Physiologic Correlations. A great variety of techniques have been applied to the study of the ERG. These include depth studies with microelectrodes (Tomita, 1976; Dowling, 1970; Brown, 1968), anatomic methods (Dowling, 1970; Kaneko and Hashimoto, 1967), pharmacologic methods (Noell, 1953), work with perfused eyes (Niemeyer, 1976), and others. It is necessary to hold certain anatomic features of the retina in mind when considering the outcomes of these methodologies and the origin of electroretinal components. A highly schematic sketch of a small section of the vertebrate retina appears in Figure 10.3. The retina is a stratified structure. Light passing the pupil at the front of the eye is transmitted through the retina, which is transparent, and is imaged on its back surface. Here, the receptor cells of the eye, the rods and cones, sit on an optically dense layer known as the pigment epithelium. Its pigment is not photosensitive pigment but among other functions acts to prevent stray light from reaching the receptors. Stimulus light is absorbed by the *photo pigment* contained in the distal parts of the receptors. It initiates activity that travels centrally through the receptor and bipolar cell layers to the ganglion cell layer and thence to the brain. There are elaborate synaptic connections within the retina, and numerous fibers course transversely through the retina. The outer plexiform layer is the layer of fibers that

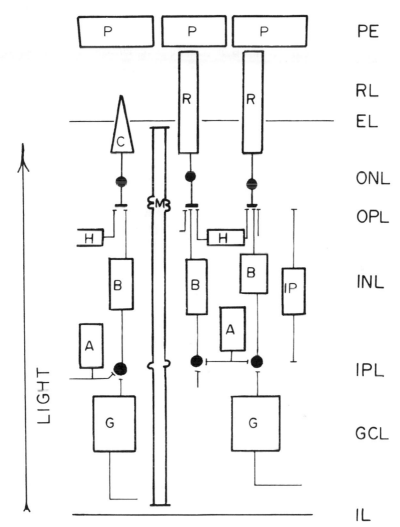

Fig. 10.3. *A schematic cross-section of the retina. This diagram depicts the principal cells and layers of the retina. Light travels to the receptors through the retina from the bottom to the top. The following layers of the retina are identified: PE, pigment epithelium; RL, receptor layer; EL, external limiting membrane; ONL, outer nuclear layer; OPL, outer plexiform layer; INL, inner nuclear layer; IPL, inner plexiform layer; GCL, ganglion cell layer; IL, internal limiting membrane. The following cell types are identified: P, pigment cell; R, rods; C, cones; H, horizontal cell; B, bipolar cell; A, amacrine cell; G, ganglion cell; M, Müller cells; IP, interplexiform cell.*

intermediates between the receptor and bipolar cells; and the inner plexiform layer is that between the bipolar and ganglion cell layers. Horizontal cells with their perikarya at the front of the outer plexiform layer send processes across the retina. Amacrine cells also send horizontal processes through the retina, but their processes extend through the inner plexiform layer. In addition to bipolar cells, a second neural cell, the interplexiform cell, extends radially through the retina. It transmits information centrifically from the inner to outer plexiform layer. Finally, a nonneural cell, the Müller cell, must also be cited because it may have special significance for electroretinography. It extends through the retina giving off numerous processes that reach into the outer and inner plexiform layers.

Considerable knowledge has been amassed regarding the transfer of information from one cell type to another, but the present concern is with their contribution to the ERG. In fact, as soon as components could be recognized in the ERG, an effort was made to assign them to definite retinal structures (Bartley, 1941). Early attempts, based on the principle that the temporal order in which retinal structures are activated should determine the latency of the components they generate, relegated short latency activity to the receptors and later activity to more proximal structures. Today, latency remains as a consideration that must be taken into account when correlating structure and function.

The first component to be seen in the ERG is the early receptor potential (Brown and Murakami, 1964; Cone, 1964). It arises with almost no latency. It is known to arise within the distal parts of the receptors and to be intimately associated with the initial photoreceptor processes. The early receptor potential gives way to the *a* wave. Its early phases are believed to arise from a more proximal part of the receptors (Brown, 1968; Dowling, 1970). Later segments of the *a* wave are probably more complicated, however, and may depict the fusion of several activities.

There is considerably more complexity of action by the time the *b* wave is underway. The *b* wave is often said to provide an indication of activity in the bipolar layer, but this does not identify the cells that generate it (Armington, 1974). The proposition that it arises from the Müller cells is an attractive one. A broad, smooth wave resembling the *b* wave has been recorded from the Müller cells of the mud puppy eye (Dowling, 1970). Müller cells are glial cells and as such generate a potential that gauges the potassium concentration in the intercellular spaces around them. Their lateral processes branch into the interplexiform layers where neural activity produces potassium change. Thus, their structure and location should render them sensitive to the complex of activity arising in the central layers of the retina. Detailed investigation of Müller cell latencies has produced some uncertainties as to their role in the *b* wave, however, and as a caution it has been suggested that the Müller cell response be termed the *m* wave (Karwoski and Proenza, 1977). The deflection that is termed the *b* wave in the human subject may be a confounding of potentials from several physiologic sources.

Contrary to denotation, the oscillatory potentials which occur during the early phases of the *b* wave do not represent true periodic activity but rather a series of discrete events. Microelectrode study has shown that they arise at differing depths within the bipolar layer (Wachtmeister and Dowling, 1978).

The *c* wave is produced by the cells of the pigment epithelium at the back of the retina. In an extensive investigation, Noell (1953) treated rats with a series of metabolic poisons and made comparisons of the destruction thus produced in the retinal tissues with the disappearance of electroretinal components. These studies implicated the pigment epithelium. More recent work has depicted the part of the pigment cells in generating the *c* wave with considerable clarity. The *c* wave is produced by a change in the extracellular potassium ion concentration secondarily to the action of the receptor cells which lie in close proximity (Oakley and Green, 1976). The slow phase of PIII (PIII is illustrated in Fig. 10.2) seen when the *c* wave is not present has been attributed to hyperpolarization of the Müller cells (Witkovsky, Dudek, and Ripps, 1975).

Not all retinal cells contribute appreciably to the ERG. The horizontal cells produce graded responses that are called S potentials, and the absence of these from the ERG may be attributed to the tangential orientation of the horizontal cells. The ganglion cells, whose axons travel across the retina and which produce spike potentials, also fail to contribute significantly to the ERG.

Most of the analysis described here is based on work with infrahuman species but can be generalized to the human eye. The importance of component analysis from a neurologic point of view is that visual disorders may affect retinal structures, and thus features of the response, differentially. The ERG thus provides a potential means of identifying the retinal source and distinguishing between various forms of blindness. As further progress is made physiologically, its value will increase.

Psychophysical Analysis of the Electroretinogram

Traditionally, psychophysics is concerned with relations between the physical properties of stimuli and visual sensation, but in the present context psychophysics refers to changes in the size and waveform of the ERG as a result of manipulating stimulus variables (Armington, 1977b).

Duplicity theory states that the retina possesses two divisions: one, the scotopic system, which functions at low levels of illumination and whose action is initiated by the retinal rods, and the other, the photopic system, which functions at high levels of illumination and whose action is driven by the cones. The activity of these two systems depends on the state of visual adaptation as well as on the properties of the stimulus. Frequently, the stimulus will activate both the rod and cone systems, and both photopic and scotopic activity will exist.

Figure 10.4, taken from an early analysis (Armington, Johnson, and Riggs, 1952) diagrams an ERG (solid line) such as can be produced by stimulating the dark adapted eye with a bright flash. The waveform, with its slightly rippled *a* and *b* waves, results from superimposed photopic and scotopic activity. A theoretical analysis resolved it into the two hypothetical constituents that are

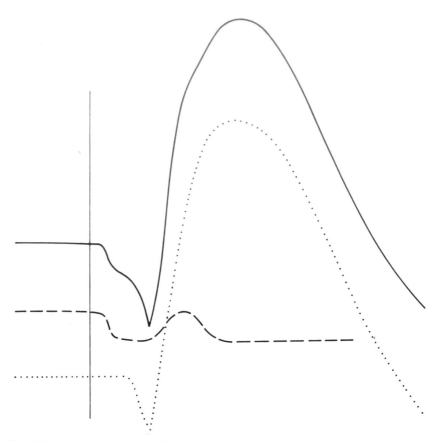

Fig. 10.4. *An analysis of the human electroretinogram. The upper tracing, drawn with a solid line, depicts the electroretinogram of the totally dark adapted eye. It appears to arise from the combination of the two parts shown by dashed and dotted lines (from Armington, J. C., Johnson, E. P. and Riggs, L. A. 1952. J. Physiol., 118, 289).*

shown by the dashed and dotted lines. These represent constituent photopic and scotopic ERGs. Thus, the *a* wave and the *b* wave are often further identified with the subscripts $_p$ and $_s$ when it is known under specific testing conditions which system generated them.

The waveform shown by the solid line in Figure 10.4 may be obtained by adding the photopic and scotopic parts together. This illustrates a property of the ERG that is characterized as *response additivity*. All of the signals that contribute to a recording add together in a simple algebraic manner to produce the resulting wave form. In actual recordings summation among the components is approximate, but the approximation frequently is close enough to be of considerable utility. Summation also takes place between potentials arising at different parts of the retina and, in the case of flickering or multiple stimulation, between successive responses that overlap. Figure 10.4 must be regarded with a degree of caution, however. Oscillatory potentials generally are superimposed on the ERG, and they produce apparent separations in the *a* and *b* waves. The ERG cannot be divided into photopic and scotopic sectors on the basis of waveforms alone. Further information, such as that based on measures of spectral sensitivity discussed below, is necessary for positive identification of photopic and scotopic activity.

Not all of the light that enters the eye is successfully imaged. Some is scattered before reaching the image and a fraction of the light that does fall in the image area is reflected back to receptors in other parts of the retina. This stray light falling on the typically large retinal area that lies outside of the image area is an effective stimulus. The receptors are remarkable because of the extended range of stimulus intensities to which they can respond. Thus, although the stray light is not intense but is substantially weaker than that in the image, it produces local activity of low amplitude over a wide region, and the sum of this activity from all of the retina produces a large recorded response. A striking example of the importance of stray light has been given by experiments where a small but strong stimulus was focused on the blind spot, the retinal region where the optic nerve fibers leave the eye and where there are no receptors (Asher, 1951; Boynton and Riggs, 1951). In these experiments, full-sized ERGs were produced even though no receptors were stimulated directly. Stray light produced ERGs that were barely distinguishable from those found in more typical recording situations.

When stimuli of moderately large diameter (e.g., with a visual angle of 60°) are imaged on the retina, the recording is triggered both by stray light and by the light forming the stimulus image. The ERG can be factored into two parts, one elicited by stray light and one by light that is imaged (Fig. 10.5). Because of its relatively high intensity, the light entering the image area produces activity with short latency. The part produced by stray light outside the image area is delayed a few milliseconds because the stimulus is less intense. When the strength of the stimulus and its area are suitably adjusted, the two parts of the response are of similar magnitude. Then the *b* wave shows a double peak, the first elicited by the imaged stimulus light, and the second by stray light. An important variable in producing this effect is the spatial extent of the stimulus flash. When the stimulus is very small, response is produced almost entirely by stray light. When, on the contrary, the stimulus is large enough to extend across most of the retina, response is produced almost entirely by direct illumination.

Stimulus Variables and ERG Measurement. The ERG has been investigated with a wide disposition of stimuli to produce differential emphasis of its properties. Only certain relevant aspects of this work can be summarized here, but much of it has been reviewed more fully elsewhere (Armington, 1974). Some means of measuring the ERG is needed to describe the systematic way in which it is related to stimulus variables. Although many forms of measurement have been attempted, simple amplitude and latency measures of the peaks have found the widest application. These are illustrated in Figure 10.6. Latency is measured from the time of stimulus onset to the beginning of the wave being

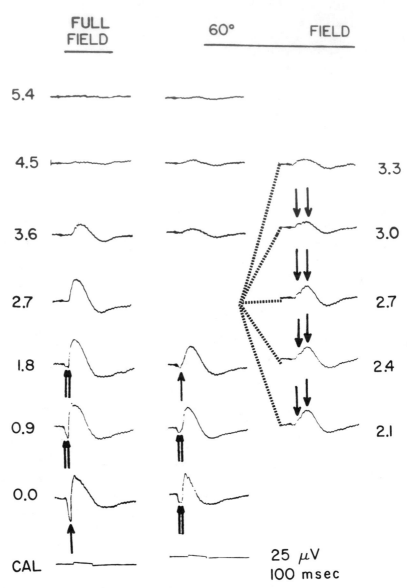

Fig. 10.5. *A comparison between electroretinograms produced by a 60° stimulus field with those produced by full-field stimulation. A range of luminances was obtained by placing neutral density filters in the light path. The dimmest stimulus had a value of 5.4 and the brightest, 0.0 units. Double b waves were obtained with a 60° field through the luminance range from 2.1 to 3.3 units (from Armington, J. C.: The Electroretinogram. Academic Press, New York, 1974).*

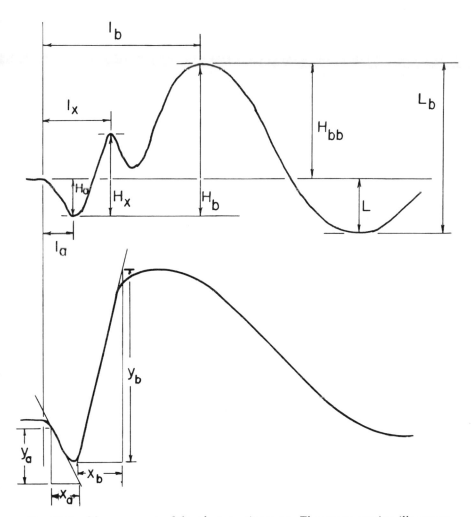

Fig. 10.6. *Measurement of the electroretinogram. The upper section illustrates amplitude and latency measurement. The lower section shows slope measurement. The following measures are identified in the upper section: I_b, implicit time of the b wave; I_x, implicit time of the X (photopic B) wave; I_a, implicit time of the a wave; H_a, amplitude of the a wave; H_x, amplitude of the X wave; H_b, amplitude of the b wave; H_{bb}, amplitude of the b wave as measured from the base line; L, amplitude of the late negative potential as measured from the base line; L_b, amplitude of the late negative potential measured from the peak of the b wave. Slope is measured by drawing a line through the changing phase of a wave and taking the ratio of the rise (y) to the run (x) of this line. Slope measures for the b wave and the a wave are illustrated. The vertical line running through both tracings marks stimulus onset.*

considered. The more common measurement made to the peak of a wave is called its implicit time or, alternately, its culmination time. Amplitude measures are frequent in electroretinography. Generally they are from the troughs to the peaks of successive waves. Occasionally, however, they are made from the baseline, defined as the level of the tracing before the stimulus is presented. Occasionally the slope of the initial phase of a wave is determined. In the case of the *a* wave this measure is believed to give an index of receptor function. The areas that lie under waves have also been measured, but the problem then arises as to the level that is to be taken as a baseline. Except for the early portion of the *a* wave, it may be assumed that several components of the ERG are superimposed, so that any one of these measures is a mixed index of the underlying activity. Nevertheless, they have proven quite practical.

Luminance. The luminance (intensity) of the stimulus is changed during the course of most testing procedures. As it is raised, the amplitude of the ERG grows and the latency is shortened. Representative data illustrating measurements of these changes as well as changes in response waveforms appear in Figure 10.7. Two plots (upper and middle curves) of *b* wave amplitude (as measured from the trough of the *a* wave) are shown as a function of luminance. The upper plot obtained when stray light was effective is more curved than the lower obtained when it was not. Amplitude-luminance plots may be more irregular than the examples shown here. In some cases, the height measurement may shift subtly from one component peak of the *b* wave to another, producing abrupt changes (Armington, 1959). Most curves in the current clinical literature have a sigmoidal form, having been obtained under stray light conditions.

The size of the response produced by the same stimulus will vary somewhat among normal subjects (Peterson, 1968) and, of course, will vary considerably with stimulus conditions. As a result the upper levels achieved by amplitude-luminance curves and their slopes will not always be the same. Thus, in any testing situation it is important to have knowledge of variation encountered among normals, based upon empirical testing with the specific conditions of interest. An analytic method has been developed for comparing response-luminance curves that reach different upper levels (Fulton and Rushton, 1978), but will not be discussed here.

Stimulus Size. The ERG grows with increases in stimulus area as well as in luminance. There are two reasons for this, the balance between them depending upon the degree to which stray light is under control. When the response is not produced by stray light, the effect of increasing stimulus area is to increase the number of active receptors. Under this condition the amplitude of the *b* wave is approximately proportional to the number of receptors stimulated (Armington, 1977a). When stray light is not under control, an increase in the area of the stimulus also produces an increase in the intensity of the stray light falling on the retinal receptors outside of the image area. The result is then complex because areal and stray light increments in the response are confounded.

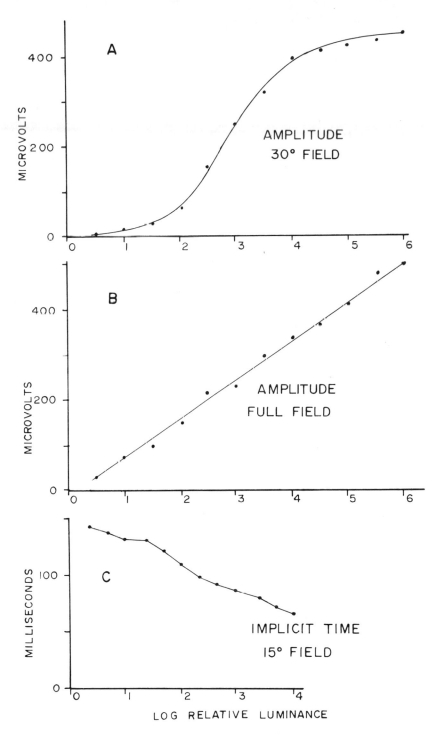

Fig. 10.7. *Luminance curves. Plot A: amplitude of the* b *wave vs luminance. This curve is typical of stimulation to the totally dark adapted eye with a stimulus field that does not fill the retina. Plot B: amplitude of the* b *wave as a function of stimulus luminance for full field stimulation. Plot C: decrease of* b *wave implicit time with increasing luminance.*

Stimulus Duration. For short periods the stimulation by a flash of light sums across time. For the photopic ERG this critical duration is approximately 10 msec and for the scotopic it extends up to 25 msec or more (Biersdorf, 1958). Thus, stimulus duration can be selected to optimize the appearance of photopic or scotopic components.

Spectral Sensitivity and Adaptation. The scotopic and photopic visual systems are named according to their operating range; the scotopic system mediates vision at low levels of illumination and the photopic at high. But they differ in other respects. An important distinguishing characteristic of these two systems is their relative sensitivity to stimuli of different wavelengths. This property is described by a function that relates the stimulus energy needed to produce a response of fixed size and character to stimulus wavelength, a function that is called a spectral sensitivity curve. When the eye adapts to darkness its overall sensitivity increases, but in addition the spectral region to which it is relatively most sensitive shifts from approximatley 555 nm to 500 nm (Fig. 10.8). Thus, photopic and scotopic response activity may be distinguished by the form of its spectral sensitivity curve. Spectral sensitivity may be determined using photochemical, psychophysical, evoked potential recording, or other procedures, as well as those of electroretinography. When the data obtained by the procedures are expressed on the same scales of measurement, they can be compared directly. Criterional analysis of the ERG is appropriate for making comparisons

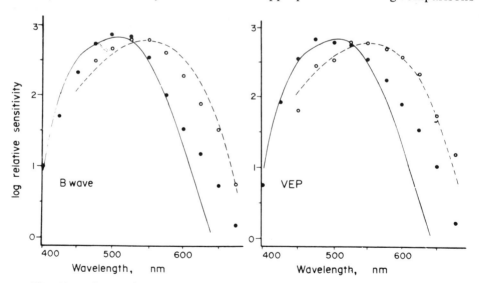

Fig. 10.8. *Spectral sensitivity of the b wave in the light and the dark adapted eye. Sensitivity in the light adapted eye is represented by the dashed lines and open circles; for the dark adapted eye by the solid lines and filled circles. The experimental points in the left plot are for the b wave of the electroretinogram; those on the right are for the evoked potential. The curves drawn through the points are standardized psychophysical functions for the light adapted and dark adapted eye (from Korth, M. and Armington, J. C. 1976. Vision Res., 16, 703. Reprinted with permission from Pergamon Press, Ltd.).*

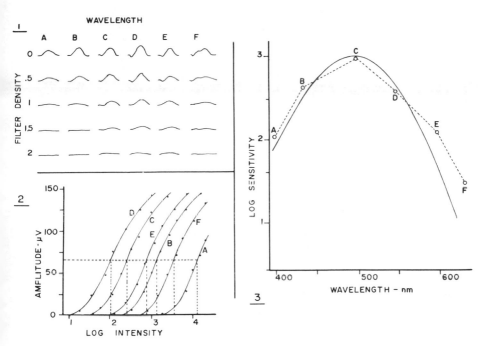

Fig. 10.9. *Steps used to determine spectral sensitivity using criterional analysis. Panel 1: First, electroretinograms are obtained that sample a range of stimulus intensities and wavelengths. The recordings shown here are typical of those found with stimulus flashes of small angular extent presented to the dark adapted eye. Panel 2: The responses are measured. Amplitude vs luminance curves are plotted from these measures. A criterion amplitude is selected. Panel 3: The reciprocal of the intensities that produce the criterion response when plotted against wavelength yield a spectral sensitivity curve. The points connected by a broken line describe the electroretinogram. A smooth scotopic psychophysical curve has been drawn through the points for comparison (from Armington, J. C.: The correlation of electrophysiological and psychophysical measures: the electroretinogram. In: Doc. Ophthalmol. Proc. Ser. ERG, VER and Psychophysics, 14th I.S.C.E.R.G. Symposium. Lawwill, T., ed. W. Junk, The Hague, 1977).*

(Armington, 1974; Armington, 1977b; Riggs, Berry, and Wayner, 1949), and may be based on response amplitudes, latencies, or other response measures. Amplitude of the scotopic *b* wave is assumed for the example illustrated by Figure 10.9.

Separation of Photopic and Scotopic Activity. Unless the eye is strongly light-adapted, both photopic and scotopic components will exist in the recordings. The sensitivity of one or the other can be selectively reduced by superimposing test stimuli on colored adaptation fields. When the eye is adapted to short wavelength (blue) light, the sensitivity of scotopic components is reduced, and the components that remain display photopic sensitivity. Adaptation to long wavelength (red) light produces the opposite effect. Figure 10.10 shows exam-

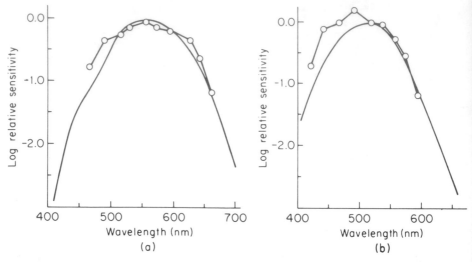

Fig. 10.10. *Spectral sensitivity of electroretinograms obtained after adapting the eye to blue (a) and red (b) light. Straight lines connect the experimental points. The smooth curves are psychophysical functions. The responses obtained with blue adaptation are photopic and those with red adaptation are scotopic (from Armington, J. C. and Thiede, F. C. 1954. J. Opt. Soc. Am., 44, 779).*

ples of spectral sensitivity curves that were obtained by superimposing test flashes upon a continuously presented colored background.

A second technique for separating photopic and scotopic components employs flicker. The photopic parts of the ERG follow rapidly flickering stimuli better than the scotopic. Stimuli flashing off and on at a rate below 4 Hz can be used to obtain strong scotopic waves, and stimuli flickering above 20 Hz to obtain photopic (Johnson and Cornsweet, 1954). An ERG having a multiple waveform in which off as well as on effects are expressed can be produced by using stimuli that flicker at a rate of approximately 15 Hz (Bornschein and Schubert, 1953).

Retinal Position. The distribution of rods and cones across the retina is not uniform. Cones are concentrated in the fovea, the small region in the center of the retina that mediates the most acute vision. The rods, on the other hand, are most concentrated 10° to 15° to the periphery (Cohen, 1975). When recording is carried out so as to isolate the action of local areas, the sensitivity of the ERG reflects these anatomic properties. The largest photopic responses are obtained when stimuli are directed to the fovea (Armington et al, 1961). At low levels of stimulation, maximum scotopic sensitivity is seen when the stimulus forms a ring around the central region and falls on the retina where the rods are most concentrated (Armington, 1976). Advantage may be taken of these spatial properties of the ERG in clinical diagnosis (Brindley and Westheimer, 1965).

RECORDING METHODOLOGY

The information that can be gained from electroretinal recording is conditioned by the recording procedures that are used. Attempts have been made to define a standard recording situation for clinical investigation, but they have not met with universal adoption because no one procedure is appropriate for testing all conditions. Protocols have been worked out for screening subjects efficiently, but they too vary widely in their specific details from laboratory to laboratory. Many innovations have been made in recording technology in recent years and this trend is likely to continue. Thus, when reporting data, it is always important to provide a complete description of the manner in which the data were collected as well as specifications of the recording assembly and adequate calibration information. The present discussion will draw attention to some of the principal features and applications of systems in current use.

A flow diagram for a typical recording situation is sketched in Figure 10.11. Regardless of the application, all recording facilities can be divided into two main sections, a stimulation system for eliciting the ERG, and a recording system for registering it. These two will be examined separately.

Stimulation Systems

Perhaps the most easily produced stimulus is an intense flash of light generated by a photoflash tube of the sort used frequently in electroencephalography. Unfortunately, the spatial and temporal distribution of light that is produced by such a device is not simply described. Hence, the responses that are obtained are neither easily interpreted nor related to the findings of others. Nevertheless, a very intense flash is useful when the concern is merely whether the retina is functional. When the ocular media are cloudy or even nearly

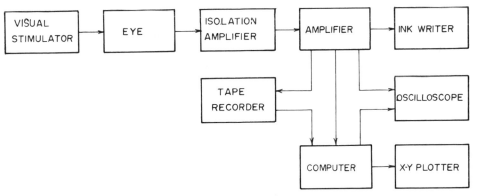

Fig. 10.11. *Elements of a system for recording the electroretinogram. Light from a visual stimulator triggers an electroretinogram. This response is then taken from the eye and passed through a protective isolation amplifier to an assembly of electronic devices used for display and analysis. The arrows indicate the direction in which information flows.*

opaque and when the retina cannot be viewed with an opthalmoscope, a strong flash may be used to test for overall retinal function. The presence of a large ERG suggests a retention of retinal function that can be detected by no other simple means. Flashes from discharge tubes, however, are of no value in testing the response of local retinal regions.

An improved stimulus may be obtained by delivery through an optical system that presents the light in so-called Maxwellian view (Armington, 1974). Stimulators of Maxwellian design present light to the eye from a source lamp through a system of lenses and other optical components. Although more complicated than a flash tube, such a stimulator is more suitable for most work because it permits better stimulus control. Figure 10.12 is a drawing of a Maxwellian system set up to produce alternating patterns on the retina. The advantage of alternation will be considered shortly. When the system is used to produce single flashes a shutter is placed in the light path. Stimulus luminance, spectral composition, duration, area, position on the retina, and other stimulus variables can be readily changed in a properly designed apparatus by inserting appropriate optical components. Changes in the size of the pupil do not change the amount of light entering the eye because the light rays form a small image as the rays enter the eye.

When Maxwellian stimulators are used to present stimuli in the form of flashes, the difficulties of stray light remain. Nevertheless, until the last decade such stimuli were used for most experimental work with the ERG and have

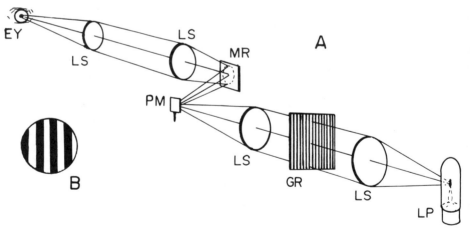

Fig. 10.12. A Maxwellian view stimulator is sketched in section A of this figure. Light from a lamp, LP, is delivered to the eye, EY, by means of lenses, LS, and mirrors, MR and PM. This particular version is designed to present alternating stimuli. The grating, GR, is imaged on the retina. Mirror, PM, is mounted on a pivot. When it turns, the position of the light and dark strip are interchanged. Neutral density filters, not shown in this figure, usually are inserted in the optical path to control luminance, and other components such as shutters, monochromators, etc., are required for specific applications. Insert B shows how the stimulus appears to the subject.

provided a body of useful information regarding spectral sensitivity (Riggs, Berry, and Wayner, 1949), dark adaptation (Johnson, 1949), color blindness (Armington, 1952; Dodt, Copenhaver, and Gunkel, 1959), and other phenomena.

Control of Stray Light. Several stimulus methods for dealing with stray light have been worked out and are now finding accelerated application. Three will be considered here: full-field stimulation, differential regional adaptation, and stimulus alternation.

Full-Field Stimulation. One way the problem of stray light can be avoided is by stimulating all of the retina at once. Full-field stimulation can be produced with a spherical screen placed about the face as shown in Figure 10.13. The interior surface of the screen is matt white and is illuminated with light that is projected from a point beyond view. When the head is in position the light fills the entire field of view. Thus, since light travels from the screen to all parts of the retina directly, stray light becomes relatively ineffective. An advantage of this method lies in its convenience and the reliability of the data produced. The stimulus enters the eyes even when the subject does not follow instructions to hold his eyes in position quite as steadily as directed. Most stimulators provide "fixation points" for the subject to look at and thus to keep his eyes properly aligned. Obviously no stimulus enters the eye with the Maxwellian view described above if the subject allows his eyes to deviate from fixation.

A serious disadvantage of full-field stimulators is that they provide no means of tracing the activity of specific retinal locations. However, they do permit investigation at several levels of adaptation. Test flashes presented over the full field may be superimposed upon a steady adaptation illumination that also is projected onto the spherical screen. Because the responses are generated by the entire retina acting as a unit, full field stimulators are most useful for screening purposes.

Regional Adaptation. When it is necessary to record from a specific location on the retina, a more sophisticated technique is required. One approach is to flood all of the retina except the area under investigation with adaptation light in an attempt to reduce the sensitivity to stray light. No adaptation, but only stimulus flashes are directed to the test area. Some finesse is required for success with this method (Brindley and Westheimer, 1965; Aiba, Alpern, and Maaseidvaag, 1967) because the luminances of the test and adaptation stimuli must be carefully balanced. If the test is too strong, its stray light will still elicit responses; if it is too weak, no response will be found because stray light from the adaptation field enters the test area, appreciably reducing local sensitivity. Biersdorf and Diller (1969) have developed a subtractive procedure that overcomes this difficulty. It is useful to detect the response of the macular area. First, an ERG is produced by delivering stimuli to the blind spot. Since the stimulus image falls where there are no receptors, this response is produced entirely by stray light. Second, an ERG is produced by delivering the same

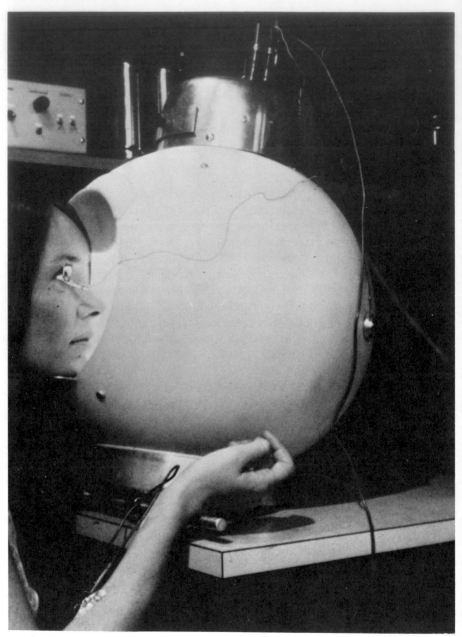

Fig. 10.13. *A ganzfeld stimulator used to stimulate all the retina directly. A stroboscope light is recessed in the housing on the top of the spherical screen. When it flashes the interior of the sphere is lighted uniformly. During actual testing the subject is supported by the chin rest and views the interior of the sphere through the port. The sphere has a hinged mount so that recording can also be performed with the subject in a reclining position (from Rabin, A. R. and Berson, E. L., 1974. Arch. Ophthalmol., 92, 59; Copyright 1974, American Medical Association).*

stimulus to the macula. It represents the combined action of stray light falling outside of the macula and of imaged light falling on the macular area. When the second ERG is subtracted from the first, the resultant represents the response of the macula alone.

Mention has already been made of the difficulty of holding an uncooperative patient's eye in proper alignment with the stimulus. This becomes particularly important when the responses of local retinal regions are under investigation. Stimulation equipment, incorporating a built-in ophthalmoscope has been assembled to allow the experimenter to view the stimulus on the retina as recording is performed (Hirose, Miyoke, and Hara, 1977). Local stimulation is produced with a laser under good visual control. The device presents an adaptation field to control stray light. A hand-held ophthalmoscopic stimulator, developed for work with the visually evoked cortical potential, is a second device of this sort that holds promise for electroretinography (Sandberg and Ariel, 1977).

Alternating Stimuli. A particularly valuable method for recording local response activity is provided by phase alternation (Riggs, Johnson, and Schick, 1964; Lawwill, 1974a and b). The eye views a recurrent pattern of checks or stripes (Fig. 10.12). Typically, the elements that make up the pattern differ in luminance (e.g. black and white stripes), but in special applications they may differ with respect to other variables such as wavelength (Riggs, Johnson, and Schick, 1966). Stimulation is produced by an interchange of the pattern elements. In Figure 10.12 this is accomplished with a mirror that is driven by an electromagnetic mechanism to displace the pattern exactly one stripe width. Since this motion is abrupt, all the bright stripes appear to become dark at the same time as the dark become bright. Excellent control of stray light is achieved because there is no change in the amount of light entering the eye when the pattern alternates. Thus, the light that scatters before reaching the retina does not fluctuate and for similar reasons there is no fluctuation in the light that is reflected from the image area. In a properly designed system, the only place where there is a change in stimulation, and thus the only place where ERGs are produced, is within the image area itself. The method is eminently suited for investigating the action of local retinal regions. Furthermore, the patterned structure of the alternating stimulus makes it possible to investigate visual acuity, resolution, and related variables. Alternating stimuli cannot be produced by equipment as simple as that used for flashes, and some extra effort is required to administer them, but the gain in the information they provide more than justifies their use.

Alternating stimuli may be produced to advantage with Maxwellian view optical systems because they produce sharply focused stimuli of known physical character on the retina. A more convenient way to produce alternating stimuli is on the screen of a television cathode ray tube, and commercial visual stimulators for doing this are now available. Cathode ray displays have important limitations, however. The pattern on their screen is never quite so sharp as that generated by a good optical system, and there is a certain graininess to it. A high-quality cathode ray tube with a uniform phosphor is essential. Another limitation is that it takes some time for the cathode ray that generates the pattern to sweep over the entire screen and thus to produce a single frame. This time, typically amounting to several milliseconds, is long enough to produce errors in latency measurement (Bartl, van Lith, and van Marle, 1978).

Recording Apparatus

Recording apparatus for work with the ERG is similar to that used for other forms of human electrophysiology, and frequently, in fact, ERGs and evoked potentials or other signals are recorded with the same apparatus. There are, however, certain special requirements to be kept in mind when recording the ERG and these are considered here.

Electrodes. The ERG is recorded between an "active" electrode over the cornea and a reference electrode on the forehead or other part of the head. Although small ERGs may be recorded under optimum conditions from electrodes on the canthi or from other electrodes attached to the skin close to the eyes (Tepas and Armington, 1962), extreme caution must be taken when examining the recordings. Recordings from such electrodes are particularly prone to disturbance from blinks and various forms of artifactual activity. These artifacts may be taken as true ERGs by the inexperienced examiner.

Wick electrodes and metallic electrodes in direct contact with the cornea have been used on occasion to obtain large response waves, but by far the most successful recordings have been made using contact lenses to support the electrode. Typically, the lens and electrode do not actually touch the cornea. A film of tears or of contact lens solution acts as a conducting bridge between the front surface of the eye and the actual metallic electrode that is embedded in the contact lens. A variety of contact lens electrodes have been worked out (Fig. 10.14). The first ones made use of a lens set a short distance in front of the cornea, with the bathing solution held between the cornea and the electrode making the actual contact (Riggs, 1941; Karpe, 1945). This type of electrode is still widely used today, but cannot be worn with comfort without local anesthetic unless individually fitted to the eye. A second common type of lens electrode is the Burian-Allen lens (Burian and Allen, 1954), actually an assembly consisting of a speculum that lightly holds a small electrode-bearing contact lens against the eye. Its advantage is the convenience with which it may be applied. However, because it fits directly against the cornea, a local anesthetic still is needed and the stimulus image on the retina may be blurred, a problem that is troublesome when administering alternating stimuli.

In recent years, increasing use has been made of soft hydrophilic contact lenses to hold the recording electrode. The pliability of the material from which they are formed lessens the problem of matching the shape of the lens to that of the eye. One design employs two lenses that are sandwiched together with an electrode wire between them (Schoessler and Jones, 1975). A second design

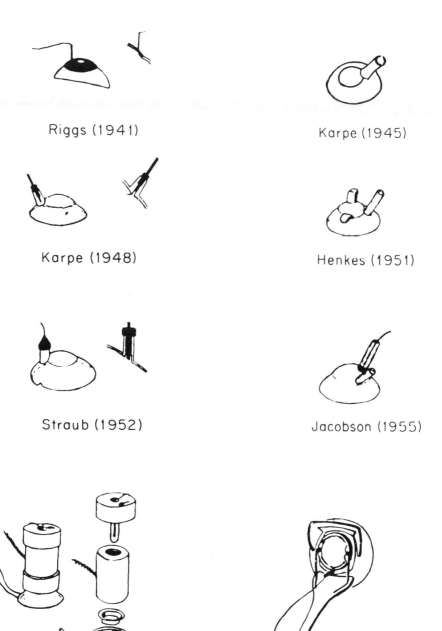

Riggs (1941)

Karpe (1945)

Karpe (1948)

Henkes (1951)

Straub (1952)

Jacobson (1955)

Dollfus-Krauthamer-Chalvignac
(1951)

Burian-Allen
(1954)

Fig. 10.14. *Various designs of contact lens electrodes (from Sundmark, E., 1959. Acta Ophthalmol. Suppl. 52, 14).*

with better optical qualities uses a soft contact lens against the eye that is overlaid with a harder scleral lens (Bloom and Sokol, 1977).

No one electrode suits all purposes. The scleral contact lens electrode individually fitted to each subject is generally preferred for research. For clinical purposes individual fittings are not possible. The electrode must be convenient to apply, comfortable, should permit a clear, unblurred, and unobstructed view of the stimulus pattern, and should establish satisfactory electrical contact over the corneal surface.

In addition to the corneal electrode, a reference electrode is required. A standard electroencephalographic electrode attached to the forehead or cheek is usually used, but in certain cases the reference is also supported in the contact lens. This is done to reduce artifacts from blinking, but also reduces the size of the signal. Generally, recording will be performed with differential amplification. Then, a third electrode attached to an ear or some other convenient point on the head will be needed.

It is important to diagnose progressive blindnesses and certain other disorders in childhood. The ERG is a useful tool for this even though the contact lens electrode presents special problems in children and they may be uncooperative in other respects. Sedation or general anesthesia are frequently used to meet this problem, but they must be employed with caution. Berson (1975) points out that anesthesia can reduce *b* wave amplitudes by at least 50 percent, and Marmor (1977) emphasizes that sedation is not always necessary on a routine basis if sufficient effort is spent attracting the cooperation of the patient.

Presentation of Recordings. After the signal has been amplified and filtered as necessary, the ERG can be displayed on a wide variety of instruments including an oscilloscope, inkwriter, or some form of recording galvanometer. A well-equipped laboratory may have several alternative methods of presenting responses. Generally, ERGs are plotted as they are recorded, but they may also be stored on magnetic tape for subsequent analysis. No matter how display is accomplished, it is important that the equipment reproduce the signals fed to it accurately. A general requirement is that the display system respond uniformly to all frequencies in the range from 0 to 120 Hz.

Special Recording Devices. The ERG is a small signal in comparison with many of the other activities that appear between the recording electrodes— especially when responses are being obtained from small local regions of the retina or when the stimulation levels are low. ERGs produced under these conditions can only be observed by stimulating the eye repeatedly and averaging the successive response waves together. Special fixed program computers known as response averagers are available for this purpose. Once programmed, general purpose minicomputers can be just as convenient as the special purposes averagers, however, their real advantage being that they can be set up to carry out a diversity of operations, including mathematical filtering, various forms of signal to noise analysis, data processing, and filing.

When the eye moves or blinks, large artifactual signals with amplitudes ranging up to several millivolts are generated. These may not occur frequently with well-trained subjects, but they are certainly a problem with the inexperienced. Subjects should always be encouraged not to blink, as no amount of averaging can adequately correct this situation, but improvement may be had using a sampling procedure together with averaging. This can be done with a minicomputer programmed to discard response epochs that occur with artifactual activity above some predetermined level. Only those responses that occur in the absence of blinks contribute to the average. In the absence of a computer, special electronic devices may be used for cleaning up recordings. Data can be passed through filters and noise-suppressing circuits. An electronic device known as a limiter may be used to clip off the tops of potentials of extreme amplitudes and a "blanking" circuit may block signal tramsission during the presence of high amplitude interference. These techniques while less effective than actually eliminating erroneous signals from recorded averages, can nevertheless prove helpful under certain circumstances. Caution must always be maintained however, as these special techniques may distort the result rather than improve it.

Electro-oculography. The techniques considered so far are those for recording the transient features of the ERG. The electro-oculogram describes changes in relatively steady resting potential during dark and light adaptation (Fig. 10.15). The information it provides may be used to supplement that produced by conventional electroretinography. The electro-oculogram is recorded by placing a pair of electrodes close to the two canthi of the eye, and these are connected to regular recording equipment. The subject is presented with two fixation points that are well separated (in different laboratories from 30 to 80 degrees of visual angle). His task is to shift his eyes periodically from one fixation point to the other. As he does this, a change in the voltage is recorded due to the change in position of the polarized eye relative to the recording electrodes. Its magnitude changes during light and dark adaptation as illustrated. These changes are reduced in retinal degenerations, some of which are briefly described below (Fishman, 1975; Arden and Fojas, 1962). In addition, the electro-oculogram has found numerous applications besides the obvious clinical ones and can be used, for example, for studying eye movements during reading.

CLINICAL ELECTRORETINOGRAPHY

The preceding discussion makes it clear that more than one technology exists for electroretinal recording; the procedures should be chosen with the purpose of the recording in mind. Much clinical work has been conducted with simple flashing stimuli and most of the work reported below is based on this. Certain of the techniques, such as stimulus alternation, have been developed too recently for widespread adoption. However, Lawwill (1974a and b, 1977) already has drawn attention to the potential of this method for evaluating visual

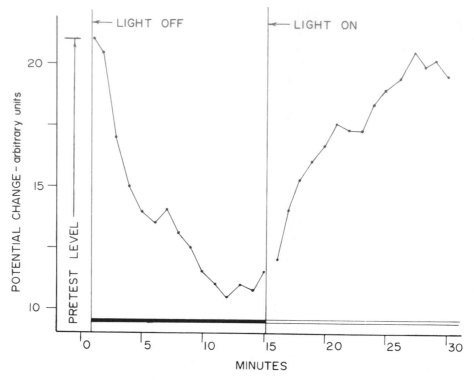

Fig. 10.15. *The electro-oculogram. This figure illustrates the temporal changes of the resting potential that are induced by light and dark adaptation. The magnitude of the changes depends upon the recording situation. A change of several hundred microvolts is representative of typical conditions.*

function. Only highlights of an extensive clinical literature will be brought forth here, after initial mention has been made of the changes that take place in the ERG with age.

Normal Development

It is well known that the human visual system is not completely formed at birth. Significant development occurs during the first year, growth being especially rapid during the first weeks following delivery. These changes are reflected in the ERG. Although just detectable at birth, its amplitude is extremely small (Zetterstrom, 1970). The latency also is somewhat longer than the ERG of the mature eye, but both photopic and scotopic components can be identified (Lodge et al, 1969). Development is rapid during the first postnatal weeks, and by a year reaches full expression. Changes beyond this point are not large, although there is a trend for *b* wave amplitude to decrease with increasing age (Peterson, 1968).

Hereditary Diseases

The ERG has found its widest application in diagnosing disorders and diseases of hereditary origin. These exist in wide variety, and even their classification has not been entirely worked out. Using full-field stimulus flashes and looking at photopic and scotopic components, Berson (1977) suggests that the ERG can be used to place hereditary retinal diseases in four functional classes:

I. Congenital disorders that involve either rod or cone function across all or nearly all of the retina.

II. Diseases that involve rod and cone function, but only in localized areas of the retina (e.g. retinitis pigmentosa in a single sector of the visual field).

III. Diseases that involve either rod or cone function across nearly all of the retina with macular degeneration.

IV. Diseases that involve both rod and cone function across nearly all of the retina and entail progressive deterioration with age.

The first three of these categories include disorders that generally are considered to be nonprogressive. The ERG is particularly valuable for diagnosis of category IV because it permits early detection before fundoscopic or other changes become apparent. The following discussion centers on categories I and IV. Problems with the macula are considered later following a section on acquired disorders.

Trichromatic color theory, buttressed by extensive physiologic research (Rushton, 1972; Riggs and Wooten, 1972), divides the photopic system into three subsystems that mediate color perception: the red or long wavelength, the green or middle wavelength, and the blue or short wavelength system. When a person is born without one or more of these systems active, he is said to be color blind: thus, the protanope lacks red sensitive cones and is red blind, the deutranope is green blind, and the tritanope is blue blind. The ERG of protanopes differs markedly from normal. When red stimuli are used, protanopes can be identified by the lack of photopic components in their response waveform (Schubert and Bornschein, 1952). However, spectral sensitivity measures are most effective in working with color blindness (Armington, 1952; Copenhaver and Gunkel, 1959). Lack of function is indicated by a lowering of the spectral curve in the region of deficiency (Fig. 10.16). The loss of a color mechanism is not always complete. In cases where there is a deficiency but not a total loss of function, the so-called color anomalies, smaller changes from normal are reported (Dodt et al, 1958; Padmos, van Norren, and Jaspers Faijer, 1978).

Night Blindness

When the scotopic system is incapable of function, the patient is said to be night blind. Present from birth and generally unaccompanied by conspicuous ophthalmoscopic changes, congenital night blindness is easily overlooked in routine examination. Nevertheless, it is a serious problem for those who are

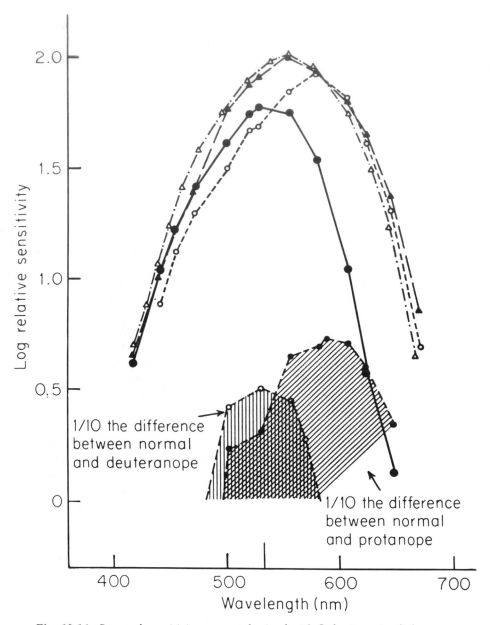

Fig. 10.16. *Spectral sensitivity curves obtained with flickering stimuli from normal and color blind subjects. The sensitivity of a normal subject is represented by filled triangles. The protanope, whose data are depicted by filled circles, has reduced long wavelength sensitivity. The deuteranope, open circles, has reduced short wavelength sensitivity. The open triangles are photopic psychophysical data (from Copenhaver, R. M. and Gunkel, R. D., 1959. Arch. Ophthalmol., 62, 55; Copyright 1959, American Medical Association).*

afflicted, some of whom, at least, mistakenly have been referred to psychiatric services for evaluation of their difficulty (Armington and Schwab, 1954). Night blindness is characterized by an inability to see at low levels of illumination, and hence an accident proneness results when travelling at night or otherwise performing under low levels of illumination. The changes that occur in the ERG with congenital night blindness are readily detected with simple stimulus flashes presented to the dark adapted eye because compared with normal, all activity is enormously reduced in amplitude. The scotopic components which generally contribute most to the flash evoked ERG are absent. The waveform of the response which is obtained varies among individuals. Examples are shown in Figure 10.17. Some ERGs have a small *a* wave followed by a conspicuous photopic *b* wave. In others, the *a* wave seems larger and the *b* wave is absent, a predominantly negative response being the result (Auerbach, Godell, and Rowe, 1969).

Oguchi's disease, a form of night blindness that is characterized by a faint, diffuse grey coloring of the fundus, presents a unique electrophysiologic picture (Gouras, 1970). Under ordinary test conditions the ERG is a negative one of very low amplitudes similar to that one seen in other forms of night blindness. Remarkably, however, if the eye is allowed to dark adapt for very long periods of time (12 hours or more), a *b* wave of large amplitude and having typical scotopic waveform appears. This *b* wave is extremely labile. A single stimulus flash is sufficient to cut down the response to a following flash unless several additional minutes of dark adaptation intervene.

Retinal Degeneration

Electroretinography finds one of its most valuable applications in detecting retinal degeneration at its earliest stages and in distinguishing progressive from nonprogressive forms (Berson, 1976). Many of these degenerations are referred to collectively as retinitis pigmentosa. Classically, retinitis pigmentosa is a progressive hereditary disease that begins in adolescence with a loss of peripheral vision accompanied by night blindness. It advances with age until if any vision remains, it is limited to the very center of the visual field. Pigmentation of the retina becomes visible with the ophthalmoscope as the disease advances. Extensive investigation during recent decades has identified a number of distinct entities that formerly fell under the heading of retinitis pigmentosa, and these may be classified according to their mode of inheritance, the functional changes that occur, ophthalmoscopic changes, the rate at which they advance, and whether or not all of the retina is afflicted (Merin and Auerbach, 1976). Both the ERG and the electro-oculogram can be used to advantage in investigating all of these cases.

The Electro-oculogram in Retinitis Pigmentosa. The standing potential whose magnitude is indicated by the electro-oculogram arises from multiple sources among which the pigment epithelium is a strong participant (Arden and Fojas, 1962). The electro-oculogram is useful for examining retinitis pigmentosa be-

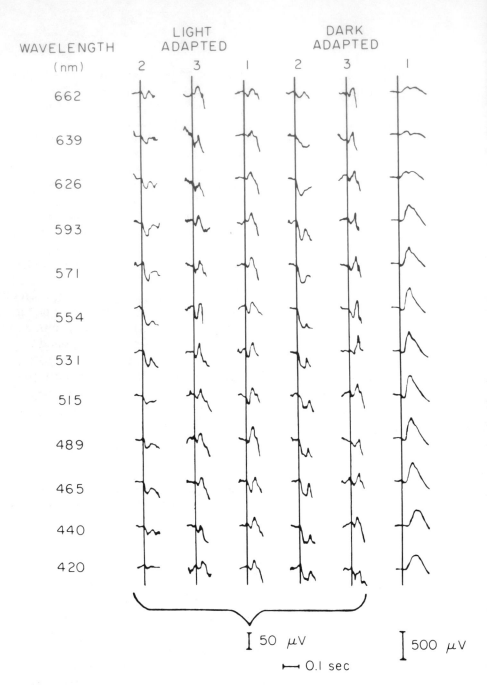

Fig. 10.17. *Electroretinograms from two night blind subjects (2,3) compared with those of a normal one (1). Responses are shown for different test wave lengths and for the dark and light adapted eye. When light adapted, one subject (3) had a response similar to that of normal. The other subject (2) exhibited a large negative potential. Dark adaptation did not change the responses of the night blind subjects appreciably whereas the responses of the normal exhibited a substantial increase. Note that a different calibration scale applies to the normal subject when dark adapted (from Armington, J. C. and Schwab, G. J., 1954. Arch. Ophthalmol., 52, 725; Copyright 1954, American Medical Association).*

cause it emphasizes the activity of this layer to a greater extent than does the typical transient ERG. In the various forms of retinitis pigmentosa, the electro-oculogram is small or even absent. In addition to the subnormality of response, the peak that occurs with light adaptation is earlier than is normal (Dayton et al, 1964). Arden and Kolb (1964) found that the sensitivity of the electro-oculogram rivaled that of the ERG in detecting retinal degenerations, but more recent work has greatly enhanced the value of the ERG. Today, the electro-oculogram should be regarded as a complement to the ERG and one that is particularly sensitive to damage of the pigment epithelium.

The Transient Electroretinogram in Progressive Retinitis Pigmentosa. All features of the ERG are profoundly depressed with the advance of retinitis pigmentosa. Early studies, made before the advent of response averaging, reported the ERG as absent (i.e. "extinguished") even in the early phases of degeneration (Karpe, 1945; Riggs, 1954). Later research (Ruedemann and Noell, 1959) has made it clear that a small response generally remains. The amplitude of the *b* wave drops off often before any other signs of incipient degeneration are noticed. The size of the response is correlated with the area of the retina that retains function (Armington et al, 1961). Using full-field stimulation, Berson (1976) has shown that there is an increase in *b* wave peak latency (implicit time) in progressive retinitis pigmentosa. It is seen well before there is any reduction in response amplitude. This increase of latency is an important sign of future retinal degeneration when testing children who for genetic reasons are suspected as likely to be afflicted later in life (Berson, 1976). Examples of ERGs in various forms of retinitis pigmentosa are shown in Figure 10.18.

Because the early receptor potential originates in the distal parts of the receptors in proximity to the pigment epithelium and because it too is reduced (Fig. 10.19), it has a special relevance for understanding retinitis pigmentosa. In humans the cones contribute most to the early receptor potential; thus, the fact that this potential is markedly affected in retinitis pigmentosa demonstrates that the disease invades the photopic as well as the scotopic system (Berson, 1976).

The local changes that take place across the retina in retinitis pigmentosa have been investigated using local stimulation (Sandberg, 1978). Not only do the pigmented areas fail to respond, but an impaired response can be demonstrated in the macular region and in other areas where visible damage is not apparent.

Acquired Retinal Degenerations. The retina may be damaged, impaired, or may deteriorate for reasons that are not hereditary. Usually, these conditions involve the periphery (which comprises most of the retina), and thus may be accompanied by night blindness. Frequently, however, the macular region— and so acute vision—is also involved. The electrophysiologic effects of these disorders generally are marked.

Traumatic injury of the retina results in decreased response, the degree of which may reflect the extent of the injury. Injury may result from many causes. Siderosis, induced by foreign intraocular metal particles, produces a progressive reduction in the amplitude of the *b* wave (Knave, 1969). The ERG may thus be of value for early diagnosis of this condition. Retinal detachments generally are accompanied by reductions in electroretinal sensitivity. It is reported that there is a correlation between this loss and the success of subsequent corrective surgery in restoring vision (Zetterstrom, 1964).

Syphilitic chorioretinitis presents symptoms and fundus changes that mimic retinitis pigmentosa. Heckenlively (1977) reports that the ERG is reduced in

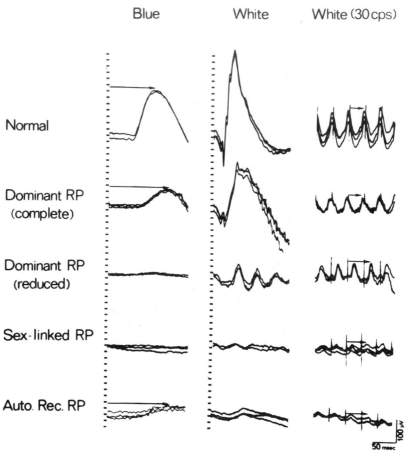

ERGs in EARLY RETINITIS PIGMENTOSA (RP)

Fig. 10.18. *Electroretinograms in early retinitis pigmentosa. Responses of a normal subject are compared with those of four children with retinitis pigmentosa. Four varieties of retinitis pigmentosa are represented. Full field stimulation was used. The responses in the first two columns were obtained with blue and with white flashes delivered to the totally dark adapted eye. Responses to flicker are shown in the third column. Implicit times are indicated over some of the tracings with arrows. An increased delay of the patients as compared with normal is evident (from Berson, E. L., 1976. Trans. Am. Acad. Ophthal. Otolaryngol., 81, 659).*

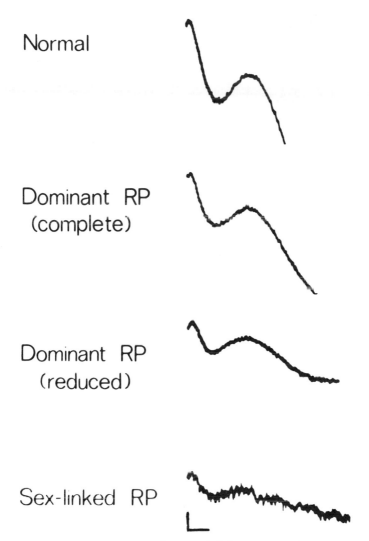

Normal

Dominant RP
(complete)

Dominant RP
(reduced)

Sex-linked RP

Fig. 10.19. Early receptor potentials recorded from a normal subject and three patients with retinitis pigmentosa. The calibration symbol signifies 0.5 msec horizontally and 50 μV vertically for the top three tracings and 0.5 msec and 20 μV for the bottom tracing. The abnormality of the early receptor potential in the three forms of retinitis pigmentosa shown is clearly evident (from Berson, E. L., 1976. Trans. Am. Acad. Ophthalmol. Otolaryngol., 81, 659).

amplitude in such cases, but not to the same degree as in true retinitis pigmentosa.

Vitamin A is essential for the formation of visual pigment and the maintenance of vision. Loss of scotopic vision and a reduction of photopic vision may be evident when there is insufficient vitamin A intake over an extended period of time. With extreme deprivation, the scotopic components of the ERG virtually disappear and photopic components are markedly reduced in amplitude (Bornschein and Vukovich, 1953). The ERG returns to normal with vitamin A therapy. Similar results have been reported for vitamin A deficiency associated with chronic alcoholism and subsequent therapy (Sandberg, Rosen, and Berson, 1977).

Other causes of retinal injury, including exposure to intense light or other radiation, tumors, ingestion of toxic substances such as wood alcohol, and side effects from clinical agents such as chloroquine, also result in *b* waves of reduced amplitude. Many of these have been reviewed by Fishman (1975).

Macular Degenerations. Diseases of the macula are singularly debilitating because they influence the parts of the retina where acuity is normally the highest. Macular lesions must be examined using stimulus techniques that are not complicated by stray light because the macula is a small part of the whole retina. Average response computers, techniques of light adaptation, and stimulus alternation are necessary for this work (Lawwill, 1974a and b). There has been a progressive evolution of methods designed to control stray light in testing macular function during the last two decades.

In early work, Gouras and his colleagues (1964) compared responses obtained simultaneously from the two eyes of each of a group of patients characterized by unilateral loss of central field vision. The patients were selected for the sharp localization of their lesion and gave essentially normal ERGs when records were obtained with full-field stimulation. In an attempt to reduce the effectiveness of stray light, dim orange flickering stimuli of limited angular extent were presented in a test area that was surrounded with weak adaptation illumination. Since all responses were small, computer averaging was employed. The response of the defective area was found to be smaller than the comparable area of the normal eye. However, differences between the two eyes could be established only when the lesions were quite large, and even under the best circumstances could be detected only if they subtended a visual angle of 7 degrees.

Subsequently Biersdorf and Diller (1969) used flickering stimuli of 4 degrees visual angle and took the ratio of response amplitudes produced by stimuli delivered to the blind spot (where only stray light is effective) to those produced by stimuli to the central area. Patients having senile macular degeneration were readily distinguished from normals. With normal macular function a response that was up to three times larger was obtained with macular stimulation than with stimulation imaged on the blind spot. In patients with severely impaired acuity (at least 20/40 to 20/800) all responses were nearly the same, regardless of stimulus location.

Lawwill (1977) has shown how alternating stimuli may be used effectively to test for reduced vision in the central field of both children and adults. Although this stimulus method requires relatively elaborate stimulus equipment as well as more care during testing, its value for diagnosing macular problems is quite clear.

Circulatory Disturbances of the Retina

Normal circulation of blood to the retina is crucial for maintaining the size and shape of the ERG. It is well-recognized that experimental interference with retinal circulation produces immediate changes in the ERG, and this has been one basis for physiologic analysis of the ERG (Granit, 1935). Experimental interruptions of circulation and their electrophysiologic effects usually are much greater than those found in the clinic. Nevertheless some changes have been described in the ERG with naturally occurring reduction of the retinal blood supply. On their basis, two hypotheses having importance for diagnostic work might be made: 1, the amplitude of the ERG is reduced to the degree that circulation is impaired and 2, waveform changes take place that are specific to the character of the circulatory impairment. Examples of ERGs obtained with simple strobe flashes and reflecting increasing degrees of impairment are shown in Figure 10.20. Amplitude changes in the *a* wave, *b* wave, or both, may occur. The following reasoning has been invoked to explain the waveform changes. If circulation to the inner layers of the retina is cut down, the *b* wave should be more reduced than the *a* wave because the latter, reflecting at least in part receptor activity, arises more distally. ERGs with negative polarity may result from a reduced blood supply to the proximal parts of the retina. In support of this reasoning Henkes (1954) and later investigators (Armington, 1974) have found that negative ERGs are characteristic of a blockage of the central retinal artery.

Glaucoma is an increase in intraocular pressure, and this disorder may be

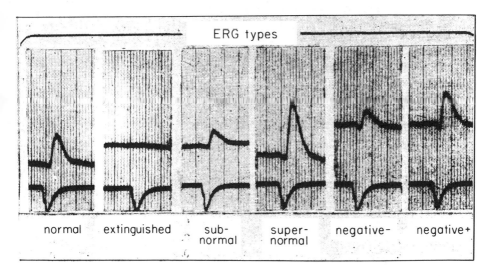

Fig. 10.20. *Electroretinograms representing increasing degrees of retinal impairment resulting from circulatory disorders. Single flashes were used for these recordings. Note that the responses have been classified according to their waveform and magnitude (from Henkes, H. E., 1953. Arch. Ophthalmol., 49, 190; Copyright 1953, American Medical Association).*

associated with a general lowering of retinal circulation. Under typical recording conditions and when the pressure has not yet risen to extreme values,
glaucoma does not produce marked electroretinal changes, but small changes in
the *b* wave have been reported (Wulfing, 1963). Moderate glaucoma, coupled
with a testing technique in which the pressure of the eye is raised to even higher
pressures through the application of external force, produces a reduction in
response that does distinguish between people with normal vision and
glaucoma (Burian, 1953). There is also some evidence that glaucoma interferes
with oscillatory potentials of the ERG (Gur and Zeevi, 1978).

Diabetes is another condition that produces changes in retinal circulation.
These changes may range from a slight dilation of the retinal vessels to actual
rupture. The *b* wave is not altered in the early phases of diabetic retinopathy,
when diagnosis is most important (Karpe, Kornerup, and Wulfing, 1958), but
the oscillatory potentials may be significantly decreased (Fig. 10.21) or even

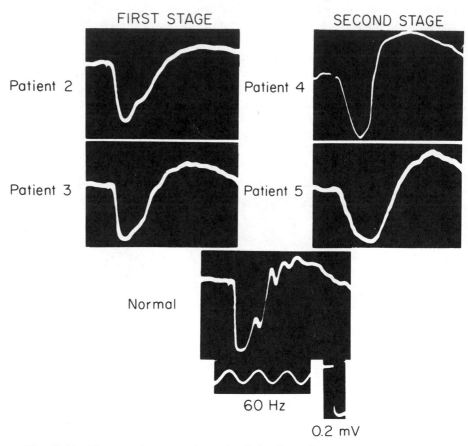

*Fig. 10.21. Electroretinograms from the dark adapted eyes of diabetic patients.
Single flashes. The retinopathy in patients 2 and 3 is less advanced than in
patients 4 and 5. Note that the oscillatory potentials characteristic of the normal
eye are markedly reduced (from Yonemura, D., Aoki, T. and Tsuzuki, K., 1962.
Arch. Ophthalmol., 68, 19; Copyright 1962, American Medical Association).*

absent (Yonemura, Aoki, and Tsuzuki, 1962). Simonsen (1968) finds a reduction of these wavelets in certain diabetic patients in whom no ophthalmoscopic changes can yet be detected. Oscillatory potentials are believed to have some prognostic value—diabetic patients with reduced oscillatory potentials have a strong disposition towards progressive deterioration of vision.

Visual Acuity

The term *acuity* pertains to the ability of the eye to resolve the detail of a stimulus pattern. Acuity may be reduced because of problems with the optical structures of the eye or because of macular deterioration. In the case of amblyopia exanopsia, for example, poor acuity is evidenced even though the optics of the eye are clear and the stimulus is sharply imaged on an apparently sound retina. Alternating stimulus patterns, which not only reduce the effectiveness of stray light but which must be in clear focus to produce optimum response, are particularly appropriate for testing acuity. In an ingenious study, Millidot and Riggs (1970) investigated the effect of placing lenses of various powers in front of an alternating set of stimulus stripes. A large response was produced when the stimulus was accurately focused on the retina (Fig. 10.22). A small refractive error resulted in a substantial reduction of response amplitude. The visually evoked cortical potential is even more critically sensitive to the sharpness of the image in the macular region, but the ERG, because it arises from an extended retinal area, is more responsive to the quality of the image over the entire test field. The ERG thus yields information that is not readily obtained by other electrophysiologic procedures.

When unpatterned stimuli are used, ERGs from amblyopic eyes appear normal, but the deficiency becomes apparent with alternating patterns (Sokol, 1978; Nadler and Sokol, 1978). Both the *b* wave and the late negative potential fall below normal in amblyopic eyes. These data point to a retinal involvement in amblyopia and thus are pertinent to the question of whether the loss of acuity has a retinal or cortical basis.

The Electroretinogram and the Visually Evoked Cortical Potential

Future neurologic research of the visual system will likely feature simultaneous recording of both these responses because together they can answer questions that neither can answer alone (Schreinemachers and Henkes, 1968). Thus, it is fitting to conclude this chapter by drawing attention to the possibilities of joint recording. Only the first steps have yet been taken. In the case of multiple sclerosis there is clear evidence for an abnormally delayed evoked potential but the evidence for changes in the ERG are still conflicting (Halliday, McDonald and Mushin, 1972; Feinsod, Abramsky, and Auerbach, 1973). Harden and Pampiglione (1977) report that combined recording of the ERG and the evoked potential is useful in the analysis of several progressive neurometabolic diseases in children. In the case of neurologic disorders, the ERG may detect occasional retinal impairments that with evoked potential recording alone might be attributed to more central causes. Although at present results obtained

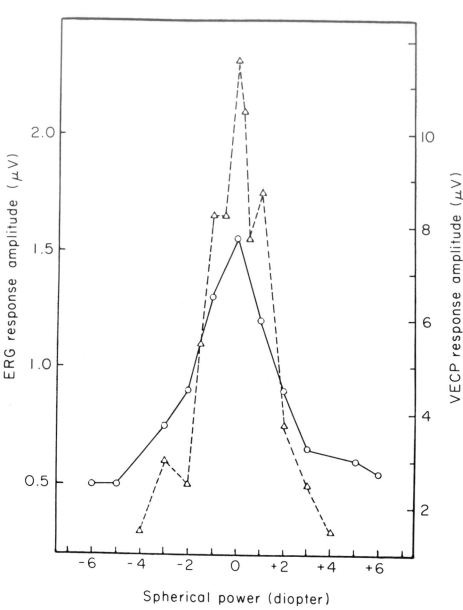

Fig. 10.22. *The amplitude of the electroretinogram and the visually evoked cortical potential as dependent upon the sharpness of the retinal image. When the retinal image is blurred by placing lenses of various powers in front of the eye, both responses become smaller (from Millodot, M. and Riggs, L., 1970. Arch. Ophthalmol., 84, 276; Copyright 1970, American Medical Association).*

with joint recording are incomplete and must be regarded as tentative, there is little doubt but that their combined use will soon be an important feature of visual diagnosis.

REFERENCES

Adrian, E. D. (1945). The electric response of the human eye. J. Physiol. (Lond.), *104:*84.

Aiba, T. S., Alpern, M., and Maaseidvaag, F. (1967). The electroretinogram evoked by the excitation of human foveal cones. J. Physiol. (Lond.), *189:*43.

Arden, G. B. and Fojas, M. R. (1962). Electrophysiological abnormalities in pigmentary degenerations of the retina. Arch. Ophthalmol., *68:*369.

Arden, G. B. and Kolb, H. (1964). Electrophysiological investigations in retinal metabolic disease: their range and application. Exp. Eye Res. *3,*334.

Armington, J. C. (1952). A component of the human electroretinogram associated with red color vision. J. Opt. Soc. Am., *42:*393.

Armington, J. C. (1959). Chromatic and short term dark adaptation of the human electroretinogram. J. Opt. Soc. Am., *49:*1169.

Armington, J. C. (1974). The Electroretinogram. Academic Press, New York.

Armington, J. C. (1976). Spectral sensitivity of low level electroretinograms. Vision Res., *16:*31.

Armington, J. C. (1977a). Visual cortical potentials and electroretinograms triggered by saccadic eye movements. In: Visual Evoked Potentials in Man: New Developments. Desmedt, J. E., Ed., p. 286, Clarendon, Oxford.

Armington, J. C. (1977b). The correlation of electrophysiological and psychophysical measures: the electroretinogram. Doc. Ophthalmol. Proc. Series, 14th ISCERG Symposium, 123.

Armington, J. C., Corwin, T. R., and Marsetta, R. (1971). Simultaneously recorded retinal and cortical responses to patterned stimuli. J. Opt. Soc. Am., *61:*1514.

Armington, J. C., Gouras, P., Tepas, D. I., and Gunkel, R. (1961). Detection of the electroretinogram in retinitis pigmentosa. Exp. Eye Res., *1:*74.

Armington, J. C., Johnson, E. P., and Riggs, L. A. (1952). The scotopic A-wave in the electrical response of the human retina. J. Physiol. (Lond.), 118:289.

Armington, J. C. and Schwab, G. J. (1954). Electroretinogram in nyctalopia. Arch. Ophthalmol., *52:*725.

Armington, J. C., Tepas, D. I., Kropfl, W. J., and Hengst, W. H. (1961). Summation of retinal potentials. J. Opt. Soc. Am., *51:*877.

Asher, H. (1951). The electroretinogram of the blind spot. J. Physiol. (Lond.), *112:*40P.

Auerbach, E., Godell, V., and Rowe, H. (1969). An electrophysiological and psychophysical study of two forms of congenital night blindness. Investig. Ophthalmol., *8:*332.

Bartl, G., van Lith, G. H. M., and van Marle, G. W. (1978). Cortical potentials evoked by a TV pattern reversal stimulus with varying check sizes and stimulus field. Brit. J. Ophthalmol., *62:*216.

Bartley, S. H. (1941). Vision: a study of its basis. Van Nostrand-Reinhold, New Jersey.

Berson, E. L. (1975). Electrical phenomena in the retina. In: Adler's Physiology of the Eye. 6th edn. Moses, R. A., Ed., p. 453, C. V. Mosby, Saint Louis.

Berson, E. L. (1976). Retinitis pigmentosa and allied retinal diseases: electrophysiological findings. Trans. Am. Acad. Ophthalmol. Otolaryngol., *81:*659.

Berson, E. L. (1977). Hereditary retinal diseases: classification with the full-field electroretinogram. Doc. Ophthalmol. Proc. Series, 14th ISCERG Symposium, 149.

Biersdorf, W. R. (1958). Luminance-duration relationships in the light-adapted electroretinogram. J. Opt. Soc. Am., *48:*412.

Biersdorf, W. R. and Diller, D. (1969). Local electroretinogram in macular degeneration. Am. J. Ophthalmol., *68:*296.

Bloom, B. H. and Sokol, S. (1977). A corneal electrode for patterned stimulus electroretinography. Am. J. Ophthalmol., *83:*272.

Bornschein, H. (1966). Slow components in the ERG. In: The Clinical Value of Electroretinography. Francois, J., Ed., p. 144, Karger, New York.

Bornschein, H. and Goodman, G. (1957). Studies on the A-wave in the human electroretinogram. Arch. Ophthalmol., *58:*431.

Bornschein, H. and Schubert, G. (1953). Das Photopische Flimmer-Elektroretinogramm des Menschen. Zeitschr. fur Biologie, *106:*299.

Bornschein, H. and Vukovich, V. (1953). Das Elektroretinogramm bei Mangelhemeralopie. Albrecht von Graefes Arch. Klin. Exp. Ophthalmol., *153:*484.

Boynton, R. M. and Riggs, L. A. (1951). The effect of stimulus area and intensity upon the human retinal response. J. Exp. Psychol., *42:*217.

Brindley, G. S. and Westheimer, G. (1965). The spatial properties of the human electroretinogram. J. Physiol., *179:*518.

Brown, K. T. (1968). The electroretinogram: its components and their origins. Vision Res., *8:*633.

Brown, K. T. and Murakami, M. (1964). A new receptor potential of the monkey retina with no detectable latency. Nature, *201:*626.

Brunette, J. R. (1972). Double A-waves and their relationship to the oscillatory potentials. Invest. Ophthalmol., *11:*199.

Burian, H. (1953). Electroretinography and its clinical application. Arch. Ophthalmol., *49:*241.

Burian, H. M. and Allen, L. (1954). A speculum contact lens electrode for electroretinography. Electroencephalogr. Clin. Neurophysiol., *6:*509.

Cohen, A. I. (1975). The retina and optic nerve. In: Adler's Physiology of the Eye, 6th edn., Moses, R. A., Ed., p. 367, C. V. Mosby, Saint Louis.

Cone, R. A. (1964). Early receptor potential of the vertebrate retina. Nature, *204:*736.

Copenhaver, R. M. and Gunkel, R. D. (1959). The spectral sensitivity of color defective subjects determined by electroretinography. Arch. Ophthalmol., *62:*55.

Dayton, G. O., Jr., Jones, M. H., Kelly, W., Limpaecher, R., and Lee, W. (1964). The electro-oculogram as a diagnostic tool in retinitis pigmentosa. J. Pediatr. Ophthalmol., *1:*9.

Dewar, J. (1877). The physiological action of light. I, II, Nature, *15:*433; 452.

Dodt, E., Copenhaver, R. M., and Gunkel, R. D. (1958). Photopischer Dominator und Farbkomponenten im menschlichen Elektroretinogramm. Pflugers Arch., *267:*497.

Dowling, J. E. (1970). Organization of vertebrate retinas. Invest. Ophthalmol., *9:*655.

Einthoven, W. and Jolly, W. A. (1908). The form and magnitude of the electrical response of the eye to stimulation by light at various intensities. Quart. J. Exp. Physiol., *1:*373.

Feinsod, M., Abramsky, D., and Auerbach, E. (1973). Electrophysiological examinations of the visual system in multiple sclerosis. J. Neurol. Science, *20:*161.

Fishman, G. A. (1975). The electroretinogram and electro-oculogram in retinal and choroidal disease. American Academy of Ophthalmology and Otolaryngology, Rochester, Minnesota.

Fulton, A. B. and Rushton, W. A. H. (1978). The human rod ERG: correlation with psychophysical responses in light and dark adaptation. Vision Res., *18:*793.

Gouras, P. (1970). Electroretinography: some basic principles. Invest. Ophthalmol., *9:*557.

Gouras, P., Armington, J. C., Kropfl, W. J., and Gunkel, R. D. (1964). Electronic computation of human retinal and brain responses to light stimulation. Ann. N.Y. Acad. Science, *115:*763.

Granit, R. (1933). The components of the retinal action potential in mammals and their relation to the discharge in the optic nerve. J. Physiol. (Lond.), *77:*207.

Granit, R. (1935). Two types of retinas and their electrical responses to intermittent stimuli in light and dark adaptation. J. Physiol. (Lond.), *85:*421.

Gur, M. and Zeevi, Y. Y. (1978). Frequency domain analysis of the human electroretinogram. Submitted for publication.

Halliday, A. M., McDonald, W. I., and Mushin, J. (1972). Delayed visual evoked responses in optic neuritis. Lancet, *1:*982.

Harden, A. and Pampiglione, G. (1977). Visual evoked potential, electroretinogram, and electroencephalogram studies in progressive neurometabolic 'storage' diseases of childhood. In: Visual Evoked Potentials in Man: New Developments. Desmedt, J. E., Ed., p. 470, Clarendon, Oxford.

Heckenlively, J. R. (1977). Secondary retinitis pigmentosa (syphilis). Doc. Ophthalmol. Proc. Series, 14th ISCERG Symposium, 245.

Henkes, H. E. (1953). Electroretinography in circulatory disturbances of the retina. I. Electroretinogram in cases of occlusion of the central retinal vein or one of its branches. Arch. Ophthalmol., *49:*190.

Henkes, H. E. (1954). Electroretinogram in circulatory disturbances of the retina. IV. Electroretinogram in cases of retinal and choroidal hypertension and arteriosclerosis. Arch. Ophthalmol., *52:*30.

Hirose, T., Miyoke, Y., and Hara, A. (1977). Simultaneous recording of electroretinogram and visual evoked response. Arch. Ophthalmol., *95:*1205.

Johnson, F. P. (1949). The electrical response of the human retina during dark adaptation. J. Exp. Psychol., *39:*597.

Johnson, E. P. (1958). The character of the B-wave in the human electroretinogram. Arch. Ophthalmol., *60:*565.

Johnson, E. P. and Cornsweet, T. N. (1954). Electroretinal photopic sensitivity curves. Nature, *174:*614.

Kaneko, A. and Hashimoto, H. (1967). Recording site of the single cone response determined by an electrode marking technique. Vision Res., *7:*847.

Karpe, G. (1945). The basis of clinical electroretinography. Acta Ophthalmol., Supp. 24, 1.

Karpe, G., Kornerup, T., and Wulfing, B. (1958). The clinical electroretinogram. VIII. The electroretinogram in diabetic retinopathy. Acta Ophthalmol., *36:*281.

Karwoski, C. J. and Proenza, L. M. (1977). Relationship between Muller cell responses, a local transretinal potential, and potassium flux. J. Neurophysiol., *40:*244.

Knave, B. (1969). Electroretinography in eyes with retained intraocular foreign bodies. Acta Ophthalmol. Supp. 100, 1.

Lawwill, T. (1974a). The bar-pattern electroretinogram for clinical evaluation of the central retina. Am. J. Ophthalmol., *78:*121.

Lawwill, T. (1974b.) Pattern stimuli for clinical ERG. Doc. Ophthalmol. Proc. Series, 11th ISCERG Symposium, 353.

Lawwill, T. (1977). Clinical applications of electroretinography. Perspect. Ophthalmol., *1:*17.

Lodge, A., Armington, J. C., Barnet, A. B., Shanks, B. L., and Newcomb, C. M. (1969). Newborn infants electroretinograms and evoked electroencephalographic responses to orange and white light. Child Dev., *40:*267.

Marmor, M. F. (1977). Unsedated corneal electroretinograms from children. Doc. Ophthalmol. Proc. Series, 14th ISCERG Symposium, 349.

Merin, S. and Auerbach, E. (1976). Retinitis pigmentosa. Survey of Ophthalmology, *20:*303.

Millidot, M. and Riggs, L. (1970). Refraction determined electrophysiologically. Arch. Ophthalmol., *84:*276.

Nadler, D. and Sokol, S. (1978). The electroretinogram and visually evoked potential of adult amblyopes in response to a pattern stimulus. Investigative Ophthalmology and Visual Science, ARVO Supplement, 293.

Niemeyer, G. (1976). Retinal physiology in the perfused eye of the cat. In: Neural Principles in Vision. Zettler, F., and Weiler, R., Eds., p. 158. Springer, New York.

Noell, W. (1953). Studies on the electrophysiology and metabolism of the retina. Project no. 21-1201-0004, Report no. 1, U.S. Air Force School of Medicine, Randolf Field, Texas.

Oakley, B., II and Green, D. C. (1976). Correlation of light-induced changes in retinal extracellular potassium concentration with C-wave of the electroretinogram. J. Neurophysiol., *39:*1117.

Padmos, P., van Norren, D., and Jaspers Faijer, J. W. (1978). Blue cone function in a family with an inherited tritan defect, tested with electroretinography and psychophysics. Invest. Ophthalmol. Vis. Sci., *17:*436.

Peterson, H. (1968). The normal B-potential in the single-flash clinical electroretinogram. Acta Ophthalmol., Supp. 99, 1.

Piper, H. (1911). Uber die Netzhautstrome. Arch. f. Physiol. (Leipz.), 85.

Riggs, L. A. (1941). Continuous and reproducible records of the electrical activity of the human retina. Proc. Soc. Exp. Biol. N.Y., *48:*204.

Riggs, L. A. (1954). Electroretinography in cases of night blindness. Am. J. Ophthalmol., *38:*70.

Riggs, L. A., Berry, R. N. and Wayner, M. A. (1949). Comparison of electrical and psycho-determinations of the spectral sensitivity of the human eye. J. Opt. Soc. Am., *39:*427.

Riggs, L. A., Johnson, E. P., and Schick, A. M. (1964). Electrical responses of the human eye to moving stimulus patterns. Science, *144:*567.

Riggs, L. A., Johnson, E. P., and Schick, A. M. L. (1966). Electrical responses of the human eye to changes in wavelength of the stimulating light. J. Opt. Soc. Am., *56:*1621.

Riggs, L. A. and Wooten, B. R. (1972). Electrical measures and psychophysical data on human vision. In: Visual Psychophysics. Jameson, D., and Hurvich, L. M., Eds., p. 690, Springer, New York.

Ruedemann, A. D., Jr., and Noell, W. K. (1959). A contribution to the electroretinogram of retinitis pigmentosa. Am. J. Ophthalmol., *47:*564.

Rushton, W. A. H. (1972). Visual pigments in man. In: Photochemistry of Vision. Dartnall, H. J. A., Ed., p. 364, Springer, New York.

Sandberg, M. A. (1978). Personal Communication.

Sandberg, M. A., and Ariel, M. A. (1977). A hand-held two channel stimulator ophthalmoscope. Arch. Ophthalmol., *95:*1881.

Sandberg, M. A., Rosen, J. B., and Berson, E. L. (1977). Cone and rod function in vitamin A deficiency with chronic alcoholism and in retinitis pigmentosa. Am. J. Ophthalmol., *84:*658.

Schoessler, J. P. and Jones, R. (1975). A new corneal electrode for electroretinography. Vision Res., *15:*299.

Schreinemachers, H. P. and Henkes, H. E. (1968). Relation between localized retinal stimuli and the visual evoked response in man. Ophthalmologica, *155:*17.

Schubert, G. and Bornschein, H. (1952). Beitrag zur analyse des menschlichen elektroretinogramms. Ophthalmologica, *123:*396.

Simonsen, S. E. (1968). ERG in diabetics. In: The clinical value of electroretinography. Francois, J., Ed., p. 403, ISCERG Symposium, Ghent 1966. Karger. New York.

Sokol, S. (1978). Patterned elicited ERGs and VECPs in amblyopia and infant vision. In: Visual Psychophysics and Physiology. Armington, J. C., Krauskopf, J., and Wooten, B. R., Eds., Academic Press, New York.

Tepas, D. I. and Armington, J. C. (1962). Electroretinograms from noncorneal electrodes. Investig. Ophthalmol., *1:*784.

Tomita, T. (1976). Electrophysiological studies of retinal cell function. Investig. Ophthalmol., *15:*169.

Wachtmeister, L. and Dowling, J. E. (1978). The oscillatory potentials of the mud puppy retina. Investig. Ophthalmol., *17:*1176.

Witkovsky, P., Dudek, F. E., and Ripps, H. (1975). Slow PIII component of the carp electroretinogram. J. Gen. Physiol., *65:*119.

Wulfing, B. (1963). Clinical electroretino-dynamography. Acta Ophthalmol., Supp. 63, 1.

Yonemura, D., Aoki, T., and Tsuzuki, K. (1962). Electroretinogram in diabetic retinopathy. Arch. Ophthalmol., *68:*19.

Yonemura, D., Masuda, Y., and Hatta, M. (1963). The oscillatory potential in the electroretinogram. Jpn. J. Physiol., *13:*129.

Zetterstrom, B. (1964). Some experience of clinical flicker electroretinography. Documenta Ophthalmol., *18:*315.

Zetterstrom, B. (1970). The electroretinogram of the newborn infant. Proceedings of the VIIIth ISCERG Symposium, Pisa, 1.

11
Visual Evoked Potentials

SAMUEL SOKOL

INTRODUCTION

Before the availability of computers the relatively large amplitude and wide topographic distribution of the human electroencephalogram prevented examination of the minute signals elicited in the occipital cortex when the visual system was stimulated by light. With the development of averaging computers, however, the visually evoked potential (VEP) can now be recorded. Further, measurement of electrical activity at the retina (Ch. 10) and occipital pole can be used as a clinical tool to detect abnormalities of the visual system and—since many neurologic diseases present with visual symptoms—can thus be useful to neurologists and neurosurgeons. The purpose of this chapter will be to review some of the fundamentals of the VEP and to illustrate its use as a diagnostic tool in the investigation of neurologic diseases. Readers interested in more detailed discussion of VEPs are referred to Perry and Childers, 1969; Regan, 1972; Thompson and Patterson, 1974; and Desmedt, 1977.

The VEP is a gross electrical signal recorded from the occipital cortex in response to a systematic change in some visual event, such as a flashing light. If an EEG electrode is taped over the occipital cortex and referenced to the ear the amplitude and latency of the waveform generated by the occipital cortex can be measured (Fig. 11.1). Fortunately for the busy clinician, commercially available equipment packages are now available which can enable one to record VEPs with a minimum of electronic experience, but the clinician still has a responsibility to carefully calibrate the equipment and to acquire adequate normative data before making clinical judgments.

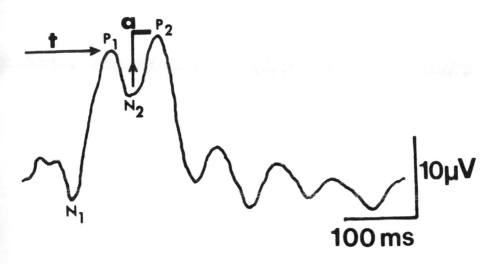

Fig. 11.1. *Flash elicited VEP. VEP was recorded with a photostimulator set at 1 flash per second. Electrode was placed 1 cm. above the inion on the midline and referenced to the right ear. Positivity is upward in this and all subsequent figures. t, implicit time; a, amplitude of P_2 component from trough of N_2. 64 flashes were presented to the subject to acquire the VEP (from Sokol, S., 1976. Surv. Ophthalmol., 21, 18).*

RECORDING THE VEP

To record the VEP the scalp is prepared in much the same way as for standard EEG recording. The skin should be cleaned and care taken to keep electrode resistance low. Goff (1974) presents an excellent discussion of the various preparatory techniques and electronic procedures employed in the recording of human evoked potentials. Electrode location is an arbitrary decision and there are different opinions as to the optimal location for clinical testing. In general, the largest amplitude signal is usually obtained 1 to 2 cm above the inion along the midline. Some prefer to use the international EEG guidelines and place the active electrode at Oz, while electrodes located at O1 and O2 have been used by others. It is preferable to use "monopolar" electrode configurations; the occipital electrode is referenced to some relatively indifferent place on the head such as the earlobe, mastoid, or midfrontal region. Bipolar electrode configurations, e.g. recording between Oz and O1, are not recommended since polarity reversals and interactions may occur at two occipital locations and VEP results will be equivocal (Goff, 1974; Michael and Halliday, 1971). Figure 11.2 shows a block diagram of how VEPs are recorded in humans.

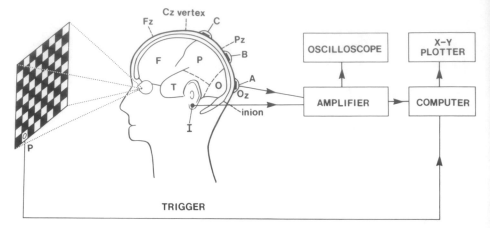

Fig. 11.2. *Schematic diagram of electrode locations and electronic equipment for recording the VEP in man. A, B, and C indicate possible locations of active electrodes. (I = indifferent location). In this example, the recording configuration is electrode A referenced to the ear (I) which is led into a differential amplifier. Other combinations include A-B, A-C, or B-C (bipolar), or C-I and B-I (monopolar). The output of the differential amplifier goes to a computer of average transients. The computer is "triggered" by a photocell (P) placed at the stimulus. This ensures a time-locked VEP. The oscilloscope can be used to monitor the ongoing VEP activity as well as provide a view of the final averaged waveform. Finally, a plotter prints out a permanent record of the VEP (from Sokol, S., 1976. Surv. Ophthalmol., 21, 18).*

ORIGINS OF THE VEP

Regardless of the placement of the electrodes, the VEP is primarily a reflection of the activity originating in the central 3 degrees of the visual field. Two factors are responsible for this. First, the nature of the anatomy of the human visual system is such that retinal projections from the central 3 degrees of the visual field are sent to the surface of the occipital lobe, while projections arising from peripheral retina are directed to regions deep within the calcarine fissure. As a result, when an electrode is taped to the back of the scalp it is located directly over cortical tissue that receives central retinal input. Secondly, there is a significant degree of foveal magnification between the human retina and visual cortex. For example, one millimeter of occipital lobe tissue receiving input from the fovea processes information from 2 minutes of visual angle at the surface of the retina, while the equivalent one millimeter of occipital cortex receiving input from retinal receptors 5 degrees from the fovea is responsible for 18 minutes of visual angle (Duke-Elder and Scott, 1971). The situation is reversed at the retina where the ERG is generated primarily by receptors outside the central 3 degrees (Ch. 10). While the VEP is mostly foveal in origin and, therefore, mainly a reflection of cone activity, it is still possible, albeit with great difficulty, to record VEPs that arise from rod receptors (Wooten, 1972).

Moreover, if large checks are used (greater than 30 minutes of arc), signals outside the central 3 degrees but not beyond 10 degrees of visual field can be recorded (Harter, 1970).

STIMULI USED TO ELICIT THE VEP

There are two general types of visual stimuli that are most often used to elicit VEPs: unpatterned flashing lights and patterned stimuli, which in clinical labs are usually checkerboards. Unpatterned flashing stimuli can be produced with a photostimulator similar to those used in standard EEG recording for photic driving. The intensity, color, and rate of stimulation of the stimulator can be varied.

Pattern stimuli can be presented in three ways. The first, a flashing patterned stimulus, is produced by placing a photostimulator behind a large photographic transparency of black and white checks (Harter and White, 1968). However, it has been pointed out by Regan (1972) and Spekreijse, van der Tweel, and Zuidema (1973) that a flashing pattern stimulus contains two parameters which change simultaneously, so that there is an abrupt increase in brightness and the presentation of a pattern. Further, it has been demonstrated that there is an interaction between the brightness and pattern change, and this produces a pattern VEP which is "contaminated" by luminance changes. To avoid luminance contamination of the VEP a pattern with a constant average luminance is presented. This can be accomplished in two ways: pattern onset-offset or pattern reversal. In pattern onset-offset the checks appear for a discrete amount of time, e.g. 500 msec, and then disappear. In order to avoid luminance changes, however, the pattern is immediately replaced by an unpatterned diffuse field of the same size with the same average luminance as previously seen in the pattern stimulus. The diffuse field remains on for the same amount of time, i.e. 500 msec, and the pattern then reappears. This onset-offset sequence is repeated for an arbitrarily chosen number of times and a VEP is recorded.

In the pattern reversal situation, checks are visible at all times. In order to maintain a constant luminance level one half of the checks increase in luminance while the other half decrease. This can be accomplished electronically by using a TV monitor to generate the checks (Arden, Faulkner, and Mair, 1977) or mechanically by having a mirror rotate so that the checks move through a distance equal to one check size (Halliday, McDonald, and Mushin, 1972, 1973b). In either case, the subject sees the checks move back and forth, and a VEP is generated. Figure 11.3 gives examples of the type of response obtained with pattern stimuli of constant luminance.

RESPONSES TO VARIOUS STIMULI

The basic description of the VEP waveform is primarily dependent on the type of stimulus that is used to generate the signal. For example, a bright

PATTERN REVERSAL

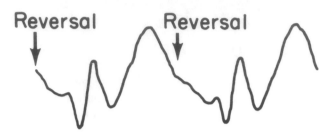

PATTERN ONSET-OFFSET

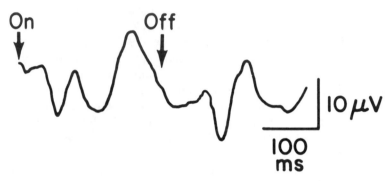

Fig. 11.3. *Pattern reversal and onset-offset VEPs. Note the difference in polarity between the second pattern reversal and the offset of the checks.*

pattern stimulus will generate VEPs with large amplitude and short latency components. Figure 11.4 shows an example of a pattern reversal VEP and demonstrates how the nature of the VEP changes with systematic change in the intensity of the stimulus.

A useful distinction that is made in VEP work is the comparison between "transient" and "steady state" VEPs. A transient VEP is produced when the stimulus is presented at a slow temporal rate. In the case of flashing stimuli, one flash every second would produce a transient VEP (Fig. 11.1), as would one alternation per second if pattern reversal is used. On the other hand, steady state VEPs are produced when stimuli are presented at a rapid temporal rate. For example, ten flashes per second of a photostimulator or alternations per second of a pattern reversal stimulus would produce steady state VEPs. The temporal rate at which VEPs change from transient to steady state varies depending on a variety of factors, but in general six to eight flashes or alternations per second represent the region of change. Figure 11.5 shows examples of transient and steady state responses using a pattern stimulus.

Whether one records transient or steady state VEPs depends on the parameter of interest. Transient VEPs have the advantage of component analysis. For example, the peak latency of a particular component can be measured from transient VEPs. Thus, in many studies of patients with neurologic disease the latency of the first major positive component (P_1) of the VEP, which occurs between 95 and 110 msec after pattern reversal, is measured as the clinical parameter of interest. When steady state VEPs are recorded specific component analysis is no longer appropriate and one then measures amplitude and phase (Regan, 1977).

Two major variables which affect the unpatterned flash elicited VEP are intensity and rate of flicker. As intensity is decreased, the peak latency of the specific components becomes longer and the amplitude is attenuated. Further, as the rate of flicker is increased and steady state VEPs are produced, the amplitude waxes and wanes and shows three peaks as a function of flicker rate (Regan, 1972). A peak occurs at 10 Hz, a second peak occurs at 13 to 25 Hz, and a third at 40 to 60 Hz. These three peaks contain different types of information and reflect different channels in the visual system. For example, Milner, Regan, and Heron (1974) reported that the middle frequency peak (13 to 25 Hz) was affected in patients with retrobulbar neuritis while in the same patients the amplitude and phase characteristics of the 40 to 60 Hz peak were normal.

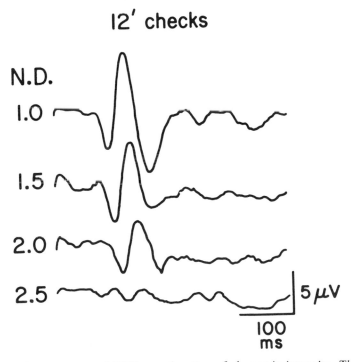

12′ checks

Fig. 11.4. Pattern reversal VEP as a function of change in intensity. The luminance of the TV monitor which produced the checks was 75 cd per m². The luminance was reduced by placing a neutral density filter in front of the subject's eye. The amount of filter neutral density (ND) in log units used to reduce the luminance is shown to the left of each record.

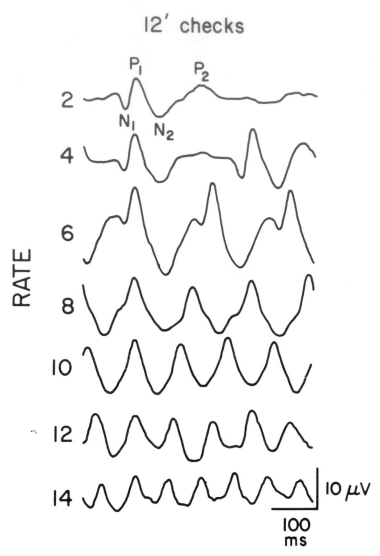

Fig. 11.5. *Pattern reversal VEPs in response to 12 minute checks for different alternation rates. Alternation rate per second is shown to the left of the records. Note the change from transient to steady state VEPs at 8 alternations per second.*

There are a number of variables that will affect the pattern VEP. The type of pattern presentation which has been previously discussed will affect the waveform morphology. Another factor that is important is the check or stripe size. Usually, the check or stripe size is expressed in minutes of visual angle at the retina. Figure 11.6 shows pattern reversal VEPs for a series of checks and stripes of increasing angular subtense. These records show that checks generate a different type of waveform than stripes, particularly with small pattern elements. Further, small checks elicit a more complex wave than large checks; for example, compare the VEPs obtained with 15 minute checks and 120 minute checks. Finally, as check size increases the peak latency for the various components shortens (Parker and Salzen, 1977a and b).

There is an interaction between check size and alternation rate of a pattern reversal stimulus which affects the amplitude (Regan, 1978). With checks smaller than 20 minutes of arc, a single peak in amplitude is found between six and seven reversals per second. If the checks are larger than 30 minutes of arc two peaks will occur at six and ten reversals per second. Regan (1978) has suggested that large checks are similar to unpatterned flashing lights and that the peak at ten reversals per second with large checks is not unlike the peak obtained with flashing lights.

Changes in check size and retinal location will affect the VEP. As stated previously, checks smaller than 30 minutes of arc elicit large signals within the central 3 degrees of the visual field. If regions outside the central 3 degrees are stimulated with small checks the VEP amplitude is significantly reduced (Harter, 1970). Large checks are necessary to elicit signals outside the central 3

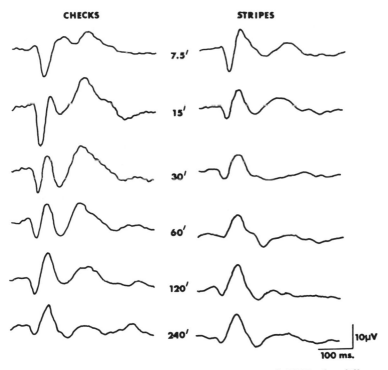

Fig. 11.6. Pattern reversal (2 alternations per second) VEPs for different size stripes and checkerboard pattern stimuli. The visual angle subtended in minutes of arc is shown in the center column. The recording electrode was located 1 cm above the inion along the midline and references to the ear.

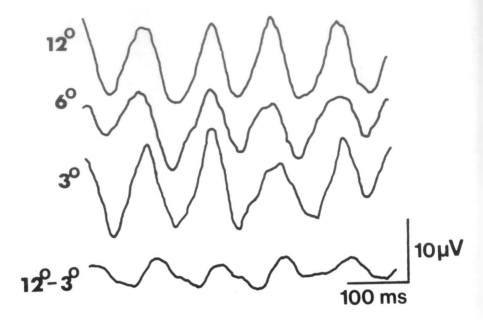

Fig. 11.7. *Pattern reversal (12 alternations per second) VEPs for 15 minute checks as a function of a decrease in field size. The field size was reduced from 12 degrees to 3 degrees without any significant change in amplitude. The bottom record was obtained when the eye was stimulated with a 12 degrees field that had the central 3 degrees blanked out (from Sokol, S., 1976. Surv. Ophthalmol., 21, 18).*

degrees and beyond 6 degrees it is difficult to elicit VEPs without a great deal of averaging. Figure 11.7 shows the effect of reducing the field size when small checks are used and demonstrates how dependent the VEP is on stimulation of central retina. If the optical quality of the pattern stimulus on the retina is poor (Fig. 11.8) the amplitude of the VEP will be attenuated (Millodot and Riggs, 1970). Consequently, when recording pattern VEPs the patient should always be appropriately refracted.

Other factors that will affect the VEP include pupil size, level of light adaptation and age of the patient. Pupil size will affect the retinal illuminance which will in turn determine the peak latency. Therefore, one must exercise caution in comparing peak latencies of a normal control group with a patient who has miotic or dilated pupils. The level of light adaptation will affect the pattern VEP. For small checks to be an effective stimulus, the pattern stimuli must be within the photopic range of visibility which is usually the case with most commercial TV monitors. Finally, the age of the patient will affect the VEP. In particular, the peak latency of the major P_1 component shortens rapidly during the 1st year of life and levels off at around 6 or 7 years of age (Sokol and Jones 1979). The latency remains stable until 60 years of age and then increases (Celesia and Daly, 1977a).

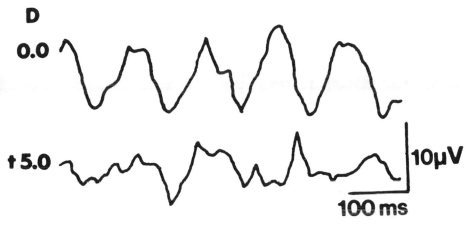

D

0.0

↑5.0

10µV

100 ms

Fig. 11.8. Pattern reversal (12 alternations per second) VEP as a function of optical clarity. VEPs were recorded from an electrode located 1 cm anterior to the inion along the midline and referenced to the right ear. Stimulus was a 12 degree field of sinusoidally alternating 15 minute checks. When a +5.00 spherical lens was placed in front of the subject's eye there was no subjective recognition of the squares (from Sokol, S., 1976. Surv. Ophthalmol., 21, 18).

USE OF THE VEP IN NEUROLOGY AND NEURO-OPHTHALMOLOGY

Long before the pattern VEP became useful as a clinical tool it was reported that the peak latency of the flash VEP was much less variable than its amplitude. DeVoe, Ripps, and Vaughan (1968) demonstrated that the peak latency provided a more reliable correlation with subjective visual function than amplitude. That is, if the intensity of a flashing light is increased the amplitude of a particular component of the VEP increases but on an irregular basis, while the peak latency to that same component decreases in an exact and orderly fashion. Further, if the same subject is tested on a number of different occasions and the same intensity is used, the amplitude can vary substantially while the peak latency will change by only a few milliseconds. Consequently, because of its low variability, it seemed that measurement of the peak latency of the VEP would have clinical relevance.

Optic Neuritis

A common problem that may arise for the neurologist is the detection of a previous attack of optic neuritis or retrobulbar neuritis, particularly if the patient is a poor historian. In the belief that the latency of the VEP depends in part on the conduction velocity of optic nerve fibers, Halliday et al (1972) recorded the pattern and flash evoked responses in 17 healthy subjects and in 19 patients with unilateral optic neuritis. They obtained a normal response to stimulation of the unaffected eye in the 19 patients, but the response evoked by pattern

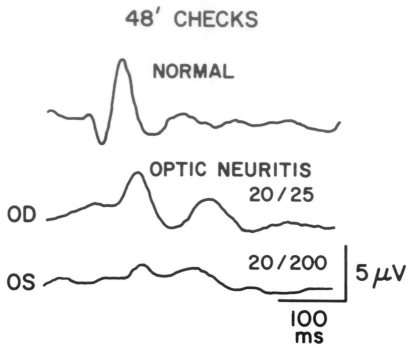

48′ CHECKS

NORMAL

OPTIC NEURITIS
20/25

OD

20/200

OS

5 μV

100
ms

Fig. 11.9. *Pattern reversal (2 alternations per second) VEP from a 12-year-old boy during recovery of a bilateral optic neuritis. Also shown for comparison is a normal VEP (upper record). Note that acuity difference between eyes is reflected in the difference in amplitude but that the peak latency is equally abnormal in both eyes.*

reversal from the affected eye was delayed. The mean latency of the response from the affected eyes increased by almost 30 percent, with halving of amplitude. This prolongation in latency persisted even after visual acuity had returned to normal. There was no comparable increase in latency of the response evoked by flash stimuli. In their later study, Asselman, Chadwick, and Marsden (1975) similarly found a delayed VEP to pattern reversal in each of 15 patients with a past history of optic neuritis, and other confirmatory reports (Fig. 11.9) have also been published (Milner et al, 1974; Bornstein, 1975).

Multiple Sclerosis

Abnormal responses to pattern stimulation in a large proportion of patients without any history of optic nerve involvement and without eye symptoms at the time of testing indicates that the evoked potential technique can reveal subclinical involvement of the visual pathways in patients with multiple sclerosis (MS). This was first clearly shown by Halliday et al (1973b) who, in view of their findings in patients with optic neuritis, evaluated the diagnostic validity of the VEP in patients with suspected multiple sclerosis. Among the 51 patients they studied, only 2 had normal latency in both eyes. Abnormal delays were uniocular in 14 cases and binocular in 35; most importantly, almost half of those with delayed response latencies had normal optic discs. Significant delays in the responses evoked by flash stimulation seemed to occur less commonly, and variability of the waveform often made it difficult to identify a particular component with certainty. Twenty-two patients in other diagnostic categories were also evaluated; only three had delayed VEPs to pattern reversal but two of these three patients had optic neuritis.

Table 11.1 presents a summary of the studies published to date in which the pattern reversal VEP has been used in the investigation of patients with MS. It should be kept in mind that, in constructing a table of this complexity, arbitrary decisions have sometimes had to be made when summarizing authors' data, but the goal has been to provide the reader with an overall picture of the wide range of stimulus conditions, electrode locations, and number of patients in the different series. Only abnormalities in peak latency have been considered.

As the data presented in the table clearly demonstrate, the peak latency of the P_1 component of the pattern reversal VEP is prolonged in a high percentage of patients with a definite diagnosis of MS. With the exception of the 13 patients studied by Regan, Milner and Heron (1976), the proportion of abnormal VEP latencies found in patients with definite MS ranges from 75 to 97 percent. However, in these cases the diagnosis has been made on clinical grounds, and it is for the evaluation of patients in the possible and probable categories that a sensitive test is required. Unfortunately, as can be seen in the table, the percentage of abnormal VEPs is both lower and more variable in these diagnostic categories. Among the reasons for this wide variability must be the large differences in stimulus conditions used. For example, the check size used ranges from 12 to 70 minutes of arc, and field size ranges from 6 degrees to 30 degrees. Further, a wide range of luminance levels have been used; indeed, the "black" squares used by Asselman et al (1975) are equal in luminance to the "white" squares used by Halliday et al (1973). Hennerici, Wenzel, and Freund (1977), in an attempt to expand on the clinical utility of the VEP, found a higher percentage of abnormal P_1 latencies when a "foveal" rectangular stimulus of 45 minutes of arc is used instead of a large checkerboard stimulus field comprised of 70 minute checks. One difficulty with comparing the results of these two stimulus conditions is that the mean luminance of the 45 minute rectangle is not constant while the mean luminance of the large checkerboard stimulus is constant. An alternative paradigm, which would be easier for other investigators to explore and would not require monitoring of fixation of small "foveal" targets, would be to use checkerboard pattern reversal stimuli, of equal field size, of large (50 minute) and small (15 minute) checks. In these stimulus conditions the mean luminance would be equal for the two check sizes and signals originating from peripheral (large checks) and foveal (small checks) ganglion cell fibers could be recorded.

The incidence with which VEPs of prolonged latency are encountered in patients with a single acute neurologic episode of uncertain etiology—but which may be the first clinical manifestation of MS—has also been investigated. Asselman et al (1975) found VEP abnormalities in 25 percent of those patients

Table 11.1. SUMMARY OF THE STIMULUS PARAMETERS, CRITERIA FOR ABNORMALITY, ELECTRODE LOCATION AND PERCENT PEAK LATENCY ABNORMALITIES OF THE P_1 COMPONENT OF PATTERN REVERSAL VEP IN PATIENTS WITH A DEFINITE, PROBABLE OR POSSIBLE DIAGNOSIS OF MULTIPLE SCLEROSIS.

Authors	Field Size Degrees	Check Size Minutes	Normal P_1 Latency msec. (±SD)	Luminance Log Candles/m² White Checks / Black Checks	"Abnormal" Criterion Standard Deviations	Electrode Location Active → Reference	% abnormal (Number of Patients) Definite MS	Probable MS	Possible MS
Halliday et al (1973)	32°	50'	103.8±4.3	2.04 / 0.93	2.5	I^a + 5 cm. → mid-frontal	97(34)	100(5)	91(12)
Asselman et al (1975)	18°	30' / 57'	90.5±4.3[b] / 97.2±4.1[c]	3.28 / 2.08	3.0	I + 5 cm → linked ears	84(31)	83(6)	21(14)
Mastaglia et al (1976)	*	*	118 (normal +2.5 SD)	*	2.5	Oz → Pz	83(23)	33(9)	33(36)
Hume & Cant (1976)	20°	40'	110.4±5.3	1.18 / *	3.0	Oz,O1,O2 → linked ears	86(7)	80(5)	50(10)
Regan et al (1976)	14°	50'	120±12	2.84 / *	2.0	I + 1 cm → mid-frontal	46(13)	*	*
Celesia & Daly (1977)	9°	15'	97.8 Range=84.6 to 118.	1.53[e]	2.5	Oz-Cz[d] / O1-P3 / O2-P4	78(29)	33(2)	60(6)

Hennerici et al. (1977)	20°	70'	102.5±2.9	1.71	3.0	I + 6 cm ↓ linked ears	81(16)	67(18)	43(23)
	0.75°	45'	120±3.5	0.46 / 2.11	3.0		94(16)	94(18)	78(23)
Matthews et al (1977)	23°	28'	100.5±4.4	2.40 / 1.58	2.5	I + 0.5 cm ↓ mid-frontal	75(61)	58(24)	38(28)
Mastaglia et al (1977)	*	*	118	*	2.5	Oz → Pz	84(40)	43(30)	22(32)
Zeese (1977)	30°	45'	103.3±3.2	*	3.0	I + 1cm ↓ mid-frontal	77(30)	*	*
Collins et al (1978)	6°	12'	99±5.5	*	2.5	Oz → Pz	78(29)	50(15)	23(7)
Nilsson (1978)	8.8°	23'	96.3±4.1	3.0–3.3 / 1.08–1.20	3.0	Oz → Fz	79(19)	90(9)	30(10)
Shahrokhi et al (1978)	8.7°	26'	102.3±5.1	2.23[f]	2.5	I + 3cm ↓ Cz	82(60)	52(46)	28(43)
Bodis-Wollner et al (1979)	4°	13'	116.8±8	1.53[e]	2.5	I + 2.5 cm ↓ temporal	90(50)	70(21)	15(32)

* Information not given; a, I represents inion; b, < 60 yrs.; c, > 60 yrs.; d, bipolar montage; e, mean space average luminance of total field; f, luminance difference between black and white checks. Note that the number of patients tested in each group is given in parentheses.

with an acute spinal cord lesion and in 46 percent of those with an isolated brainstem lesion whom they studied. However, neither Halliday et al (1973b) nor Matthews et al (1977) found prolonged VEP latencies in patients with an isolated brainstem disturbance.

The diagnosis of MS depends on clinical or laboratory evidence for the presence of multiple lesions in the central nervous system, and the optic nerve is one of the commonest sites to be involved in that disorder. Measurement of the latency of the response evoked by pattern stimulation provides an objective means of identifying lesions of the visual pathways, even when they are subclinical. Accordingly, when patients presenting with clinical evidence of a single lesion of the nervous system—and especially one below the level of the foramen magnum—are being evaluated, VEP studies provide a means of establishing the presence of multiple lesions by permitting the detection of clinically silent pathology in the visual system.

The pathophysiologic basis of the VEP changes described above remains uncertain. Direct experimentation has shown that a complete conduction block may result from extensive demyelination of central nerve fibers, while conduction velocity is slowed in less severe and less extensive demyelinating lesions. This suggests that delay in the latency of VEPs may reflect a reduced conduction velocity in damaged visual fibers, although some of the prolongation in latency may also be due to delay at the cortical or retinal level. Amplitude changes presumably reflect in large part a complete conduction block in damaged fibers.

Other Optic Nerve Abnormalities Affecting the VEP

VEP abnormalities have also been reported in patients with Leber's hereditary optic neuropathy. Dorfman et al (1977) measured pattern reversal VEPs in two brothers with this disorder, during the active phase of the disease. No abnormalities were found prior to the onset of visual symptoms, but subsequently there was a progressive prolongation of VEP latency, and a less consistent reduction in amplitude of the response until eventually VEPs could no longer be measured. No abnormalities were found in asymptomatic family members, including the presumed carrier of the disorder. These findings suggest that VEP measurement is not an effective means of screening individuals at risk of developing this disorder, although it may be a useful means of following the progression of the condition.

Patients with ischemic optic neuropathy (Asselman et al, 1975; Hennerici et al, 1977; Ikeda, Tremain, and Sanders, 1978), or tropical amblyopia (Asselman et al, 1975) may also have delayed VEPs. VEP abnormalities have also been reported in patients with glaucoma. Cappin and Nissim (1975), for example, recorded steady state pattern VEPs from glaucoma patients with field defects and found latency abnormalities that correlated with the degree of field loss. Huber and Wagner (1978) recorded transient pattern reversal evoked potentials in glaucoma patients and found abnormal peak latencies. Unfortunately, the peak latencies of a control group with presumably normal pupil diameter were compared to the peak latencies from glaucoma patients who had miotic pupils from glaucoma medication. Since pupil size can affect peak latency, their results are somewhat equivocal.

Compressive Lesion of the Anterior Visual Pathways

As indicated above, the evoked potential method provides a sensitive means of detecting subclinical lesions of the optic nerve, and consequently is being increasingly applied to the early diagnosis of multiple sclerosis. A prolongation of the latency of the potential evoked in the occipital cortex by pattern stimulation is not, however, specific to multiple sclerosis and optic neuritis, and compressive lesions of the anterior visual pathways produce similar abnormalities.

Halliday et al (1976) studied the VEPs elicited by pattern reversal in 19 patients with compression of the optic nerve, chiasm or radiation. Four of these patients had orbital tumors, two had craniopharyngiomas and eight had pituitary tumors. Abnormalities were found in 18 of these cases, even when there were no clinical signs of visual impairment, such as abnormalities of visual acuity, fields, or fundoscopic appearance; the single case with a normal response was a patient with an intracranial cavernous hemangioma of the left orbit. The character of the changes encountered was somewhat different from that seen in patients with primary demyelinating disease; the latency of the response was increased in only 4 instances, but in 6 other patients the response was abolished completely and latency measurements could not be made. Therefore, the latency of the VEP is prolonged by compressive lesions, but only at an early stage. Moreover, even when there was an increase in latency, it was generally much smaller in patients with compressive lesions than in those with demyelinating disease. For example, Halliday et al (1976) found that the latency was not delayed more than 20 msec beyond the upper limit of the normal range, while in optic neuritis and multiple sclerosis the mean delays were between 35 and 45 msec and the actual delays in individual cases ranged up to 100 msec. In addition, the VEPs in the patients with compressive lesions showed a much higher incidence of waveform abnormalities than in patients with demyelinating disorders, and asymmetry of the VEP was especially characteristic of patients with a tumor arising in the region of the sella turcica. Such changes cannot, however, be regarded as pathognomonic of the underlying lesion. In several cases abnormal responses were recorded from the clinically normal eye, suggestive that the evoked potential technique may permit detection of subclinical damage to optic nerve fibers in this clinical context as well as in patients with demyelinating disease.

The pathophysiologic basis of the VEP abnormalities found in patients with compressive lesions remains unclear. It seems reasonable to assume, however, that such changes relate, at least in part, to demyelination of nerve fibers in the anterior visual pathways, secondary to compression.

Primary Neuronal Diseases

Most of the reports of VEPs in primary neuronal diseases have been based on flash elicited VEPs. Lee and Blair (1973) found an initial increase in the amplitude of the flash VEPs in Creutzfeldt-Jakob disease. As the disease progressed, the latency increased and amplitude decreased. Ellenberger, Petro, and Ziegler (1978) found abnormal flash VEP amplitudes and normal peak latencies in Huntington's disease. Friedman et al (1978) report that the amplitude of flash VEPs are abnormal in Menkes' disease. Harden and Pampiglione (1977) found abnormal flash VEPs in childhood storage diseases; these included Tay-Sachs, Santavuori, Bielschowsky-Jansky, and Spielmeyer-Vogt disease. Normal VEPs were found in metachromatic leukodystrophy and mucopolysaccharidoses. Finally, in one of the few studies using pattern stimuli Bodis-Wollner and Yahr (1978) found abnormal peak latencies in Parkinson's disease.

Field Defects

Early investigations of field defects using the VEP were conducted with flash stimuli and the correlation between the VEP and subjective results was unreliable, in part because of the inherent large variability of VEPs with flashing stimuli (Copenhaver and Beinhocker, 1963; Vaughan, Katzman, and Taylor, 1963; Kooi, Guvener, and Bagchi, 1965). More recently, it has been found that the pattern VEP shows a better correlation with subjective visual fields than do flash elicited VEPs (Regan and Heron, 1969; Wildberger et al, 1976; Barrett et al, 1976; Blumhardt, Barrett, and Halliday, 1977).

Barrett et al (1976) found a "paradoxical" lateralization of the VEP when right and left hemifields were stimulated with pattern stimuli. Based upon partial decussation of retinal fibers one would predict that the largest amplitude monocular VEP would be found over the hemisphere contralateral to the hemifield tested. VEPs were recorded from a transverse chain of 5 electrodes, 5 centimeters up from the inion. One of the electrodes was located along the midline, and the remaining pairs were placed 5 and 10 centimeters lateral to the midline electrode over each hemisphere. Contrary to the prediction, the largest amplitude VEP occurred over the hemisphere ipsilateral to the hemifield tested. The authors suggest that this paradox is due to the fact that the cortical generator dipoles for pattern stimuli are transversely oriented at locations on the medial and posteromedial surface of the cortex. As a result electrodes placed over the ipsilateral hemisphere will detect voltage changes more readily than electrodes over contralateral hemisphere, even though the contralateral hemisphere is the anatomic destination of visual input from the hemifield which is stimulated. Blumhardt et al (1977) confirmed this hypothesis by testing a patient with a complete homonymous hemianopia subsequent to a subtotal right occipital lobectomy. Using full field stimulation, VEPs were still recordable over the ablated "ipsilateral" hemisphere. Further, when hemifield stimulation was used there was no VEP from the scotomatous half field and the intact half field responses were similar to the full field responses.

Blumhardt et al (1977, 1978) offer a number of suggestions which are critical to proper VEP field testing. First, a transverse chain of monopolar electrodes referenced to a midfrontal indifferent location is necessary. Bipolar configurations and references other than midfrontal will result in artifactual distortions of the VEP and misinterpretation of the field defect. Electrodes placed further laterally than the International EEG O1 and O2 locations are recommended, rather than a single midline electrode, to increase the amount of information obtained and also to avoid the effects that a macula-splitting hemianopia will have on the VEP recorded from the midline.

Hemifield VEP testing can reveal field defects that may go undetected with subjective techniques. For example, Halliday et al (1976) found two patients, one with a sphenoidal wing meningioma and the other with a pituitary tumor, with abnormal VEPs in the absence of a field defect.

Regan and Milner (1978) have recently pointed out difficulties that may arise if one attempts to evaluate the visual fields with VEPs. They note that a lower amplitude pattern VEP recorded from stimulation of one retinal location relative to another does not necessarily indicate the presence of a field defect, particularly if only one electrode position is used. Further, they find that there is wide variation in topographic distribution in control subjects without pathology, especially with small (3 to 6 degrees) fields. Therefore, the use of multiple electrode locations does not completely solve the problem. The same limitations also apply to flicker VEPs according to Regan and Milner. For example, the VEPs from a specific quadrant can be normal for one flicker frequency and "abnormal" for another frequency. Their conclusion is similar to that of Blumhardt et al; namely, that several electrode locations and flicker frequencies should be used to detect field defects. Whether the VEP can be reliably used on large groups of patients to reveal field defects that would not be found using subjective techniques must await further investigation.

CONCLUDING COMMENT

The purpose of this chapter has been to introduce the reader to the methodology of recording VEPs, and to illustrate the clinical utility of this technique in patients with certain categories of neurologic disease. The method, particularly with pattern stimuli, currently provides the most sensitive means of detecting subclinical lesions of the optic nerve, and its application in this regard may enable a diagnosis of MS to be made at an earlier time than otherwise. VEP abnormalities are not specific to any particular disorder, however, and are certainly not pathognomonic of MS since abnormalities are, for example, also encountered in patients with compressive lesions of the anterior visual pathways. The character of the changes seen in patients with compressive lesions—abnormal peak latency, atypical waveform, and a reduced amplitude—is different from that seen in primary demyelinating disease, in which waveforms are typically of prolonged latency but normal morphology and amplitude. These differences, however, are not sufficiently distinctive to permit these two diagnostic possibilities to be distinguished in individual cases on electrophysiologic grounds. Clearly, therefore, the clinical significance of an abnormal VEP will depend very much on the context in which the examination has been performed.

There is now increasing interest in the use of VEP techniques to evaluate the visual fields, and some evidence that defects may thereby be detected when they are not readily apparent using standard clinical tests. Further studies are necessary, however, before the value of evoked potential methods can be established in this regard.

The establishment of additional parameters in VEP analysis may further increase the utility of the VEP in neurologic diagnosis. Currently, most workers arbitrarily select and use one check size at one intensity and contrast level (Table 11.1) and the effect of varying these parameters has not been fully explored. For example, measurements of VEP amplitude and peak latency as function of different check sizes may be of value in providing information with regard to the processing of spatial information by different visual channels. Further exploration of these parameters may also help to more accurately delineate various neurologic diseases (Hennerici et al, 1977; Celesia and Daly, 1977b; Collins, Black, and Mastaglia, 1978; Hoeppner and Lolas, 1978).

ACKNOWLEDGEMENTS

The author is supported in part by National Eye Institute research grant EY00926 and Career Development Award EY70725.

REFERENCES

Arden, G. B., Faulkner, D. J., and Mair, C. (1977). A versatile television pattern generator for visual evoked potentials. In Visual Evoked Potentials in Man: New Developments, Desmedt, J. E., Ed., p. 90. Clarendon Press, Oxford.

Asselman, P., Chadwick, D. W., and Marsden, C. D. (1975). Visual evoked responses in the diagnosis and management of patients suspected of multiple sclerosis. Brain, *98:*261.

Barrett, G., Blumhardt, L., Halliday, A. M., Halliday, E., and Kriss, A. (1976). A paradox in the lateralization of the visual evoked response. Nature, *261:*253.

Blumhardt, L. D., Barrett, G., and Halliday, A. M. (1977). The asymmetrical visual evoked potential to pattern reversal in one half field and its significance for the analysis of visual field defects. Br. J. Ophthalmol., *61:*454.

Blumhardt, L. D., Barrett, G., Halliday, A. M., and Kriss, A. (1978). The effect of experimental "scotomata" on the ipsilateral and contralateral responses to pattern reversal in one half-field. Electroencephalogr. Clin. Neurophysiol., *45:*376.

Bodis-Wollner, I., and Yahr, M. D. (1978). Visual evoked potential measurements in Parkinson's disease. Brain, *101:*661.

Bodis-Wollner, I., Hendley, C. D., Mylin, L. H., and Thornton, J. (1979). Visual evoked potentials and the visuogram in multiple sclerosis. Ann. Neurol., *5:*40.

Bornstein, Y. (1975). The pattern evoked responses (VER) in optic neuritis. Albrecht Von Graefes Arch. Klin. Exp. Ophthal., *197:*101.

Cappin, J. M. and Nissim, S. (1975). Visual evoked responses in the assessment of field defects in glaucoma. Arch. Ophthalmol., *93:*9.

Celesia, G. G. and Daly, R. F. (1977a). Effects of aging on visual evoked responses. Arch. Neurol., *34:*403.

Celesia, C. G. and Daly, R. F. (1977b). Visual electroencephalographic computer analysis (VECA): A new electrophysiologic test for the diagnosis of optic nerve lesions. Neurology, *27:*637.

Collins, D. W. K., Black, J. L. and Mastaglia, F. L. (1978). Pattern-reversal visual evoked potential: method of analysis and results in multiple sclerosis. J. Neurol. Sci., *36:*83.

Copenhaver, R. M. and Beinhocker, G. D. (1963). Objective field testing: occipital potentials evoked from small visual stimuli. J.A.M.A., *186:*767.

Desmedt, J. E. (1977) (ed.). Visual Evoked Potentials in Man: New Developments. Clarendon Press, Oxford.

DeVoe, R. G., Ripps, H., and Vaughan, H. G. (1968). Cortical responses to stimulation of the human fovea. Vision Res., *8:*135.

Dorfman, L. J., Nikodkelainen, E., Rosenthal, A. R., and Sogg, R. L. (1977). Visual evoked potentials in Leber's Hereditary Optic Neuropathy. Ann. Neurol., *1:*565.

Duke-Elder, S. and Scott, G. I. (1971). System of Ophthalmology: Vol. II, The Anatomy of the Visual System. Henry Kimpton, London.

Ellenberger, C., Petro, D. J., and Ziegler, S. B. (1978). The visually evoked potential in Huntington disease. Neurology, *28:*95.

Friedman, E., Harden, A., Koivikko, M., and Pampiglione, G. (1978). Menkes' disease: neurophysiological aspects. J. Neurol. Neurosurg. Psychiatry, *41:*505.

Goff, W. R. (1974). In: Bioelectric Recording Techniques. Part B, Electroencephalography and Human Brain Potentials, Thompson, R. F. and Patterson, M. M., Eds., p. 101. Academic Press, New York.

Halliday, A. M., McDonald, W. I., and Mushin, J. (1972). Delayed visual evoked response in optic neuritis. Lancet, *1:*982.

Halliday, A. M., McDonald, W. I., and Mushin, J. (1973a). Delayed pattern evoked responses in optic neuritis in relation to visual acuity. Trans. Ophthalmol. Soc. U.K., *93:*315.

Halliday, A. M., McDonald, W. I., and Mushin, J. (1973b). Visual evoked response in diagnosis of multiple sclerosis. Br. Med. J., *4:*661.

Halliday, A. M., Halliday, E., Kriss, A., McDonald, W. I., and Mushin, J. (1976). The pattern-evoked potential in compression of the anterior visual pathways. Brain, *99:*357.

Harden, A. and Pampiglione, G. (1977). Visual evoked potential, electroretinogram, and electroencephalogram studies in progressive neurometabolic "storage" diseases of childhood. In: Visual Evoked Potentials in Man: New Developments, Desmedt, J. E., Ed., p. 470. Clarendon Press, Oxford.

Harter, M. R. (1970). Evoked cortical responses to checkerboard patterns: effects of check size as a function of retinal eccentricity. Vision Res., *10:*1365.

Harter, M. R., and White, C. T. (1968). Effects of contour sharpness and check size on visually evoked cortical potentials. Vision Res., *8:*701.

Hennerici, M., Wenzel, D., and Freund, H. J. (1977). The comparison of small size rectangle and checkerboard stimulation for the evaluation of delayed visual evoked responses in patients suspected of multiple sclerosis. Brain, *100:*119.

Hoeppner, T. and Lolas, F. (1978). Visual evoked responses and visual symptoms in multiple sclerosis. J. Neurol. Neurosurg. Psychiatry, *41:*493.

Huber, C., and Wagner, T. (1978). Electrophysiological evidence for glaucomatous lesions in the optic nerve. Ophthal. Res., *10:*22.

Hume, A. L., and Cant, B. R. (1976). Pattern visual evoked potentials in the diagnosis of multiple sclerosis and other disorders. Proc. Austral. Assoc. Neurol., *13:*7.

Ikeda, H., Tremain, K. E., and Sanders, M. D. (1978). Neuro-physiological investigation in optic nerve disease: combined assessment of the visual evoked response and ERG. Br. J. Ophthalmol., *62:*227–239.

Kooi, K. A., Guvener, A. M., and Bagchi, B. K. (1965). Visual evoked responses in lesions of the higher optic pathways. Neurology, *15:*841.

Lee, R. G., and Blair, R. D. G. (1973). Evolution of EEG and visual evoked response changes in Jakob-Creutzfeldt disease. Electroencephalogr. Clin. Neurophysiol., *35:*133.

Mastaglia, F. L., Black, J. L., and Collins, D. W. K. (1976). Visual and spinal evoked potentials in diagnosis of multiple sclerosis. Br. Med. J., *2:*732.

Mastaglia, F. L., Black, J. L., Cala, L. A., and Collins, D. W. K. (1977). Evoked potentials, saccadic velocities, and computerized tomography in diagnosis of multiple sclerosis. Br. Med. J., *1:*1315.

Matthews, W. B., Small, D. G., Small, M., and Pountney, E. (1977). Pattern reversal evoked visual potential in the diagnosis of multiple sclerosis. J. Neurol. Neurosurg. Psychiatry, *40:*1009.

Michael, W. F., and Halliday, A. M. (1971). Differences between the occipital distribution of upper and lower field pattern-evoked responses in man. Brain Res., *32:*311.

Millodot, M., and Riggs, L. A. (1970). Refraction determined electrophysiologically: responses to alternation of visual contours. Arch. Ophthalmol., *84:*272.

Milner, B. A., Regan, D., and Heron, J. R. (1974). Differential diagnosis of multiple sclerosis by visual evoked potential recording. Brain, *97:*755.

Nilsson, B. Y. (1978). Visual evoked responses in multiple sclerosis: comparison of two methods for pattern reversal. J. Neurol. Neurosurg. Psychiatry, *41:*499.

Parker, D. M. and Salzen, E. A. (1977a). The spatial selectivity of early and late waves within the human visual evoked response. Perception, *6:*85.

Parker, D. M. and Salzen, E. A. (1977b). Latency changes in the human visual response to sinusoidal gratings. Vision Res., *17:*1201.

Perry, N. W. and Childers, D. C. (1969). The Human Visual Evoked Response. Charles C Thomas, Springfield.

Regan, D. (1972). Evoked Potentials in Psychology, Sensory Physiology and Clinical Medicine. Wiley, New York.

Regan, D. (1977). Steady-state evoked potentials. J. Opt. Soc. Am., *11:*1475.

Regan, D. (1978). Assessment of visual acuity by evoked potential recording: ambiguity caused by temporal dependence of spatial frequency selectivity. Vision Res., *18:*439.

Regan, D. and Heron, J. R. (1969). Clinical investigation of lesions of the visual pathway: a new objective technique. J. Neurol. Neurosurg. Psychiatry, *32:*479.

Regan, D. and Milner, B. A. (1978). Objective perimetry by evoked potential recordings: limitations. Electroencephalogr. Clin. Neurophysiol., *44:*393.

Regan, D., Milner, B. A., and Heron, J. R. (1976). Delayed visual perception and delayed visual evoked potentials in the spinal form of multiple sclerosis and in retrobulbar neuritis. Brain, *99:*43.

Shahrokhi, F., Chiappa, K. H., and Young, R. R. (1978). Pattern shift visual evoked responses. Arch. Neurol., *35:*65.

Spekreijse, H., van der Tweel, L. H., and Zuidema, T. H. (1973). Contrast evoked responses in man. Vision Res., *13:*1577.

Sokol, S. (1976). Visually evoked potentials: theory, techniques and clinical applications. Surv. Ophthalmol., *21:*18.

Sokol, S. and Jones, K. (1979). Implicit time of patterned evoked potentials in infants: an index of maturation of spatial vision. Vision Res., *19:*747.

Thompson, R. F. and Patterson, M. M. (eds.) (1974). Bioelectric Recording Techniques. Part B, Electroencephalography and Human Brain Potentials. Academic Press, New York.

Vaughan, H. G., Katzman, R., and Taylor, J. (1963). Alterations of visual evoked response in the presence of homonymous visual defects. Electroencephalogr. Clin. Neurophysiol., *15:*737.

Wildberger, H. G. H., van Lith, G. H. M., Wijngaarde, R., and Mak, G. T. M. (1976).

Virtually evoked cortical potentials in the evaluation of homonymous and bitemporal visual field defects. Br. J. Ophthalmol., *60:*273.

Wooten, B. R. (1972). Photopic and scotopic contributions to the human visually evoked cortical potential. Vision Res., *12:*1647.

Zeese, J. A. (1977). Pattern visual evoked responses in multiple sclerosis. Arch. Neurol., *34:*314.

12

Brainstem Auditory Evoked Potentials in Neurology: Methodology, Interpretation, Clinical Application

JAMES J. STOCKARD, JANET E. STOCKARD, and FRANK W. SHARBROUGH

INTRODUCTION

If one could record directly from several different levels of the subcortical auditory pathway in man, one would see in the first 10 milliseconds (msec) following an appropriate acoustic stimulus a series of potentials corresponding to the sequential activation of peripheral, pontomedullary, pontine, and midbrain portions of the pathway (Fig. 12.1). As shown diagrammatically in Figure 12.1, when these acoustic nerve and brainstem potentials are volume-conducted to surface recording electrodes at the vertex and earlobe, they form a composite series of vertex-positive and vertex-negative waves known as brainstem auditory evoked potentials (BAEPs). The peak-to-peak amplitudes of the BAEPs recorded from the scalp are, at most, only about one one-

370

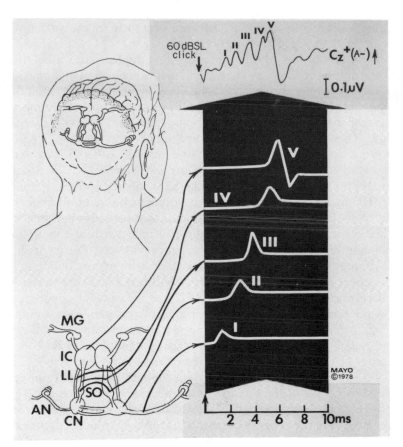

Fig. 12.1. Concept of volume conduction of short-latency auditory evoked potentials to surface electrodes. Click is delivered at first arrow and BAEPs are plotted earlobe-negative-up (A-↑). Potentials that are largely generated in or near the indicated brainstem auditory structures are reflected in the "far-field" composite response shown at top right. Abbreviations: AN—auditory nerves; CN—cochlear nuclei; SO—superior olives; LL—lateral lemnisci; IC—inferior colliculi; MG—medial geniculates. The individual BAEPs are probably generated largely in tracts rather than nuclei, and the one-to-one electroanatomic correspondence suggested by the figure is an oversimplification (see text) (modified from Stockard, J. J., Stockard, J. E. and Sharbrough, F. W., 1978. American Journal of EEG Technology, 18, 177).

hundredth the amplitude of the ongoing spontaneous EEG activity and, therefore, must be extracted from this and other noise by the use of computer averaging techniques. The vertex-positive (earlobe-negative) representations of the eighth nerve action potential and the four successive BAEPs are usually designated as waves I through V, respectively, and plotted vertex-positive-up (earlobe-negative-up) as in the convention of Jewett and Williston (1971). Figure 12.1 oversimplifies some of these concepts; it must be kept in mind that the precise depth correlates of the BAEPs are presently unknown but are much more complex than suggested by the Figure.

Jewett and Williston (1971) were the first to fully describe the human BAEPs and interpret them as such, although Sohmer and Feinmesser (1967) actually recorded them earlier and recognized the possibility of their brainstem origin. Sohmer, Feinmesser, and Szabo (1974) were the first to report selective alterations of different BAEPs by various types and loci of posterior fossa pathology. These clinicopathologic correlations with specific BAEP abnormalities were extended over the next three years by others (Starr and Achor, 1975; Stockard et al, 1976; Starr, 1976; Starr and Hamilton, 1976; Stockard and Rossiter, 1977; Gilroy et al, 1977). On the basis of such studies, it appears that waves I, III, and V primarily represent volume-conducted electrical activity from the acoustic nerve, pons, and midbrain, respectively, and that the latencies between these three potentials indirectly reflect neural conduction in the corresponding segments of the central auditory pathway. For example, wave I to wave III interpeak latency (I-III IPL) is a measure of conduction in the more caudal segment of the brainstem auditory pathway—acoustic nerve and pontomedullary portion—while the III-V IPL is a measure of conduction in the more rostral pontine and midbrain portions of the pathway. Another basic BAEP parameter of central auditory conduction, introduced in the study of Starr and Achor (1975), is based on the relative amplitudes of BAEPs, but this parameter is of limited clinical utility for reasons to be discussed.

This chapter describes the utility and the limitations of BAEPs in neurologic diagnosis. Proper use of the test in clinical neurology requires a full appreciation of the technical, physiologic, otologic, and pharmacologic factors which may alter BAEPs in the absence of neurologic disease (Stockard, Stockard, and Sharbrough, 1978b). Therefore, the first portion of this chapter will deal with these "non-neurologic" factors, which are not analyzed elsewhere in the literature. Identification of BAEP components and clinical interpretation of BAEPs will then be discussed in subsequent sections against this background of their normal variability. Only the vertex-positive BAEPs are emphasized in this chapter, but the vertex-negative BAEPs (waves I_N, III_N, and V_N) are equally reproducible and important in our clinical BAEP applications.

METHODS AND MATERIALS

We routinely use a click intensity 60 dB above the patient's hearing threshold (60 dBSL), as determined at the time of testing for each ear, and present these clicks monaurally at a rate just above 10 per second to avoid an integral factor of 60 Hz. The other ear is masked with white noise of variable intensity (depending on audiogram), at least 40 dBHL. The clicks are generated by passing 0.1 msec square pulses through shielded headphones (Telephonics TDH-39 or Telex 1470) with the polarity that produces rarefaction clicks. The bipolar EEG activity recorded from vertex (Cz) to earlobe ipsilateral (A_i) to acoustic stimulation is filtered (-6 dB points 100 Hz and 3 kHz) and amplified

(5×10^5) with Grass P511J amplifiers and the activity time-locked to the stimulus is sampled at 25-100 kHz over the first 10.24 msec following the stimulus (Grass Model 10 or Nicolet CA-1000 signal averagers). Peak latencies are measured to the nearest 10–40 μsec and peak-to-peak amplitudes to the nearest 10 nanovolts using digital cursors. At least two separate trials/averages of 2,000 to 4,000 responses are recorded and superimposed per ear and these four separate trials are put into the four quandrants of the computer memory. The decision as to how many responses per trial to average is determined, in part, by the degree of intertrial variability in interpeak latencies: the I-III, III-V and I-V IPLs should not vary by more than 80 μsec between trials at the most, and the waveforms should superimpose closely. This basic protocol for routine clinical use usually gives such highly reproducible waves I, III, and V that the patient can be disconnected after four trials of 2,000 clicks and the data analyzed in detail with digital latency and amplitude cursors while still in the computer memory. When using instruments that allow addition of the various sections of memory (additive transfer), more trials incorporating fewer samples per trial are recorded from each ear, e.g., four separate averages of 1,000 responses. If the above criteria for intertrial reproducibility are met, the results of individual trials are then added, and latency and amplitude measurements are made from the composite plot. This provides a true average of averages and a correspondingly higher signal-to-noise ratio (proportional to the square root of the total number of samples). Audiograms are obtained prior to testing when feasible, and patients are sedated if there is prominent EMG artifact in the EEG input. (We found no effect of chloral hydrate in doses up to 2 g., p.o., or of sleep itself on BAEPs and routinely sedate adult patients with 1 g., p.o., of this drug. Sohmer, Gafni, and Chisin, 1978, found no BAEP effects from sleep induced by other sedatives.)

NORMATIVE DATA AND CRITERIA FOR ABNORMALITY

Figure 12.2 shows a typical recording of BAEPs from a normal subject, gives our upper limits of normal for the I-II, I-III, III-V, and I-V IPLs and also shows the normative IPL values between the vertex-negative peaks I_N, III_N, and V_N for 50 young adults with normal audiograms (mean age 28 years, SD=3, range 19-42). Prolongation of these IPLs beyond the 99 percent tolerance limit (TL) represents the only criterion for BAEP abnormality that is routinely employed because of the low interindividual variability of these IPLs. Interpeak latencies involving the other waves show low intraindividual variability, but sufficient variability (in the standard recording derivation) among individuals in cross-sectional studies of a normal population that they are probably diagnostically useful only in longitudinal studies of certain individuals who have well-defined waves II, IV, VI, and VII to begin with (Stockard and Rossiter, 1977). Figure 12.3 shows the normal values for the relative amplitudes of the IV/V complex and wave I when employing three different periaural "reference" sites. These so-called "reference" sites are, of course, highly active with

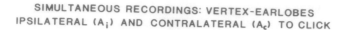

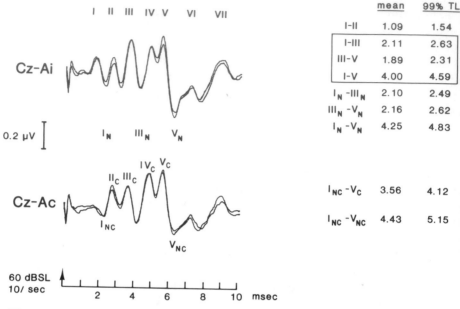

Fig. 12.2. Latency norms for young adult population described in text. In this and all subsequent figures, two independent averages of 2,048 responses from the same ear are superimposed to show intertrial reproducibility, and the original data were photographed directly to make the illustrations. TL: upper tolerance limit (modified from Stockard, J. J., Stockard, J. E. and Sharbrough, F. W., 1978. American Journal of EEG Technology, 18,177).

respect to BAEPs and this is reflected in the amplitude differences resulting from minor displacements of the recording site about the ear. When all such factors affecting relative amplitude are controlled in a way to be discussed, a IV/V:I amplitude ratio in response to 60 dBSL monaural stimulation of less than 0.5 is suggestive of central auditory dysfunction when an earlobe "reference" is used (although this also represents a tolerance limit below which 1 percent of normal subjects will fall). We recommend the earlobe as the periaural recording site for BAEPs because of the cleaner recordings and larger waves I it affords (Stockard et al, 1978b). Placement on the medial surface of the lobe reduces artifact.

Although norms for interpeak latency and relative amplitude are given in Figures 12.2 and 12.3 for a population of young adults with an equal sex distribution, each laboratory should define its own normal values and make them specific for age and sex. There are only a few major determinants of IPL, and in the absence of CNS immaturity or hypothermia, abnormal IPL prolongation usually reflects a pathologic disturbance of central auditory conduction. In contrast, there are many factors that markedly affect relative BAEP amplitudes,

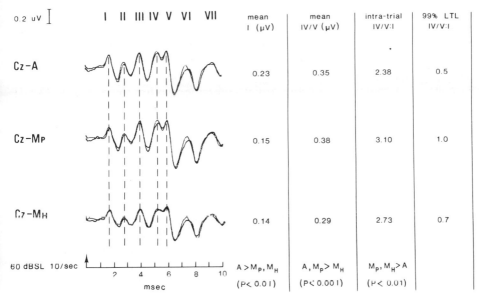

Fig. 12.3. *Relative amplitude values for same normal population as in Fig. 12.2. Simultaneous recordings between vertex and earlobe (A), mastoid process (M_p), and high mastoid (M_h)—the latter point 4.0 cm above M_p—ipsilateral to monaural click. LTL: lower tolerance limit (modified from Stockard, J. J., Stockard, J. E., and Sharbrough, F. W., 1978. American Journal of EEG Technology, 18, 177).*

and these factors must be rigorously controlled if normative amplitude criteria are to be employed. The morphology of BAEPs is highly variable and not readily quantified, and, therefore, has not proven useful in defining abnormality (Chiappa, Gladstone, and Young, 1979). The most common morphologic changes seen in abnormal BAEPs, such as the decrease in terminal negativity of the IV/V complex (downslope of wave V), can usually be quantified in terms of relative amplitude changes. Although there is a close interdependence of the latency and amplitude of a given BAEP component, the former has proven more useful diagnostically. Therefore, the nonpathologic factors affecting IPL will be emphasized in the following analysis of the normal variability of BAEPs.

NON-NEUROLOGIC FACTORS INFLUENCING IPL AND RELATIVE AMPLITUDE OF BAEPs

Temperature

Moderate hypothermia prolongs the IPLs of human BAEPs and this can lead to diagnostic error in BAEP interpretation, if not recognized. As determined in neurologically and audiometrically normal patients subjected to hypothermia during cardiopulmonary bypass, the upper limit of normal for the

I-IV/V IPL at normothermia is exceeded at an esophageal temperature of about 32° C and that for the I-III and III-IV/V IPLs at about 28° C (Stockard, Sharbrough, and Tinker, 1978). This degree of hypothermia (32° C) is not uncommon in cases where there is impaired thermoregulation and the effects of body temperature should, therefore, be kept in mind when interpreting BAEPs from patients prone to develop hypothermia. Hyperthermia has the opposite* BAEP effects, but one patient with multiple sclerosis (MS) whom we studied had prolonged IPLs at 40° C (nasopharyngeal) but not at 37°, the hyperthermia in that case being due to a febrile illness.

Age

Below the age of about 2 years, interpeak latencies are prolonged relative to adult values and vary inversely with age (Hecox, 1975; Salamy, McKean, and Buda, 1975; Starr et al, 1977). This change is not linear with age and reaches its maximum in the 32-34 week conceptional age (C.A.) as shown by Starr et al (1977), when I-IV/V IPL will change by as much as 0.4 msec per week (Fig. 12.4). The average decrease for prematures is about 0.15 msec per week from 26 weeks C.A. (I-IV/V ~ 7 msec) to term (I-IV/V ~ 5 msec). Up to age 6 months, the absolute latency of wave I is prolonged due to immaturity of the peripheral auditory apparatus as well (Hecox, 1975). Advancing age was reported by Rowe (1978) to prolong the I-III IPL by about 0.2 msec in a comparison of subjects over 50 years of age (mean = 61 years) with a group averaging 25 years of age, but sex ratio and audiometric configuration of his subjects were not controlled for.

Sex

Females have significantly shorter III-V and I-V IPLs than males (Stockard et al, 1978b). This difference might be related to shorter anatomic distances in the corresponding segments of the auditory pathway, in view of the smaller average brain size of females as compared to males. For example, small differences in pathway length from cochlea to midbrain could well account for the observed 0.1–0.2 msec difference in I-V IPL between the sexes. Females also have shorter stimulus-to-peak latencies and higher amplitude BAEPs, on average, and this again may relate to smaller head/brainstem size. Other factors may instead be responsible but, whatever the explanation of this sex difference, it is worthwhile to have separate IPL norms for males and females just as it is desirable to have them for age. In our experience, norms based on two major age groups (under and over 50) for each sex have proven adequate in routine neurologic applications in adults.

---

* Slight IPL decreases are normally seen in man and cats (Jones, Stockard, and Weidner, 1979) with mild hyperthermia.

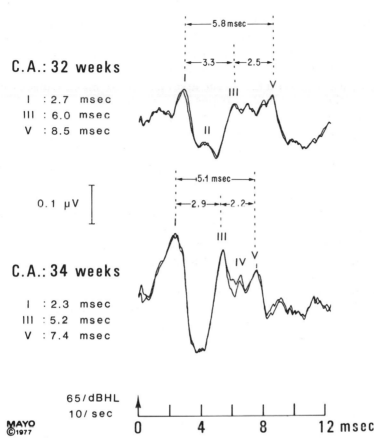

C.A.: 32 weeks

I : 2.7 msec
III : 6.0 msec
V : 8.5 msec

0.1 μV

C.A.: 34 weeks

I : 2.3 msec
III : 5.2 msec
V : 7.4 msec

65/dBHL
10/sec

MAYO
©1977

0   4   8   12 msec

Fig. 12.4. *Decrease in poststimulus and interpeak BAEP latencies in a normal premature infant between the conceptional ages (C.A.) of 32 weeks and 34 weeks. With stimulation at 10 per second, all seven vertex-positive waves of the response can usually be resolved, if a long enough sweep is employed (bottom tracings). Note the shorter latency of wave IV relative to III and V than is usually seen in adults; this is common in neonates, and the field properties of this pattern make it distinguishable from a bifid wave III, which it resembles somewhat (from Stockard, J. J., Stockard, J. E. and Sharbrough, F. W., 1978. American Journal of EEG Technology, 18,177).*

Audiogram Shape

In a study of patients with sensorineural hearing loss, Coats and Martin (1977) found an abrupt increase in the latency of wave I (which is the surface correlate of the auditory nerve action potential) at 50-60 dB 4 to 8 kHz hearing loss; this abrupt increase in wave I peak latency was not paralleled by a similar increase in wave V latency and thus the I-V IPLs in these subjects were shorter than in those with normal audiograms. The authors attributed the increase in wave I latency in these patients to selective loss of a population of auditory nerve fibers which have a high threshold for acoustic stimulation and which contribute to the earlier of the two peaks of the nerve action potential. With moderately high intensity stimuli, this first peak of the auditory nerve action potential is usually reflected on the surface as the peak of wave I in subjects with normal hearing. With loss of the first peak due to high-frequency cochlear hearing loss, the second peak of the nerve action potential—which is generated by a population of nerve fibers responding to lower intensities of acoustic stimulation—becomes the peak of wave I as reflected in the BAEPs, and the I-V IPL decreases. Theoretically, then, lesser degrees of I-III and I-V IPL prolongation might signify retrocochlear pathology in patients with high-frequency hearing loss than in patients with normal audiograms.

We recommend obtaining an audiogram, when possible, prior to recording BAEPs in neurologic applications of the test, to control for these peripheral auditory factors. High-frequency hearing losses are usually associated with increased IV/V:I amplitude ratios, partly because the portion of the subcortical auditory pathway generating wave V takes origin from more apical regions of the cochlea than that generating wave I (Don and Eggermont, 1978), and the latter are relatively spared in high-frequency sensory hearing loss. Flat conductive hearing losses are essentially equivalent to reductions in stimulus intensity in terms of their BAEP effects, and are associated with unchanged or slightly decreased IPLs (Fig. 12.5) and increased IV/V:I amplitude ratios, unless compensated for by increasing stimulus intensity.

Stimulus Phase

The initial phase of the click (rarefaction vs condensation) becomes an important determinant of BAEP latencies in patients with significant high-frequency hearing loss and in neonates. Rarefaction (R) clicks are produced by initial movement of the headphone transducer away from the tympanic membrane, and condensation (C) clicks result from initial displacement toward it. A given auditory neuron is likely to respond only during the period when the basilar membrane is displaced toward the scala vestibuli, i.e., during the rarefaction phase of the acoustic stimulus, and this may account largely for the lesser absolute latencies and better resolution of BAEPs elicited by R as compared to C clicks in most cases (Stockard et al, 1978b). We have found that wave V changes less than waves I to IV with changes in click phase, suggesting that the pathways generating this component do not have the same cochlear origins as those generating the earlier waves. Differences in BAEP latency as a function of phase also suggest that the more apical portions of the cochlea mature earlier than the basal portion—the former are largely responsible for the C vs R differences in BAEPs that are so prominent in newborns (Fig. 12.6) although they can be striking in some normal adults as well (Fig. 12.7). The common practice in many electrodiagnostic laboratories is to alternate the polarity of stimuli (and, therefore, the phase of the clicks) to minimize electrical and stimulus artifacts. This results in partial cancellation of R/C out-of-phase BAEP components and distortion of the response, particularly in newborns and

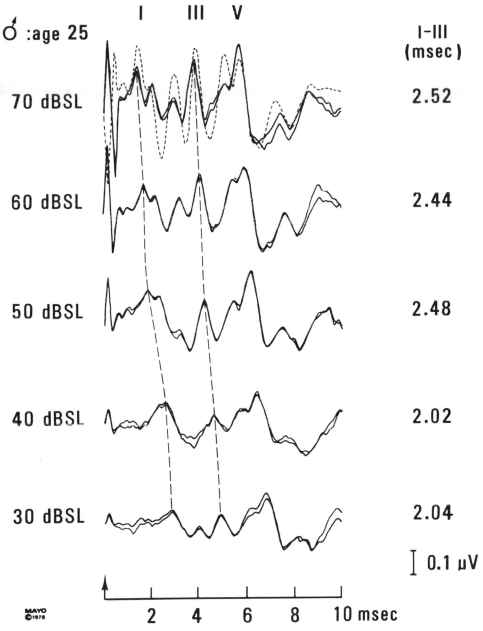

Fig. 12.5. Decrease in I-III IPL with decreasing stimulus intensity in an audiometrically and neurologically normal subject. Note that decrease occurs between 50 and 40 dBSL as the result of an abrupt increase in the latency of wave I as a second constituent peak becomes predominant at lower intensities. Dotted lines in top tracing show response to condensation clicks, all others being to rarefaction clicks (initial phases of the acoustic waveform). See Stockard et al (1979a) for details.

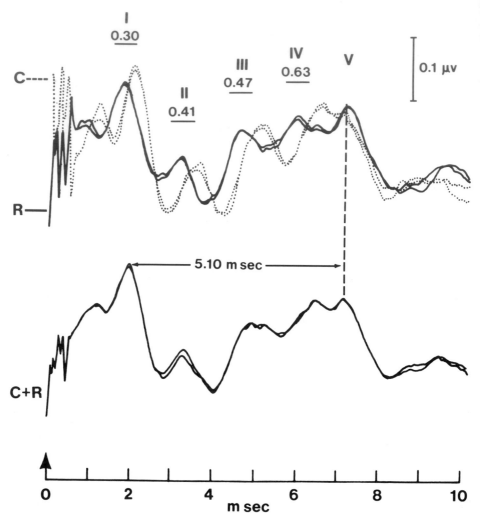

Fig. 12.6. *Effects of click phase on BAEPs from a normal neonate. The underlined values are the differences in msec between the absolute latencies of waves I through IV when elicited by condensation (C) and rarefaction (R) clicks, respectively. The latency of wave V is the same in response to both phases of click and therefore the indicated phase differences for the earlier waves give the C:R differences in IPL between any given component and wave V; for example, the I-V IPL in response to R clicks is 0.30 msec longer than that elicited by C clicks. The averaging effect of alternating R/C clicks can be seen in the bottom tracings, in which the R and C trials above were added by the computer (C + R).*

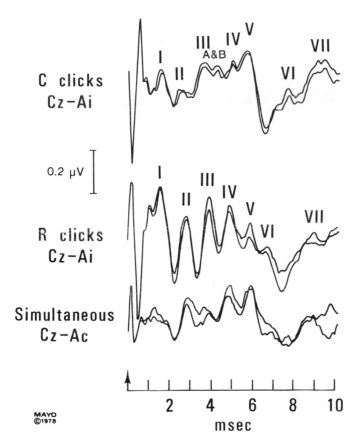

Fig. 12.7. *Extreme example of alteration of BAEP waveform by change in acoustic stimulus from rarefaction (R) to condensation (C) clicks. Note bifid wave III with R clicks and change in relative amplitudes of waves IV and V with C clicks. Recorded from normal subject.*

in adults with high-frequency hearing loss. Because of the lesser vulnerability of wave V to such effects (possibly due, in part, to its different origin on the cochlear membrane), wave I is attenuated more by the use of alternating R/C clicks and the IV/V:I amplitude ratio increases with use of alternating-phase as compared to single-phase clicks. We recommend use of R clicks in routine BAEP applications, although alternating R/C clicks may sometimes be necessary to minimize artifact and clicks with a predominant C phase sometimes elicit better BAEPs (Fig. 12.5, top).

Stimulus Intensity

IPLs are relatively independent of click intensity but those involving wave I usually decrease slightly at lower intensities. As shown in Figure 12.5, this is largely due to an increase in wave I peak latency, as an earlier-firing population

♂ age: 38

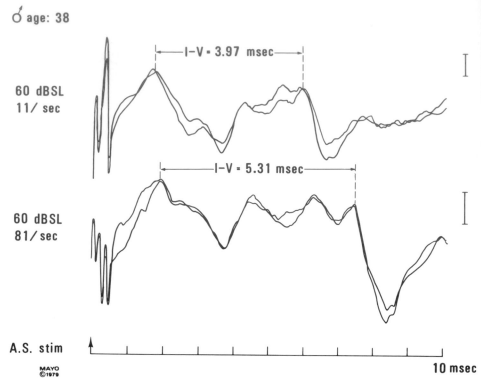

60 dBSL
11/ sec

⊢——I–V = 3.97 msec——⊣

60 dBSL
81/ sec

⊢——I–V = 5.31 msec——⊣

A.S. stim

MAYO
©1979

10 msec

Fig. 12.8. Rate-dependent IPL abnormality in patient with definite MS, but no clinical evidence of brainstem involvement. Condensation clicks. Cal: 0.1 µV.

of auditory nerve fibers drops out at low intensities. Shortening of IPLs has been reported before in the literature for sensorineural hearing losses (Coats and Martin, 1977), but not with reduction in stimulus intensity—which is effectively the same as a conductive hearing loss. As can be seen in Figure 12.5, decreasing stimulus intensity also results in increasing IV/V:I amplitude ratio, and the great intensity-dependence of wave I contributes to the considerable variability of relative amplitude ratios. Unless markedly reduced for our routine intensity or showing a clear trend in sequential, technically equivalent recordings, IV/V:I amplitude ratios are used to define abnormalities in our lab only when intensity series such as that shown in Figure 12.5 are performed.

Stimulus Rate

Increasing stimulus rate increases the poststimulus latencies of all BAEP components and also increases the IPLs (Rowe, 1978; Stockard et al, 1978b). Our criterion for rate-dependent abnormality is that there be a prolongation of I-V IPL by more than 1.3 msec to a value greater than 5.3 msec * (Fig. 12.8),

---

* This applies to condensation clicks only, because rate-phase interactions make rate-dependent IPL changes with rarefaction clicks more variable (Stockard et al, 1979).

giving our 99 percent tolerance limits for both I-V IPL change and the I-V IPL attained as a function of increasing the click rate from 10 to 81 per second. By decreasing interstimulus interval, Robinson and Rudge (1977) unmasked latency abnormalities in 57 percent of their MS patients who had "low-amplitude" waves V. Hecox et al (1979) have demonstrated rate-dependent abnormalities in head trauma and hypoxic encephalopathy as well as MS. However Chiappa et al (1979) mention that increasing click rate from 10 per second to only 30 per second has no value and this has been our experience as well; they also found no value in increasing rate to 70 per second. Faster rates (more than 80 per second) have proven most useful in eliciting rate-dependent abnormalities in our experience, but use of such rapid rates of stimulation is self-defeating in some cases because of the associated loss of BAEP resolution and interpretability. Yagi and Kaga (1979) have reported a different type of pathologic rate change—selective disappearance of BAEPs at high click rates; this must be interpreted cautiously since similar findings obtain in some normal subjects. Newborns normally show greater rate-dependent IPL changes than adults (Stockard et al, 1979a) and each lab should have age-specific rate norms for the very young.

"Reference" Site *

Changing the periaural recording site to the ear contralateral (A_c) to acoustic stimulation usually produces a decrease in the II-III IPL and increase in IV-V IPL (Stockard et al, 1978b). The statement by Starr and Achor (1975) that BAEP latency is not affected by the choice of these electrode arrays is incorrect—most subjects show decreased peak latencies of waves III and IV and increased peak latencies of waves II and V in $Cz-A_c$ as compared to $Cz-A_1$ derivations. Relative amplitudes of BAEPs are highly dependent on ear reference site and even minor changes in the site ipsilateral to acoustic stimulation will alter the IV/V·I amplitude ratio (Fig. 12.3). The use of a periaural "reference" contralateral to the ear being stimulated acoustically also changes relative BAEP amplitudes markedly and results in selective attenuation of wave III and the ear—negative peak of wave I in most cases (Fig. 12.9). Periaural sites are highly active with respect to BAEPs and interaction of BAEP activity at these sites with that at the vertex results in complex latency, amplitude and morphology changes for all BAEPs (Stockard et al, 1978b).

Drugs

Interpeak latencies are relatively resistant to pharmacologic insults when secondary temperature effects of the intoxication are controlled. Of especial importance clinically is the fact that IPLs are little affected by most nonspecific CNS depressants. The BAEPs shown in Figure 12.10 were recorded from a

---

* Cephalic and even nuchal sites are active references because of the significant BAEP activity that can be recorded there when they are themselves referenced against a truly indifferent site, such as the ankle (Stockard et al, 1978b).

neurologically and audiometrically normal patient undergoing general anesthesia with isoflurane, an agent which produces true electrocerebral silence at concentrations required for surgical anesthesia in some patients. All BAEPs are well-preserved and have normal IPL despite the absence of any spontaneous EEG activity or clinical evidence (on reflex testing) of CNS function. The amplitude of wave IV/V is reduced relative to wave I in the tracings obtained during anesthesia, compared with those recorded before and afterward. The isomer of isoflurane, enflurane, does produce temperature-independent prolongation of IPL unlike most nonspecific CNS depressants (Jones, Stockard, and Henry, 1978). Other general anesthetics or adjuvant agents that we have studied, including halothane, meperidine, nitrous oxide, barbiturates, and diazepam, have not significantly altered human IPLs in clinically used dosages or concentrations. Acute ethanol intoxication has been reported to prolong IPLs (Squires, Chu, and Starr, 1978), but this may have been, at least in part, a temperature effect in view of the propensity of ethanol to lower core temperature and the difficulty of reproducing these findings when temperature is controlled (Jones and Stockard, 1979). Temperature effects would not account for all residual IPL changes seen in the nonintoxicated state following chronic ethanol intoxication (Chu, Squires, and Starr, 1978); we have seen similar IPL prolongations in chronic (but not acute) diphenylhydantoin intoxication. High doses of many nonspecific CNS depressants, including most general anesthetics, reduce the amplitudes of the latest BAEPs relative to earlier ones before IPLs are significantly prolonged. Drugs affecting specific neurotransmitters involved in the generation and modulation of BAEPs, e.g., serotonin (Bhargava and McKean, 1977) and acetylcholine (muscarinic receptors), alter relative amplitudes of BAEPs and will undoubtedly be shown to affect IPLs as well.

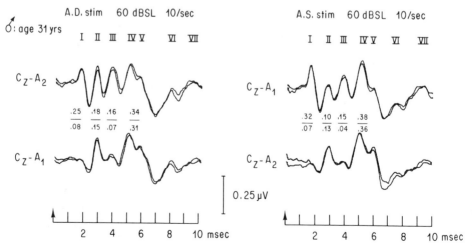

Fig. 12.9. *Amplitudes of different BAEP components as recorded simultaneously in Cz-A$_i$ and Cz-A$_c$ derivations. The amplitude values are in μV and pertain only to the recordings from this one subject, who shows more severe attentuation of waves I and III and lesser latency effects in C$_z$-A$_c$ than most.*

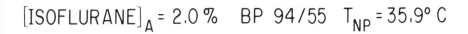

$[ISOFLURANE]_A = 2.0\%$ BP 94/55 $T_{NP} = 35.9°\,C$

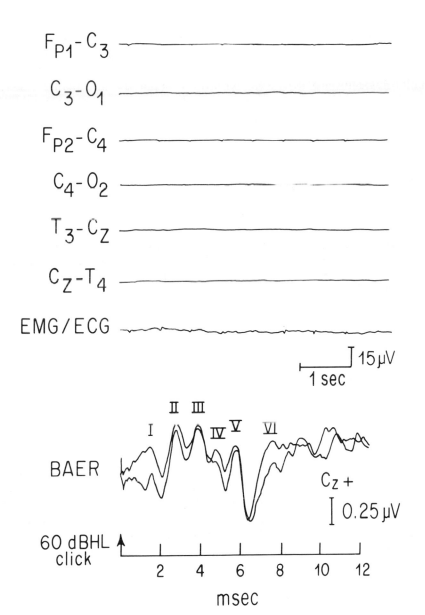

Fig. 12.10. BAEPs recorded from a surgical patient anesthetized with isoflurane, an inhalational agent that produces electrocerebral silence (upper traces) in the strict sense at concentrations near those required for surgical anesthesia. Latencies of waves I through V are not significantly different from those obtained during the unanesthetized state in this patient. The only difference from the control tracings is reduction of the amplitudes of waves IV/V, VI and VII in the anesthetized state, the latter two waves usually being abolished by deep anesthesia.

Stimulus Mode

Binaural stimulation produces higher-amplitude waves III through V at all stimulus intensities than monaural stimulation and, because of the monaural contribution to wave I but binaural contribution to waves IV and V, binaural stimulation logically produces a higher IV/V:I amplitude ratio than monaural stimulation at a given stimulus intensity. Binaural stimulation should be avoided in routine clinical applications because monaural abnormalities are common in neurologic disease and may otherwise be masked by the response from the normal ear (Stockard et al, 1978b). Separate monaural stimulation of each ear also allows for comparison of interaural asymmetries in IPL, and thus may indicate abnormality even when BAEPs from each ear are within normal limits when considered separately. Interaural I-V IPL differences greater than 0.5 msec are abnormal assuming proper identification of components and technically optimal recordings. When monaural stimulation is employed, masking of the non-stimulated ear is important to prevent cross-hearing and the spurious resultant BAEPs. In the presence of significant interaural hearing asymmetries, failure to mask the good ear when stimulating the bad is capable of cross-evoking BAEPs from the good ear even when only moderate click intensities are used (Fig. 12.11).

Filter Settings

These affect relative amplitudes more than interpeak latencies and, in diagnostic applications, should remain fixed at the values used when collecting each laboratory's normative data. The ideal bandpass for clinical purposes is probably 100 Hz to 3000 Hz or higher. A low-frequency filter of much less than 100 Hz allows EMG, EEG and other extraneous signals into the average, and a cutoff much higher than 100 Hz distorts the low-frequency BAEP components (Jewett and Williston, 1971). A high-frequency cutoff of at least 3000 Hz is necessary to resolve the highest-frequency components of the BAEP; settings of less than 1,000 Hz increase the apparent latencies of the BAEPs and decrease their resolution (Jewett and Williston, 1971). Increases in high-pass filter above 100 Hz markedly reduce IV/V:I amplitude ratio because of the longer duration of wave IV/I than I (Stockard et al, 1978b). High-pass filtering at 30 Hz or lower is needed in audiologic BAEP applications.

Signal-to-noise Characteristics

The signal-to-noise ratio increases with increasing sample size in rough proportion to the square root of the number of samples (Cooper, Osselton, and Shaw, 1974), but the ratio of the variability of the signal to the variability of the noise does not change with increasing sample size. Because, when recording BAEPs, the range of variability of the noise remains about three orders of magnitude greater than the range of variability of the signal, the inherent (Gaussian) variability of the signal is undetectable (Jewett and Williston, 1971). Dif-

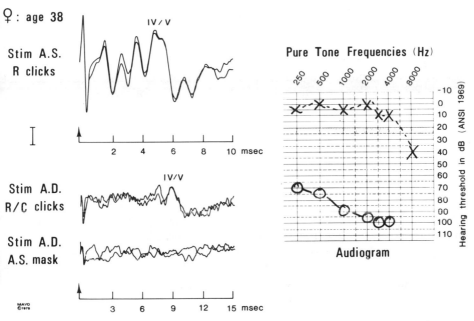

Fig. 12.11. *Top and middle tracings show BAEPs elicited from left and right ears, respectively, by 70 dBHL clicks in patient with 70 to 100 dB hearing loss in right ear for all frequencies tested. Bottom tracing shows elimination of prolonged low-amplitude IV/V complex elicited by right ear stimulation when left ear is masked with 40 dBHL white noise. This indicated that BAEPs seen in middle tracings were actually arising from cross-stimulation of the left ear (by bone conduction). Alternating R/C clicks were used on the affected ear in this case to minimize stimulus artifact and "ringing." X (O): left (right) ear thresholds. Cal: 0.1 μV.*

ferences in the averages that result from separate trials are thus best attributed to variations in the noise or to systematic variations in the signal such as those discussed above. The greatest source of noise and noise-variability in routine recordings is muscle artifact. Even moderate amounts of muscle (EMG) artifact can invalidate the use of relative amplitude criteria and prevent resolution of BAEP peaks. The EEG should, therefore, not be sampled when it contains EMG or other artifact that is visible on the oscilloscope.

IDENTIFICATION OF COMPONENTS

Proper identification of the different BAEPs is obviously crucial to the diagnostic use of interpeak latencies in lesion detection and localization. It is important that the method used to identify the different waves should not be self-verifying, e.g., that wave V not be identified on the basis of its being the fifth vertex-positive wave following the stimulus (which it often is not), or by virtue of its having the latency of the "normal" wave V (absolute latencies vary greatly with peripheral conductive hearing loss and changes in effective stimulus intensity), or because it is the highest-amplitude component (waves I or III may be in normals). There are more valid ways of distinguishing the different waves, but it must be kept in mind that abnormal BAEPs may not always respond the way normal BAEPs do to the following maneuvers for identification of components.

Wave V

In normals, wave V is the most reliable component and usually consists of a prominent positivity followed by a long, sharp negative deflection that results in a positive-to-negative shift of the BAEP baseline to below a horizontal "equipotential" line bisecting the earlier peaks. This sudden negative baseline shift appears to be the termination of a slow wave which has waves II, III, and IV superimposed on its rising phase. Even in the presence of brainstem pathology, identification of wave V may be possible because of certain other characteristics—its relative resistance to very high rates of stimulation (100 per second), and, especially, its resistance to very low stimulus intensities. Even within 10 dB of the subjective hearing threshold (and sometimes even just below it), the characteristic terminal negativity of wave V can usually still be recognized, while earlier waves are lost in the noise. A confusing normal variant, in which the greatest negative downslope follows the peak of wave VI, can be recognized and interpreted correctly if simultaneous Cz-A_c recordings are obtained (Fig. 12.7, middle tracings). As seen at the bottom of Figure 12.7, the V_N downslope usually assumes a greater amplitude and more normal configuration in the Cz-A_c derivation when recorded as a normal variant in Cz-A_i. This pattern, like so many BAEP waveform variations, can appear as a function of one click phase only (Fig. 12.7). If this pattern is not recognized, wave VI may be mistaken for a wave V with prolonged latency.

Wave IV

This component is usually easy to identify after wave V has been recognized because it and wave V tend to form a complex biphasic wave in vertex to ipsilateral (to the clicks) ear electrode derivations. It is normal to have either: (1) a completely fused wave IV/V with a peak latency appropriate to either IV or V (or intermediate); (2) separate peaks with either IV or V higher (can vary in same subject); or (3) a skewed peak which consists primarily of a wave IV with only a small inflection on its downslope for wave V, or, conversely, a predominant wave V with a small inflection on its upslope representing wave IV. Different morphologic variants of the IV/V complex can occur in the same subjects in the same recording session as a function of slight changes in a number of technical variables (Fig. 12.12), or between recording sessions in the same subjects tested with similar methods. These inter- and intrasubject varia-

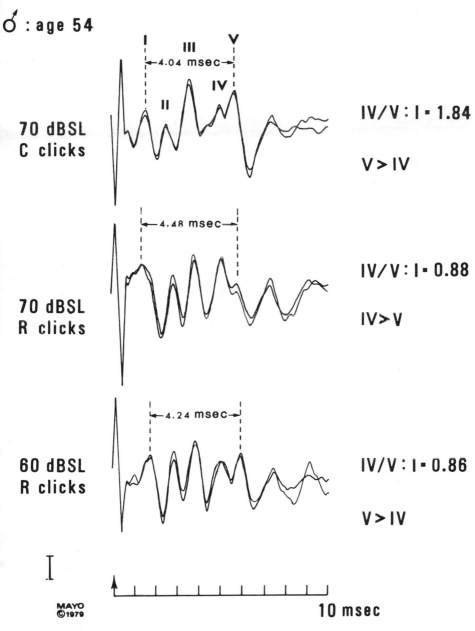

ⓓ : age 54

70 dBSL
C clicks

I III V
←4.04 msec→
II IV

IV/V : I = 1.84

V > IV

70 dBSL
R clicks

←4.48 msec→

IV/V : I = 0.88

IV > V

60 dBSL
R clicks

←4.24 msec→

IV/V : I = 0.86

V > IV

I

MAYO
©1979

10 msec

Fig. 12.12. BAEP latency, amplitude, and waveform changes resulting from alteration of stimulus intensity and phase. The three sets of BAEP tracings were obtained from the same normal subject in the same recording session with only the click phase being changed between the top and middle tracings, and only the intensity being changed between middle and bottom tracings. Note that I-V IPL and relative amplitudes of waves IV and V and of IV/V and I all change markedly with change from condensation (C) to rarefaction (R) clicks. Decrease of R click intensity by 10 dB again reverses configuration of IV/V complex. Cal: 0.1 μV.

tions in the morphology of the IV/V complex have no clinical significance. Most of the problems of peak definition resulting from variability of the IV/V complex are avoided when the vertex-negative waves are employed also, as we do routinely. Combinations of vertex-positive to III_N or V_N peaks, e.g., I-V_N, also help in this regard. If one relies on only Cz-positive waves, a simple technique which usually resolves waves IV and V when other measures fail is the use of an ear reference contralateral to the ear being stimulated; this usually decreases the latency of wave IV and increases that of wave V, although there is individual variability in the extent to which this occurs. Use of single click phase and faster, longer sampling also help resolve IV.

Wave III

This component is usually attenuated in vertex to contralateral ear derivations while wave II is relatively preserved (Fig. 12.9). If wave IV has already been recognized, this attenuation between two peaks (II and IV) is useful for identifying wave III. Some normal subjects have a bifid wave III which is associated with a normal I-V IPL. As with the various configurations of wave IV and V, the bifid III may be related to the initial phase (R or C) of the click stimulus, as seen in Figures 12.7 and 12.12. In infants and some adults, wave IV may normally fall closer to III than to V and give the appearance of a bifid wave III. In contrast to waves IV and V, II and III tend to fuse in Cz-A_c recordings, the latency of III decreasing and that of II increasing. In some patients, a II/III complex forms in the vertex-to-contralateral-ear derivation and this may itself help to identify these two waves in the ipsilateral ear derivation, just as splitting of the IV/V complex with the contralateral ear reference may help to identify the complex in the routine derivation.

Wave II

As shown in Figure 12.9, wave II is relatively spared by employing a contralateral ear reference and the amplitude of its negative downslope may even increase in amplitude. As can be seen in Figures 12.2 and 12.9, among the early BAEPs, it is the positive upslope (ascending limb) of wave II which shows the least alteration by changing from the vertex-ipsilateral ear to vertex-contralateral ear derivation. The vertex-positive peak of wave I is usually truncated by going to the contralateral ear as a reference, and thus wave II stands out in most vertex-contralateral ear recordings as a peak resembling that which occurs near the same latency in the ipsilateral ear derivation but which is preceded and followed by two attenuated peaks (I and III), as seen in Figures 12.2 and 12.9.

Wave I

It is important to identify wave I because it is the electrophysiologic benchmark from which more proximal brainstem auditory conduction must be assessed. It is ideally suited for this purpose because of its retrocochlear yet extra-axial locus of generation in the acoustic nerve—peripheral auditory factors will tend to affect it and the later BAEPs similarly, while it will be less affected than the BAEPs by central nervous system disorders such as multiple sclerosis. As mentioned, wave I identification is facilitated by simultaneous vertex-contralateral ear recording as shown in Figures 12.2 and 12.9. The ear-negative activity which mainly comprises wave I is lost in the contralateral ear derivation, but some residual far-field positivity of wave I persists at the vertex even when the periaural "reference" ipsilateral to stimulation is eliminated (Streletz et al, 1977). The easiest way to enhance resolution of wave I in the usual recording derivation is to increase stimulus intensity and decrease stimulus rate. When these measures fail, recording from vertex to an external auditory canal (EAC) reference electrode will allow resolution of wave I (if present) under even the most difficult recording conditions (Stockard et al, 1978b). Electrical and acoustic noise and EMG artifact may be difficult to reduce in many acute medical situations and therefore an EAC reference electrode should be available. Mechanical (click) and electrical stimulus artifacts and cochlear microphonics may all be distinguished from wave I by their complete polarity inversion with reversal of stimulus polarity. Use of alternate-polarity stimuli may sometimes be necessary to resolve wave I when high-intensity clicks are employed since, in addition to the increased stimulus artifact, the latency to wave I will decrease and the artifact may overlap wave I when single-polarity stimuli are used.

CLINICAL INTERPRETATION OF BAEPs IN NEUROLOGIC DIAGNOSIS

The neurologic applications in which BAEPs have proven most useful are: (1) the evaluation of the etiology and reversibility of coma; (2) the diagnosis of multiple sclerosis; and (3) the early detection and localization of posterior fossa tumors. The interpretation of BAEPs in these three clinical contexts will, therefore, be discussed and illustrated here.

Coma

BAEPs may provide useful diagnostic or prognostic information in the differentiation of metabolic from structural causes of brainstem dysfunction. As mentioned earlier, and as shown in Figure 12.10, human BAEPs are relatively resistant to metabolic insults and—of especial importance—are little affected by most nonspecific CNS depressants. As an example of this, Figure 12.13 shows the normal BAEPs recorded from a 33-year-old comatose female who had had a respiratory arrest of unknown cause and duration. On admission, she had fixed midposition pupils and no spontaneous or reflex activity at any level of the CNS, including the brainstem level. Her EEG showed long, complete suppressions of spontaneous activity for up to 18 minutes with occasional

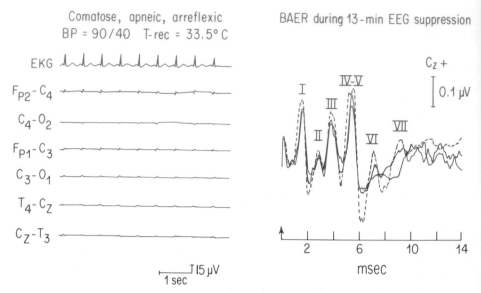

Fig. 12.13. *Normal BAEPs from a comatose patient who met clinical criteria for "brain death" and had a burst suppression pattern in the EEG. The normal brainstem evoked potentials suggested a metabolic etiology for the brainstem dysfunction in this case rather than structural damage on the basis of anoxia (see text). The dashed tracing indicates the average BAEP waveform recorded from the same patient after complete neurologic recovery had occurred. Esophageal temperature was 35.8°C. (from Stockard, J. J. and Sharbrough, F. W. 1979. Unique contributions of short-latency auditory and somatosensory evoked potentials to neurologic diagnosis. In: Clinical Uses of Cerebral, Brainstem and Spinal Somatosensory Evoked Potentials. Desmedt, J. E., Ed., p. 231. Karger, Basel).*

bursts of unreactive, low-amplitude polymorphic delta activity lasting several seconds. During periods of suppression, there was no visible response to auditory, somatosensory, or photic stimuli in the unaveraged EEG. However, the BAEPs recorded at this time (Fig. 12.13) were normal from both ears, and, in the face of this degree of clinical brainstem dysfunction, suggested some type of metabolic process; drug intoxication seemed to be the most likely cause in this case. The patient recovered completely over the next 96 hours and massive CNS depressant overdose, mainly with gluthethimide, was indeed determined to be the etiology of the coma. Even had this been known initially, the EEG and clinical data could still have been consistent with cerebral and brainstem damage resulting from anoxia at the time of the arrest. Normal BAEPs, on the other hand, would be highly unlikely with a structural lesion sufficient to eliminate all cephalic reflexes and spontaneous respiration. Intact BAEPs in the presence of less global brainstem dysfunction do not necessarily imply a metabolic or otherwise reversible coma—we have recorded completely normal BAEPs from patients rendered irreversibly comatose by structural lesions involving the midbrain tegmentum, or by diffuse bilateral cerebrocortical damage.

When clinical evidence of pontine and medullary activity is absent, IPL abnormalities or the absence of waves III and IV/V in the presence of wave I suggest widespread structural damage as the cause of the brainstem dysfunction, with a correspondingly poor prognosis. No BAEPs at all (including wave I) has a similarly poor prognosis but requires more cautious interpretation since technical or otologic problems have then to be excluded. Absence of either all BAEPs or of all except wave I are the two common patterns seen in patients with brain death, but we have also observed a third pattern in which waves I and II are preserved (Fig. 12.14). Lesser degrees of abnormality or no BAEP abnormality will be seen in cerebrocortical death cases where there is no damage to the brainstem auditory pathways.

In other cases, where coma results from brainstem lesions and the EEG is noncontributory, BAEPs can provide information about the structural nature and extent of the lesion. The patient whose cochlear microphonic is shown in Figure 12.15 had no BAEPs yet only a mildly abnormal EEG, as seen in Figure 12.16. This previously healthy patient was admitted 5 hours after suddenly losing consciousness during a chiropractic manipulation of his neck. He had been artificially ventilated and his blood pressure supported with intravenous

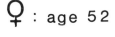

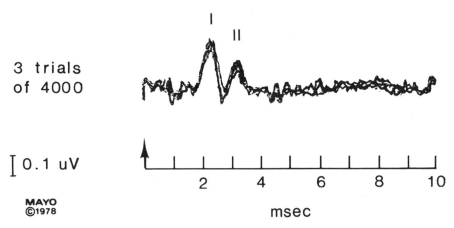

Fig. 12.14. *Preservation of wave II as well as wave I in case of complete brain death. The patient expired 2 hours after this recording and was found at postmortem to have complete necrosis of the pons and upper medulla which included the cochlear nuclei. Simultaneous electro-cochleographic recordings and attenuation of this second peak along with the first in Cz-A$_c$ and Cz-ankle recordings suggested that the second peak was originating in the auditory nerve (N$_2$ of the compound action potential). This recording was obtained with 80 dBHL 10 per second alternating R/C monaural clicks; the second wave was not resolved when intensities below 60 dBSL were employed, consistent with it being the extra-axial (nerve) component of wave II.*

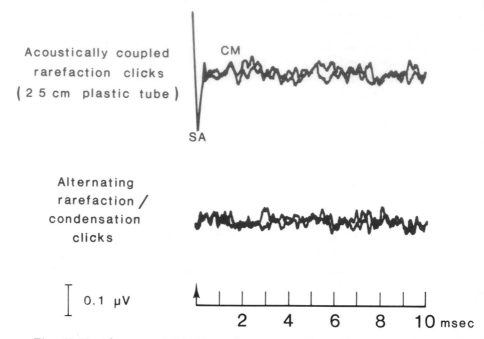

Acoustically coupled
rarefaction clicks
(2 5 cm plastic tube)

CM

SA

Alternating
rarefaction /
condensation
clicks

0.1 µV

2   4   6   8   10 msec

Fig. 12.15. *Absence of BAEPs and presence of cochlear microphonic in rhombencephalic death due to vertebrobasilar thrombosis. Loss of wave I correlated with infarction of the eighth nerves found at postmortem. Preservation of cochlear microphonic (CM) reflects greater resistance of cochlea to ischemia and ruled out conduction or end-organ failure as the etiology of the BAEP loss in this case. As shown, CM was distinguished from stimulus artifact by acoustic coupling through a length of tubing (25 cm) which delayed CM by about three-quarters of a millisecond with respect to the electrical stimulus artifact (SA). CM was distinguished from wave I by its inversion with reversal of stimulus polarity and disappearance when alternating-polarity stimuli were used (modified from Stockard, J. J., Stockard, J. E. and Sharbrough, F. W. 1978. American Journal of EEG Technology, 18,177).*

vasopressors throughout the interim until his BAEPs and EEG were recorded. At the time of testing, he was unresponsive to deep pain, had no spontaneous respirations, and showed no spontaneous or reflex movements except for continuous vertical ocular bobbing. There were no oculocephalic, caloric, corneal, or gag reflexes and no deep tendon reflexes in the extremities. Despite this, his pupils reacted normally to light, indicating that midbrain pathways were intact. In the absence of any history from relatives of aural or auditory problems, and of any clinical or radiologic evidence of otologic abnormalities, the absence of BAEPs under technically optimal recording conditions suggested rhombencephalic death, despite the EEG. The patient subsequently became profoundly hypotensive despite an intravenous dopamine infusion and had numerous cardiac arrhythmias, and a subsequent EEG showed electrocerebral silence. The patient expired 24 hours later and autopsy revealed acute thrombosis of the upper cervical and intracranial portions of the vertebral arteries with extension into the basilar artery and resultant infarction of the entire brainstem up to the level of the midbrain. Absence of wave I was therefore, presumably due to eighth nerve ischemia, and the presence of the cochlear microphonic reflects the relative resistance of the cochlea to ischemia for short periods (5 hours in this case).

BAEPs may thus suggest the reversibility of coma even when the EEG is flat, as in cases of drug overdose. Conversely, they can suggest the irreversibil-

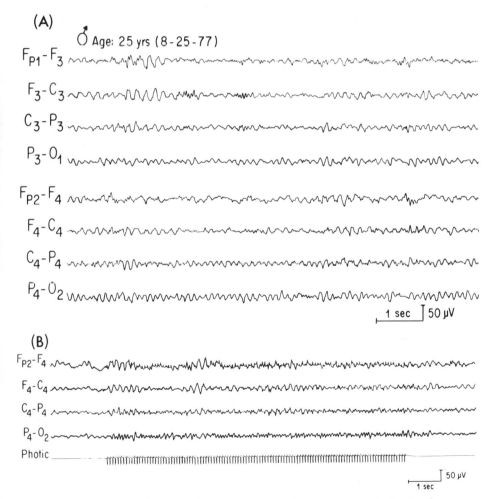

Fig. 12.16. *Mildly abnormal EEG in patient with rhombencephalic death syndrome and no BAEPs is shown in A. The segment shown represents the maximal abnormality recorded at this time, excessive anterior theta and beta activity. In addition to a normal posteriorly predominant 9 Hz alpha rhythm that attenuated symmetrically with passive eye opening, there was also a good, bilaterally symmetric driving response to photic stimulation shown over the right occipital region only in B.*

ity of an unresponsive state when the EEG is still relatively normal, by suggesting that there is widespread structural brainstem damage. BAEPs have also been shown to have prognostic value in post-traumatic coma (Greenberg et al, 1977).

Demyelinating Disease

A common diagnostic problem facing neurologists is whether the signs and symptoms attributable to a single CNS lesion are the first manifestation of MS. If a separate region of the CNS can be shown by evoked potentials to be involved—even though that involvement is not apparent from the history or physical findings—a diagnosis of MS receives some support. This use of BAEPs to identify subclinical lesions requires that the one manifest clinically be clearly outside the brainstem. For example, a patient presenting with the sole complaint of diplopia and in whom examination reveals only an internuclear ophthalmoplegia has a brainstem lesion irrespective of whether or not the BAEPs are abnormal; even if abnormalities are found, they are no more than confirmatory. Certain BAEP abnormalities could argue against MS in such a case but none would establish it, since the electrophysiologic and clinical abnormalities could easily be reflecting the same lesion. It would be more appropriate to test visual and spinal evoked potentials in such a case, since an abnormality of these would provide evidence of multiple lesions or at least of a diffuse process. Thus, only when the single CNS lesion can be clinically localized to outside the brainstem, i.e., to the cerebrum or spinal cord, will BAEPs be of diagnostic value in MS—and then only when they are abnormal. ("Cerebellar" signs and symptoms do not allow the primary lesion to be localized outside the brainstem since they may reflect involvement of cerebellar projections in the stem.)

We have studied 135 patients with clinical evidence of a single nonbrainstem CNS lesion who were referred for BAEPs, in an attempt to find a second subclinical lesion that would suggest the diagnosis of MS. Eighty-four of these patients had unilateral optic neuritis as their primary lesion and 51 had an acute or subacute thoracic or lumbar myelopathy which was of unknown etiology, was associated with a normal myelogram, and had no specific antecedents such as infection. These patients developed their symptoms and were tested between the ages of 21 and 46, were predominantly female (91F:44M) and had no significant audiometric abnormalities or subjective auditory complaints. The patients were divided into three groups: Group A consisted of patients tested during their first attack of symptoms and signs attributable to a nonbrainstem lesion, i.e., with a single lesion in time and space; Group B comprised patients tested after remission and re-exacerbation of symptoms and signs attributable to a nonbrainstem lesion, i.e., with a single lesion in space only; and Group C consisted of patients who were tested during their first attack of symptoms and signs specific for an optic nerve lesion (8 patients) or a spinal cord lesion (7 patients) but who had in addition a vague history of a nonspecific symptom not attributable either to the primary lesion or to the brainstem and which had no objective correlates, e.g., mild monocular "blurring of vision" which had never interfered with daily function, was recalled only on specific questioning, and was now associated with a normal eye examination, in those with a myelopathy.

Groups A to C thus reflected an increasing probability of having MS on clinical grounds, although there was objective evidence for only a single lesion in each group and none of these groups met the clinical criteria for classification in even the "probable MS" category of McAlpine, Lumsden, and Acheson (1972). In Figure 12.17 the height of the diagonal lines in each group shows the prevalence of BAEP abnormalities involving interpeak latency prolongation, which we consider a more definitive abnormality than relative amplitude reduction. Rate-dependent abnormalities (Fig. 12.8) were excluded from this analysis. The percentages at the lower right of each bar indicate the proportion of patients with BAEP abnormalities in each group who went on to develop clinically definite (McAlpine et al, 1972) MS within 1 to 3 years of testing.

As expected, the prevalence of BAEP abnormalities (all of which reflected subclinical lesions) increased with the factors indicating multiplicity of lesions

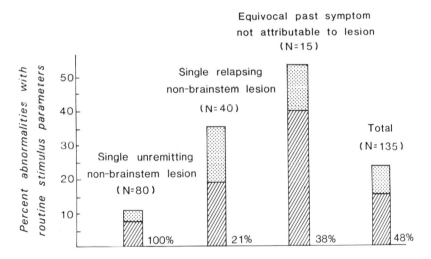

Fig. 12.17. Prevalence of BAEP abnormalities at the time of initial testing in 3 groups of patients in whom the question of MS was raised but who had objective evidence for only optic neuritis or myelopathy. The percentages at the lower right of each bar indicate the proportion of patients with BAEP abnormalities who went on to develop clinically definite MS (McAlpine et al, 1972) within 1 to 3 years of testing. The portion of each bar enclosing diagonal lines indicates the proportion of BAEP abnormalities involving interpeak latency prolongation, the stippled portion representing the relative amplitude abnormalities (IV/V:I <0.5 in Cz-A$_i$, <0.7 in Cz-M). All 80 patients in group A (left) were followed for 3 years, while patients in the other two groups were followed for only 1 to 2 years.

in time (Group B) or suggesting multiplicity in time and space (Group C). In each group, however, the BAEP abnormality was the first objective evidence of multiple lesions and, as such, helped to establish the diagnosis in these cases. All nine patients with BAEP abnormalities in Group A went on to develop clinically definite MS within 3 years of testing, although 13 (16 percent) of the patients without BAEP abnormalities did also. In Groups B and C, 21 and 38 percent of those with BAEP abnormalities developed clinically definite MS in the period of follow-up, while none of those with normal BAEPs did so. Of the total population of patients with isolated nonbrainstem lesions, thirty-one (23 percent) had BAEP abnormalities and these abnormalities accurately predicted the development of clinically definite MS in one to three years in 15 (48 percent) of the patients having them. There was no statistically significant difference in the accuracy of the different types of BAEP abnormality (latency vs amplitude) in predicting the subsequent development of MS over this period of follow-up, although the inclusion of absent waves IV/V or absent III and IV/V (with intact I) probably increased the reliability of amplitude criteria in this study. Of the 104 patients not having BAEP abnormalities, 13 (12 percent) developed definite MS over one to three years. Thus, patients with single nonbrainstem CNS lesions in this study were 4 times more likely to develop clinically definite MS within this time period than were similar patients without BAEP abnormalities at initial testing, a highly significant difference (p<0.001, chi-square analysis): The absence of an initial BAEP abnormality had no predictive value with regard to the subsequent development of MS and cannot therefore be used to "rule out" this diagnosis, as the indication for referral so often reads.

Three patients with well-documented MS whom we studied had only a wave I from one ear with no subsequent BAEPs despite optimal control of technical variables (Fig. 12.18). While it is conceivable that in each of these cases there was demyelination of the small portion of the proximal eighth nerve covered by "central" myelin, there was no audiometric evidence for eighth nerve involvement and the patients could still hear well on the affected side. We speculate that the "block" in conduction as reflected in the BAEPs occurred in projections from the ipsilateral cochlear nucleus and mainly in the subpopulation of brainstem auditory tracts which subserves BAEP generation. The cochlear nuclei themselves would, of course, be spared by any demyelinating lesion and, therefore, this finding suggests that wave II reflects axonal conduction in auditory tracts rather than synaptic activation within brainstem auditory nuclei.

This would be consistent with our clinical experience that BAEPs are more sensitive to white matter diseases than grey matter diseases involving the brainstem. Our experience of patients with progressive supranuclear palsy (PSP), a disease in which nuclei of the pontine and midbrain tegmentum degenerate but white matter is spared (Steele, Richardson, and Olszewski, 1964), and those with central pontine myelinolysis (CPM), a demyelinating lesion of the pons in which axis cylinders and brainstem nuclei are spared (Adams, Victor, and Mancall, 1959), can be used to illustrate this point. We have studied BAEPs in 3 patients with PSP and found them to be within normal limits despite an

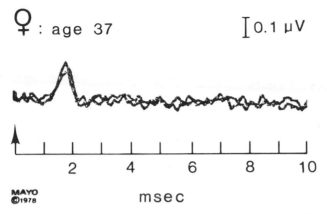

♀ : age 37   ⊥0.1 µV

2   4   6   8   10

MAYO
©1978   m s e c

Fig. 12.18. Wave I only in patient with definite MS in response to 10 per second 60 dBSL monaural click stimulation. At higher intensities, N_2 of the compound auditory nerve action potential became apparent as revealed by simultaneous electrocochleographic recording but at no intensity was any intra-axial wave II activity seen, i.e. far-field activity with appropriate latency that was not at tenuated in Cz-A_c derivations or seen in Cz-ankle recordings.

advanced stage of the disease with complete ophthalmoplegia, obtundation, and severe corticobulbar tract signs; in contrast, all the patients with CPM (1 pathologically proven, 2 highly likely on clinical grounds) that we studied, had marked BAEP abnormalities (Stockard and Sharbrough, 1979). In Wernicke's encephalopathy, the predominantly grey matter lesions have a periventricular distribution in the brainstem, somewhat similar to that of white matter lesions in brainstem MS. Yet BAEPs have been normal in Wernicke's cases in our experience, no matter how severe the brainstem dysfunction (Fig. 12.19), but abnormal in approximately one-third of all our MS patients, many of whom had no clinical evidence of brainstem dysfunction. Such comparisons are made with the realization that the nature of the lesions rather than their predilection for tracts or nuclei may account largely for observed differences in the prevalence of associated BAEP abnormality. For example, brainstem gliomas are associated with a very high (greater than 90 percent) prevalence of BAEP abnormality, but this may be because they grow slowly and infiltrate widely before they cause clinical decompensation, and thus there is a better chance that they will have involved the auditory pathway by the time BAEPs are tested. Moreover, they exert prominent pressure effects on areas of the brainstem they do not involve directly, increasing the likelihood of indirect involvement of the auditory pathway. In contrast, patients with brainstem infarcts come very quickly to BAEP testing because of the sudden onset of a conspicuous neurologic deficit and, in accord with the improbability of a given infarct (if small) involving the brainstem auditory pathway, BAEPs are normal more often than not if the lesion is embolic. Brainstem infarcts associated with hemorrhage or edema are more likely to be associated with BAEP abnormality as are those, of course, involving the anterior inferior cerebellar artery and other vessels directly perfusing brainstem auditory structures. Occlusion of the posterior inferior cerebellar artery is not associated with BAEP abnormality in our experience.

Posterior Fossa Tumors

The diagnostic application of BAEPs with the greatest therapeutic implications is the early detection of posterior fossa tumors. We have previously reported BAEP abnormalities in 12 of 15 consecutive patients who proved to

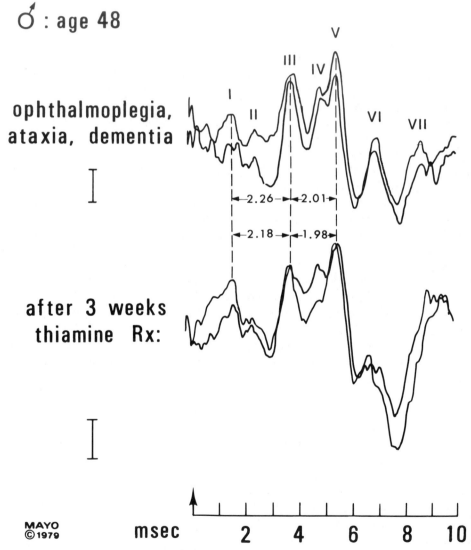

Fig. 12.19. *Normal BAEPs before and after treatment in 48-year old male with Wernicke's encephalopathy. Cals: 0.1 μV.*

have infratentorial neoplasms (Stockard, Stockard and Sharbrough, 1977). In 2 of these patients, who had no neurologic signs, BAEP abnormalities first indicated the presence of an intracanalicular acoustic neuroma in one and a fourth ventricular ependymoma in the other; in these patients, the test led directly to the performance of contrast studies that would not have otherwise been performed, and to subsequent removal of the tumors at surgery. In subsequent screening of 307 patients with equivocal or negative findings on clinical examination and non-invasive radiologic studies who were referred for the test to "rule out a brainstem lesion," 9 (2.9 percent) had BAEP abnormalities consistent with intra-axial (5 patients) or extra-axial (4 patients) posterior fossa tumors that were subsequently confirmed. None of the other 298 cases without BAEP abnormality have yet (average 1 year follow-up) shown evidence of posterior fossa lesions. Several of these cases and others demonstrating the BAEP patterns associated with intra-axial and extra-axial posterior fossa tumors will now be discussed.

Intra-axial Tumors. Prolongation of the III-V interpeak latency suggests disturbance of central auditory conduction within the brainstem. In the case of tumors, this is usually the result of an intrinsic brainstem lesion although it may also be the result of an extra-axial lesion compressing the stem. Prolongation of both the I-III and III-V IPLs from the same or both ears is suggestive of multilevel disturbance of conduction in the brainstem auditory pathway and, when the I-II IPL is normal, this is the pattern often seen with infiltrating, multilevel gliomas (Fig. 12.20).

Figure 12.20A shows the BAEPs from one ear of a patient who was admitted to hospital with the isolated symptom of severe orthostatic dizziness. Examination was unremarkable except for a marked drop of blood pressure on standing and mild gait ataxia, which was initially attributed to her orthostatic dizziness. A sweat test revealed anhidrosis and a diagnosis of Shy-Drager syndrome was made. CT scan with and without contrast was equivocal but screening BAEPs indicated a multilevel intrinsic brainstem lesion (Fig. 12.20A, top). The patient accordingly had a rhombencephalogram that confirmed the presence of an intrinsic pontine and midbrain lesion, and this ultimately proved to be a glioma. Following irradiation of the area, her gait ataxia improved as did brainstem auditory conduction as reflected in the BAEPs—the I-V IPL decreased from 5.48 to 4.79 msec with right monaural stimulation and from 5.61 to 4.80 msec with left monaural stimulation. The IV/V:I amplitude ratio increased from well below to well above unity from each ear (mastoid reference employed). These changes are shown for the left ear at the bottom of Figure 12.20A.

Figure 12.20B shows the BAEPs in a similar case but one in which they indicated progression rather than regression of the intrinsic brainstem tumor. The patient was a 13-year-old female referred for evaluation of intermittent left facial myokymia of 6 months' duration. Apart from the myokymia, she was asymptomatic and had no neurologic signs. All studies except for the BAEPs were normal or noncontributory, including CT scans with and without contrast,

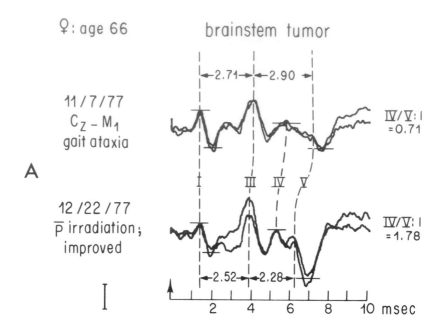

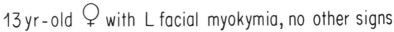

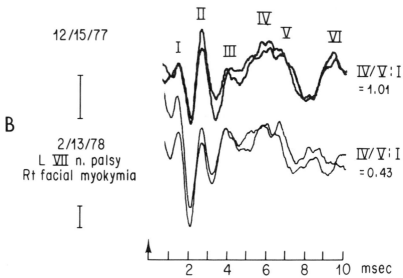

Fig. 12.20. *Serial BAEP studies in two cases of brainstem glioma described in text. Cals: 0.1 μV.*

isotope brain scan, skull tomograms, electronystagmogram, audiogram, blink reflex and facial nerve conduction studies. EMG showed only left facial myokymia, and a rhombencephalogram was indeterminate because the tonsils were down in the foramen magnum and dye could not be passed into the posterior fossa. This study was interpreted as consistent with either an Arnold-Chiari malformation or a posterior fossa mass lesion, and the BAEP findings favored the latter. After one month, the patient began to show evidence of clinical deterioration—left lower motor neuron facial weakness and bilateral facial myokymia—and BAEPs showed a parallel electrophysiologic worsening (Fig. 12.20B, bottom) that was reflected only in a decrease in the IV/V:I amplitude ratio. CT scans were still normal at this time as were short latency (5 to 25 msec) somatosensory evoked potentials. The patient proved to have a pontine glioma.

The pattern of "multilevel" disturbance shown in Figure 12.20A could probably result from a lesion at one level, given the complexity of BAEP generation, but we have not seen it. Certainly, no BAEP pattern is specific for lesion type; this one reflects only the extent of the lesion, whether due to infiltrating glioma as in the above cases, to multifocal lesions as in MS or patchy vertebrobasilar infarctions, or to compression of multiple levels of the brainstem auditory pathway by intrinsic or extrinsic tumors. In the case of tumors extrinsic to the brainstem, however, there are usually clues in the BAEP pattern to the extra-axial location of the lesion, as will now be discussed.

Extra-axial Tumors. The ability of extra-axial tumors to produce BAEP abnormalities usually associated with intrinsic brainstem lesions (i.e. III-V IPL prolongation) is well-illustrated in the case of large cerebellopontine angle (CPA) tumors which compress the stem. This secondary BAEP abnormality can be of diagnostic value if recognized; when produced by an angle tumor it usually consists of a prolongation of the III-V or IV-V IPL from the ear *contralateral* to the lesion, without an associated I-III IPL prolongation from that ear (Fig. 12.21). In contrast, the most common BAEP abnormalities found ipsilateral to such lesions (Fig. 12.22) are absence or abnormality of wave I due to involvement of the eighth nerve and/or cochlear blood supply, and absence or abnormality of all waves after I or even after II (Fig. 12.22A, B, C). This last observation (Fig. 12.14) indicates that a part of wave II is generated in the proximal auditory nerve. Wave I or wave III may be selectively absent even though wave IV/V and III or wave IV/V and I are present (Fig. 12.22D). When both waves I and III are elicited from the ear ipsilateral to the lesion, the most common single abnormality is I-III IPL prolongation (Fig. 12.22E). This, like the other patterns from the ipsilateral ear, may develop before any "hard" clinical signs or radiologic abnormality, and we have yet to observe normal BAEPs from an ear ipsilateral to a CPA lesion, but as with almost any neurologic diagnosis * would not exclude it on the basis of normal BAEPs. The III-V IPL on the side of the lesion is often normal even when the III-V or IV-V

---

* Brainstem death can be excluded if all BAEPs are normal.

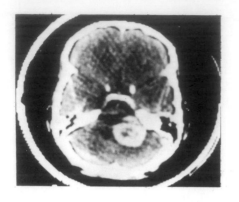

Pre-op contrast CT scan

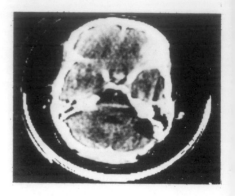

Post-op contrast CT scan

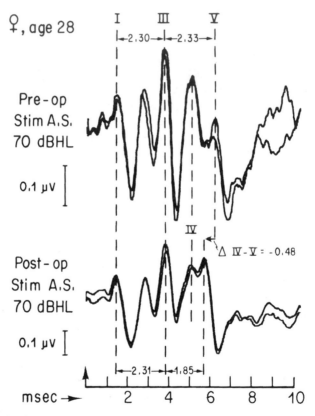

Fig. 12.21. *Effects of brainstem compression and decompression on the BAEPs elicited from the ear contralateral to an extra-axial posterior fossa tumor. Fourth ventricle can be seen to be displaced to the left in the pre-op CT scan and returns to midline following tumor removal as seen in the post-op scan. Such lesions produce "crossed" BAEP abnormalities consisting of a late (in the III-V segment) abnormality from the ear contralateral to the tumor that is due to brainstem compression, and an early, I-III segment abnormality on the side of the lesion (abnormal I and absent III in this case, Fig. 12.22D). There was no clinical or CT evidence of increased intraventricular pressure.*

IPL from the contralateral ear is prolonged; these are usually cases where there is not enough brainstem compression to cause "notching" of the brainstem against posterior fossa structures on the side opposite to the lesion. This observation suggests that generation of wave V is mainly contralateral to the stimulated ear and at a level rostral to that where IV is generated. All of our electroanatomic correlations (Fig. 12.21) suggest a primarily pontine origin for wave IV.

With severe compression below the midpontine level, the latencies of both waves IV and V from the ear contralateral to the lesion may be prolonged relative to waves I, II and III. As shown in Figure 12.21, BAEP effects of brainstem compression reverse with decompression of the posterior fossa and tumor removal. Such BAEP changes can be diagnostically helpful in cases where there is a question of whether cranial nerve deficits contralateral to an extra-axial posterior fossa tumor that has been localized with the CT scan are an indirect effect of the lesion—due to stem compression against the contralateral side of the posterior fossa—or are direct effects from extension of the lesion around the stem or from a second, contralateral lesion. In the case shown in Figure 12.21, for example, there was bilateral trigeminal nerve dysfunction that was equally prominent on the side contralateral to as on the side ipsilateral to the lesion. The BAEP findings, however, were consistent with a single right CPA lesion involving the acoustic nerve and compressing the brainstem, thereby accounting for the left sided cranial nerve signs. At surgery, a right acoustic neuroma was found compressing the brainstem and, following its removal, the left-sided cranial nerve deficit and IV-V IPL prolongation from the left ear did indeed resolve (Fig. 12.21).

In many cases in which there is an extra-axial tumor compressing the brainstem, the resultant displacement of midline structures can be visualized on CT scan, as in Figure 12.21. However, there may be sufficient brainstem compression to produce the characteristic BAEP abnormality seen in Figure 12.21 before there is CT evidence of such compression. We recently studied a patient with neurofibromatosis who had had subtotal resection of a left acoustic neuroma 7 years earlier (1970). When she presented in late 1977 with progressive right-sided cranial nerve (V, VII-IX) deficits, it was suspected that she now had a right acoustic neuroma. The BAEPs from her right ear, however, did not reveal any of the patterns shown in Figure 12.22 that occur ipsilateral to such lesions. Instead, they showed the pattern seen from the ear contralateral to the acoustic neuroma in Figure 12.21—normal waves I, II, III, and IV but an abnormal wave V which was prolonged in latency relative to wave III and had an abnormal, bifid morphology (Fig. 12.23) that was unrelated to any technical variables, an initial consideration. No BAEPs could be elicited from the left ear because of the previous eighth nerve transection on that side at the time of the earlier surgery. CT scanning was noncontributory because it showed no right acoustic neuroma and only residual tumor tissue in the left CPA; most importantly in view of the new right-sided cranial nerve deficits, the CT scan of the posterior fossa revealed no evidence of brainstem compression by the residual left-sided tumor (Fig. 12.23). Despite the absence of structural evidence of such

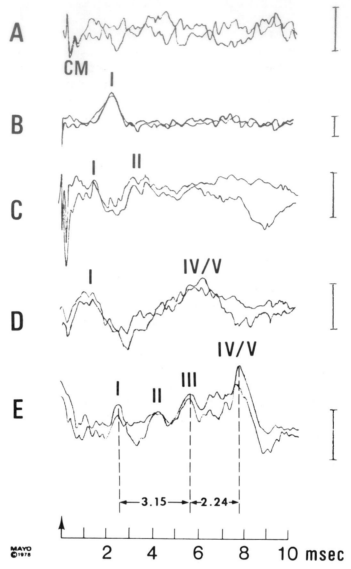

Fig. 12.22. Five different BAEP patterns that may be elicited from the ear ipsilateral to confirmed cerebellopontine angle tumors. One additional pattern, related to D above, is selective absence of wave I (K. H. Chiappa, personal communication). In three of the examples above, the BAEP abnormality shown was the first (C) or only (B, E) objective evidence for CPA lesions. Lesions were: A—large intracanalicular acoustic neurilemmoma which extended into CPA and compressed brainstem, resulting in false localization clinically. B—small petrous ridge meningioma compressing extracanalicular portion of eighth nerve and pontomedullary junction of brainstem. C—aneurysmal dilatation of tortuous basilar artery impinging on most proximal portion of eighth nerve resulting in segmental demyelination of nerve at its entrance into the brainstem. D—large extracanalicular acoustic neurilemmoma resulting in severe pontine compression and bilateral cranial nerve deficits (cf. Fig. 12.21). E—small cholesteatoma involving eighth nerve at its entrance into CPA. Cals: 0.1 μV.

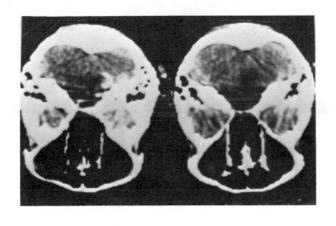

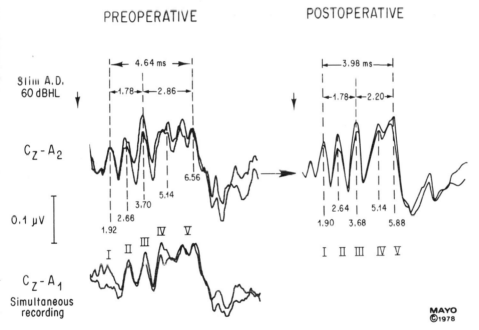

PREOPERATIVE   POSTOPERATIVE

Fig. 12.23. *BAEPs in 63-year-old female with recurrent left acoustic neurilemmoma. Patient had neurofibromatosis and was, therefore, thought to have a second, right acoustic neuroma when she presented with rapidly progressive right-sided cranial nerve deficits and no clinical evidence to suggest that these were due to brainstem compression. CT scans without (left) and with (right) contrast showed residual left neuroma, unchanged in appearance from that of three years earlier, and showed no evidence of either right-sided lesion or stem compression. All BAEPs could be resolved from right ear and identified with aid of simultaneous $Cz–A_c$ recording as shown. These revealed normal I-III segment and prolonged III-V with abnormal wave V, arguing against right acoustic neuroma and suggesting instead stem compression from left. Normal post-op BAEPs at right.*

compression, the BAEPs from the right ear indicated considerable functional compression of the pons, sufficient to prolong the III-V IPL by over half a millisecond. They thus suggested that the new, right-sided cranial nerve deficits were all due to stem compression from the left side rather than direct involvement by any right-sided lesion. Surgical exploration of the left CPA revealed a large regrowth of left acoustic neurilemmoma compressing the pons, the tumor mass being considerably greater than suggested by the contrast CT scan. Following removal of the recurrent left-sided tumor, the right-sided cranial nerve deficits disappeared and the III-V IPL from the right ear reverted to normal (Fig. 12.23), as expected.

CONCLUDING COMMENT

The most important clinical applications of BAEPs in adult neurology are dealt with above—evaluation of the cause and reversibility of coma, the early diagnosis of multiple sclerosis, and detection (and crude localization) of posterior fossa tumors. BAEP abnormalities are, of course, not specific for any type of brainstem pathology and occur with a wide variety of other neurologic syndromes as described in references cited in the Introduction. We have encountered a significantly ($p < 0.05$) increased prevalence of I-V IPL prolongation in three neurological syndromes in which involvement of the subcortical auditory pathway was not expected: hereditary sensorimotor neuropathy (Fig. 12.24), sleep apnea (Fig. 12.25) and spastic dysphonia (Sharbrough, Stockard and Aronson, 1978). These preliminary findings are noted here so that BAEP abnormalities encountered in these syndromes will not be misinterpreted as necessarily reflecting a second lesion or disease process. In only one of these syndromes is the basis for BAEP abnormality reasonably clear and that is the I-III IPL prolongation in certain polyneuropathies, which presumably reflects involvement of the eighth cranial nerve as well as peripheral nerve. (Note the wide I-II separation but normal II-III IPL in Fig. 12.24). However, we have also noted a temporarily increased III-V IPL in a patient with well-documented inflammatory cranial polyneuritis (but associated long-tract signs that reversed with recovery) and borderline III-V IPLs (Fig. 12.24, left ear) in some cases of hereditary sensorimotor neuropathy, suggesting that the mechanism of the BAEP changes may be more complex than simple extra-axial involvement of primary auditory neurons.

The finding of BAEP abnormality in some patients with sleep apnea is of particular interest to us because of the reported associations between sudden infant death syndrome (SIDS) and sleep apnea (Shannon, Kelly, and O'Connell, 1977) and SIDS and brainstem gliosis (Takashima et al, 1978). The only infant in whom we have obtained screening BAEPs who subsequently went on to die a "crib death" had no retrocochlear BAEP abnormality, but we hope that others with access to large populations of infants at high risk for SIDS will systematically evaluate the possibility of some sort of premonitory BAEP pro-

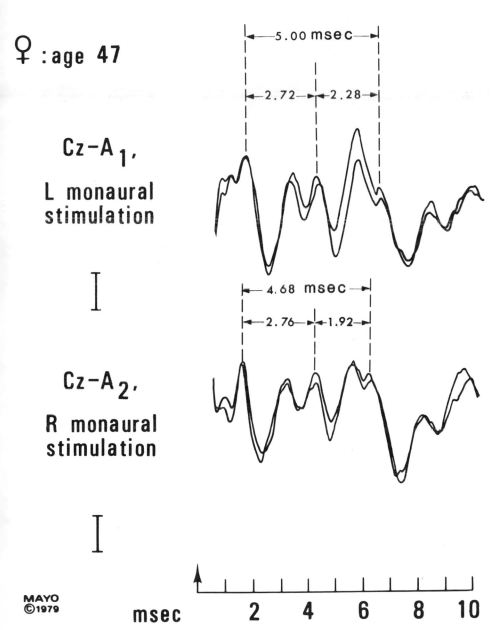

Fig. 12.24. *Bilateral I-III IPL prolongation in an audiometrically normal patient with a predominantly demyelinating type of hereditary sensorimotor neuropathy (HSMN). The patient was diagnosed as having Charcot-Marie-Tooth disease 26 years earlier at the age of 21 and all studies, including EMG, nerve conductions, and nerve and muscle biopsies were consistent with the diagnosis of HSMN. BAEPs were performed because of an 18-month history of "dizzy spells" that were sometimes vertiginous in nature. Cal: 0.1 μV.*

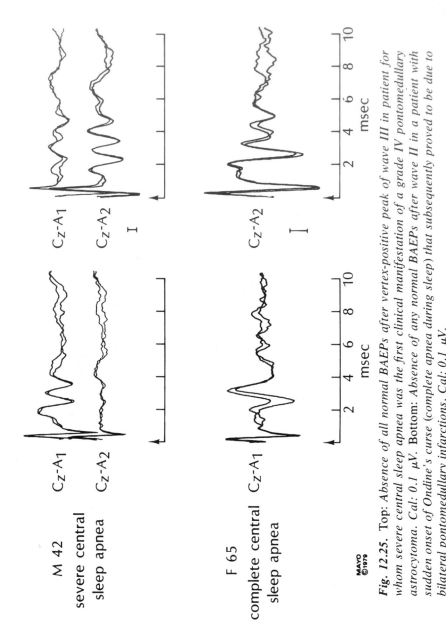

Fig. 12.25. Top: *Absence of all normal BAEPs after vertex-positive peak of wave III in patient for whom severe central sleep apnea was the first clinical manifestation of a grade IV pontomedullary astrocytoma. Cal: 0.1 μV.* Bottom: *Absence of any normal BAEPs after wave II in a patient with sudden onset of Ondine's curse (complete apnea during sleep) that subsequently proved to be due to bilateral pontomedullary infarctions. Cal: 0.1 μV.*

file in potential victims of this syndrome. All four patients (two shown in Fig. 12.25) with central sleep apnea and abnormal BAEPs whom we studied proved to have intrinsic brainstem lesions (Stockard et al, 1979b). The BAEP abnormalities in some adults with spastic dysphonia are of unknown significance but raise the possibility that organic brainstem and/or cranial nerve dysfunction underlies the syndrome in a subset of afflicted patients.

The findings of unexpected BAEP abnormalities in such syndromes illustrates both the potential value and potential danger of using BAEPs as the independent variable in neurologic investigations. BAEPs are themselves highly dependent on a number of physiologic and technical variables, which must themselves be controlled and minimized before statistical criteria of "abnormality" can be meaningfully applied. As an example of suboptimal control of physiologic variables, the I-V IPLs reported as abnormal by Gilroy and Lynn (1978) in 3 cases of olivopontocerebellar atrophy are within our normal limits for age-matched, sex-matched controls when their methods are employed. The upper limit of normal for I-V IPL of less than 4.2 msec could conceivably have been valid for the young female controls in that study, but was probably too low for the male and elderly female patients to whom it was applied. As an example of inadequate control of technical variables, Hashimoto, Ishiyama, and Tozuka (1979) overlooked the profound BAEP effects seen in normal subjects (Fig. 12.9) when using a periaural reference contralateral rather than ipsilateral to acoustic stimulation. They attributed the differences in these two recording derivations to asymmetric involvement of the brainstem by lesions, when the observed asymmetries were actually predictable from the recording derivations employed (Stockard et al, 1978b). In one case with normal BAEPs (their Case 4), abnormality was interpreted on the basis of the normal field effect seen in the contralateral ear derivation, and it was erroneously concluded that the sensitivity of the test to pathology had been increased. A number of other errors in defining BAEP abnormalities have been pointed out by Chiappa et al (1979), who themselves failed to control for several physiologic variables (age, sex, audiogram) and for click phase, a major technical determinant of the normal "waveform variations" they described (cf. Figs. 12.7 and 12.12). Rowe (1978) probably also overestimated the "intrinsic variability" of BAEPs by not minimizing certain extrinsic (mainly technical) factors, but appropriately emphasized the importance of prior knowledge of normal variability to any clinical BAEP applications.

Clearly, the normal variability of BAEPs requires analysis rather than mere description. Uncritical tabulation of numerical ranges and pattern variations can conceal reducible, methodologic sources of BAEP variation which decrease the sensitivity of the test to pathologic variations. Analysis of the non-pathologic factors in BAEP variability reveals that most of those factors, if recognized, can be largely controlled or controlled for (Stockard et al, 1978b). Proper attention to technical details and patient characteristics will greatly reduce normal BAEP variability but will not eliminate it, and each lab should operationally define that irreducible BAEP variability for itself, with the methods intended for use on patients. We hope that these considerations of normal BAEP variation and the principles of abnormal BAEP interpretation put forth earlier will be of value to other neurologists in their applications of this promising new tool.

REFERENCES

Adams, R. D., Victor, M., and Mancall, E. L. (1959). Central pontine myelinolysis: a hitherto undescribed disease occurring in alcoholic and malnourished patients. Arch. Neurol. Psych., *81:*154.

Bhargava, V. K. and McKean, C. M. (1977). Role of 5-hydroxytryptamine in the modulation of acoustic brainstem (far-field) potentials. Neuropharmacology, *16:*447.

Chiappa, K. H., Gladstone, K. J., and Young, R. R. (1979). Brainstem auditory evoked responses: studies of waveform variation in 50 normal human subjects. Arch. Neurol., *36:*81.

Chu, N. S., Squires, I. C., and Starr, A. (1978). Auditory brainstem potentials in chronic ethanol intoxication and alcohol withdrawal. Arch. Neurol., *35:*596.

Coats, A. and Martin, J. (1977). Human auditory nerve action potentials and brainstem evoked responses. Arch. Otolaryngol., *103:*605.

Cooper, R., Ossleton, J. W., and Shaw, J. C. (1974). EEG Technology. 2nd edn., p. 163. Butterworths, London.

Don, M. and Eggermont, J. (1978). Analysis of click-evoked brainstem potentials in man using high-pass noise masking. J. Acoustical Soc. Am., *63:*1984.

Gilroy, J., Lynn, G. E., Ristow, G. E., and Pellerin, R. J. (1977). Auditory evoked brainstem potentials in a case of "locked-in" syndrome. Arch. Neurol., *34:*492.

Gilroy, J. and Lynn, G. E. (1978). Computerized tomography and auditory-evoked potentials. Use in diagnosis of olivopontocerebellar degeneration. Arch. Neurol., *35:*143.

Greenberg, R. P., Martin, D. J., Becker, D. P., and Miller, J. D. (1977). Evaluation of brain function in severe human head trauma with multimodality evoked potentials. J. Neurosurg., *47:*150.

Hashimoto, I., Ishiyama, Y., and Tozuka, G. (1979). Bilaterally recorded brainstem auditory evoked responses. Their asymmetric abnormalities and lesions of the brainstem. Arch. Neurol., *36:*161.

Hecox, K. (1975). Electrophysiologic correlates of human auditory development. In: Infant Perception, Cohen, L. B. and Salapetek, P., Eds., Vol. 2, p. 151. Academic Press, New York.

Hecox, K., Lastimosa, C., Mokotoff, B., and Sandlin, R. (1979). Effects of increasing stimulus rate on brainstem auditory evoked responses. Arch. Neurol., in press.

Jewett, D. L. and Williston, J. S. (1971). Auditory evoked far-fields averaged from the scalp of humans. Brain, *94:*681.

Jones, T. A. and Stockard, J. J. (1979). Temperature-dependence of acute ethanol effects on brainstem auditory evoked potential latencies. Electroencephalogr. Clin. Neurophysiol., in press.

Jones, T. A., Stockard, J. J., and Henry, K. R. (1978). Temperature-independent alteration of brainstem auditory evoked responses by enflurane. Society for Neuroscience Abstracts, *4:*154.

Jones, T. A., Stockard, J. J., and Weidner, W. J. (1979). The effects of temperature and acute ethanol intoxication on brainstem auditory evoked potentials in the cat. Electroencephalogr. Clin. Neurophysiol., in press.

McAlpine, D., Lumsden, C. E., and Acheson, E. D. (1972). Multiple Sclerosis: A Reappraisal. 2nd edn., p. 202. E. and S. Livingstone, Edinburgh.

Robinson, K. and Rudge, P. (1977). Abnormalities of the auditory evoked potentials in patients with multiple sclerosis. Brain, *100:*19.

Rowe, M. J. (1978). Normal variability of the brainstem auditory evoked response in young and old adult subjects. Electroencephalogr. Clin. Neurophysiol., *44:*459.

Salamy, A., McKean, C., and Buda, F. (1976). Maturational changes in auditory transmission as reflected in human brainstem potentials. Brain Res., *96:*361.

Shannon, D. C., Kelly, D. H., and O'Connell, K. (1977). Abnormal regulation of ventilation in infants at risk for sudden-infant-death-syndrome. N. Engl. J. Med., *14:*747.

Sharbrough, F. W., Stockard, J. J., and Aronson, A. E. (1978). Brainstem auditory-evoked responses in spastic dysphonia. Trans. Am. Neurol. Assoc., *103:*198.

Sohmer, H. and Feinmesser, M. (1967). Cochlear action potentials recorded from the external ear in man. Ann. Otol. Laryngol. Rhinol., *76:*427.

Sohmer, H., Feinmesser, M., and Szabo, G. (1974). Sources of electrocochleographic responses as studied in patients with brain damage. Electroencephalogr. Clin. Neurophysiol., 237:663.

Sohmer, H., Gafni, M., and Chisin, R. (1978). Auditory nerve and brainstem responses: comparison in awake and unconscious subjects. Arch. Neurol., *35:*228.

Squires, K. C., Chu, N., and Starr, A. (1978). Acute effects of alcohol on auditory brainstem potentials in humans. Science, *201:*174.

Starr, A. (1976). Auditory brainstem responses in brain death. Brain, *99:*543.

Starr, A. and Achor, L. J. (1975). Auditory brainstem responses in neurological disease. Arch. Neurol., *32:*761.

Starr, A. and Hamilton, A. E. (1976). Correlation between confirmed sites of neurological lesions and abnormalities of far-field auditory brainstem responses. Electroencephalogr. Clin. Neurophysiol., *41:*595.

Starr, A., Amlie, R. N., Martin, W. H., and Sanders, S. (1977). Development of auditory function in newborn infants revealed by auditory brainstem potentials. Pediatrics, *60:*831.

Steele, J. C., Richardson, J. C., and Olszewski, J. (1964). Progressive supranuclear palsy. Arch. Neurol., *10:*333.

Stockard, J. E., Stockard, J. J., Westmoreland, B. F., and Corfits, J. F. (1979a). Normal variation of brainstem auditory evoked potentials as a function of stimulus and subject characteristics. Arch. Neurol., *36:*823.

Stockard, J. J. and Rossiter, V. S. (1977). Clinical and pathologic correlates of brainstem auditory response abnormalities. Neurology, *27:*316.

Stockard, J. J. and Sharbrough, F. W. (1979). Unique contributions of short-latency auditory and somatosensory evoked potentials to neurologic diagnosis. In: Clinical Uses of Cerebral, Brainstem and Spinal Somatosensory Evoked Potentials, Desmedt, J. E., Ed., p. 231. Karger, Basel.

Stockard, J. J., Rossiter, V. S., Wiederholt, W. C., and Kobayashi, R. M. (1976). Brainstem auditory-evoked responses in suspected central pontine myelinolysis. Arch. Neurol., *33:*726.

Stockard, J. J., Sharbrough, F. W., and Tinker, J. A. (1978a). Effects of hypothermia on the human brainstem auditory response. Ann. Neurol., *3:*368.

Stockard, J. J., Stockard, J. E., and Sharbrough, F. W. (1977). Detection and localization of occult lesions with brainstem auditory responses. Mayo Clin. Proc., *52:*761.

Stockard, J. J., Stockard, J. E., and Sharbrough, F. W. (1978b). Nonpathologic factors influencing brainstem auditory evoked potentials. Am. J. EEG Technol., *18:*177.

Stockard, J. J., Sharbrough, F. W., Staats, B. A., and Westbrook, P. R. (1979b). Brainstem auditory evoked potentials in sleep apnea. Electroencephalogr. Clin. Neurophysiol., in press.

Streletz, L. J., Katz, L., Hohenberger, M., and Cracco, R. Q. (1977). Scalp recorded auditory evoked potentials and sonomotor responses: an evaluation of components and recording techniques. Electroencephalogr. Clin. Neurophysiol., *43:*192.

Takashima, S., Armstrong, D., Becker, L., and Bryan, C. (1978). Cerebral hypoperfusion in the sudden infant death syndrome. Brainstem gliosis and vasculature. Ann. Neurol., *4:*257.

Yagi T. and Kaga K. (1979). The effect of click repetition rate on the latency of the auditory evoked brain stem response and its clinical use for a neurologic diagnosis. Arch. Otorhinolaryngol., *222:*91.

13

Scalp-Recorded Somatosensory Evoked Potentials

DENIS R. GIBLIN

INTRODUCTION

It was just over 30 years ago that Dawson (1947a) showed that somatosensory evoked potentials (SEPs) were fairly well localized to the scalp overlying the somatosensory cortex of the cerebral hemisphere contralateral to applied stimuli; Dawson gave reasons to believe that they were not artifactual in nature but were generated in the underlying brain. A few years later he (Dawson, 1954) went on to describe an ingenious method of automatic averaging of scalp potentials, which greatly facilitated recording of the SEP: the potentials evoked by successive stimuli added or summated while random potentials tended to cancel out. Other methods were devised (Debecker and Desmedt, 1964; Desmedt, Debecker, and Manil, 1965) but the dramatic expansion of research in this field followed the introduction of compact commercially available computers, specifically adapted to electrophysiologic purposes, in the early 1960s.

METHODS

Subjects are examined, either lying down or sitting in a comfortable chair with a head rest, in a quiet room that may have to be shielded if there is a great deal of electrical interference. The subject is instructed to relax to minimize artifact from muscle, to move as little as possible, and not to talk during recording periods. Desmedt (1971) emphasizes that the temperature of the stimulated limb should be monitored and maintained above 34° C by gentle warming if necessary, so that the deep temperature is 35° -36° C.

Stimulus

Usually brief electrical square-wave pulses (100 to 500 μsec) are applied through metal electrodes placed on the skin over the nerve trunk, or through ring electrodes on the fingers (Dawson, 1956; Debecker and Desmedt, 1964). The skin should be washed or swabbed with ether or other fat solvent and the electrodes smeared with conducting jelly. It is probably unnecessary to abrade the skin but, because skin impedance and resistance is relatively high and may change as a result of stimulation, it is desirable to use a constant-current stimulator isolated from ground, such as was introduced by Allison, Goff, and Brey (1967), and to monitor the current periodically with a current probe. Placing the grounding electrode on the limb proximal to the stimulation site helps to decrease stimulus artifact.

The cathode should be placed over the nerve trunk proximal to the anode, and its position adjusted so that the paresthesiae evoked by a stimulus of a given intensity are maximal. The cathode is then fixed in position and the limb firmly supported.

Satisfactory SEPs can be recorded with stimulation of almost any nerve trunk at various levels in the limb. The greatest experience is with stimulation of the median or ulnar nerves with the cathode placed just proximal to the wrist, or with digital stimulation. Desmedt et al (1966a) have warned that, when investigating patients with suspected median nerve pathology, stimulating electrodes must be applied to the distal phalanges of the fingers since more proximal sites in the digits will evoke impulses in fibers travelling in the radial nerve and give misleading results. Veale, Mark, and Rees (1973) found that the duration of the stimulus pulse affects the proportion of sensory and motor fibers excited. Very brief pulses of the order of 10 μsec, applied to the ulnar nerve at the wrist, excited impulses in both sensory and motor axons, whereas pulses of 1 msec or longer preferentially excited sensory fibers. Stimulation rates of 0.5 to 1 per second are convenient, but potentials with latencies greater than 100 msec will be attenuated; if only the earliest components of the response are of concern, higher rates are permissible.

The application of electric shocks to nerve or skin is certainly not a physiologic mode of sensory stimulation and a number of authors, beginning with Halliday and Mason (1964), have investigated the use of mechanical stimulation. To be effective, mechanical stimuli must be applied abruptly so that impulses are initiated in a number of mechanoreceptive fibers within a brief time. Sears (1959) showed that brisk taps delivered to a fingernail evoked recordable action potentials in digital nerve and in the median or ulnar nerves proximally, and Halliday and Mason (1964) showed that satisfactory cerebral evoked responses could be recorded to such stimuli. Methodologic problems with mechanical stimulation include control of stimulus intensity and provision of a signal indicating the occurrence of the stimulus, which is fundamental to any averaging method. Using as a stimulus abrupt changes of skin temperature, Duclaux et al (1974) have recorded potentials over the contralateral parietal area, but as yet this new technique has not been employed clinically.

Recording Arrangements

The recording of nerve action potentials with electrodes on the skin (Dawson and Scott, 1949) or needle electrodes (Desmedt, 1971) is a standard procedure in clinical neurophysiology and is discussed briefly in Chapter 7.

Potentials are recorded from the scalp using silver EEG electrodes filled with conducting jelly and fixed in place with collodion, or with fine needles placed subcutaneously. Electrodes may be placed using the 10-20 system conventional in electroencephalography and this has advantages, particularly for investigating the distribution of responses over the scalp (Goff et al, 1962, 1969, 1977). Giblin (1964) and others have found that the SEP when stimulating nerves of the upper extremity is usually maximally recorded by an electrode placed 7 to 8 cm from the midline, 2.5 cm behind a line connecting the vertex with the external auditory meatus; this is believed to approximately overlie the "hand" region of the postcentral gyrus and is generally between C3 and P3 or C4 and P4 of the 10-20 system. Records from electrodes only a short distance from this placement often showed diminished amplitude or altered configuration of the SEP (Fig. 13.1). The corresponding site, optimal for recording responses from leg stimulation, falls on the same coronal plane but 2 to 3 cm from the midline (i.e. 2 to 3 cm behind and 2 to 3 cm lateral to the vertex electrode, Cz). Preliminary recording from an array of electrodes, clustered in the vicinity of these placements, allows the one best showing the response to be selected.

It is now widely accepted that so-called monopolar or referential recording is generally preferred to bipolar recording. Ideally, the reference electrode should not itself record cerebral potentials evoked by the stimulus nor potentials generated by muscle or structures in the orbit, whether time-locked to the stimulus or not. There is probably no reference site that meets the ideal, for Cracco and Cracco (1976) have recently reported that all electrodes on the head pick up early potentials generated subcortically. Goff et al (1969) prefer to use the earlobe contralateral to the applied stimulus, while Desmedt (1971) and his colleagues routinely employ as reference an electrode on the upper forehead, and Giblin (1964) employed an electrode 7 cm anterior to the one over the postcentral gyrus or on the midline.

A serious hazard in SEP recording is contamination of the records by muscle potentials that may be present more or less continuously. A somewhat different problem are myogenic potentials which appear to be time-locked to the stimulus and thus have to be differentiated from potentials of cerebral origin. First reported by Bickford et al (1964), they were most prominent with auditory but seen also with visual and somatosensory stimulation. The myogenic responses evoked by median nerve stimulation were investigated by Cracco and Bickford (1968) and found to consist of potentials similiar in latency

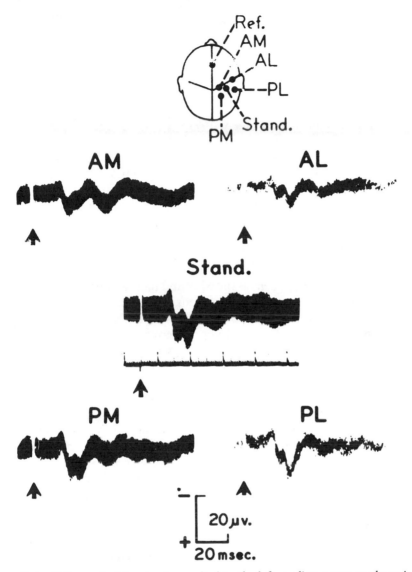

Fig. 13.1. *SEPs evoked by shocks applied to the left median nerve at the wrist and recorded by scalp electrodes in the vicinity of the hand area of the right postcentral gyrus. The "standard" electrode is 7 cm lateral to the midline and placed as in Figure 13.3. AM and PM are 4 cm, and AL and PL 10 cm lateral to the midline. AM and AL are 3 cm anterior to PM and PL. In each case the reference electrode is on the midline 7 cm anterior to the vertex. Shocks were applied at the same time in each sweep, indicated by the arrow, and the responses were revealed by photographic superimposition of 100 consecutive sweeps. In this and subsequent figures, an upward deflection indicates that the potential at the active electrode is negative with respect to the reference. The records are from the same subject as those seen in Figure 13.3 and the similarity of the response recorded by the "standard" electrode is evident. P22 and P30 are of similar amplitude in the response recorded from the standard electrode and PM, but P22 predominates in the record from AM while P30 is the larger component at PL (from Giblin, D. R. 1964. Ann. N.Y. Acad. Sci., 112, 93).*

but different in distribution from the SEP, being largest over scalp muscles. They were markedly enhanced by active contraction of the muscle but could usually be eliminated by having the subject relax, as with random muscle activity. Stimulation of digital nerve rather than median nerve at the wrist had no advantage (Calmes and Cracco, 1971).

Given the relatively small amplitude (5 to 10 μV), particularly of the early components of the SEP, amplifiers with a low noise level, at least comparable to the size of the signal (Desmedt, 1971) are required. The overall frequency response of the system should extend from 1 or 2 Hz to 1,000 or even 3,000 Hz without attenuation. A high-frequency response of this order and also an averager with a bin-width not exceeding 100 to 200 μsec (i.e. 5 to 10 bins per msec) is required if the early SEPs which have rapid rise times and brief durations are to be recorded accurately (Desmedt et al, 1974); insertion of a 100 Hz filter having a sharp (24 dB per octave) roll-off markedly decreased the amplitude of the initial negative component of the SEP and increased the apparent latency of its onset by 4 msec. Too short a time constant, on the other hand, will distort the later slow potentials of the SEP. A reasonably reliable test of the performance of the recording and amplifying system as a whole may be obtained by feeding a calibration pulse (e.g. a square-wave of 5 μV and 20 to 50 msec duration) into the input stage and treating it in exactly the same way as the cerebral records.

The small amplitude SEPs recorded from the scalp may be revealed in the presence of the often larger potentials in the background by high-speed analog-to-digital conversion of the recorded potentials and computer-averaging of this digital information. The subject of computer techniques applied to clinical neurophysiology has been reviewed by Halliday (1968).

The improvement in signal-to-noise ratio with averaging is proportional to the square root of the number of responses averaged. It must be recognized that large random potentials, even though they occur infrequently, may still appear with diminished amplitude in the final record. Some idea of this background activity may be obtained by averaging the potentials recorded from the electrodes in the usual way but without delivering the stimulus. Another control is to apply the stimulus but add and subtract successive responses (Schimmel, 1967). The reproducibility of the response may be judged by superimposing a number of records obtained under the same circumstances.

The choice of sweep duration or time following the stimulus which is averaged depends on the purpose of the experiment—30 to 50 msec may be used if the latencies of the earliest components are of interest, while 500 msec or more are required to show the later components. The final record may be displayed on an oscilloscope and photographed or written out using an X-Y plotter. Most English and European investigators have used the convention that a potential, negative at the active electrode with respect to the reference, is represented by an upgoing deflection in the final record, while the opposite convention has often been used in American laboratories. The former has the advantage of yielding records comparable to those of classical neurophysiology.

DESCRIPTION OF THE SEPs RECORDED IN MAN

Papers from a number of laboratories in Europe and America, which gave detailed descriptions of SEPs, were published during the 1960s (Allison, 1962; Goff et al, 1962; Shagass and Schwartz, 1964; Debecker and Desmedt, 1964; Desmedt et al, 1965; Giblin, 1964; Bergamini et al, 1965). There was a considerable measure of congruity in the results and they have been confirmed in later papers by these and many other authors.

The SEPs most frequently described are those evoked by shocks applied to the contralateral median or ulnar nerves at the wrist; the usual configuration of this response, recorded in healthy adults from an electrode over the "hand" area of the postcentral gyrus with shocks giving potentials of close to maximal amplitude, will, therefore, be described. The first component of the response is a brief negative potential with onset at 14 to 16 msec and a peak at 17 to 20 msec after the stimulus (Figs. 13.2 and 13.3; see also Table 13.1). As was first noted by Allison (1962) and Goff et al (1962), this component is sometimes preceded by a small-amplitude positive potential which peaks at 14 to 15 msec; since it is now generally agreed that this potential is of subcortical origin it will be described in the section concerned with afferent pathway.

The initial negative potential is followed by a positive potential which almost always exceeds it in amplitude. While the range of peak latencies for the initial negative potential is narrow and the standard deviation of its mean is remarkably small considering that no correction is made for differences in conduction pathway (i.e. arm length) between individuals, the range of peak latencies given in the literature for the first positive potential is considerably greater, roughly 21 to 32 msec (Table 13.2). The observations of Giblin (1964)

Table 13.1. LATENCIES, IN MILLISECONDS, OF COMPONENTS OF CEREBRAL RESPONSE EVOKED IN 25 HEALTHY SUBJECTS BY SHOCKS TO CONTRALATERAL MEDIAN NERVE AT THE WRIST

	V-Configuration of Early Components (18 Subjects)			W-Configuration of Early Components (7 Subjects)		
	Mean	S.D.	Range	Mean	S.D.	Range
Onset	16.14	1.08	14–18	15.50	0.87	14.5–17
Early potentials, in sequence						
Initial negative	19.39	0.93	18–21	18.29	0.57	17.5–19
First positive	26.78	2.24	23–31	22.14	0.04	22–23
Second negative	—	—	—	26.14	1.22	24–27
Second positive	—	—	—	30.71	1.50	29–33
Later waves						
Negative wave	36.00	4.31	30–45	39.57	1.99	38–42
Positive wave	45.29	5.27	39–55	49.33	7.84	41–60

(From Giblin, D. R. 1964. Annals of the New York Academy of Sciences, 112, 93.)

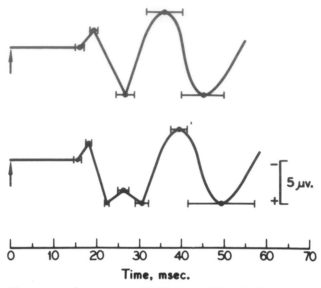

Fig. 13.2. *The two configurations of SEPs evoked by shocks to the contralateral median nerve at the wrist in a group of 25 healthy subjects. The curves were constructed using the mean peak latencies shown in Table 13.1 and the horizontal bars represent one standard deviation on either side of the mean. Upper curve is the V configuration recorded in 18 of the subjects, and the lower curve is the W configuration recorded in 7 subjects and shows two early positive components, P22 and P30 (from Giblin, D. R. 1964. Ann. N.Y. Acad. Sci., 112, 93).*

suggest an explanation for this; he found that while records of 18 of 25 healthy subjects showed a single positive potential with peak latencies ranging from 23 to 31 msec (mean 26.8 msec, SD 2.2 msec), the records of the remaining 7 subjects showed two distinct brief positive potentials within this same range (Table 13.1). Mean peak latencies of these early positive components were 22.1 and 30.7 msec, with an intervening negative-going peak at 26.1 msec, and the range of latencies for each of these components was exceedingly narrow. In these subjects, the two potentials were either of similar amplitude so that the early part of the SEP had the configuration of a W, or the first or second was predominant so that the other appeared as a notch on its ascending or descending limb. To explain these findings, Giblin suggested that, in all subjects, both positive peaks at 22 and 31 msec are generated in the somatosensory cortex (where their foci are separated by a few centimeters—see Fig. 13.1); both are recorded by electrodes on the scalp in some subjects, but in the majority they merge to give a single positive wave whose peak latency is intermediate between the two.

Following this single or double early positive component there is another negative-going wave which peaks between about 30 and 40 msec; it is a consistent feature of the response but in some cases it barely reaches the isopotential line. This in turn is followed by an equally consistent positive deflection which peaks between 40 and 50 msec. When the first positive potential is single or

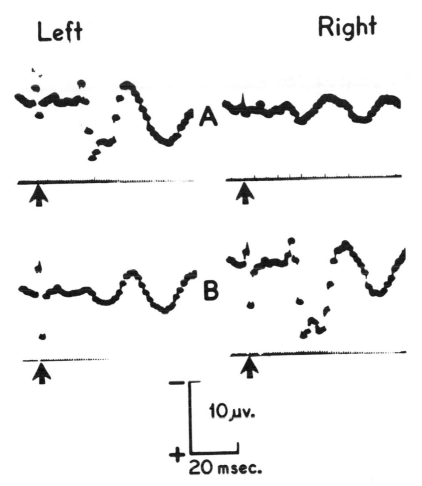

Left   **Right**

A

B

10 μv.

20 msec.

Fig. 13.3. *SEPs of a healthy subject with the W configuration. Responses were recorded simultaneously from electrodes over the left and right hemispheres. The active electrode is 7 cm lateral to the midline, 2.5 cm behind a line connecting vertex and external auditory meatus, and the reference electrode is 7 cm anterior to it. Upper records, A, show responses evoked by shocks just greater than motor threshold applied to the right median nerve at the wrist and lower records, B, are those recorded when similar shocks were applied to the left median nerve. Each record is the averaged response to 110 stimuli. In this subject, responses recorded from the hemisphere contralateral to the stimulus are virtually identical. Ipsilateral responses were seldom seen with this recording arrangement but here are identical in latency to the contralateral SEPs indicating that they are recorded by volume conduction (from Giblin, D. R. 1964. Ann. N.Y. Acad. Sci., 112, 93).*

Table 13.2. LATENCIES (MEAN AND STANDARD DEVIATION) OF SEP * FROM STIMULATION OF CONTRALATERAL MEDIAN NERVE AT THE WRIST

	N20	P25	P30	N35	P45	N55	P80	N140	P190
Goff et al 1977, N = 12	21.3 ± 2.1	24.4 ± 1.9	28.6 ± 3.4	34.5 ± 4.8	45 ± 5	55 ± 6	80±7	140 ± 13	192 ± 16
Giblin, 1964 W form, N = 7	18.3 ± 0.6	22.1 ± 0.04	30.7 ± 1.5	39.6 ± 2.0	49 ± 8				
V form, N = 18	19.4 ± 0.9		26.8 ± 2.2	36.0 ± 4.3	45 ± 5				
Broughton et al 1969, N = 10	19.1 ± 1.5	25.6 ± 4.4		34.5 ± 4.1	44 ± 3	64 ± 7	89±11	128 ± 15	199 ± 30
Lüders et al † 1970, N = 16	17.6 ± 0.2	23.7 ± 0.4		32.7 ± 0.5	42 ± 0.4	54 ± 0.8	93±5	122 ± 3	214 ± 10
Bergamini et al 1965, N = 10	16.6 ± 1.3		27.3 ± 3.9	35.8 ± 3.9	46.2 ± 5	57 ± 3	70±5		
Domino et al 1965, N = 20	19.2 ± 0.8	24.3 ± 0.7		31.3 ± 0.6	47 ± 0.4	79 ± 7			

* Latencies of components shown in Figs. 13.5a, b.
† Group with ages 19–29 years.

slightly notched, and particularly when relatively long analysis times are used, this and the positive peak at 40 and 50 msec may again give the early part of the response a bifid or W-shaped appearance. Unfortunately, this has sometimes given rise to confusion with the earlier W of Giblin.

Between these relatively early potentials, and the large-amplitude negative-positive potentials recorded maximally at the vertex, most authors describe a negative component peaking between about 50 and 70 msec and a positive one peaking at about 80 to 95 msec (the N55 and P80 components of Goff et al, 1977). They are clearly more variable in both amplitude and latency than earlier components and may be absent in the records of any one individual. The late waves, seen best in monopolar records from the vertex (N140 and P190 of Goff), also vary in latency but generally have the largest amplitudes of any component of the SEP. Still later negative and positive waves out to 500 msec are often seen; indeed Kusske et al (1975) and Rush et al (1976) recorded slow oscillations, time-locked to the stimulus, from 500 to 3,500 msec, largest at vertex, central, and frontal locations and with frequencies of stimulation between 1 and 3 pulses per second.

Although there is reasonably good agreement about the data concerning the sequence of components and their latencies (Table 13.2) there has not in the past been any uniformity of nomenclature. It is probable that no system of nomenclature can be entirely satisfactory but the system suggested by Vaughan (1969) and recommended by the Committee on Methods at the International Symposium on Evoked Potentials in Man (Brussels, 1974) is the best presently available and will be used in this chapter. In this system, each component is named by its polarity and mean latency or range of latencies.

SEPs recorded from any one individual during a session lasting several hours or at sessions separated widely in time are remarkably consistent if stimulus intensities are comparable, and any difference can be accounted for by minor variations in electrode placement. Similarly, only minor differences in the configuration of responses are seen when shocks are applied at different sites on the same limb; the onset of the response to shocks applied to the median nerve at the elbow is, however, 3 to 5 msec earlier than when shocks are applied to the same nerve at the wrist, while that evoked by stimulating digital nerves (proximal phalanx) has its onset 2 to 3 msec later (Giblin, 1964). Calmes and Cracco (1971), comparing stimulation at wrists and fingers, found each component of the response to have a roughly similar difference in latency.

Comparison of the responses of the right and left hemispheres evoked by stimulation of the contralateral median nerves shows that, for components occurring during the first 50 msec at least, the responses are usually indistinguishable (Giblin, 1964).

When the responses evoked in different subjects by stimulation of nerves in the arm are compared, it is evident that the same basic sequence of potentials is recorded. The considerable differences in configuration sometimes encountered are largely accounted for by differences in the relative amplitudes of the various components. Peak latencies of adjacent negative and positive components may overlap but those of successive negative or positive components do not (Table 13.2). There is, therefore, seldom any ambiguity about the identity of a component even when, as sometimes occurs, a neighboring component fails to appear in the record.

Studies of the SEPs recorded in the healthy neonate and subsequent changes with age have been reported in a series of papers by Desmedt and his colleagues (Manil et al, 1967; Desmedt and Manil, 1970; Desmedt, Brunko, and Debecker, 1976), by Hrbek and colleagues (1968, 1969, 1973), and by Laget et al (1973a, b, c, 1976), to which the interested reader is referred. Lüders (1970) has studied the effect of age on the SEP in an adult population. Forty subjects divided into groups by age were studied. Latencies showed few significant differences or trends, but the N35 component decreased while the N55 increased with age.

Responses evoked by stimulation of nerves of the lower extremity have been less often investigated than those evoked from the arm. The response to shocks applied to the medial or lateral popliteal nerves at the level of the knee does not show an initial negative component but rather a single positive potential beginning 25 msec after the stimulus and reaching a peak at 35 msec; it is followed by large negative and positive peaks at 43 and 61 msec respectively (Giblin, 1964). The results reported by Tsumoto et al (1972) and illustrated in Figure 13.4 and Table 13.3 are very similar.

THE DISTRIBUTION OF SEPs OVER THE SCALP

Dawson (1947a) found the early potentials of the SEP to be quite localized to scalp locations presumed to overlie the postcentral gyrus contralateral to the stimulated limb, 7 cm lateral to the midline for the upper extremity and close to the midline for the leg. Debecker and Desmedt (1964) similarly showed localization of the positive potential (peak 25 to 30 msec) evoked by mechanical stimu-

Table 13.3. PEAK LATENCIES OF COMPONENTS OF SEP EVOKED BY SHOCKS TO CONTRALATERAL LATERAL POPLITEAL NERVE AT THE KNEE (N = 41)

Peak Latency (msec)	Mean	S.D.
P_1	34.3	±2.0
N_1	44.8	±3.3
P_2	55.6	±4.7
N_2	74.2	±5.6
P_3	98.5	±7.3
N_3	126.0	±15.0
P_4	203.5	±16.6

(From Tsumoto, T., Hirose, N., Nonaka, S. and Takahashi, M., 1972. Electroencephalography and Clinical Neurophysiology, 33:379.)

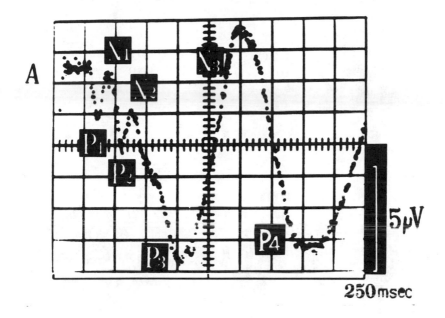

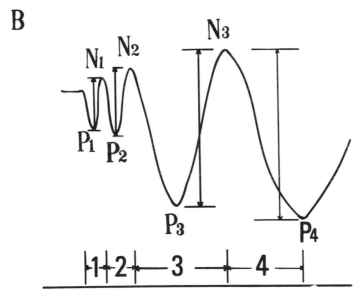

Fig. 13.4. *SEPs evoked by shocks just greater than motor threshold applied to the lateral popliteal nerve at the level of the knee and recorded from an electrode on the midline 2 cm posterior to the vertex with an earlobe reference. A is a typical response recorded in a healthy subject and is the averaged response to 100 stimuli. B is a schema of the SEP, indicating its four components. Their amplitudes are measured from P_1 to N_1, from P_2 to N_2, from P_3, to N_3, and from N_3 to P_4 respectively (from Tsumoto, T., Hirose, N., Nonaka, S. and Takahashi, M. 1972. Electroencephalogr. Clin. Neurophysiol., 33, 379).*

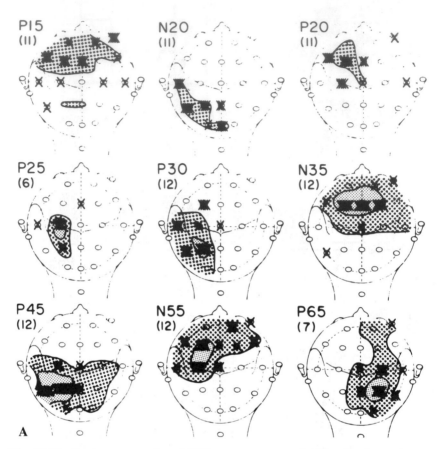

Fig. 13.5A. *Scalp topography of SEP components evoked by shocks applied to the right median nerve at the wrist. Electrodes were placed according to the 10:20 system. Isopotential maps were constructed using records from 12 healthy subjects. The number in brackets under each component is the number of subjects in whom that component was recorded. Crosses indicate electrode sites at which the component was 90% or more of maximal amplitude in any subject while fine stippling indicates 75% or more of maximal amplitude and coarse stippling indicates regions where it was 50–75% of maximal. Note that the N20 and P25 components have the most restricted distributions. P30 and P45 are largest over the posterior region of the hemisphere contralateral to the stimulus. These are of neural origin while components P65, N70 and P100 were thought to be of myogenic origin. The N140 and P190 are the vertex potentials and they and later components are symmetrically distributed across the midline (from Goff, G. D., Matsumiya, Y., Allison, T., and Goff, W. R. 1977. Electroencephalogr. Clin. Neurophysiol., 42, 57).*

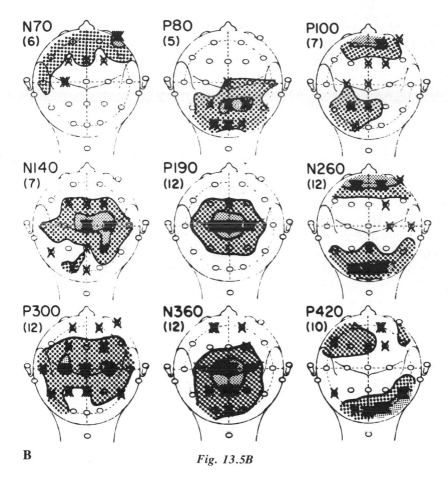

B

Fig. 13.5B

lation of a finger over the "hand" area, and neither they nor Dawson recorded evoked potentials over the ipsilateral hemisphere.

Localization of components earlier than 50 msec of the response to median nerve stimulation to the contralateral posterior quadrant of the head was confirmed by Giblin (1964), who also observed differences in the fields of the early positive potentials at 22 and 30.7 msec. Figure 13.1 shows that they appear with similar amplitudes at the electrode 7 cm from the midline, while an electrode a few centimeters anterior and medial to this recorded only P22, and P30 was the larger at an electrode more laterally and posteriorly situated.

Goff and his colleagues have, over the years, made an extensive study of the scalp topography of evoked responses in man (Goff et al, 1962, 1969, 1977). Maps based mainly on records from 12 subjects, with electrodes placed according to the 10-20 system and referred to the earlobe contralateral to the stimulus, are summarized in Figure 13.5a and b and require little comment. Early components N20, P25 and P30 are well localized to the posterior quadrant contralateral to the stimulated side as is P45, although its field is more diffuse. N20 and P25 have the most localized fields which are almost identical and within the larger fields of P30 and P45.

It is of practical importance, as Goff et al point out, that the P3 and P4 electrode sites are within the 75 percent range for components N20, P31, P48, and the posterior neurogenic component P100; and within the 50 percent range for the vertex potentials N140 and P190. If a single electrode placement of the 10-20 system is to be used to record the SEP evoked by stimulation of the upper extremity, P3 or P4 would appear to be the appropriate choice.

It should be emphasized that responses evoked by stimulation of any of the nerve trunks of the upper extremity and at any level from finger to axilla have the same distribution on the scalp (Desmedt et al, 1966a, b; Desmedt and Noël, 1973). Recording from a coronal chain of electrodes, Manil and Ectors (1966) showed that stimulation of the index and fifth fingers evoked SEPs of similar appearance and that both showed phase-reversal between electrodes 6 and 9 cm lateral to the midline.

Potentials ipsilateral to the stimulated upper limb were not found by Dawson (1947a) or by Debecker and Desmedt (1964). Goff et al (1962) found ipsilateral early potentials, similar to those seen contralaterally, only occasionally, while the bipolar records of Larson, Sances, and Christenson (1966) showed only relatively late ipsilateral potentials.

When early potentials are recorded by scalp electrodes over the ipsilateral hemisphere with latencies nearly identical to those of the contralateral SEP, it is probable that they are generated in the contralateral hemisphere and recorded at a distance by volume conduction. This is not necessarily the case with the later potentials (see below) and does not explain the findings of Tamura (1972) that ipsilateral potentials (after P14) had peak latencies 4.5-6.5 msec greater than presumably comparable components recorded contralaterally. Stimulation of the unaffected upper limbs in three patients with unilateral cerebral lesions gave similar results, while neither contralateral nor ipsilateral potentials were seen when the affected arm was stimulated. Latency differences between contralateral and ipsilateral potentials were noted also by Cracco (1972b). These observations are compatible with the hypothesis that the potentials recorded over the ipsilateral hemisphere are generated within that hemisphere and are a consequence of potentials evoked by the afferent volley in the contralateral hemisphere, with subsequent transmission of impulses via an interhemispheric pathway. Tamura's findings that stimulation of the affected arm in his patients evoked neither ipsilateral nor contralateral cerebral potentials is against the alternative hypothesis that ipsilateral potentials were evoked by impulses in an uncrossed pathway having a slightly greater conduction time. A functionally ipsilateral pathway is probably responsible for later waves recorded ipsilaterally, however, as is indicated by the findings of Hazeman, Olivier, and Fischgold (1969), although crossing and recrossing at a subcortical level cannot be excluded. Hazeman et al studied six patients who had undergone hemispherectomy; the earliest potential recorded over the remaining hemisphere when shocks were applied to the ipsilateral hand was a positive potential with a peak at 100 msec, seen in two patients, while a negative potential with a mean latency of 144 msec was recorded in five and a positive potential with a peak at 240 msec was recorded in four (Fig. 13.6). These late waves have the latencies

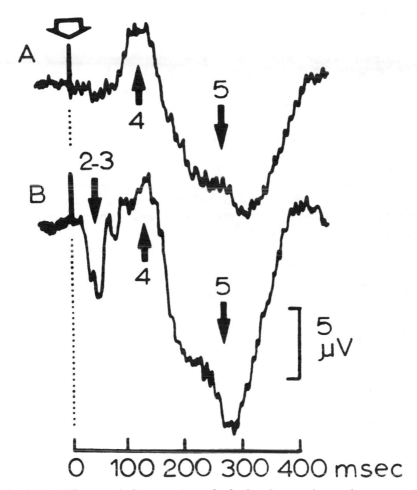

Fig. 13.6. *SEPs recorded in a patient who had undergone hemispherectomy. B, is the response evoked by shocks to one finger contralateral to the remaining hemisphere and has a normal configuration. The upper record, A, shows potentials recorded from the same scalp electrodes when shocks were applied to a finger of the ipsilateral hand. Early components, labelled 2-3, are absent in this response but negative and positive components with peak latencies of about 140 and 300 msec (labelled 4 and 5) are seen and resemble those evoked by contralateral stimuli. These late potentials must have been generated in the remaining hemisphere, presumably by impulses in a functionally ipsilateral afferent pathway (from Hazemann, P., Olivier, L., and Fischgold, H. 1969. C. R. Acad. Sci. [D] (Paris), 268:195, as modified by Desmedt, J. E., 1971, in: Handbook of Electroencephalography and Clinical Neurophysiology, Remond, A. (Ed.) 9:55).*

of the vertex potentials. Similar results are reported by Saletu, Itil, and Saletu (1971), and results reported by Laget et al (1973a), who studied 56 children ranging in age from 3 days to 14 years, may also be interpreted in this way.

As would be expected, the SEPs evoked by shocks to nerve trunks of the lower extremity are maximal at scalp electrodes over the postcentral gyrus closer to the midline than those of the upper extremity (Dawson, 1947a; Giblin, 1964). Maps similar to those of Goff et al for the upper extremity may be found in the paper of Tsumoto et al (1972).

THE AFFERENT PATHWAY OF SEPs IN MAN

The afferent pathway responsible for SEPs evoked by upper limb stimulation was first discussed by Dawson in 1950 and further investigated by him in 1956. He noted that shocks applied to the fingers, which subjects were just able to perceive, evoked a detectable cerebral response. Shocks applied to the median or ulnar nerves at the wrist which gave rise to a just detectable action potential, recorded percutaneously at the elbow, evoked an SEP whose initial phase was 35 percent of maximal amplitude. Stronger shocks were required to excite motor fibers in the nerve and at motor threshold the action potential at the elbow was 50 percent and the cerebral response 85 percent of their maximal amplitudes (Dawson, 1956).

The findings of Dawson relating stimulus intensity to sensory and motor thresholds and to afferent volley and cerebral response have been confirmed by many workers (Debecker and Desmedt, 1964; Giblin, 1964; Debecker, Desmedt, and Manil, 1965). It seems, therefore, that the SEP depends on impulses in large, rapidly conducting myelinated afferents, presumably cutaneous and joint afferents.

The afferent pathway of the SEP and its maturation has been studied particularly by Desmedt and his colleagues (Desmedt et al, 1970, 1973). Stimulating the fingers and recording at multiple sites along the limb up to the brachial plexus at the supraclavicular region, they found that in the adult the corticopetal volley travelled at a very consistent velocity of the order of 65 m per second (Fig. 13.7A), reaching the brachial plexus at about 12 msec (Desmedt et al, 1973). Assuming that this velocity is maintained between this point and the cuneate nucleus, a distance of about 20 cm, the volley would be expected to arrive at the cuneate at about 15 msec. The latency of the onset of the SEP (N_1 component) in this subject was at about 19 msec and the authors conclude that, even taking into account synaptic delays, conduction velocity in the central pathway must be slower than in the periphery; it was estimated in this case as 56 m per second. Markedly slower velocities are found in young children; peripheral conduction velocity in the normal full-term neonate is between 20 and 34 m per second, but it increases rapidly during the first few months of life and reaches values in the adult range by 12 to 18 months. By contrast, conduction velocity of the central pathway is estimated to be only 7.5 m per second in the newborn (Fig. 13.7C) increasing to 21 m per second in a child 7.5 months of age (Fig. 13.7B) and attaining velocities in the adult range only at age 5 to 7 years.

As mentioned before, a small, inconsistent, positive potential peaking at 14 to 15 msec was noted as early as 1962 by Allison and by Goff et al, in records from the scalp. Cracco (1972a) found it more consistently and reported that it had a peak latency of 13 to 17 msec following shocks to the median nerve at the wrist and a much wider distribution over the scalp than the negative and positive potentials which followed it (N18.5, P25). Cracco found that it was unaffected by changes in tension of neck and scalp muscles, and concluded that it was almost certainly of intracranial origin and that—given its short latency and wide distribution—its generator was probably subcortical. A positive potential

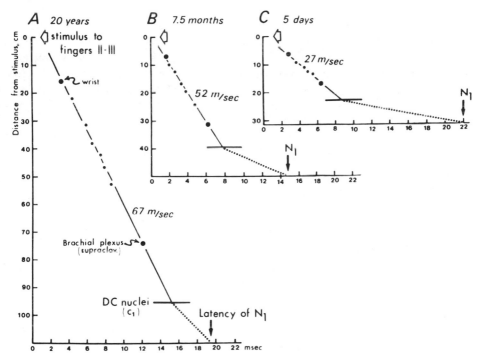

Fig. 13.7. Graphs representing peripheral and central conduction velocities of the afferent volley evoked by shocks applied to two fingers and showing the effect of age. The ordinate represents the distance travelled from the site of stimulation and is in the same scale in each graph. The large dots represent arrival of the volley at the wrist and brachial plexus and the smaller dots recording at other sites along the limb. Conduction velocities in the periphery are indicated and are linear throughout the limb. The arrival of the volley at the cuneate nucleus is indicated by horizontal lines and is estimated by assuming that conduction velocity in the periphery is maintained between brachial plexus and the nucleus. Conduction velocities in the central pathway were then estimated using the latency to onset of the initial negative potential of the SEP, indicated by arrows. This was 56 m per second in the adult (A), 21 m per second in a child of 7.5 months (B) and only 7.5 m per second in the neonate (C) (from Desmedt, J. E., Noël, P., Debecker, J., and Namèche, J. 1973. In: New Developments in Electromyography and Clinical Neurophysiology, Desmedt, J. E., Ed., Vol. 2, p. 52, Karger, Basel).

with a latency of about 17 msec following natural stimulation of the contralateral hand was recorded by Ervin and Mark (1964) from electrodes in the nucleus ventralis posterolateralis (VPL) of thalamus. Again, Pagni (1967) reported that a large positive potential whose latency was "about 13-16 msec" was recorded from this nucleus after shocks to the contralateral median nerve at the wrist, and similiar results were reported by Larson and Sances (1968), Haider, Ganglberger and Groll-Knapp (1972) and Fukushima, Mayanagi, and Bouchard (1976). It seems likely that, since the P15 component is nearly identical in latency, it represents the potential generated in VPL and recorded from the scalp, and thus identifies the arrival of the corticopetal volley at this last relay on the central pathway.

Further information concerning the central afferent pathway is provided by the important recent papers of Cracco and Cracco (1976) and by Jones (1977). The former authors, recording from the vertex with the unstimulated contralateral hand or knee as reference, describe three positive potentials, the first having its onset 6.5 to 9.0 msec and its peak 9 to 11.4 msec following shocks to the median nerve at the wrist, the second with onset 10 to 12.4 msec and peak 10.7 to 13.4 msec, and the third with onset 12.0 to 14.4 and peak at 14.0 to 16.5 msec (Fig. 13.8). Only this last was seen in records from the vertex with ear as reference and it is clearly identifiable as the P15 potential discussed above. The first two were recorded with similar amplitude by an electrode anywhere on the head—nose, inion, and ear, as well as vertex with a noncephalic (e.g. hand) reference—indicating that the entire head is isopotential for these potentials.

The first potential, P9, has the same peak latency as the negative potential recorded over the median nerve, 2 cm proximal to the axilla, with the contralateral hand as reference. This is in good agreement with the data of Desmedt et al (1973), Matthews, Beauchamp, and Small (1974), and Jones (1977). Cracco and Cracco concluded that their P9 potential was a volume-conducted potential generated by the afferent volley at or just proximal to the brachial plexus, and Jones similarly concluded that his N9 potential was the electrical field of a dipole generated by the advancing wave of depolarization in a nerve trunk in the region of the brachial plexus.

While the origins of the P9 and P15 potentials of Cracco can thus be identified with considerable confidence, there are as yet insufficient data to locate the origin of the intervening positive potential with a peak at 11 to 13 msec. Presumably, it too is the volume-conducted field of a positive-negative dipole with its positive pole rostrally situated, somewhere between the brachial plexus and the thalamus and, to the present author, the cuneate nucleus appears a probable location. Jones (1977) found two negative peaks between N9 and N14 with latencies of 11 and 13 msec, and tentatively ascribed their origins to cervical roots and spinal cord respectively, but this would appear not to apportion sufficient time to synaptic transmission in the cuneate nucleus and propagation of the volley in the medial lemniscus.

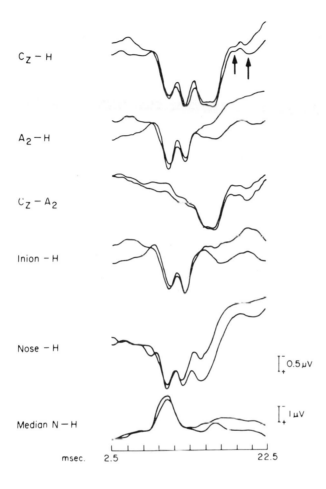

Fig. 13.8. *Far field potentials generated subcortically by impulses initiated by shocks applied to the right median nerve at the wrist and recorded by electrodes on the vertex (Cz), right ear (A2), inion, nose, and right axilla with an electrode on the dorsum of the contralateral (left) hand (H) as reference. The third record is the vertex with right ear reference for comparison. Each record is the summated response to 1,024 or 2,048 stimuli delivered at 10 per second. Note the short analysis time. Early positive potentials with peak latencies of 9.9 and 12.0 msec are seen in records from vertex, right ear, nose and inion with hand reference and are isopotential at all these cephalic locations and therefore not seen in the Cz-A2 record. The third potential, P15, appears in records from the vertex with either right ear or hand reference. The lowest trace shows that the P9.9 component recorded from electrodes on the head with hand reference corresponds to a negative-going component recorded from the axilla, suggesting that it is generated by the afferent volley in the brachial plexus (from Cracco, R. Q. and Cracco, J. B. 1976. Electroencephalogr. Clin. Neurophysiol., 41, 460).*

SEP CHANGES IN NEUROLOGIC DISORDERS

Reports of SEP recordings in patients with a variety of neurologic disorders have been reviewed by Halliday (1967c), Desmedt, (1971), and Desmedt and Noël (1973, 1975).

Peripheral Nerve Lesions

SEPs were first studied in patients with abnormalities of peripheral nerves by Giblin (1960, 1964). The response was completely abolished in the most severely affected, while in the milder cases it was frequently of reduced amplitude, altered morphology and/or prolonged latency, even when no sensory deficit could be demonstrated clinically (Fig. 13.9). Similar results were reported by Bergamini et al (1965), who studied 13 patients with peripheral neuropathies of diverse etiology. Amplitudes of SEPs were usually and often profoundly decreased and the morphology was so altered that some components could not be identified. They calculated the mean latency of each SEP component in the records of their group of patients as a whole and found them to be approximately 8 to 12 msec greater than latencies of corresponding components in healthy subjects. It seems, then, that the evoked potential method may provide a fairly sensitive indication of abnormality of conduction in peripheral nerve, since SEPs may be clearly abnormal when clinical examination fails to reveal sensory deficit. Moreover, SEPs can sometimes be recorded even when nerve action potentials cannot be detected in the limbs, and thus permit conduction velocity measurements to be made.

The findings reported by Desmedt and his colleagues in a series of papers are concerned for the most part with patients having a lesion of a single peripheral nerve. When shocks were applied to the distal phalanx of second or third fingers of patients with compression of the median nerve at the wrist (carpal tunnel syndrome), Desmedt et al (1966a, b) recorded SEPs which in configuration resembled those evoked from the unaffected fifth finger but were delayed in onset by 7 to 15 msec. Records from such a patient (Fig. 13.10) show SEPs with onsets of 40 and 25 msec respectively, while with stimulation of the median nerve above the wrist SEPs had a latency of 24 msec. In this patient, the afferent volley recorded from the median nerve at the wrist, evoked by stimulating the third finger, was highly desynchronized and consisted of a series of small potentials ranging in latency from 9 to 20 msec compared with the normal well-synchronized action potential with a latency of about 2 msec. The authors comment on the discrepancy between the conduction delay to the wrist of 7 msec for the fastest fibers in the nerve and the total delay of 16 msec in the onset of the SEP, and suggest that temporal summation of the desynchronized afferent volley may be occurring in the cortex, that is, that the cortex may be able to "operate as an integrator in the time dimension" (Desmedt, 1971). To the present author, the relatively normal configuration of the response recorded by Desmedt makes this seem unlikely, but temporal summation at dorsal col-

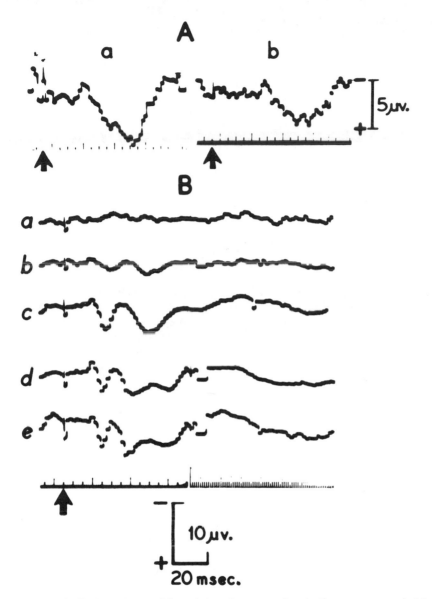

Fig. 13.9. *SEPs in patients with peripheral neuropathy. A: Response recorded in a patient recovering from acute polyneuropathy; he noted dysesthesiae but had no sensory deficit on examination. Aa is the response to strong shocks to the contralateral median nerve at the wrist and Ab that to stimulation of two fingers. Both responses are delayed compared to normal and corresponding components differ by 7 msec (normal 2 to 3 msec). B: SEPs recorded in a patient with severe but distal sensory loss, evoked by shocks of increasing intensity applied to the median nerve at the elbow. Ba: without stimulus; Bb shocks at sensory threshold, Bc at motor threshold, Be at twice motor threshold. In Be, the initial negative component has a normal latency but the two succeeding positives have delayed peaks. Note that with increasing stimulus intensity the latency of the second positive peak shortens progressively (from Giblin, D. R. 1964. Ann. N.Y. Acad. Sci.,112, 93).*

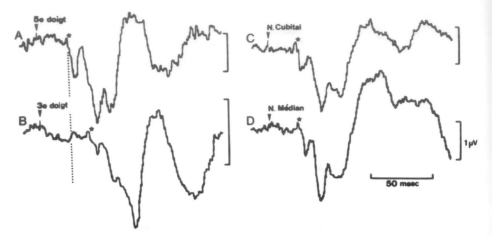

Fig. 13.10. SEPs in a patient with carpal tunnel syndrome: all records are from the same electrode over the contralateral hand area of postcentral gyrus. A: Response to stimuli applied to the distal phalanx of the fifth finger. B: Response to stimuli applied to the distal phalanx of the middle finger. C and D responses to shocks to the ulnar and median nerves respectively applied just proximal to the wrist. The peak latencies of the initial negative components (indicated by stars) are 25 msec in A, 23 msec in C and D, and 40 msec in B, i.e. conduction times from finger to wrist were 17 msec for the median and 2 msec for the ulnar nerves. Voltage calibration for each record is 1 μV. Note that despite its small amplitude, the response in B is relatively normal in configuration (from Desmedt, J. E., Franken, L., Borenstein, S., Debecker, J., Lambert, C. and Manil, J. 1966. Rev. Neurol. 115, 255).

umn and thalamic relays might serve to both "boost" the afferent volley finally delivered to the cortex and account for the greater-than-expected delay in SEP onset.

Comparable delays of 1.6 and 1.9 msec respectively in afferent volley at the wrist and the SEP of normal configuration were recorded in a patient with a partial lesion of the median nerve at the wrist (Desmedt and Noël, 1973) while in a patient whose median nerve had been severed by trauma, studied four months after nerve suture, the SEP evoked by strong shocks to the distal phalanx of the third finger has its onset 57.5 msec after the stimulus (Desmedt et al, 1966b). Latency to onset of SEPs evoked from the fifth finger and the median nerve at the wrist had normal values of 23.5 msec and 22.5 msec respectively. No action potential at the wrist could be recorded from stimulation of the third finger but, using the conduction time of 35 msec over the distance of 19 cm from finger to wrist, they estimated the conduction velocity in the regenerating nerve fibers to be 5.4 m per second.

Using the latencies to onset of the SEPs evoked by shocks applied at various sites along the limb, Desmedt (1971) was able to calculate conduction velocity of the afferent volley in the upper limb of a child with advanced metachromatic leukodystrophy, and showed it to be slowed. The same technique was used by Noël (1973) in a study of sensory nerve conduction in the upper limb in diabetic patients to estimate conduction velocity in patients whose neuropathy was so advanced that sensory nerve action potentials were not recordable. Again, applying the method to a patient with an old lesion of the ulnar nerve at the elbow, Desmedt and Noël (1973) were able to demonstrate that conduction velocity was slowed across the affected segment of the nerve. Similar findings of delayed onset, altered configuration and reduced amplitude of SEPs in patients with peripheral nerve lesions have since been reported by a number of authors.

There are to date only a few reports of the use of SEP recording to investigate patients with proximal lesions of the brachial plexus or lesions of the lumbosacral plexus or spinal roots, even though the recording of SEPs should prove to be of particular diagnostic value in such a context. For example, in a patient who had suffered ischemic damage to the brachial plexus secondary to trauma, Desmedt and Noël (1973) were able to show that conduction was markedly slowed, not only distally but well proximal to the axilla, and the same authors reported in 1975 delayed SEPs from stimulation of the femoral nerves in a patient with Hodgkin's disease with presumed involvement of spinal roots.

Lesions of the Spinal Cord

The earliest reports concerning SEPs recorded in patients with lesions of the spinal cord are those of Giblin (1960, 1964) and of Halliday and Wakefield (1963). The lesions were diverse but the electrophysiologic observations correlated well with the type of sensory deficit found by clinical examination. The conclusions reached by these authors were identical, and were confirmed by Larson et al (1966). When shocks were applied to a limb in which appreciation of pin prick and temperature alone was diminished or lost, the SEPs recorded were entirely normal in form, latency, and amplitude. By contrast, stimulation of a limb in which appreciation of joint position sense was more than mildly impaired evoked either no recognizable cerebral response or SEPs which were markedly abnormal in configuration and of prolonged latency. Figure 13.11 shows records obtained from a patient with a spinocerebellar degeneration, with lesions of the spinal cord but complete sparing of peripheral nerves. Appreciation of pain and temperature was normal but joint position sense was moderately impaired in the upper and severely impaired in the lower extremities. Nerve action potentials, recorded at the knee following stimulation of the anterior tibial nerve at the ankle and at the elbow following stimulation of the median nerve at the wrist, were of normal amplitude and latency. SEPs could not be recorded to shocks applied to any nerve trunk in the lower extremities, while those evoked from nerves of the upper extremities were markedly abnormal, even with intense stimulation—a low amplitude positive wave of indefinite onset beginning 30 msec or more after the stimulus. Similar records were obtained by Halliday and Wakefield from patients with varying loss of joint position sense but preservation of pin prick and temperature, two of whom had demyelinating disease. Of greater interest, however, are three of

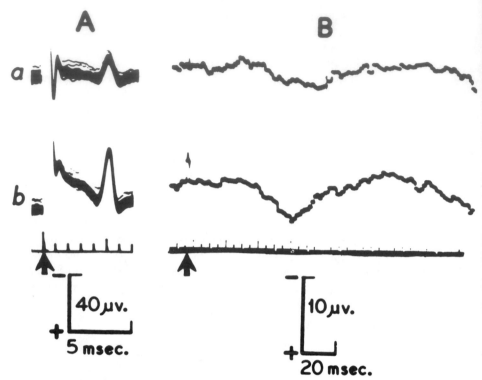

Fig. 13.11. *Abnormal SEPs recorded in a patient with a progressive degenerative disease involving the long tracts of the spinal cord but sparing peripheral nerves. Joint position sense was moderately impaired in the upper and severely impaired in the lower extremities but appreciation of pin and temperature was intact. Upper records, a, are responses to shocks applied to the median nerve at the wrist at just greater than motor threshold, and b are responses to shocks three times greater in intensity. A are records of the compound action potentials recorded percutaneously from the median nerve at the elbow and are normal in appearance. B are SEPs recorded from the contralateral parietal hand area and consist of shallow positive waves with onset at about 30 msec and peaks about 65 msec after the stimulus (from Giblin, D. R. 1964. Ann. N.Y. Acad. Sci., 112, 93).*

their patients who had shown impaired joint position sense but had either partially or almost completely recovered; the SEPs evoked from the affected limbs were in each case extremely small and abnormal.

These observations suggested that the pathways in the spinal cord utilized by impulses ultimately transmitted to the contralateral sensory cortex and giving rise to the SEP are ipsilateral to the stimulated limb, presumably in the dorsal columns but perhaps also including the dorsolateral pathway which joins the medial lemniscus in the lower medulla. Furthermore, since the SEPs evoked by stimulation of a limb in which appreciation of pain and temperature was severely impaired were indistinguishable from normal—at least with regard to those components in the first 100 msec (Giblin, 1960, 1964) or 180 msec (Halliday and Wakefield, 1963) following the stimuli, it seems that impulses in pain and temperature fibers, ascending in the anterolateral quadrant of the spinal cord opposite the stimulated limb, make no contribution to the SEP. Although not confirmed by pathologic examination, the reports of Larson et al (1966) and of Namerow (1969), that SEPs were normal and unchanged when evoked from limbs in which loss of pain and temperature sense had been produced by percutaneous anterolateral cordotomy, are additional evidence for these conclusions.

Two of the patients in whom Halliday and Wakefield found SEPs to be absent or markedly abnormal and who showed bilateral impairment of joint position sense alone had been diagnosed as suffering from demyelinating disease; similar results in larger series of patients with this illness have been reported by Baker et al (1968), Namerow (1968a and b), Desmedt and Noël (1973), Colon et al (1977), and others. Delayed latency of the onset of the SEP, often very marked (Fig. 13.12) was noted by Desmedt and Noël (1973) in all cases when joint position sense was impaired in a limb but also in the great majority of cases when it was intact. The collective results indicate that, in patients suspected of having demyelinating disease, recording SEPs may be of value in diagnosis; particularly in patients without symptoms or findings of any disorder of somatic sensation, increased latency or other aberration of their SEPs may provide evidence of multiple lesions of the nervous system. Early in the course of the illness, however, SEP recording appears of limited value; Matthews (1978) found abnormal SEPs in only four of 39 patients presenting with acute unilateral retrobulbar neuritis, a percentage of whom might be expected to have multiple sclerosis. The usefulness of recording SEPs over the cervical spine in patients with suspected multiple sclerosis is considered separately in Chapter 14.

Application of SEP recording to the investigation of patients with spinal cord injury has been reported by Perot (1973) and by Rowed, McLean, and Tator (1978). As expected, no SEPs are recorded by stimulation of nerves entering the spinal cord below the level of the lesion in patients judged clinically to have a complete lesion. Preservation of SEPs, or their reappearance during the week following injury, indicates a favorable prognosis (Rowed et al, 1978). In a rather unique clinical situation, Bergamini et al (1967) used SEP recording to establish that, in a pair of Siamese twins fused in the lumbosacral region, the peripheral nervous systems were completely independent.

Abnormal SEPs are to be expected in clinical situations in which both peripheral nerves and central pathways are known to be affected. In Friedreich's ataxia, for example, Bergamini et al (1966) showed that nerve action potentials were either absent or conducted slowly, and SEPs were delayed or not recordable. In a patient studied by Desmedt and Noël (1973, 1975) both peripheral and central conduction velocities were estimated; no action potentials could be recorded from the median nerve at the wrist, even when strong shocks were applied to the fingers, but these evoked an SEP with onset latency of 37.8 msec, while stimulation at the level of the axilla evoked a response with

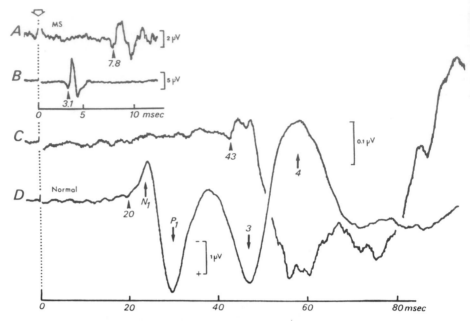

Fig. 13.12. *SEPs recorded from a female patient aged 41 years with longstanding multiple sclerosis and from a normal adult subject for comparison. Shocks were applied to the index and middle fingers. A and B are sensory action potentials recorded in the patient from median nerve at the axilla (A) and wrist (B) and indicate a maximum conduction velocity within the normal range. C and D are SEPs recorded from the contralateral parietal hand projection area. In the patient's record (C) the onset latency of the initial negative component is delayed by 23 msec compared with the normal (D) and the amplitude of the response as a whole is markedly diminished (note the different calibrations). (From Desmedt, J. E. and Noël, P. 1973. In: New Developments in Electromyography and Clinical Neurophysiology, Desmedt, J. E., Ed., Vol. 2, p. 352, Karger, Basel.)*

onset at 23.2 msec. Using this latency difference, the authors calculated the conduction velocity in the limb to be 31.5 m per second and, assuming a similar rate between axilla and spinal cord, they calculated an overall central velocity from cord to cortex of 20 m per second or about one-third that expected in the adult.

Lesions of the Brainstem and Diencephalon

The results of investigation of patients with lesions in these locations have confirmed and extended those obtained in patients with lesions of the spinal cord. In patients showing unilateral impairment of pain and temperature sense only, SEPs recorded when stimulating the affected limbs were normal and generally identical to those evoked by stimulation of the unaffected limbs. This was the case in four patients with infarction of the lateral portion of the medulla

(Wallenberg syndrome) reported by Alajouanine et al (1958), in a patient of Nakanishi, Shimada, and Toyokura (1974) and in two patients of Noël and Desmedt (1975), and in similar patients with a laterally placed lesion of the mesencephalon which spared the medial lemniscus. By contrast, SEPs are (as would be expected) frequently abnormal in patients with brainstem lesions involving the medial lemniscus. For example, in a patient with "locked-in" syndrome due to pontine infarction studied by Noël and Desmedt (1975), even strong stimulation of the median nerves at the wrist evoked SEPs with greatly delayed onsets (33 and 45 msec) and consisting of positive waves of small amplitude and peaks at 52 and 60 msec; the usual initial negative component was absent from the responses. This was tentatively attributed to a block in conduction of some of the fibers of the medial lemniscus and to slowed conduction in others, with desynchronization of the afferent volley. Similar SEP abnormalities were also found in patients with vascular lesions of the thalamus and although the extent of the lesions in these patients was not confirmed pathologically, there seems no reason to doubt that they involved the ventral-basal relay nucleus (VPL) and probably its afferent (medial lemniscus) and efferent (thalamo cortical projection fibers) connections. These obervations, therefore, confirm those of Domino et al (1965) that cryogenic lesions in this region virtually abolished cerebral potentials evoked by stimulation of the contralateral limbs.

In patients showing congenital indifference to pain without clinical evidence of any other disorder of the nervous system, the site of the lesion is unknown but SEPs are reportedly normal (Alajouanine et al, 1958; Halliday, 1967c).

Lesions of the Cerebral Hemisphere

The earliest reference to SEPs recorded in patients with cerebral lesions is that of Alajouanine et al (1958), in which it is stated that responses were absent from the damaged hemisphere in five patients with parietal lesions. In a study of 41 patients with predominantly unilateral cerebral lesions, Giblin (1960, 1964) found in 33 the expected correlation between the results of clinical sensory examination and SEP recordings. In 23 of these patients who had no sensory deficit, normal SEPs were recorded, while in 10 patients with moderate or severe cortical sensory loss SEPs were virtually abolished in the affected hemisphere. If the SEP was discerned at all in patients with cortical lesions, the latency of the initial negative component was normal while later components were lost or greatly diminished in amplitude (Fig. 13.13). The remaining eight patients exhibited a discrepancy between the clinical findings and SEP data. In one, a boy with infantile hemiplegia but no demonstrable sensory loss, SEPs were barely detectable over the damaged hemisphere. In the other seven, clinical examination showed typical somatosensory deficits of cortical type due to lesions which spared the primary receiving area, while stimulation of the affected limbs evoked normal responses in the damaged hemisphere. In these latter patients the sensory threshold to electrical stimulation was increased and fluctuated markedly, and SEPs close to maximal amplitude were recorded with

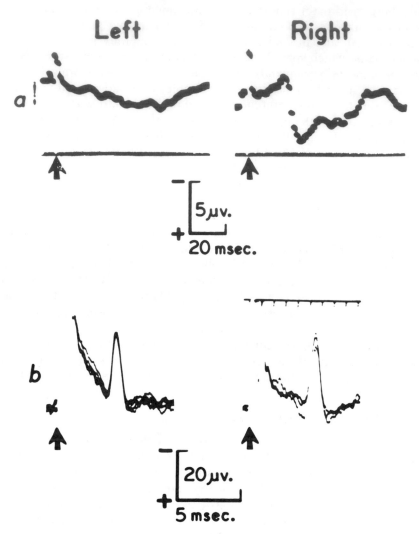

Fig. 13.13. *SEPs in a patient with cerebral vascular disease. The patient was a 45-year-old man with a presumed infarct in the left cerebral hemisphere. No SEPs could be seen in records from the left hemisphere at the first examination. The above records were made 3 weeks later when cortical sensory deficit in the right arm was moderately severe. Lower records, b, show the afferent volleys evoked by strong shocks to the right and left median nerves at the wrist, recorded at the elbow. The upper records, a, show corresponding SEPs recorded from the contralateral parietal regions. Normal SEPs were recorded from the right hemisphere while those recorded from the left hemisphere are markedly attenuated, but a small initial negative deflection with a normal peak latency of 20 msec can just be discerned (from Giblin, D. R. 1964. Ann. N.Y. Acad. Sci., 112, 93).*

shocks that were not perceived. All but one of these patients show the phenomenon of inattention with bilateral simultaneous tactile stimulation.

Responses from the damaged hemisphere were either absent or of reduced amplitude but normal latency in 15 of 21 patients with parietal lesions studied by Laget, Mamo, and Houdart (1967). All but one patient of this group showed sensory deficits of cortical type and three had focal seizures. In six other patients, however, SEPs were greater in amplitude over the abnormal hemisphere, especially the negative component with a peak latency of 100 to 160 msec. Only three of these patients had any sensory impairment but all had experienced focal sensory seizures, and augmentation of the SEP was, therefore, related by the authors to this feature of the clinical presentation.

There have been a number of other reports concerning the correlation of SEP abnormalities with clinical sensory disturbances in patients with cortical lesions, but more detailed discussion of this aspect is unnecessary here. Some comment is, however, required concerning the use of SEPs in the evaluation of unresponsive, comatose patients with regard to the prognosis for ultimate recovery.

Two patients who survived for five months after cardiac arrest are reported by Brierley et al (1971); in each, the EEG was "isoelectric" and no SEPs could be recognized in records from the scalp. Pathologic examination confirmed that the neocortex was severely damaged, maximally in the occipital and parietal regions. Fifty unconscious, unresponsive patients having "isoelectric" EEGs were studied by Trojaborg and Jørgensen (1973). No cerebral potentials were evoked by somatosensory stimuli in 31, all of whom had lost their cranial nerve reflexes and ultimately failed to survive. By contrast, cranial nerve reflexes and cerebral responses to somatic and visual (flash) stimulation were present in the other 19 patients, some of whom did recover. The SEPs recorded in these patients consisted only of the P15 and N20 components, suggesting that no components reflecting postsynaptic potentials of cortical neurones were generated by the thalamocortical afferent volley. SEP techniques may, therefore, be of some prognostic value in such clinical circumstances, although this awaits more adequate and complete demonstration.

Hysterical Anesthesia

Seven patients with hysterical anesthesia were studied by Alajouanine et al (1958), who obtained normal SEPs by stimulating the nerves of the anesthetic limb. This was confirmed by Bergamini and Bergamasco (1967), and by Halliday and Mason (1964), who also found no change in SEPs to electrical or mechanical stimuli during hypnotically induced anesthesia. However, Levy and Behrman (1970), and Levy and Mushin (1973) studied 9 patients and found that cerebral potentials, evoked by either weak or strong shocks applied to anesthetic regions of the skin, were significantly smaller in amplitude than those evoked by comparable stimuli applied to unaffected regions, suggesting "inhibition of receptor sensitivity." There were no differences in the responses evoked by strong shocks applied to nerves of affected and unaffected limbs, but weak shocks near threshold for sensation evoked smaller SEPs from the affected than the unaffected limb. The authors concluded that this latter finding implicated a centrally acting inhibitory mechanism.

SEPs of Enhanced Amplitude

Abnormally large SEPs have been recorded in patients with myoclonus and epilepsy (Dawson, 1947b; Kugelberg and Widén, 1954; Halliday, 1967a, b, c; Sutton and Mayer, 1974; Giblin, unpublished observations), especially if the recordings are made at a time that the myoclonic jerking is occurring. Such enhanced responses are not invariable and are not pathognomonic of the disorder, and SEPs are of normal or only slightly enhanced amplitude in patients with benign essential myoclonus (Halliday and Halliday, 1970). SEPs of enhanced amplitude may also be found in patients with photosensitive epilepsy, in whom light flashes evoked massive bilateral myoclonus or generalized seizures (Broughton, Meier-Ewert, and Ebe, 1969). The significance of these greatly enhanced SEPs in some patients with myoclonus is at present obscure. It does not reflect any disturbance in somatic sensation since none is present. Presumably, it does reflect a loss of inhibitory mechanisms normally operating in the CNS and indeed reveals how powerfully these serve to restrict cortical excitation by the afferent volley in healthy subjects.

Recording of evoked responses has been found to be of value in diagnosis in pediatric neurology by Harden et al (1973) and Pampiglione and Harden (1973), who report that both SEPs and visual evoked potentials of markedly increased amplitude characterize children with late-infantile onset ceroid lipofuscinosis, and the latter remain above normal in amplitude despite disappearance of the electroretinogram.

SEPs of larger amplitude than normal have also been found on the side of a previous craniotomy (Giblin, 1964), and occasionally on the side of a brainstem (Halliday and Wakefield, 1963; Halliday, 1967c) or parietal lobe lesion (Laget et al, 1967). Enhanced SEPs have also been reported in hyperthyroidism (Takahashi and Fugitani, 1970), and following administration of tri-iodothyronine to volunteers (Straumanis and Shagass, 1977), while SEPs with enlarged late components (peak latencies between 200 and 500 msec) have been reported in some patients with Down's syndrome (Bigum, Dustman, and Beck, 1970; Straumanis, Shagass, and Overton, 1973). Such findings seem to have little immediate diagnostic relevance and will not be considered further.

CLINICAL USES OF SEP RECORDING

From the preceding sections of this chapter, it is clear that scalp-recorded SEPs may be abolished in patients with lesions at any level of the nervous system—from peripheral nerve to somatosensory cortex—that give rise to anesthesia or severe impairment of joint position sense in the stimulated limb. With a lesion involving the afferent path from peripheral nerve to thalamus, the characteristic feature of the SEPs, if they are detectable, is a delay in their onset, while in patients with a lesion of the somatosensory cortex of the postcentral gyrus the SEP may be greatly reduced in amplitude but its latency to onset is normal. In patients with sensory loss of "cortical" type, but in whom shocks to the affected limb evoke SEPs of normal latency, configuration and amplitude, the lesion is likely to be posteriorly placed in the parietal lobe, sparing the primary somatosensory cortex; such a finding may indicate a relatively favorable prognosis for recovery of sensory function.

SEP recording can be used to identify and/or localize peripheral nerve lesions, especially when nerve action potentials cannot be recorded peripherally. The technique also permits the definition of lesions involving the spinal roots, limb plexuses, and proximal portion of the peripheral nerves—that is, of lesions involving parts of the peripheral nervous system that are too inaccessible to be investigated by more routine neurophysiologic procedures.

With regard to the central nervous system, the method can be applied to the detection of clinical silent lesions in patients with suspected multiple sclerosis, and this can help to establish the diagnosis by providing evidence of multiple lesions. Moreover, in patients with sensory disturbances due to central pathology, the SEP findings can help to localize the lesion to the cortex or subcortical regions, and in the latter circumstances can help to define the extent to which lemniscal fibers are involved. In conjunction with other electrophysiologic evoked potential techniques, it may also be of value in determining the prognosis for ultimate recovery of unresponsive, comatose patients, but its place in this regard awaits adequate definition.

REFERENCES

Alajouanine, Th., Scherrer, J., Barbizet, J., Calvet, J., and Verley, R. (1958). Potentiels évoqués corticaux chex des sujets atteints de troubles somesthésiques. Rev. Neurol., *98:*757.

Allison, T. (1962). Recovery functions of somatosensory evoked responses in man. Electroencephalogr. Clin. Neurophysiol., *14:*331.

Allison, T., Goff, W. R., and Brey, J. H. (1967). An isolated constant-current stimulator for use with man. J. Appl. Physiol., *22:*612.

Baker, J. B., Larson, S. J., Sances, A., and White, P. T. (1968). Evoked potentials as an aid to the diagnosis of Multiple Sclerosis. Neurology, *18:*286.

Bergamini, L. and Bergamasco, B. (1967). Cortical Evoked Potentials in Man. Charles Thomas, Springfield, Ill.

Bergamini, L., Bergamasco, B., Fra, L., Gandiglio, G., and Mutani, R. (1967). Diagnostic recording of somatosensory cortical evoked potentials in man. Electroencephalogr. Clin. Neurophysiol., *22:*260.

Bergamini, L., Bergamasco, B., Fra, L., Gandiglio, G., Mombelli, A. M., and Mutani, R. (1965). Somatosensory evoked cortical potentials in subjects with peripheral nervous lesions. Electromyography, *5:*121.

Bergamini, L., Bergamasco, B., Fra, L., Gandiglio, G., Mombelli, A. M., and Mutani, R. (1966). Résponses corticales et périphériques évoquées par stimulation du nerf dans la pathologie des cordons postérieurs. Rev. Neurol., *115:*99.

Bickford, R. G., Jacobson, J. L., Thane, D., and Cody, R. (1964). Nature of average evoked potentials to sound and other stimuli in man. Ann. N.Y. Acad. Sci., *112:*204.

Bigum, H. B., Dustman, R. E., and Beck, E. C. (1970). Visual and somatosensory evoked responses from mongoloid and normal children. Electroencephalogr. Clin. Neurophysiol., *28:*576.

Brierley, J. B., Adams, J. H., Graham, D. I., and Simpsom, J. A. (1971). Neocortical death after cardiac arrest. Lancet, *2:*560.

Broughton, R., Meier-Ewert, K. and Ebe, M. 1969. Evoked visual, somatosensory and retinal potentials in photosensitive epilepsy. Electroencephalogr. Clin. Neurophysiol., *27:*373.

Calmes, R. L., and Cracco, R. Q. (1971). Comparison of somatosensory and somatomotor evoked responses to median nerve and digital nerve stimulation. Electroencephalogr. Clin. Neurophysiol., *31:*547.

Colon, E. J., Notermans, S. L. H., Vingerhoets, H. M., Kap, J., and de Weerd, J. (1977). Cortical and cervical somatosensory evoked responses in demyelinating diseases. Eur. Neurol. *15:*124.

Cracco, R. Q. (1972a). The initial positive potential of the human scalp-recorded somatosensory evoked response. Electroencephalogr. Clin. Neurophysiol., *32:*623.

Cracco, R. Q. (1972b). Traveling waves of the human scalp-recorded somatosensory evoked response. Electroencephalogr. Clin. Neurophysiol., *33:*557.

Cracco, R. Q., and Bickford, R. G. (1968). Somatomotor and somatosensory evoked responses: median nerve stimulation in man. Arch. Neurol., *18:*52.

Cracco, R. Q., and Cracco, J. B. (1976). Somatosensory evoked potentials in man: far field potentials. Electroencephalogr. Clin. Neurophysiol., *41:*460.

Dawson, G. D. (1947a). Cerebral responses to electrical stimulation of peripheral nerve in man. J. Neurol. Neurosurg. Psychiatry, 10:134.

Dawson, G. D. (1947b). Investigations on a patient subject to myoclonic seizures after sensory stimulation. J. Neurol. Neurosurg. Psychiatry, *10:*141.

Dawson, G. D. (1950). Cerebral responses to nerve stimulation in man. Br. Med. Bull., *6:*326.

Dawson, G. D. (1954). A summation technique for the detection of small evoked potentials. Electroencephalogr. Clin. Neurophysiol., *6:*65.

Dawson, G. D. (1956). The relative excitability and conduction velocity of sensory and motor nerve fibres in man. J. Physiol., *131:*436.

Dawson, G. D. and Scott, J. W. (1949). The recording of nerve action potentials through skin in man. J. Neurol. Neurosurg. Psychiatry, *12:*259.

Debecker, J. and Desmedt, J. E. (1964). Les potentiels évoqués cérébraux et les potentiels de nerf sensible chez l'homme. Acta. Neurol. Belg., *64:*1212.

Debecker, J., Desmedt, J. E., and Manil, J. (1965). Sur la relation entre le seuil de perception tactile et les potentiels évoqués de l'écorce cérébrale somato-sensible chez l'homme. C. R. Acad. Sci., Paris, *260:*687.

Desmedt, J. E. (1971). Somatosensory cerebral evoked potentials in man. In: Handbook of Electroencephalography and Clinical Neurophysiology, Vol. 9, Cobb, W. A., Ed., p. 55. Amsterdam, Elsevier.

Desmedt, J. E. and Manil, J. (1970). Somatosensory evoked potentials of the normal human neonate in REM sleep, in slow wave sleep and in waking. Electroencephalogr. Clin. Neurophysiol., *29:*113.

Desmedt, J. E. and Noël, P. (1973). Average cerebral evoked potentials in the evaluation of lesions of the sensory nerves and of central somatosensory pathways. In: New Developments in Electromyography and Clinical Neurophysiology, Desmedt, J. E., Ed., Vol. 2., p. 352. Basel, Karger.

Desmedt, J. E. and Noël, P. (1975). Cerebral evoked potentials. In: Peripheral Neuropathy, Dyck, P. J., Thomas, P. K. and Lambert, E. H., Eds., Vol. 1, p. 480. Philadelphia, Saunders.

Desmedt, J. E., Brunko, E., and Debecker, J. (1976). Maturation of the somatosensory evoked potentials in normal infants and children with special reference to the early N1 component. Electroencephalogr. Clin. Neurophysiol., *40:*43.

Desmedt, J. E., Debecker, J., and Manil, J. (1965). Mise en évidence d'un signe électrique cérébral associé à la détection par le sujet d'un stimulus sensoriel tactile. Bull. Acad. Roy. Med. Belg., *5:*887.

Desmedt, J. E., Brunko, E., Debecker, J. and Carmeliet, J. (1974). The system bandpass required to avoid distortion of early components when averaging somatosensory evoked potentials. Electroencephalogr. Clin. Neurophysiol., *37:*407.

Desmedt, J. E., Noël, P., Debecker, J., and Namèche, J. (1973). Maturation of afferent conduction velocity as studied by sensory nerve potentials and by cerebral evoked potentials. In: New Developments in Electromyography and Clinical Neurophysiology, Desmedt, J. E., Ed., Vol. 2, p. 52. Basel, Karger.

Desmedt, J. E., Franken, L., Borenstein, S., Debecker, J., Lambert, C. and Manil, J. (1966a). Le diagnostic des ralentissements de la conduction afférente dans les affections des nerfs périphériques: intérêt de l'extraction du potentiel évoqué cérébral. Rev. Neurol., *155:*255.

Desmedt, J. E., Manil, J., Borenstein, S., Debecker, J., Lambert, C., Franken, L., and Danis, A. (1966b). Evaluation of sensory nerve conduction from averaged cerebral evoked potentials in neuropathies. Electromyography, *6:*263.

Domino, E. F., Matsuoka, S., Waltz, J., and Cooper, I. S. (1965). Effects of cryogenic thalamic lesions on the somesthetic evoked response in man. Electroencephalogr. Clin. Neurophysiol., *19:*127.

Duclaux, R., Franzén, O., Chatt, A. B., Kenshalo, D. R., and Stowell, H. (1974). Responses recorded from human scalp evoked by cutaneous thermal stimulation. Brain Res., *78:*279.

Ervin, F. R. and Mark, V. H. (1964). Studies of the human thalamus: IV. Evoked Responses. Ann. N.Y. Acad. Sci., *112:*81.

Fukushima, T., Mayanagi, Y., and Bouchard, G. (1976). Thalamic evoked potentials to somatosensory stimulation in man. Electroencephalogr. Clin. Neurophysiol., *40:*481.

Giblin, D. R. (1960). The effect of lesions of the nervous system on cerebral responses to peripheral nerve stimulation. Electroencephalogr. Clin. Neurophysiol., *12:*262.

Giblin, D. R. (1964). Somatosensory evoked potentials in healthy subjects and in patients with lesions of the nervous system. Ann. N.Y. Acad. Sci., *112:*93.

Goff, G. D., Matsumiya, Y., Allison, T., and Goff, W. R. (1977). The scalp topography of human somatosensory and auditory evoked potentials. Electroencephalogr. Clin. Neurophysiol., *42:*57.

Goff, W. R., Rosner, B. S., and Allison, T. (1962). Distribution of cerebral somatosensory evoked responses in normal man. Electroencephalogr. Clin. Neurophysiol., *14:*697.

Goff, W. R., Matsumiya, Y., Allison, T., and Goff, G. D. (1969). Cross-modality comparisons of averaged evoked potentials. In: Average Evoked Potentials: Methods, Results and Evaluations. NASA. SP-191. Donchin, E., and Lindsley, D. B., Eds., p. 95. US Govt. Printing Office, Washington, D.C.

Haider, M., Ganglberger, J. A., and Groll-Knapp, E. (1972). Computer analysis of subcortical and cortical evoked potentials and of slow potential phenomena in humans. Confin. Neurol., *34:*224.

Halliday, A. M. (1967a). Cerebral evoked potentials in familial progressive myoclonic epilepsy. J. R. Coll. Physicians. Lond., *1:*123.

Halliday, A. M. (1967b). The electrophysiological study of myoclonus in man. Brain, *90:*241.

Halliday, A. M. (1967c). Changes in the form of cerebral evoked responses in man associated with various lesions of the nervous system. Electroencephalogr. Clin. Neurophysiol. Suppl., *25:*178.

Halliday, A. M. (1968). Computing techniques in neurological diagnosis. Br. Med. Bull., *24:*997.

Halliday, A. M. and Halliday, E. (1970). Cortical evoked potentials in benign essential myoclonus and progressive myoclonic epilepsy. Electroencephalogr. Clin. Neurophysiol., *29:*106.

Halliday, A. M. and Mason, A. A. (1964). The effect of hypnotic anaesthesia on cortical responses. J. Neurol. Neurosurg. Psychiatry, *27:*300.

Halliday, A. M. and Wakefield, G. S. (1963). Cerebral evoked potentials in patients with dissociated sensory loss. J. Neurol. Neurosurg. Psychiatry, *26:*211.

Harden, A., Pampiglione, G., and Picton-Robinson, N. (1973). Electroretinogram and visual evoked response in a form of 'neuronal lipidosis' with diagnostic EEG features. J. Neurol. Neurosurg. Psychiatry, *36:*61.

Hazemann, P., Olivier, L., and Fischgold, H. (1969). Potentiel évoqués somesthésique ipsilatéral enregistré au niveau du scalp chez l'homme hémisphèrectomisé. C. R. Acad. Sci. (Paris), *268:*195.

Hrbek, A., Hrbková, M. and Lenard, H.-G. (1968). Somatosensory evoked responses in newborn infants. Electroencephalogr. Clin. Neurophysiol., *25:*443.

Hrbek, A., Hrbková, M., and Lenard, H.-G. (1969). Somatosensory auditory and visual evoked responses in newborn infants during sleep and wakefulness. Electroencephalogr. Clin. Neurophysiol., *26:*597.

Hrbek, A., Karlberg, P., and Olsson, T. (1973). Development of visual and somatosensory evoked response in preterm newborn infants. Electroencephalogr. Clin. Neurophysiol., *34:*225.

Jones, S. J. (1977). Short latency potentials recorded from the neck and scalp following median nerve stimulation in man. Electroencephalogr. Clin. Neurophysiol., *43:*853.

Kugelberg, E. and Widén, L. (1954). Epilepsia partialis continua. Electroencephalogr. Clin. Neurophysiol., *6:*503.

Kusske, J. A., Burke, B. L., Dill, R. C., Porter, R. W., and Verzeano, M. (1975). Somatosensory evoked responses and slow potential oscillations in human scalp recordings. Physiol. Behav., *15:*241.

Laget, P., Mamo, H., and Houdart, R. (1967). De l'intérêt des potentiels évoqués somesthésiques dans l'étude des lésions du lobe pariétal de l'homme. Neuro-Chirurgie (Paris), *13:*841.

Laget, P., Raimbault, J., and Thieriot-Prevost, G. (1973a). Premiers résultats à propos des potentiels évoqués somesthésiques (P.E.S.) homolatéraux chez l'enfant. C. R. Soc. Biol. (Paris), *167:*421.

Laget, P., Raimbault, J., and Thieriot-Prevost, G. (1973b). L'évolution des potentiels évoqués somesthésiques chez le nourrisson normal durant les deuz premiers mois de la vie. C. R. Soc. Biol. (Paris), *167:*649.

Laget, P., Raimbault, J., and Thieriot-Prevost, G. (1973c). L'évolution du potentiel évoqué somesthésique (P.E.S.) chez l'enfant normal âgé de 61 jours à 7 ans. C. R. Soc. (Paris), *167:*831.

Laget, P., Raimbault, J., D'Allest, A. M., Flores-Guevara, R., Mariani, J., and Thieriot-Prevost, G. (1976). La maturation des potentiels évoqués somesthésiques (PES) chez l'homme. Electroencephalogr. Clin. Neurophysiol., *40:*499.

Larson, S. J. and Sances, A. (1968). Averaged evoked potentials in stereotaxic surgery. J. Neurosurg., *28:*227.

Larson, S. J., Sances, A., and Christenson, P. C. (1966). Evoked somatosensory potentials in man. Arch. Neurol., *15:*88.

Levy, R. and Behrman, J. (1970). Cortical evoked responses in hysterical hemianaesthesia. Electroencephalogr. Clin. Neurophysiol., *29:*400.

Levy, R. and Mushin, J. (1973). The somatosensory evoked response in patients with hysterical anaesthesia. J. Psychosom. Res., *17:*81.

Lüders, H. (1970). The effects of aging on the wave form of the somatosensory cortical evoked potential. Electroencephalogr. Clin. Neurophysiol., *29:*450.

Manil, J. and Ectors, M. (1966). Etude des potentiels cérébraux évoqués par la stimulation des divers doigts de la main chez l'homme normal. C. R. Soc. Biol. (Paris), *160:*1327.

Manil, J., Desmedt, J. E., Debecker, J., and Chorazyna, H. (1967). Les potentiels cérébraux évoqués par la stimulation de la main chez le nouveau-né normal. Rev. Neurol., *117:*53.

Matthews, W. B. (1978). Somatosensory evoked potentials in retrobulbar neuritis. Lancet, *1:*443.

Matthews, W. B., Beauchamp, M., and Small, D. G. (1974). Cervical somatosensory evoked responses in man. Nature, *252:*230.

Nakanishi, T., Shimada, Y., and Toyokura, Y. (1974). Somatosensory evoked responses to mechanical stimulation in normal subjects and in patients with neurological disorders. J. Neurol. Sci., *21:*289.

Namerow, N. S. (1968a). Somatosensory evoked responses in multiple sclerosis. Bull. Los Angeles. Neurol. Soc., *33:*74.

Namerow, N. S. (1968b). Somatosensory evoked responses in multiple sclerosis patients with varying sensory loss. Neurology, *18:*1197.

Namerow, N. S. (1969). Somatosensory evoked responses following cervical cordotomy. Bull. Los Angeles. Neurol. Soc., *34:*184.

Noël, P. (1973). Sensory nerve conduction in the upper limbs at various stages of diabetic neuropathy. J. Neurol. Neurosurg. Psychiatry, *36:*786.

Noël, P. and Desmedt, J. E. (1975). Somatosensory cerebral evoked potentials after vascular lesions of the brain-stem and diencephalon. Brain, *98:*113.

Pagni, C. A. (1967). Somatosensory evoked potentials in thalamus and cortex of man. Electroencephalogr. Clin. Neurophysiol. Suppl., *26:*147.

Pampiglione, G. and Harden, A. (1973). Neurophysiological identification of a late infantile form of 'neuronal lipidosis.' J. Neurol. Neurosurg. Psychiatry, *36:*68.

Perot, P. L. (1973). The clinical use of somatosensory evoked potentials in spinal cord injury. Clin. Neurosurg., *20:*367.

Rowed, D. W., McLean, J. A. G., and Tator, C. H. (1978). Somatosensory evoked potentials in acute spinal cord injury: prognostic value. Surg. Neurol., *9:*203.

Rush, J. L., Kusske, J. A., Porter, R. W., and Verzeano, M. (1976). Driving of slow oscillations in the human somatosensory system. Electroencephalogr. Clin. Neurophysiol., *41:*168.

Saletu, B., Itil, T. M., and Saletu, M. (1971). Evoked responses after hemispherectomy. Confin. Neurol., *33:*221.

Schimmel, H. (1967). The (±) reference: accuracy of estimated mean components in average response studies. Science, *157:*92.

Sears, T. A. (1959). Action potentials evoked in digital nerves by stimulation of mechanoreceptors in the human finger. J. Physiol. (Lond.), *148:*30P.

Shagass, C. and Schwartz, M. (1964). Recovery functions of somatosensory peripheral nerve and cerebral evoked responses in man. Electroencephalogr. Clin. Neurophysiol., *17:*126.

Straumanis, J. J. and Shagass, C. (1977). Effects of lithium, triiodothyronine and propranolol on human somatosensory evoked potentials. Psychopharmacol. Bull., *13:*58.

Straumanis, J. J., Shagass, C., and Overton, D. A. (1973). Somatosensory evoked responses in Down Syndrome. Arch. Gen. Psychiatry, *29:*544.

Sutton, G. G. and Mayer, R. F. (1974). Focal reflex myoclonus. J. Neurol. Neurosurg. Psychiatry, *37:*207.

Takahashi, K. and Fujitani, Y. (1970). Somatosensory and visual evoked potentials in hyperthyroidism. Electroencephalogr. Clin. Neurophysiol., *29:*551.

Tamura, K. (1972). Ipsilateral somatosensory evoked responses in man. Folia Psychiatr. Neurolog. Jap., *26:*83.

Trojaborg, W. and Jørgensen, E. O. (1973). Evoked cortical somatosensory in patients with "isoelectric" EEGs. Electroencephalogr. Clin. Neurophysiol., *35:*301.

Tsumoto, T., Hirose, N., Nonaka, S., and Takahashi, M. (1972). Analysis of somatosensory evoked potentials to lateral popliteal nerve stimulation in man. Electroencephalogr. Clin. Neurophysiol., *33:*379.

Vaughan, H. G. (1969). The relationship of brain activity to scalp recordings of event-related potentials. In: Average Evoked Potentials: Methods, Results, Evaluations. NASA SP-191. Donchin, E. and Lindsley, D. B. (Eds.), p. 45. US Govt. Printing Office, Washington, D.C.

Veale, J. L., Mark, R. F., and Rees. S. (1973). Differential sensitivity of motor and sensory fibres in human ulnar nerve. J. Neurol. Neurosurg. Psychiatry, *36:*75.

14

The Cervical Somatosensory Evoked Potential in Diagnosis

W. B. MATTHEWS

INTRODUCTION

The ability to record the electrical activity of the human spinal cord would clearly be of potential value in the understanding of normal physiology and in the diagnosis of disease. In the experimental animal, where stimulation of the dorsal roots and recording from the surface or substance of the spinal cord present no difficulty, evoked potentials have long been known (Gasser and Graham, 1933), but these conditions are far removed from the clinical context. Magladery et al (1951), although mainly concerned with evoked potentials in the spinal roots and in reflex activity, also recorded potentials from the lumbar spinal cord using lumbar puncture needles in normal volunteers. Pool (1946) recorded spontaneous activity and also the discharges accompanying reflex flexor spasm from the surface and possibly the substance of the isolated spinal cord in a paraplegic patient. The first indication that spinal cord potentials might be recorded from the body surface was that of Liberson and Kim (1963), who described a potential evoked by sensory stimulation that could be recorded from the posterior surface of the neck. With advances in averaging techniques, workers at a number of centers have embarked on the exploration of the spinal somatosensory evoked potential (SEP), and indeed the method is available to anyone with standard recording equipment. In this chapter attention will be paid particularly to the possible clinical applications of the method but some preliminary consideration of the nature of the potentials is necessary.

TECHNIQUE

Stimulation techniques have varied little, the method commonly employed being bipolar electrical surface stimulation of the main mixed nerve trunks in the upper and lower limbs, sensory nerve or cutaneous stimulation being reported only occasionally. Shimoji et al (1972) used needle electrodes inserted into the nerve trunks but without obvious advantage. The duration of the stimulus has usually been 0.1 or 0.2 msec, but the intensity has been more variable. Matthews, Beauchamp, and Small (1974) used, on the median nerve, a stimulus of approximately three times the sensory threshold and showed that stronger stimuli did not significantly alter the characteristics of the evoked response recorded from the skin of the neck. In many reports stimuli of equivalent strength have been used; for example, Cracco (1973) used the muscle twitch of the thenar muscles as his criterion, a point which implies a closely similar stimulus intensity. Ertekin (1976a, b), however, used supramaximal stimuli, while Shimoji et al (1972) did not standardize their mode of stimulation but used stimuli of "varying intensity." They showed that increasing intensity did not alter the latency of the response but did increase the amplitude. The number of potentials averaged has ranged up to 8,192 (Cracco, Cracco, and Graziani, 1975) and frequency has usually been one or two per second. There is no evidence that variations in the nature of the stimulus have been responsible for any of the discrepancies observed in the resulting SEP. The siting of the recording electrodes is, however, of paramount importance.

Recording from the surface of the body has the obvious advantages of being atraumatic and readily repeatable, but the disadvantage that the potential is of low amplitude and has an uncertain relationship to the underlying electrical events in the spinal cord. Additional problems that may arise relate to the presence of muscle artifact, particularly in spastic patients, and, in the dorsal region, to a large EKG artifact. The use of depth electrodes, either epidural (Shimoji, Higashi, and Kano, 1971) or intrathecal (Ertekin, 1976a) has the disadvantages of requiring skilful placing of the electrodes, of causing some discomfort to the patient, and of being potentially hazardous. Accordingly, these procedures could scarcely be used in the monitoring of the progress of disease. The potentials recorded are, however, of higher amplitude and presumably more closely related to physiologic activity in the spinal cord. The technique of Shimoji et al (1971) is that of epidural puncture with a Tuohy needle through which a polyethylene tube is passed, and through which, in turn, are passed the stainless steel recording electrodes. Ertekin's (1976a, b) intrathecal electrode is a needle advanced in the midline towards the spinal cord until the appropriate segmental muscles contract in response to electrical stimulation via the needle.

NORMAL RESULTS

It is immediately obvious that different recording techniques have produced results that are difficult to reconcile. Shimoji, Matsuki, and Shimizu (1977), using epidural recording with a reference electrode in a neighboring intraspinous ligament, obtained similar results from stimulation of nerve trunks in the upper and lower limbs. The immediate segmental response was a positive spike (P_1) followed by negative (N_1) and positive (P_2) deflections and then by a less constant negative one (N_2). Peak latencies were measured from P_1 ("central latency") and not from the stimulus, which makes comparison with the results of other workers difficult, but in an earlier paper (Shimoji et al, 1972) peak latencies for SEP from stimulation of the ulnar nerve at the elbow were given as 7.0 msec for P_1, 10.6 msec for N_1, and 24.6 msec for P_2. These authors do not describe, even with epidural recording, any potential more rostral than the T11 segment after stimulation of a lower limb nerve trunk. Also using the epidural method with a subcutaneous reference electrode, Caccia, Ubiali, and Andreussi (1976) recorded a negative potential in the cervical region after stimulation of the median nerve at the wrist. The mean onset latency is given as 9.6 msec and from their figure the peak latency in the example given is approximately 14 msec. Later components were not described and recordings do not appear to have been made in the cervical region with stimulation of nerve trunks in the lower limb, although thoracic recordings were performed in two subjects.

Ertekin (1976a, 1978) recording from the surface of the cord and the epidural space, with a neighboring subcutaneous reference electrode, found that the waveform recorded varied greatly with the position of the electrode tip in relation to the spinal cord. He found a triphasic segmental response in both lumbar and cervical regions but gave no clear account of latencies. For comparison with surface recordings, the peak latency of the negative deflection illustrated as evoked in the cervical region from stimulation of the median nerve at the elbow is approximately 10 msec, but is preceded by a large positive wave. Ertekin (1976b) was also able to identify a wave recordable with increasing latency rostral to the site of entry of the stimulus. Calculation indicated a conduction velocity of this potential within the spinal cord of 37 m per second.

Cracco (1973), in his original description of surface recording, reported that stimulation of the median nerve evoked a mainly negative potential recordable over the cervical spine. The peak latency of this deflection appeared to increase with more rostral placing of the recording electrode, and naturally it was at first hoped that here was a relatively simple method of measuring conduction velocity in a sensory pathway in the cervical spinal cord. Stimulation of nerve trunks in the lower limbs also evoked a potential of increasing latency at more rostral recording sites, but of such low amplitude that measurement was difficult. Matthews et al (1974) were unable to confirm that the latency of the cervical SEP from median nerve stimulation increased at more rostral levels and this observation has since been confirmed in a very large number of subjects. This was disappointing but in children (Cracco et al, 1975) and in some adults, using a central frontal reference electrode (Jones and Small, 1978), it is possible to demonstrate a "travelling wave" at least superficially comparable to the nerve action potential so useful in peripheral clinical neurophysiology. The conduction velocity calculated from these findings in the adult is, however, much faster than that derived from the intrathecal recordings of Ertekin, being of the order of 60–65 m per second.

The spinal SEP that has been most extensively studied, because of the relative ease with which it can be elicited, is that recordable over the neck following median nerve stimulation at the wrist. Those who have employed depth electrodes have expressed doubts as to the value of surface recordings and some have, indeed, failed to detect SEPs by this method, but this is probably the result of using closely approximated bipolar recording electrodes rather than a "far field" recording technique. The cervical SEP using a midfrontal reference electrode is shown in Figure 14.1. In most normal subjects it is possible to identify all the components illustrated but the amplitude, although not the latency, of the different deflections alters according to the segmental level of the recording electrode. The components of this complex waveform have been labelled by Jones (1977) as N9, N11, N13, N14. The latencies of these components are naturally influenced by the length of each subject's arm (Small, Matthews, and Small, 1978) and the range of normal values must take account of this. For purposes of exploring the relationship of these potentials to function within the central nervous system the latency measured from N9 is probably more valuable. In my own laboratory normal values of latency from N9 to N13 are 4 ± 0.9 msec (mean ± 2 SD) and from N9 to N20, the presumed early cortical response, 9.7 ± 1.6 msec. The amplitude of the main peak of N13 seldom reaches 4 μV, and if it is less than 1 μV it cannot be reliably distinguished from background noise.

The relation of these surface-recorded SEPs to those recorded from depth electrodes is not immediately clear. The negative potential recorded by Caccia et al (1976) from the epidural space can be identified with N13 and their illustration even shows some indication of N11 and N14. The N_1 potential of Shimoji et al (1972) is also probably N13 as the latency from the elbow is approximately that seen in surface recording. Jones (1977) concluded that certain of the poten-

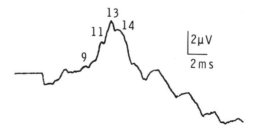

Fig. 14.1. *The normal SEP from stimulation of the median nerve at the wrist recorded from immediately rostral to the seventh cervical spine with a midfrontal reference electrode. 128 sweeps averaged. In this and subsequent figures an upward deflection is negative.*

tials recorded from intrathecal electrodes by Ertekin (1976a) also correspond with N11 and N13 and this is in conformity with the apparent latency of the negative component illustrated.

The lumbar SEP resulting from stimulation of the nerve trunks of the lower limb has been less extensively studied. The ideal reference electrode appears to be the inferior angle of the scapula. From stimulation at the level of the knee two negative components of the SEP can be recognized, N10 with maximum amplitude over the cauda equina and N14 at the level of the T12 vertebra. N14 was thought by El-Negamy and Sedgwick (1978) to be equivalent to N11 in the cervical region.

The practical difficulties of detecting SEPs above the lower dorsal spine following stimulation of the nerve trunks in the legs have not been fully overcome. Jones and Small (1978), stimulating the posterior tibial nerve at the ankle and using a midfrontal reference electrode, were able to provide figures for normal peak latency of SEP at different vertebral levels but, apart from T12 to L2, the mean amplitude of the potentials was below 1 μV.

ORIGIN OF THE SPINAL SEP

Evidence as to the origin of the components of the spinal SEP derived from the study of patients with lesions of the nervous system will be considered in a subsequent section. The origin of the evoked potentials recordable from the surface of the spinal cord in animals can legitimately be compared with intrathecal and epidural recordings in man. In both there is a segmental potential related to the arrival of the stimulus in the cord, followed or accompanied by a potential recordable with reducing amplitude and increasing latency over more rostral segments. The former is likely to arise from activity within postsynaptic neurons and the latter must be related to conduction of afferent impulses in ascending tracts in the spinal cord. Cracco and Evans (1978) have demonstrated in the cat that spinal cord compression above the site of entry of the stimulus causes reduction in amplitude and increased latency of the latter potential. Happel, LeBlanc, and Kline (1975) have emphasised that the ascending pathways probably contain very few axons of primary sensory neurons and that the rapid decline in amplitude may be due to polysynaptic conduction. These same authors also examined, in the experimental animal, the most important matter of the relation between potentials recorded from the skin and those from the surface of the spinal cord. They found that, while the two were certainly related, latencies of surface-recorded potentials were *shorter* than those directly recorded and they discussed possible explanations involving the mode of conduction through tissues remote from the site of origin of the potentials. This finding is in agreement with the different estimates of conduction velocity in the human spinal cord derived from surface and depth electrodes.

The main component of the spinal SEP as recorded in the neck from stimulation in the arm is, however, of fixed latency and cannot arise in the same way. Wiederholt and Iraqui-Madoz (1977) and Wiederholt (1978) have reported a series of experimental studies on subcortical SEPs in the experimental animal. They have identified, by means of selective brain section, the origin of subcortical components that appear to arise from fixed generating sites in the posterior columns of the spinal cord, the posterior column nuclei and medial lemniscus, and the thalamus and possibly the cerebellum. The precise relevance of these findings to human physiology is not yet clear but they are important as demonstrating that complex wave forms can be derived from the combined evoked activity of a number of subcortical centers.

When considering the origin of surface-recorded spinal SEPs it is of course first necessary to be certain that they are derived from activity within the nervous system and do not result from reflexly or otherwise induced muscle activity. From personal observation voluntary contraction of the neck muscles abolishes the response rather than enhancing it as would be expected if the potentials were myogenic. This has been confirmed by El-Negamy and Sedgwick (1978) who were also able to obtain recordings of the potential during complete muscle relaxation and light anaesthesia.

From topographic studies in normal subjects, Jones (1977) concluded that N9 arose within the brachial plexus. A potential of somewhat shorter latency can be recorded from the skin over the plexus in the supraclavicular fossa and N9 therefore appears to be generated rather more distally, probably at the level of the axilla. Similar considerations of amplitude relative to the recording site led El-Negamy and Sedgwick (1978) to conclude that N11 originates within the spinal cord and they believed that the dorsal horn was the most probable generating site. N13 and N14 have been speculatively assigned to the dorsal column nuclei and the thalamus.

In most experiments stimulation has been confined to mixed nerve trunks. Shimoji et al (1977) were unable to record spinal SEPs after intense stimulation, presumably cutaneous, of the fifth toe, and suggested that muscle afferents were the important component of the peripheral stimulus. However, El-Negamy and Sedgwick (1978) recorded the cervical SEP after stimulation of digital nerves and concluded that low-threshold cutaneous afferents were almost the sole contributors to the effective stimulus. They also concluded that a major contribution from antidromic impulses in motor fibers was improbable.

CLINICAL APPLICATIONS

Many authors, after describing their results in experimental animals or in man, have commented on the possible clinical value of recording the spinal SEP and yet actual diagnostic use of the technique has been limited. There are excellent reasons for this as there can be no justification for the use of high-cost technology to establish a diagnosis that could be better achieved with the neurologist's traditional pin and tuning fork.

Depth-Recorded SEP

The elaborate and invasive nature of epidural and intrathecal recording methods are such that there could be no indication for their use unless they provided information not obtainable by other means. It has not been shown that this is so. Using the intrathecal method Ertekin (1978) recorded from 30 subjects of whom 13 appear to have had clinical evidence of spinal cord disease. Few diagnostic details are given, however, and it seems that no correlation between clinical evidence of disease and presumed abnormalities of spinal SEP could be established. Ertekin eventually concluded that surface recording, despite obvious disadvantages, is likely to be clinically more useful.

Epidural recording was used in the study of cervical spondylotic myelopathy by Matsukado et al (1976). The cervical SEP following median nerve stimulation was graded according to degree of abnormality and correlated with the prognosis following operative decompression of the cervical canal. The major abnormality encountered was reduction in amplitude and eventual abolition of the initial negative deflection N_1, probably identical with N13 in surface recording. Abnormalities in later components were also described. The degree of abnormality of SEP was not related to the severity of the preoperative clinical state. A normal cervical SEP or minor abnormalities were found to indicate a good postoperative result, whereas with severe abnormalities the outlook was unfavourable. This result is certainly interesting but it is doubtful whether a gross abnormality of the cervical SEP should be regarded as a strong contra-indication to surgery. If this could indeed be established it would be a valuable clinical contribution as patients could be spared a fruitless and unpleasant operation.

Caccia et al (1976) used epidural recording in the cervical and thoracic regions. In radicular lesions affecting the upper and lower limbs the amplitude of the appropriate cervical or thoracic SEP on the affected side was, in general, lower than on the unaffected side with no significant change in latency. This again was an interesting observation but could not be regarded as an essential diagnostic manoeuvre in the cases described. The results in spinal cord disease were less clear-cut. Excluding one case attributed to myelitis of "Landry type" in whom no SEP could be recorded and where polyneuritis must be suspected, seven patients were examined. The authors drew a distinction between the results in patients with compression of the spinal cord and those with intrinsic disease. In the former the SEP recorded above the level of the lesion was present but reduced in amplitude, whereas in intrinsic myelopathy the SEP was normal. This conclusion is not strictly supported by their own observations as in a patient with multiple sclerosis (MS) the amplitude of the potential was much reduced and in a patient with syphilitic myelitis no potential could be recorded above the lesion. If SEPs arise from activity in ascending pathways in the spinal cord, the potentials are perhaps more likely to be influenced by the degree to which conduction in the pathways is interrupted than by the pathology of the responsible lesion.

Surface-Recorded SEP

The diagnostic possibilities of surface-recorded SEPs have been more extensively explored, particularly those of the cervical potential evoked by stimulation of the median or ulnar nerve. An immediate obstacle to the widespread use of this technique is the difficulty of defining the limit of normality. This problem was solved with regard to the visual evoked potential of the form usually examined, that evoked by pattern reversal, by selecting a prominent and relatively constant component of the response, the P100, and defining the limits of its normal amplitude and, in particular, latency. Such an enviably simple solution has not proved possible with the cervical SEP, largely because the major abnormalities encountered are changes in amplitude and in the shape of the complex potential rather than prolongation of latency, although this also occurs. The experienced observer may learn to recognize waveforms considered to be "abnormal" but to do so without clearly defined criteria would lead to the errors of routine clinical electroencephalography where reports and opinions are based almost entirely on notoriously fallible visual inspection. Mastaglia, Black and Collins (1976) attempted to use latency of the main peak (N13) as a major criterion and regarded any value in excess of 15.4 msec as abnormal. They did not, however, allow for arm length, although this has a considerable and systematic effect on the latency of the response to stimulation of the nerve at the wrist. Small et al (1978) regarded as abnormal a latency in excess of 2.5 SD above the mean normal latency for the subject's arm length (Fig. 14.2). In order to eliminate the effect of arm length, latency may be measured from N9 which arises from the brachial plexus, and El-Negamy

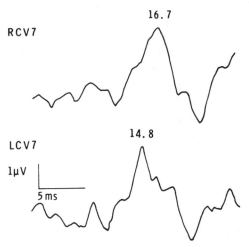

Fig. 14.2. *Recordings from immediately rostral to the seventh cervical spine (CV7) of cervical SEP from stimulation of the right and left median nerves in a man with definite MS, but without sensory abnormalities in the upper limbs. The potential from the right side is of normal form and amplitude but prolonged latency (from Small, D. G., Matthews, W. B. and Small, M. 1978. J. Neurol. Sci., 35, 211).*

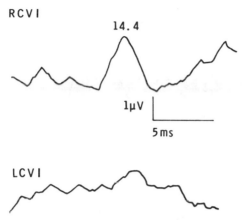

Fig. 14.3. *Absence of cervical SEP from stimulation of the left median nerve with a normal potential from the right in a man with definite MS but without sensory signs in the upper limbs. Recordings made from immediately rostral to the second cervical spine (CVI) with a midfrontal reference electrode (from Small, D. G., Matthews, W. B. and Small, M. 1978. J. Neurol. Sci., 35, 211).*

(1978) paid particular attention to increased latency between N9 and N11 as evidence of abnormality. This is certainly a reasonable assumption but from personal experience and from inspection of his published recordings it is often not possible positively to identify the low-amplitude late potentials as N11 or any other component of the normal response. Absence of SEPs is clearly abnormal (Fig. 14.3) and in practice any potential of less than 1 μV can usually be shown to be random by averaging two series of potentials at the same recording session. Both these criteria, latency and amplitude, are susceptible of measurement but do not cover the considerable proportion of recordings of potentials clearly different in shape from the normal and, therefore, perhaps legitimately to be regarded as abnormalities difficult to express as measurements. Small et al (1978) recognized one such pattern in which N13 was absent with apparent preservation of N11 and N14 (Fig. 14.4). The diagnostic value of the cervical SEP is considerably increased if the short latency scalp potential, N20, is recorded simultaneously.

Multiple Sclerosis. The main diagnostic application of spinal SEPs has been in MS (Small, Beauchamp, and Matthews, 1974; Small, 1976; Mastaglia et al, 1976; Small, Beauchamp, and Matthews, 1977; Small et al, 1978). The particular value of evoked potential techniques in this disease lies in the possibility of demonstrating abnormalities in the absence of relevant clinical symptoms or signs. Such abnormalities, already recognized in the visual system, can be presumed to be due to "silent" plaques, not detectable by conventional clinical examination. Multiple lesions can, therefore, be demonstrated in patients with clinical evidence of a single lesion or even in those who appear to have made a complete recovery. A positive diagnosis may spare the patient unpleasant in-

LCV I

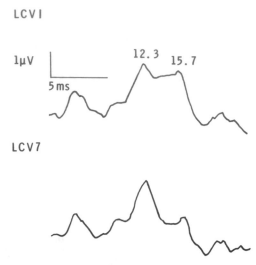

LCV7

Fig. 14.4. *Absence of N13 with preservation of the other components of the cervical SEP after stimulation of the left median nerve in a man with definite MS. Recordings were made from immediately rostral to the second and seventh cervical spines (CV1 and CV7) (from Small, D. G., Matthews, W. B. and Small, M. 1978. J. Neurol. Sci., 35, 211).*

vestigations and it is to be hoped that early diagnosis may eventually be of value in allowing early treatment.

Using the criteria of abnormality described above, Mastaglia et al (1976) found that 57 percent of 52 patients with definite, probable, or possible MS had abnormal cervical SEPs from median nerve stimulation. Of 17 patients in the definite category, 16 had abnormal potentials. Using both SEPs and visual evoked potentials they found abnormalities in 69 percent of their patients, SEP being the more sensitive test. In the Oxford series the proportion of abnormalities of the SEP was found to be as high as 75 percent in the first 60 patients and 89 percent in those in the definite category (Small et al, 1974; Small, Beauchamp, and Matthews, 1977). With larger numbers of patients this fell to 59 percent (Small et al, 1978), and 69 percent in the definite category. In patients severely disabled with MS the cervical SEP was invariably abnormal. More than half (56 percent) of the abnormalities found were from stimulation of the median nerve in arms where there were no sensory symptoms or signs, apparently revealing silent plaques. The cervical SEP was found to be a more sensitive index of abnormality than the cerebral N20. When combined with the recording of visual evoked potentials, abnormalities were found in 86 percent of 74 patients in the three diagnostic categories of MS.

A disappointing finding was that the techniques may prove to be less valuable than was at first hoped in the early diagnosis of MS. SEPs were normal in 15 of 18 patients with an acute neurologic episode, other than optic neuritis, suggestive of the onset of MS. Three of these patients are known to have developed MS and in two of them cervical SEPs were normal in the initial episode. Retrobulbar neuritis is a common presenting symptom of MS but a proportion of these patients never develop clinical evidence of multiple lesions. A reliable prognostic test would be invaluable and it was at first hoped that abnormalities in the cervical SEP might distinguish those patients who would later develop MS. This hope has not been fulfilled. Of 39 patients with isolated retrobulbar neuritis, only 4 had abnormal SEPs, 1 of whom later developed MS within the period of observation as have 2 of those with a normal SEP (Matthews, 1978). The investigation is not, therefore, capable of making this distinction, either because it is insensitive or, more probably, because patients with retrobulbar neuritis who will later develop MS do not often have plaques within sensory pathways in the cervical spinal cord or brainstem at the time of their visual symptoms.

Additional important roles for evoked potential studies, including the cervical SEP, would be to monitor the progress of MS and to assess the results of treatment. Matthews and Small (1979) made regular serial recordings in a small series of patients and found that in those who did not relapse during the period of observation the SEP, whether normal or abnormal, remained stable. In patients with active relapsing and remitting disease the cervical SEP was labile in that it fluctuated between normality and abnormality. These changes were not random, as a specific abnormal waveform sometimes persisted for several months before reverting to normal. There was, however, no relation between fluctuation in the SEP and clinical relapse or remission. In a larger series of patients examined less frequently the potentials became more abnormal with the passage of time in the majority of those who had sustained one or more relapses involving the spinal cord, but here again the abnormalities could not be closely related in time with the clinical relapse and remission was not accompanied by return of SEP to normal values.

The basis of the use of evoked potentials in the diagnosis of MS lies in the persistence of electrophysiologic abnormality in the absence of clinical signs. This property is incompatible with the use of these techniques in monitoring the course of the disease where indications of activity and recovery are required. El-Negamy (1978) has described a return towards normality following dorsal column stimulation in the treatment of MS but the significance of these changes must be in doubt in view of the absence of similar change in patients recovering spontaneously from severe relapse involving sensory tracts in the spinal cord. A further complicating factor is that the cervical SEP in MS is much influenced by increase in body temperature, normal potentials sometimes becoming abnormal and slightly abnormal SEP being abolished (Matthews, Read, and Pountney, 1978). These observations were made with increases in oral temperature of 0.5 to 1° C and the effect of smaller changes are unknown. If conclusions on the acute effect of treatment on function of the nervous system in MS are to be drawn from changes in cervical SEPs ideally core temperature should be recorded.

The value of SEP recording in MS, therefore, lies in diagnosis—in the detection of clinically silent plaques—and the use of multiple evoked potential techniques is clearly more likely to demonstrate multiple lesions. In addition it is to be hoped that the study of evoked potentials in MS will throw light on the ways in which the disease affects nervous function. At present their use has only served to emphasize the paradox of complete recovery of function with persistent lesions which can now be shown to be the cause of persistent but symptomless electrophysiologic disturbances.

Other Conditions. Much less is known of the diagnostic possibilities of the surface-recorded spinal SEP in other conditions. Koivikko, Lang, and Falck (1976) reported prolonged latency of the main negative peak on stimulating the affected arm in one patient with cervical rib and one with a cervical root lesion. Bilateral abnormalities were found in a patient with syringomyelia. Their normal value for peak latency was 15.8 msec, and it is difficult to interpret their results. El-Negamy (1978) examined nine patients with spondylotic cervical myelopathy and found a normal N9, as might be expected from its origin in the brachial plexus, and reduced amplitude and prolonged latency of the later components or their complete absence.

Personal results in a variety of conditions included the following:

1. Normal results in four cases of motor neuron disease (ALS) with prominent spinal cord symptoms. Sensory tract involvement is often seen at autopsy in this disease in spite of the absence of sensory signs but no electrophysiologic abnormality was found.
2. Normal cervical and cortical SEPs in two cases of clinically isolated cerebellar degeneration. These patients were examined because of the possibility that some components of the cervical potential might arise from the cerebellum.
3. Six cases of syringomyelia were examined, with inconsistent results. In two patients, one with unilateral and one with bilateral loss of pain and thermal sensation in the arm, cervical and cortical SEPs were normal. In two with bilateral sensory loss the latency of N13 was prolonged on one or both sides, with normal amplitude and normal N20. In two more seriously affected patients, in one of whom postural sense was also affected, cervical SEPs were absent, apart from N9, and N20 was greatly delayed or absent. From these results it was evident that severe loss of those forms of sensation conveyed through the spinothalamic tracts could exist with a normal cervical SEP.
4. Eleven cases of cervical spondylotic myelopathy were examined, the results in seven being grossly abnormal. In general N9 could be identified followed by delayed, distorted low-amplitude potentials. N20 was either greatly delayed or absent. In three patients with little or no clinical evidence of involvement of the upper limbs, SEPs were either normal or in one instance showed unilateral absence of the main peak (N13) as the only abnormality. In one patient in whom the spinal cord was compressed by osteophytes at the T1 level, SEPs were normal.
5. From a variety of spinal cord lesions examined, a number can be selected as illustrating the value and limitations of the technique. In a patient with

a cervical cord medulloblastoma producing a severe lesion with absence of postural sense in the lower limbs but only blunting of pain sensation in one arm, SEPs were entirely normal. Normal responses were also obtained in a patient with an infarct in the territory of the anterior spinal artery in the cervical region, causing loss of pain and thermal sensation but no change in modalities carried by the posterior columns. In an elderly woman who proved to have a meningioma extending from C4 to C6, cervical SEPs were abnormal bilaterally but could not be distinguished from the pattern seen in spondylotic myelopathy, the original clinical diagnosis (Fig. 14.5).

6. In three patients with myoclonic epilepsy of nonprogressive type and one patient with myoclonus due to Creutzfeldt-Jakob disease, cervical SEPs were normal. These patients were examined because of the large amplitude cerebral SEP reported in certain forms of myoclonic epilepsy (Halliday, 1967).

In the diagnosis of the nature of the disease process, therefore, the cervical SEP is of limited value, perhaps restricted to the detection of clinically unsuspected lesions in MS. The technique clearly cannot be used in isolation to distinguish MS from spondylotic myelopathy, for example (Fig. 14.5), or even to separate organic from hysterical sensory loss in view of the normal results in syringomyelia. A more extended role in the localization of lesions of the nervous system may be found.

The examination of the early component N9 arising from the brachial plexus might be expected to contribute to the differentiation of plexus from cervical root lesions and similar possibilities exist with regard to the lumbar potentials.

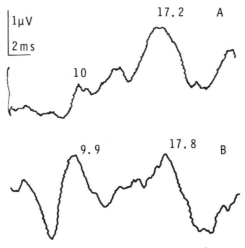

Fig. 14.5. *Cervical SEP recorded from A, a woman with a cervical meningioma, and B, a man with spondylotic cervical myelopathy, showing a similar pattern of preservation of N9 followed by a delayed low amplitude potential, presumed to be N13.*

As far as the central nervous system is concerned, important uses would be in the localization of spinal cord lesions and in the prognosis of paraplegia. It is known that the surface recorded spinal SEP cannot be detected above a complete spinal cord lesion when the stimulus enters below the lesion (personal observation; El-Negamy, 1978). There is, of course, no difficulty in determining the level of such a lesion on clinical grounds and to be useful the method should be capable of localizing incomplete lesions. The technical difficulties of recording in the upper thoracic and cervical regions with stimulation of the nerves in the legs is an immediate obstacle as minor changes in amplitude or latency, or even absence of EP, could not with certainty be regarded as abnormal. The cervical SEP following median nerve stimulation can be used in the investigation of cervical cord lesions. El-Negamy (1978) has shown that in severe lesions, either complete or partial, the expected abnormalities are found. The most promising line of investigation would be the examination of acute paraplegia in an attempt to distinguish complete from partial lesions at this stage, with possibly important prognostic implications. A different approach is suggested by the experimental observations of Cracco and Evans (1978) that with bipolar electrodes bridging a complete lesion of the spinal cord and stimulation entering at a lower level, a positive potential is recorded at the upper electrode. Whether characteristic changes could be found by surface recording in partial lesions in man is not yet known.

In three patients in a personal series a brainstem lesion, localized on clinical grounds, has been accompanied by a normal cervical SEP and a much delayed N20 (Fig. 14.6). This pattern was also present in a fourth patient originally thought to have hysterical hemiplegia but who later developed signs that were clearly organic.

The study of clinical cases has thrown some further light on the origin of the fixed latency cervical SEP from median nerve stimulation. The response may be very abnormal in the absence of sensory loss, but where such loss is present the results strongly indicate that it is impulses conveyed in the posterior columns of the spinal cord that are at some point in their course concerned in the production of the potential. The fact that an entirely normal cervical response can accompany a much delayed cortical response with a lesion clinically localizable to the brainstem suggests that all components of the spinal SEP may originate within the spinal cord or medulla rather than from the suggested sites of the thalamus and cerebellum. So far no pathologic studies have been published. In a single personal observation a patient with mild MS died of an incidental subarachnoid haemorrhage. Virtual absence of cervical SEPs from one arm was found to be associated with a plaque involving the posterior horn at the appropriate level with slight encroachment on the posterior columns, this being the only lesion of the sensory pathways (Esiri and Matthews, unpublished observations). Examination of this material is proceeding but the observation at least confirms that abnormalities of the spinal SEP can arise from anatomic abnormalities of the sensory pathways at a cervical spinal cord level.

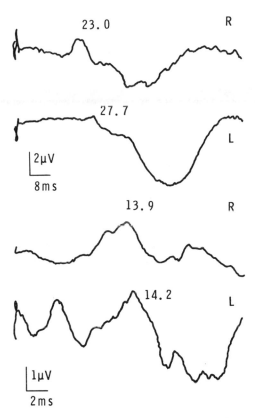

Fig. 14.6. *The upper two records are of the cortical SEP from stimulation of the right and left median nerves, and the lower two show the cervical SEP recorded simultaneously. The cervical potentials are normal but the cortical potential from the left median nerve is much delayed. There was clinical evidence of a lesion, of undetermined cause, in the right side of the medulla, apparently delaying conduction to the cortex.*

REFERENCES

Caccia, M. R., Ubiali, E. and Andreussi, L. (1976). Spinal evoked responses recorded from the epidural space in normal and diseased humans. J. Neurol. Neurosurg. Psychiatry, *39:*962.

Cracco, J. B., Cracco, R. Q. and Graziani, L. J. (1975). The spinal evoked potential in infants and children. Neurology, *25:*31.

Cracco, R. Q. (1973). Spinal evoked response: peripheral nerve stimulation in man. Electroencephalogr. Clin. Neurophysiol., *35:*379.

Cracco, R. Q. and Evans, B. (1978). Spinal evoked potential in the cat: effects of asphyxia, strychnine, cord section and compression. Electroencephalogr. Clin. Neurophysiol., *44:*187.

El-Negamy, E. H. M. (1978). Subcortical somatosensory evoked potentials studied in man. Thesis: University of Southampton.

El-Negamy, E. and Sedgwick, E. M. (1978). Properties of a spinal somatosensory evoked potential recorded in man. J. Neurol. Neurosurg. Psychiatry, *41*:762.

Ertekin, C. (1976a). Studies on the human evoked electrospinogram. I: The origin of the segmental evoked potentials. Acta Neurol. Scand., *53*:3.

Ertekin, C. (1976b). Studies on the human evoked electrospinogram. II: The conduction velocity along the dorsal funiculus. Acta Neurol. Scand., *53*:21.

Ertekin, C. (1978). Comparison of the human evoked electrospinogram recorded from the intrathecal, epidural and cutaneous levels. Electroencephalogr. Clin. Neurophysiol., *44*:683.

Gasser, H. S. and Graham, H. T. (1933). Potentials produced in the spinal cord by stimulation of the dorsal roots. Am. J. Physiol., *103*:303.

Halliday, A. M. (1967). The electrophysiological study of myoclonus in man. Brain, *90*:241.

Happel, L. T., LeBlanc, H. J. and Kline, D. G. (1975). Spinal cord potentials evoked by peripheral nerve stimulation. Electroencephalogr. Clin. Neurophysiol., *38*:349.

Jones, S. J. (1977). Short latency potentials recorded from the neck and scalp following median nerve stimulation in man. Electroencephalogr. Clin. Neurophysiol., *43*:853.

Jones, S. J. and Small, D. G. (1978). Spinal and subcortical evoked potentials following stimulation of the posterior tibial nerve in man. Electroencephalogr. Clin. Neurophysiol., *44*:299.

Koivikko, M. J., Lang, A. H. and Falck, B. (1976). Diagnostic possibilities for the nuchal evoked potential. Acta Neurol. Scand., *54*:192.

Liberson, W. T. and Kim, K. C. (1963). The mapping out of evoked potentials by stimulation of median and peroneal nerves. Electroencephalogr. Clin. Neurophysiol., *15*:721.

Magladery, J. W., Porter, W. E., Park, A. M. and Teasdale, R. D. (1951). Electrophysiological studies of nerve and reflex activity in normal man. IV: The two neurone reflex and identification of certain action potentials from spinal roots and cord. Bull. Johns Hopkins Hosp., *88*:499.

Mastaglia, F. L., Black, J. I. and Collins, D. W. K. (1976). Visual and spinal evoked potentials in diagnosis of multiple sclerosis. Br. Med. J., *3*:732.

Matsukado, Y., Yoshida, M., Goya, T. and Shimoji, K. (1976). Classification of cervical spondylosis or disc protrusion by preoperative evoked spinogram. J. Neurosurg., *44*:435.

Matthews, W. B. (1978). Somatosensory evoked potentials in retrobulbar neuritis. Lancet, *1*:443.

Matthews, W. B. and Small, D. G. (1979). Serial recording of visual and somatosensory evoked potentials in multiple sclerosis. J. Neurol. Sci., *40*:11.

Matthews, W. B., Beauchamp, M. and Small, D. G. (1974). Cervical somatosensory evoked responses in man. Nature, *252*:230.

Matthews, W. B., Read, D. J. and Pountney, E. (1978). The effect of raising body temperature on visual and somatosensory evoked potentials in patients with multiple sclerosis. J. Neurol. Neurosurg. Psychiatry, *42*:250.

Pool, J. L. (1946). Electrospinogram (ESG): Spinal cord action potential recorded from a paraplegic patient. J. Neurosurg., *3*:192.

Shimoji, K., Higashi, H. and Kano, T. (1971). Epidural recording of spinal electrogram in man. Electroencephalogr. Clin. Neurophysiol., *30*:236.

Shimoji, K., Matsuki, M. and Shimizu, H. (1977). Wave-form characteristics and spatial distribution of evoked spinal electrogram in man. J. Neurosurg., *46*:304.

Shimoji, K., Kano, T., Higashi, H., Morioka, T. and Henschel, E. O. (1972). Evoked electrograms recorded from epidural space in man. J. Applied Physiol., *33*:468.

Small, D. G. (1976). Peripherally evoked spinal cord potentials in neurological diagnosis. In: Scientific Aids in Hospital Diagnosis. Nicholson, J. P., Ed., p. 155. Plenum Press, New York.

Small, D. G., Beauchamp, M. and Matthews, W. B. (1974). Subcortical somatosensory evoked responses in man. In: Proceedings of the International Symposium on Cerebral Evoked Potentials in Man. Desmedt, J. E., Ed. (in press).

Small, D. G., Beauchamp, M. and Matthews, W. B. (1977). Spinal evoked potentials in multiple sclerosis. Electroencephalogr. Clin. Neurophysiol., *42:*141.

Small, D. G., Matthews, W. B. and Small, M. (1978). The cervical somatosensory evoked potential (SEP) in the diagnosis of multiple sclerosis. J. Neurol. Sci., *35:*211.

Wiederholt, W. C. (1978). Recovery function of short latency components of surface and depth recorded somatosensory evoked potentials in the cat. Electroencephalogr. Clin. Neurophysiol., *45:*259.

Wiederholt, W. C. and Iraqui-Madoz, V. J. (1977). Far field somatosensory potentials in the rat. Electroencephalogr. Clin. Neurophysiol., *42:*456.

15
Electronystagmography

ROBERT A. SCHINDLER and VIVIAN WEIGEL

INTRODUCTION

One of the most common medical complaints is the vague reference by many patients to "dizzy spells," a complaint that invariably poses problems for diagnosis and treatment. Care must be taken to distinguish vertigo, a hallucination of motion, most often described as falling, turning, or spinning, from lightheadedness or syncopal attacks. True vertigo invariably connotes a disturbance of either the central or peripheral vestibular system and is associated with a jerk nystagmus.

Taking an accurate history from the vertiginous patient is difficult, since the exact sensations felt during an attack are usually recalled imprecisely. The physician can observe the patient's eye movements during an attack or during visual and vestibular stimulation by various means, and may then be able to draw some conclusions concerning the anatomic location of the patient's disorder. Certain eye movements usually indicate a peripheral (inner ear) vestibular disorder, while others are characteristic of a central nervous system pathology.

In particular, jerk nystagmus, which is the repetitive slow deviation of the eye toward one side, followed by the rapid or saccadic movement of the eye back to the center gaze, is characteristic of vestibular disorders. Clinical evaluation can be misleading, however, because visual fixation can reduce jerk nystagmus by as much as 90 percent of its intensity in the absence of fixation. Moveover, certain brain lesions, as well as drugs, impair or abolish visual suppression of nystagmus, and these phenomenon cannot be demonstrated unless the nystagmus is seen both with and without visual fixation.

Frenzel glasses, 20-diopter lenses mounted together with two small lights in a goggle-like frame that fits snugly against the patient's head, have been used to abolish patient fixation, but they do not completely eliminate it.

Fortunately, nystagmography has progressed since 1880 from the mechanical and optic techniques originally employed to the electrical method that is now widely used clinically to provide the physician with a permanent record of eye movements, with the patient's eyes both open and closed, in light and/or in darkness. The electronystagmogram (ENG) is a permanent tracing of eye movement that can be examined at leisure, can be compared with previous or subsequent tests, and can allow quantitative measurements of nystagmus intensity to be made.

The eye can be regarded as a dipole, with the cornea acting as a positive pole and the retina as a negative pole. The potential difference between the two poles is normally at least 1 mV. This corneoretinal potential creates an electrical field in the front of the head that changes its orientation with eyeball rotation. Electrodes placed on the skin can detect these electrical changes which, when amplified, can drive a writing instrument, making a tracing of the eye movements. When the eyes are at midposition there is a "resting" voltage between the electrodes that serves as a baseline. By convention, the recording system is such that horizontal eye movements produce an upward pen deflection when the eyes move to the right, and a downward deflection when they move to the left. Vertical eye movements are recorded on a separate channel; upward movement causes the pen to deflect upward, and downward eye movement produces a downward pen deflection.

PHYSIOLOGY

The maintenance of equilibrium depends on the complex interaction between the visual-oculomotor, vestibular, and somatosensory systems (Fig. 15.1). The vestibular end organ consists of three semicircular canals oriented at 90° to each other. Each has an ampulla containing a crista and vestibular sensory epithelium (type I and II hair cells). The sensory hair cells lie on the crista and project into the lumen of the endolymphatic space (Fig. 15.2). The hairs, the kinocilium and the stereocilia of each cell, are imbedded in a gelatinous mass, the cupula, which fills the ampulla and thereby prevents free flow of endolymph through it.

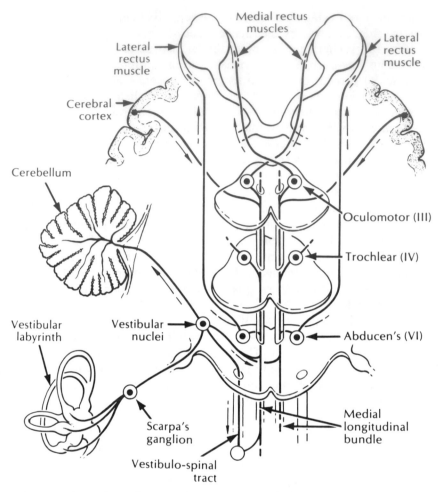

Fig. 15.1. *Central vestibular pathways (from English, G.M. 1976. Otolaryngology. A Textbook, Harper & Row, Hagerstown, Maryland).*

In the healthy ear, the semicircular canals function in angular acceleration, each canal working in consort with its counterpart in the opposite ear. Gravitational and linear acceleration are perceived by the otolith organ, the macula of the utricle. Here, hair cells, similar in structure to those in the semicircular canals, are covered by an otolithic membrane into which the kinocilium and stereocilia are imbedded. The otolithic membrane is a gelatinous mass packed with calcium carbonate crystals called otoconia. Endolymph flows freely through the healthy utricle and hair cell activation is achieved by shearing forces produced by the otolithic membrane relative to the surface of the hair cells. The function of the other otolith organ, the saccule, is uncertain, but it may also function in linear acceleration.

The orientation of the kinocilium and stereocilia on the surface of the hair

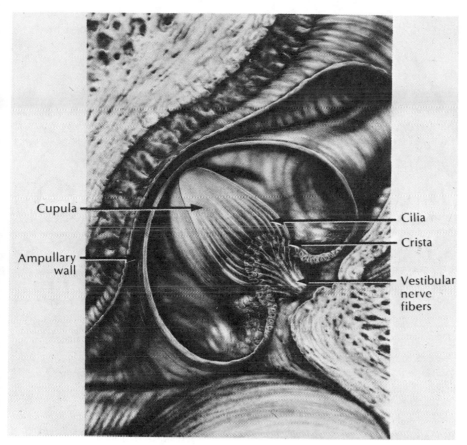

Fig. 15.2. Structural anatomy of the ampullated end of the horizontal semicircular canal (from English, G. M. 1976. Otolaryngology. A Textbook, Harper & Row, Hagerstown, Maryland).

cell determines how that particular cell will respond to displacement of the cilia by either the cupula or otolithic membrane. A bending of the cilia toward the kinocilium results in an increase in the resting discharge rate of the afferent neuron innervating that cell; displacement of the hairs away from the kinocilium decreases the neural discharge rate (Fig. 15.3). The distribution of these cells on the cristae and utricular macula determines how that sense organ responds to shearing movements by the cupula and otolithic membrane.

The orientation of hair cells in the crista is uniform with all cells polarized in the same direction. In the horizontal or lateral semicircular canal the kinocilia face the utricle. In the posterior and superior canals the kinocilia face away from the utricle. Thus, movement of endolymph and bending of the cupula toward the utricle (utriculopetal displacement) increases the resting discharge rate of afferent neurons in the horizontal crista, while decreasing the discharge rate in vestibular nerve fibers from the posterior and superior cristae. Cupular

Utriculofugal Displacement   Utriculopetal Displacement

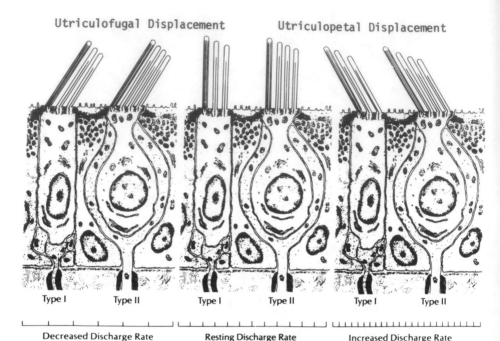

Type I   Type II   Type I   Type II   Type I   Type II

Decreased Discharge Rate   Resting Discharge Rate   Increased Discharge Rate

Fig. 15.3. *Diagram illustrating the effect of utriculofugal and utriculopetal displacement of cilia on the resting discharge rate of afferent vestibular neurons (from English, G. M. 1976. Otolaryngology. A Textbook, Harper & Row, Hagerstown, Maryland).*

displacement away from the utricle (utriculofugal displacement) decreases the activity in fibers from the horizontal crista while increasing the response of those from the posterior and superior canal cristae. On the utricular macula, hair cell kinocilia are oriented toward a central axis, while in the macula of the saccule the kinocilia are oriented toward the organ's periphery and away from its central axis.

These physiologic details permit the neural response produced by cupular movement and otolithic membrane shearing to be predicted, and help to explain the effect of caloric stimulation. With the patient positioned so the horizontal canal is perpendicular (vertical) to the ground, cooling of the endolymph in the region of the ampulla increases its relative specific gravity and produces a downward (utriculofugal) deflection of the cupula, thereby decreasing the resting discharge rate. Conversely, hot water irrigation of the ear canal warms the fluid near the ampulla, reverses the direction of the endolymph flow, and produces a utriculopetal deflection of the cupula which increases neuronal activity. The ampulla, in effect, acts as a switch, increasing or decreasing vestibular neuronal responses.

The central integration of these peripheral vestibular responses in the brain stem gives rise to the characteristic jerk nystagmus seen with caloric irrigations and peripheral vestibulopathies. The direction of the nystagmus can often be

Table 15.1. EYE MOVEMENT SYSTEMS TESTED BY ENG

Eye Movement Systems	ENG Tests
Saccadic	Calibration (refixation)
	Optokinetic (fast phase)
	Caloric (fast phase)
Smooth pursuit	Tracking
	Optokinetic (slow phase)
Vergence	Patient looks from near to far; not routinely tested
Non-optic reflex	Caloric
	Positional
	Rotational
Position maintenance	Fixation
	Gaze—right and left

helpful in determining the site of involvement. Destruction of the vestibular nerve on one side will evoke the same pattern of nystagmus as is seen with cold water caloric stimulation. Both produce a reduction in afferent neural activity on the involved side and a jerk nystagmus which beats toward the opposite ear. Since all peripheral vestibular responses are suppressed by visual fixation, ENG can be a useful means of detecting nystagmus which may only be present when the eyes are closed or in a darkened room.

The use of ENG is much broader than its application to vestibular stimulation. It may be applied to the study of eye movement systems, each of which may be tested during an ENG examination (Table 15.1). Lesions in the cerebellum, brainstem and vestibular apparatus may produce abnormal eye movements which can be recorded by electronystagmography.

ELECTRONYSTAGMOGRAPHIC EQUIPMENT

The corneoretinal potential, at 1 mv, has an axis that coincides closely with the visual axis. Eye movement changes the voltage only slightly—about 20 μV per degree. The electronystagmograph must be able to detect such minute voltage changes, amplify them about 20,000 times without distortion, and record them without interference.

Electrodes

The electrodes detect the voltage changes generated by eye movements. Only silver/silver chloride electrodes are recommended for electronystagmographic recordings because they do not polarize as easily as other metal electrodes; they have the highest stability and the lowest impedance of any readily obtainable electrode. The skin must be cleansed and is sometimes abraded before attaching the electrodes, and an electrolyte solution (electrode jelly or paste) is placed between the electrode and the skin to reduce the electrical impedance of the dry epidermis.

The placement of the electrodes depends on the sophistication of the equipment used. Since most nystagmus is horizontal or horizonto-rotatory, physicians may choose to use inexpensive, one-channel electronystagmographs in their offices, in which case three electrodes are used to measure horizontal eye movements. They are placed just lateral to the outer canthi, with the ground attached to the forehead, usually between the eyes, as in Figure 15.4. These electrodes should be as close to the eyes as possible, but sufficiently far away that they do not move when the patient blinks. In older patients or in those with folds of loose skin around the eyes, electrodes will have to be placed further away. If a machine with more than one channel is used, vertical eye movements may be recorded as well by placing electrodes above the eyebrow and on the ridge of bone just beneath the eye (Fig. 15.4). If a

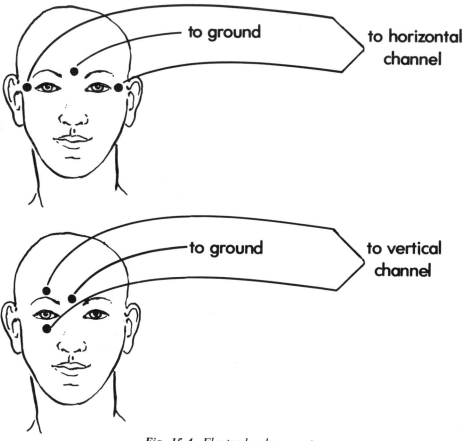

Fig. 15.4. Electrode placement.

patient has one blind eye, the quality of the ENG record may be improved if the electrodes are placed so that only the movement of the good eye is recorded. In this case, one electrode is placed on the bridge of the nose next to the good eye, and the other is located in the usual position, lateral to the outer canthus of the good eye. Disconjugate eye movements can be detected by recording from each eye on a separate recording channel.

Recording Arrangements

The ENG amplifies and displays on graph paper the small voltage changes picked up by the electrodes. The voltage changes caused by eye movements are fed to a signal conditioner which filters out extraneous parts of the signal and delivers the significant parts to the preamplifier where the voltage of the input signal is boosted. The power amplifier converts this voltage into electric current used to drive the output transducer, a galvanometer that transforms electric current into pen position. The paper drive moves the paper under the pen at a fixed rate of speed, usually 10 mm per second, making a permanent record of the input signal. Although nystagmographs are designed specifically to record eye movements, general purpose recorders may be used, usually after being modified. A complete discussion of specifications for electronystagmographs will not be entered into here; such information is readily available in any number of books and manuals on electronystagmography. The examination is usually performed with the patient on an examining table that can be adjusted so that he can be placed in either a sitting or supine position.

Vestibular Stimulators

Water Caloric Irrigators. Caloric irrigators are used routinely to stimulate the vestibular system. Both water and air caloric irrigators are available, although water caloric irrigators are widely preferred as the stimulus can be readily controlled and calibrated.

The water caloric stimulus has long been standardized as 250 cc of water, at 30° C and 44° C, that is introduced into the external auditory canal over a 30 second time period. Two irrigations of each ear are performed, once at 30° C and once at 44° C, the temperature of the water flowing from the irrigator tip being the important one. The irrigator consists of two water reservoirs capable of maintaining the water at the desired temperatures, a calibrated delivery system that consistently delivers 250 cc of water to the ear, and a timing system that controls the duration of water flow.

Caloric irrigators operate by either gravity or direct pumping, and the latter is the preferred system because temperature control of the water at the irrigating tip is not always adequate with a gravity flow system.

The disadvantages of using water to irrigate the external ear are that it can be messy, that it increases the danger of electrical shock, and that it is contraindicated for patients with a tympanic membrane perforation, myringotomy tubes, external otitis, or mastoid cavities. These disadvantages are eliminated by using warm and cool air for caloric irrigations or by using a closed-flow water caloric system.

Air Caloric Irrigators. One way of avoiding the problems involved with exposing the external auditory canal to water is by using air caloric stimulation. Air from the standard office air supply or from an air pump is forced through a Peltier thermoelectric device that generates or absorbs heat as a function of current flow through a series of semiconductor elements. The temperature sensing thermistor must be located near the irrigating tip since air loses thermal energy much more readily than water as it transverses the length of the irrigating tube. The transfer of thermal energy between air and tissue is considerably less efficient than between water and tissue; a greater volume of air than of water is therefore needed to generate a caloric stimulus of similiar intensity. Capps and others (1973) have found that 8 liters of air at 24° C or 50° C, delivered into the external auditory canal over a 60-second period, will elicit responses equal to those of 30° C and 44° C water stimulation.

Despite the advantages of air caloric irrigation systems, they are not widely accepted by clinicians who feel that air irrigation elicits less reliable responses than water irrigation. Nevertheless, they are useful when irrigation with water is prohibited. In such circumstances the condition requiring the use of air (e.g. a tympanic membrane perforation) will alter the amount of thermal energy reaching the labyrinth, thereby making the stimulation of the abnormal labyrinth different from that of the normal side. A quantitative comparison between responses of the two ears is, therefore, invalid, and all that can be determined is whether or not there is a vestibular response at all.

Closed-Flow Water Caloric System. There are a number of disadvantages to conventional water irrigating systems. The tester is required to catch the water in a basin as it dribbles from the ear, making the test awkward to perform; the examination may be unnecessarily time-consuming if the irrigating reservoir is small; and many patients dislike having water in their ears. Similarly, testing with an air caloric irrigator is disadvantageous because of its variable results, and is also often objected to by patients because of the acoustic stimulation that results.

Foti and Foti (1977) described a relatively new method of caloric stimulation, called a closed-flow water caloric system, which is a viable alternative to both water and air caloric stimulation. Closed-flow irrigating systems range from moderately sized table model systems to small, battery controlled, easily portable recirculating pumps. Both use a very thin, durable, flexible membrane which forms a hermetic seal when placed in the external auditory canal. This earmold portion is connected to a recirculating pump which controls flow, pressure, temperature, and irrigating time. The balloon portion of the earmold probe expands under pressure of the test fluid to conform to the canal and tympanic membrane. There is a hole at the dimpled tip of the probe to prevent injury or pain at the tympanic membrane when fully expanded. This hole serves to evacuate the trapped air between the tympanic membrane and the expanding probe. A thin, calibrated string allows for objectively ascertaining whether or not the probe is fully expanded to the tympanic membrane. The portable model allows for testing in emergency rooms and in operating rooms. Indeed, perhaps its most valuable use is in the evaluation in the emergency room of comatose patients with craniocerebral injuries. Such patients can be tested clinically for the presence of an oculovestibular response without exposing them to any risk of contaminating the cerebrospinal fluid.

The nonportable closed-flow caloric systems allow for simultaneous stimulation of both external auditory canals (as would using two of the portable systems together). The assumption is that, with normal labyrinths, no nystagmus, and, therefore, no patient "dizziness" will result when both ears receive exactly the same thermal stimulus at the same time. If nystagmus is recorded after such testing, each ear should be tested separately in order to determine whether the difference in nystagmus produced indicates pathology or is within normal limits.

Visual Stimulators

Fixation Points. A display of fixation points, which may be spots or lights, is needed in order to calibrate the ENG recording system and for gaze and saccadic testing. Eye movement calibrators are available commercially, and consist of a frame to hold the patient's head steady at a distance of usually three feet from an array of lights that can be illuminated by the tester in various sequences. Calibrating points of 10°, 20°, and 30° in both the horizontal and vertical planes are desirable. The formula for computing the distance from center of a fixation point at the desired angle of gaze is $X = 2Y \sin \theta$ (Fig. 15.5).

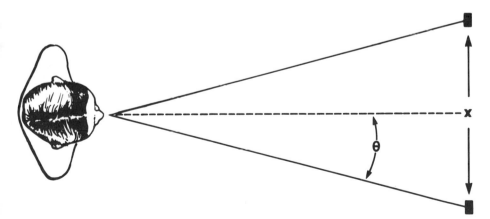

Fig. 15.5. Method of calculating distance between fixation points for desired angle of gaze from center. The distance can be calculated from the equation $x = 2y \sin \theta$, x, distance between two fixation points; y, distance from patient to fixation point; θ, angle of lateral gaze from center.

Moving Target. A moving visual target is used for assessing the tracking abilities of the patient. An easy method of constructing such a target is by using a pendulum with the string attached to the ceiling and a brightly colored or shiny object attached to its end. This target is moved through a 30° visual angle at a peak velocity of 40° per second. Alternatively, a metronome may be used, a brightly colored dot being placed on the bar of the metronome which is set between larghetto and largo. Some authorities object to such methods since the movements of the target are not purely horizontal, and prefer to use a moving light reflected on a wall opposite the patient by a projector.

Optokinetic Stripes. Optokinetic testing is performed during the ENG examination by using a small motor-driven optokinetic drum that can be made to rotate at several different speeds. It is important that the speed of the drum remain constant at the set speed when the direction of the drum rotation is reversed. Optokinetic drums should be capable of attaining a maximum speed of at least 120° per second since Morissette, Abel, and Barber (1974), and others, have ascertained that significant pathologic conditions can be detected only when high optokinetic speeds are used. Optokinetic drums that rotate in front of the patient or those that rest over the patient's head, completely surrounding his visual field, may be used, as well as devices that project large optokinetic stripes on a screen opposite the patient. These latter devices are portable, and can be turned to project either horizontal or vertical stripes, as well as stimuli other than optokinetic patterns.

PREPARATIONS FOR TESTING

The ears should be examined for tympanic membrane perforations or other abnormalities such as mastoid cavities, cholesteatomas, or external canal infections. Such findings should be confirmed by an otologist, and water caloric testing should not be performed. Any excessive accumulation of cerumen or other debris should be removed before caloric irrigation.

The patient should be questioned carefully about any recent consumption of alcohol or drugs, since some patients fail to follow instructions to abstain from 48 to 72 hours before testing, depending on the drugs concerned. Additional history should be taken regarding neck or back injury and/or surgery as these conditions might limit the examination by excluding positional tests.

No ENG recording can be obtained from patients with nonfunctioning retinae, because the corneoretinal potential is absent. Even when such a potential is present, ENG recordings on blind patients cannot provide quantitative data because of the impossibility of accurately calibrating the nystagmograph, although a crude calibration can be performed by having the patient hold out his arms with thumbs extended and asking him to "look" back and forth from one thumb to the other.

THE ENG TEST

Calibration

The electronystagmograph is first calibrated so that 1° of eye movement is equal to one millimeter of pen deflection on the ENG graph paper. The patient is asked to look at fixation points placed 10°, 20° and 30° from the center in both the horizontal and vertical planes as the technician adjusts the gain controls. Figure 15.6 shows a standard DC calibration tracing. Horizontal and vertical tracings will look identical; AC system tracings will reflect pen drifts back toward the baseline. Calibration should be repeated frequently during the test-

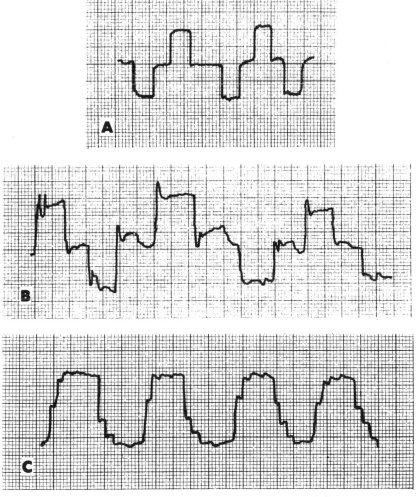

Fig. 15.6. A. *Normal calibration—by convention upward deflection represents eye movement to the right and downward to the left; B. Ocular dysmetria; C. Calibration undershoots or hypometric saccades.*

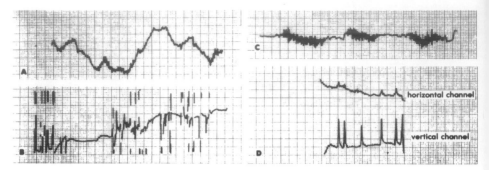

Fig. 15.7. *Artifacts. A. Baseline shift and 60 Hz "hum" caused by poor electrode contact, by a ground loop or uncommon ground, or by unusually intense radiation from nearby equipment; B. Broken electrode wire; C. Muscle potential from contraction of facial or neck muscles; D. Eye blink artifacts.*

ing procedure, since patient alertness will change the magnitude of the corneoretinal potential, and should certainly be checked before each major test and before and after each caloric irrigation.

A number of electric artifacts may obscure the tracing, and some of these are shown in Figure 15.7. In addition, a number of non-nystagmic eye movements, called "square waves," occur in many patients, but are most pronounced with nervous, apprehensive patients, who should be encouraged to relax. Such waves may, however, indicate brainstem-cerebellar pathology. Large, random eye-movements generally are seen with children or with uncooperative patients, and again greater relaxation must be obtained. Slow, sinusoidal eye swings are a sign of patient drowsiness, and may be due to heavy sedation or organic brain damage.

Gaze Testing

Gaze testing is accomplished by having the patient gaze at the center point, then 30° right, 30° left (and 30° upward, and 30° downward gaze if vertical nystagmus is recorded) both with eyes open and with eyes closed in each gaze position while a record of eye movement is obtained (Fig. 15.8). It is necessary to alert the patient during gaze testing with the eyes closed since nystagmus usually becomes weaker and may disappear when the patient is not actively performing concentration tasks. Many normal people have a physiologic gaze nystagmus if the eyes are deviated more than 30° to the left or right, and the angle of gaze must, therefore, be carefully controlled.

Tests for Spontaneous Nystagmus

After calibration and gaze testing, and before the patient is moved, tests for spontaneous nystagmus are performed. The patient is first asked to hold a blank sheet of white paper approximately four inches from his eyes, in order to

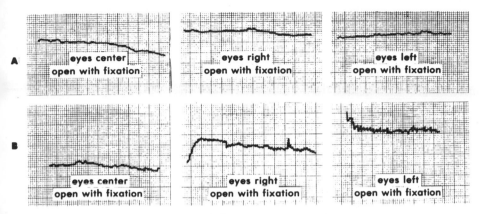

Fig. 15.8. A. Gaze test result in normal subject. B. Gaze nystagmus.

reduce visual stimulation from the rest of the room, and to keep his eyes open without visual fixation while a further record of eye movement is obtained. Alertness must be maintained by a concentration task. After recalibration, the patient is tested in a darkened room with his eyes open, then with his eyes closed.

Calibration is again performed and the patient is then asked to keep his eyes closed as he moves into various head and body positions, in order to see how postural changes affect the recorded eye movements. The patient's eyes may be taped closed in order to reduce movements from the eyelids and to insure that they are not opened during this portion of the examination. The exact order in which tests are performed may vary, but the basic positions are recumbent (with the patient's head flat); body turned to the right (the head should be kept level with the body by using a small pillow beneath the patient's head); head turned to the right (the pillow is removed so that the head is flat); body to the left; head to left; head extended back (with the head back far enough to arch the neck); and sitting up. Each position should be maintained for 60 seconds while a record of eye movement is obtained.

Positioning Tests

The Hallpike-Dix maneuvers are used for positioning tests. The seated patient is made to lie down suddenly, with his head hanging unsupported below the horizontal, and to maintain the position for approximately 40 seconds during which the eye movements are recorded. After the test has been repeated with the eyes closed, the patient is asked to sit up and allowed to rest for 15 to 30 seconds. The test is then repeated with the head back and turned to the right; then, after the rest period, with the head back and turned to the left. If nystagmus is produced by any such maneuvers, those that elicited the nystagmus are repeated since a vital characteristic of the Hallpike-Dix response is its fatigability with repeated elicitation.

Tracking and Optokinetic Tests

The patient is asked to smoothly track a horizontally moving object with his eyes while the recording is continued. This tracking is performed first with both eyes, then with the right eye alone, and finally with the left eye only. During the monocular tracking test, the patient must keep both eyes open while the technician covers one, since closing the eye not used for tracking may cause muscle artifacts to appear on the recording.

The optokinetic (OPK) test is performed by having the patient sit under or in front of an optokinetic drum, or by moving an OPK stimulus horizontally on a wall or screen before the patient's eyes. The optokinetic stimulus is moved both to the left and to the right, using velocities of 20°, 60°, 80°, 100°, and 120° visual angle per second. Vertical optokinetic responses can also be obtained at this time, if desired. Optokinetic nystagmus is an involuntary response and appears when the subject focuses on the stimulus pattern. If the patient is asked to count the stripes, a tracking response is usually obtained instead of a true OPK response (Fig. 15.9).

Caloric Testing

The caloric test is performed either with the patient sitting, head tilted back at 60°, or, more commonly during ENG testing, with the patient supine, head ventroflexed 30° so that the lateral semicircular canals are in the vertical plane perpendicular with the plane of the floor. The positioning of the lateral semicircular canal is crucial since it is the canal maximally stimulated by caloric irrigation. It is important for the patient to understand that lightheadedness or vertigo may occur during the test in normal subjects, but will not continue for

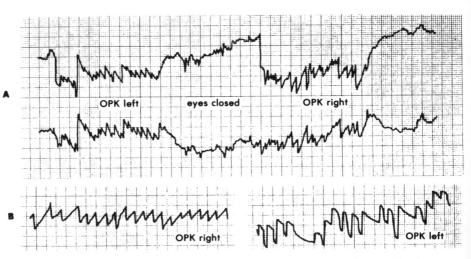

Fig. 15.9. A. Normal optokinetic nystagmus. B. Asymmetric optokinetic responses.

longer than one or two minutes. A careful record should be made of any symptoms that persist.

If no nystagmus is elicited by using 30° and 44° C water irrigations, ice water may be used to determine whether vestibular function is present or not in the nonresponsive ear or ears. The patient is asked to turn his head so that the irrigated ear faces upward as the last 2 cc of ice water is placed. After 20 seconds, the patient's head is slowly turned to the opposite side, allowing the water to run out, and then the head is returned to the usual caloric test position. The amount of ice water used varies: as little as 2 cc of ice water can be used for this purpose, and although up to 30 cc have been used by some workers, more than 5 cc is not recommended. For all practical purposes, the irrigated labyrinth (or its CNS connections) can be considered as nonfunctional if no nystagmus results from stimulating the ear with 5 cc of water. Irrigation with 30 cc of ice water may be used in the comatose patient to test the vestibulo-oculomotor connection similiar to the "doll's eyes" nystagmus. Air caloric irrigations are performed in the same manner as water calorics with air at temperatures of 24° C and 50° C. If no responses result from such irrigations, a Dundus-Grant coiled copper tube attached to the air hose and sprayed with ethyl chloride can be used to cool the air to about 14° C.

INTERPRETATION AND CLINICAL APPLICATION OF ENG TEST RESULTS

Gaze Testing

Nystagmus caused by peripheral vestibular lesions is nearly always horizontal or horizontal-rotatory, is direction-fixed (most often toward the normal side), is suppressed by ocular fixation, and is strongest when the gaze is toward the fast phase of the nystagmus. Since peripheral nystagmus results from an acute unilateral lesion that causes an unbalance in the normal input arising from the two labyrinths, this nystagmus will lose intensity with time due to central compensation. The terms *first, second and third degree* gaze nystagmus relate to Alexander's Law: nystagmus resulting from an acute peripheral lesion beats strongest when the eyes gaze in the direction of the quick component, less strongly with center gaze, and with least activity when the gaze is in the opposite direction to the fast component. Nystagmus present in all three directions is called *third degree,* that seen with straight gaze and with gaze in the direction of the fast component is called *second degree,* and that seen only with the gaze in the direction of the fast component is called *first degree* nystagmus. Third degree nystagmus is converted to second, and then first degree nystagmus as the CNS compensatory mechanisms become effective with time.

Spontaneous nystagmus can be defined as a nystagmus that is present with the eyes open or closed, is direction-fixed, and has an intensity that does not change (or varies only slightly) with changes in head and body positions. Nystagmus that varies in intensity with position changes or that disappears in one or more positions may be called direction-fixed positional nystagmus or latent spontaneous nystagmus. Spontaneous jerk nystagmus, when strictly defined, is always pathologic. Both spontaneous and direction-fixed positional nystagmus can result from either peripheral or central lesions; the direction of the nystagmus is not necessarily of localizing value.

Nystagmus caused by CNS lesions may be horizontal, vertical, oblique, or rotatory, may vary considerably in amplitude, and usually declines slowly, if at all, with time. It may be enhanced by visual fixation and is usually not suppressed by it. Horizontal CNS nystagmus usually beats in the direction of the gaze—i.e. right beating with gaze to the right and left beating with gaze to the left (Fig. 15.8B).

Bilateral horizontal gaze nystagmus is the most common form of CNS nystagmus, with the nystagmus usually beating in the direction of gaze. It is usually seen only when the patient's eyes are open, although occasionally it may be enhanced or occur only with the eyes closed. The finding suggests a brainstem lesion but provides no information about its pathologic basis. Only CNS lesions produce gaze nystagmus which is abolished by eye closure. Gaze nystagmus of low amplitude and high velocity may be obvious to the clinical observer, yet difficult to discern on the ENG tracing. Separate eye recordings help to show this nystagmus since the abducting eye has stronger nystagmus than the adducting eye.

Rebound nystagmus, described by Hood, Kayan, and Leech (1973), is a horizontal gaze nystagmus associated with chronic cerebellar system disease. It can be seen on both clinical examination and with ENG testing. It is characterized by the appearance of nystagmus that is not present on center gaze but develops into a right beating nystagmus on right gaze and reverses to a left beating nystagmus as the eyes move from right gaze back to center gaze. Similarly, a left beating nystagmus appears on left gaze and becomes right beating when the eyes return to center gaze. Accordingly, when examining patients with gaze nystagmus due to suspected CNS pathology, lateral gaze should be observed for 20 seconds and center gaze should then be examined before gaze in the opposite direction, so that rebound nystagmus is not overlooked.

Periodic alternating nystagmus (PAN) is a persistent, horizontal-rotatory nystagmus that alternates in direction at regular intervals which may be as short as 1 minute or as long as 6 minutes, but which is constant for individual patients. The nystagmus begins beating weakly in one direction, builds up to a peak level, declines, and stops. This cycle is then repeated with nystagmus beating in the opposite direction and so on. This periodic alternating nystagmus may be seen with eyes open or closed, but it is usually enhanced with fixation and with alertness. Although not of specific diagnostic significance, periodic alternating nystagmus indicates a central disturbance, probably in the cerebellomedullary region (Barber, 1973; Money, Myles, and Hoffert, 1974).

Upbeating vertical nystagmus, seen with upward or downward gaze or in the primary position, is clinically important since it indicates an acquired lesion, either from drug intoxication or posterior fossa disease. Downbeating vertical nystagmus, especially when seen with lateral gaze, suggests strongly that the medullary or medullo-cervical region is the site of the responsible lesion. Causes of such pathology include Arnold-Chiari malformation, medullary infarction, and brainstem encephalitis.

Congenital nystagmus, which appears at birth or shortly thereafter in an otherwise normal individual, is important to recognize since it should not be confused with other varieties of nystagmus that are of pathologic significance. The nystagmus may be pendular or jerk type, or both, varying with gaze direction or position. Congenital nystagmus is usually distinctive for each patient. Nystagmus that is pendular is usually congenital or secondary to blindness, but may be seen with a patient who has multiple sclerosis. Care must be taken to differentiate congenital nystagmus from lesional or drug-induced gaze nystagmus. The distorted character of the eyes open nystagmus strongly suggests a congenital origin. Congenital nystagmus will also have a null point at which nystagmus sharply declines or stops as the patient's eyes move slowly from about 30° right lateral gaze to 30° left lateral gaze. At the null point, the right beating nystagmus seen with 30° right gaze will stop, after declining as the eyes move to the center, and then to the left. As the eyes continue to move to the left, the nystagmus will become left beating. Another feature of congenital nystagmus is that it is rarely vertical, usually being horizontal or horizontal-rotatory. Thus, congenital nystagmus on upward gaze is virtually always horizontal, not vertical. (Persistent vertical nystagmus on upward gaze indicates a pathologic or drug-induced condition.) Congenital nystagmus can also be identified by its reduction or abolition on convergence (eye fixation at 6 feet will allow nystagmus to be clearly seen, but, with fixation at 2 feet, the nystagmus declines and may disappear for a few seconds). Since variability is the main trademark of congenital nystagmus, checks for null point, upward gaze and convergence effect will help to determine whether the nystagmus is, indeed, congenital or not.

Internuclear ophthalmoplegia results from a medial longitudinal fasciculus lesion between the 3rd and 6th nerve nuclei in the brainstem. Internuclear ophthalmoplegia is often found in patients with multiple sclerosis but may also be due to other discrete lesions, e.g. vascular lesions. Internuclear ophthalmoplegia presents with two distinguishing patterns: delay in movement of the adducting eye with lateral gaze, and nystagmus only in the abducting eye. Medial rectus muscle weakness from defective innervation is responsible for the adduction lag which is ipsilateral to the side of the lesion. ENG recording from each eye separately is the easiest way to identify internuclear ophthalmoplegia.

Saccadic Testing

Saccadic testing is performed as the patient moves his eyes left and right, looking at the lights or dots used for calibrating the ENG machine. Normal individuals can move their eyes rapidly and stop precisely on target, although some consistently undershoot or overshoot the target slightly, reaching it by making one or two small corrective saccades, or by moving the eyes to the target in one slow movement called a glissade.

Ocular dysmetria is an abnormal saccadic eye movement characterized by the patient's eyes overshooting (hypermetric saccades) or undershooting (hypometric saccades) the target consistently for 150 to 200 msec before fixating on the target itself. Unilateral overshoots are more common than overshoots in both directions. Ocular dysmetria accompanies diseases of the cerebellum or its neural connections and is the ocular counterpart of past-pointing. Both result from the inability of the impaired cerebellar hemispheres to control smooth integration of body muscles that function in agonist-antagonist relationship. Figures 15.6B and 15.6C illustrate ocular dysmetria seen as calibration overshoot and undershoot. The finding must be clearly and consistently seen throughout the ENG recording whenever saccadic movements are elicited for calibration before they are regarded as abnormal.

Saccadic slowing, eye movement slower than 188° per second, indicates basal ganglia disease, especially when associated with an inability to perform vertical—particularly downward—saccadic movements.

Internuclear ophthalmoplegia presents on saccadic testing as a rounding of one side of the upper plateau of the saccade, caused by the lag of the adducting eye. Separate recordings for each eye should be taken to confirm the diagnosis if such rounding is seen repeatedly.

In evaluating saccadic movements it is important to consider whether apparent abnormalities are due to superimposition of spontaneous or congenital nystagmus on the saccades; to a drug effect, especially when ocular dysmetria is a finding; or to eye blink artifacts. Eye blinks superimposed on saccades may resemble calibration overshoot on the ENG recording using bitemporal leads; the vertical channel is particularly helpful in distinguising them since blinks will appear as spikes, whereas calibration overshoots will not show up at all.

Positional Testing

Positional nystagmus that is present when the eyes are open is always abnormal, but many normal people have horizontal positional nystagmus in one or more head positions if examined with the eyes closed. This nystagmus may be direction-fixed or direction-changing (but will not change direction within a given head position); it may be persistent or intermittent. Barber and Wright (1973), who tested 112 normal people and found nystagmus in at least one head position in 92 of them, established the following criteria of abnormality for positional nystagmus that is present when the eyes are closed:

1. It changes direction within a given head position;
2. It is persistent in three or more positions;
3. It is intermittent in four or more positions; and/or
4. The slow-phase eye speed of the three strongest consecutive beats exceeds 6° per second in any head position.

Ninety-five percent of their 112 normal subjects failed to meet any of these criteria.

Direction-fixed or direction-changing positional nystagmus that is present with the eyes open and continues as long as the head position is maintained is good evidence of pathology within the posterior fossa if positional, alcohol-induced nystagmus has been excluded.

The site of lesion cannot be determined with certainty from the direction of direction-fixed positional nystagmus, although the nystagmus usually beats toward the normal side, especially in patients with vestibular neuronitis. Such nystagmus is usually found in patients with peripheral pathology but may occur with CNS disease. Usually direction-changing positional nystagmus will beat toward the down ear in lateral head and body positions (geotropic) if the nystagmus has a peripheral origin. Ageotropic (beats away from the down ear) direction-changing positional nystagmus suggests a central lesion unless alcohol has been taken within 6 to 24 hours of testing (Fig. 15.10). Also indicative of a CNS lesion is nystagmus that changes direction within a given head or body position, or during one of the Hallpike-Dix maneuvers. This nystagmus often beats geotropically, declines to nothing, then, after a few seconds, beats in the opposite direction.

Positioning Tests

Neither vertigo nor nystagmus result from the Hallpike-Dix manuevers in normal subjects with open eyes, but a few nystagmoid beats are sometimes seen on the ENG tracing if the eyes are closed while recording.

Benign paroxysmal positioning nystagmus is most often seen with the Hallpike-Dix maneuvers and is important to identify since it localizes the lesion laterally and nearly always indicates harmless inner ear disease. The nystagmus appears most often in either head hanging right (HHR) or left (HHL) positions, rarely in both. It beats in a horizontal-rotatory pattern toward the down ear, when this is the ear with the responsible peripheral vestibular lesion. Frequently, nystagmus beating in the opposite direction will be seen briefly when the patient sits up after performing the Hallpike-Dix maneuvers that provoked nystagmus. Benign paroxysmal positioning nystagmus always is (1) delayed in onset for 5 to 20 seconds after the patient's head is positioned; (2) transient, lasting only 30 seconds or less; (3) accompanied by vertigo which lasts as long as the nystagmus; and (4) fatigable, becoming weaker with each successive repetition of the maneuver. When benign paroxysmal positioning nystagmus is recorded by ENG, the nystagmus appears to beat in an "unexpected" direction—i.e. left beating in HHR and right beating in HHL.

The Hallpike-Dix maneuvers may also provoke positional nystagmus which is not rotatory, has no measurable latency, gives the patient little or nor vertiginous sensations, and does not fatigue with repetition of the test. This nystagmus may be horizontal, oblique, or vertical and is important because it strongly indicates significant CNS disease, although unidirectional positional

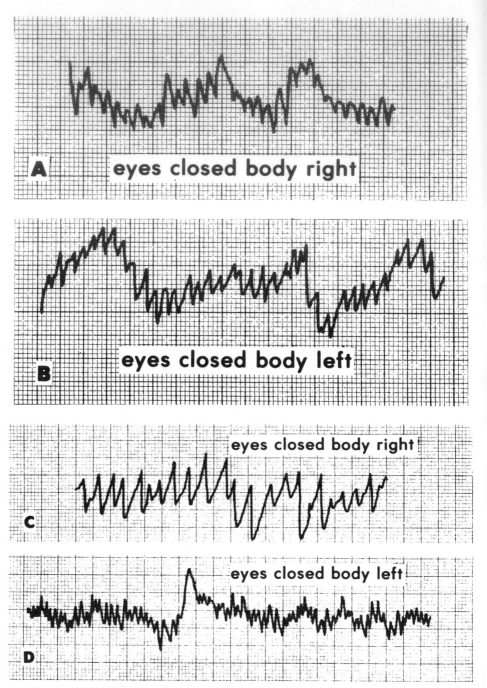

Fig. 15.10. A. Geotropic right beating positional mystagmus seen in body right position; B. Geotropic left beating positional nystagmus seen in body left position; C. Ageotropic left beating positional nystagmus seen in body right position; D. Ageotropic right beating positional nystagmus seen in body left position.

nystagmus caused by an acute unilateral peripheral vestibular lesion may also be intensified by the Hallpike-Dix maneuvers.

Tracking

Most normal individuals or patients with peripheral (end-organ) vestibular disease are able to visually track a moving object with little or no eye deviation from it, although this ability declines somewhat with age. A patient with brainstem disease involving the pursuit system will track a moving object imperfectly, producing saccadic movements instead of a smooth tracking record. As the eye repeatedly falls behind the movement of the target and catches up again with a saccade, a "cogwheeling" effect is recorded (Fig. 15.11, III)

Disorganized and disconjugate pursuit also indicates brainstem pathology. Monocular leads will allow the ENG tracing to show disconjugate eye movements, recording movement in one eye while the other remains momentarily stationary or drifts aimlessly. Bitemporal leads will record this type of eye movement as slow, wandering, inaccurate tracking. Disorganized pursuit may also be seen as rapid overshoots to both right and left (blinks should be ruled out by observing the vertical channel tracing), or as a completely ataxic tracking record that is impossible to identify as tracking at all (Fig. 15.11, IV).

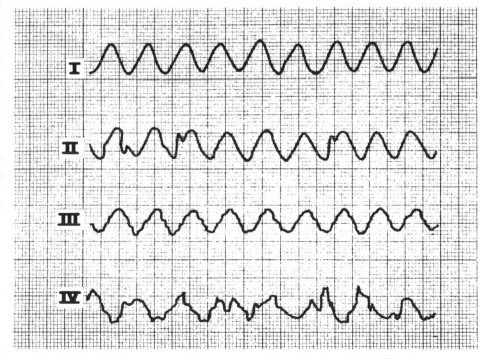

Fig. 15.11. *Benitez eye tracking patterns (from Benitez, J. T. 1970. Laryngoscope, 80, 834.*

Benitez' (1970) classification of tracking is useful, and his findings regarding the localizing information derived from the test are worth reviewing here. Pattern I is a smooth sinusoidal tracing; Pattern II is a slightly irregular, sinusoidal curve with a few periodic non-nystagmic movements appearing intermittently on it; Pattern III is a sinusoidal curve with fast saccadic movements superimposed on it; and Pattern IV is completely ataxic, so that the sinusoidal curve is lost and the pursuit eye movements are disorganized. These patterns are shown in Figure 15.11.

Optokinetic Test

A normal optokinetic (OPK) response is symmetrical, that is, the OPK nystagmus intensity will be the same for both left beating and right beating nystagmus provoked by a stimulus moving at a given speed to the right and left. OPK nystagmus is usually symmetrical, even when a unilateral peripheral lesion is present. A decidedly asymmetrical OPK response denotes a CNS abnormality without indicating laterality (Fig. 15.9B).

Brainstem pathology is indicated by nystagmus that does not increase in intensity with increasing stimulus velocities, but instead remains stable or declines in intensity. In this case, the nystagmus is symmetrical but is not appropriate to the stimulus speeds used.

In the presence of a strong spontaneous nystagmus or direction-fixed positional nystagmus, the OPK responses sometimes reflect a directional preponderance in the direction of the spontaneous nystagmus. This should not be considered as an abnormal OPK response. Drugs can affect the OPK response, making it appear abnormal, but a more common problem is patient suppression of the OPK response by staring through the drum or looking under it, by allowing it to become a blur or by tracking the stimulus.

Caloric Test Results

As with the OPK test, symmetry of responses is the expected finding in normal subjects. Three parameters of the caloric response are measured: duration, frequency, and velocity of the slow component of the induced nystagmus, the latter being the most important of the three. Duration of the nystagmus is the time that elapses from the beginning of the irrigation until the nystagmus ceases. Peak nystagmus frequency is the average frequency of beats per second within the 10-second interval in which the caloric nystagmus is most intense (usually about 60 seconds after the beginning of the irrigation). Calculating slow-component velocity is simple if the machine has been calibrated so that 1° of eye movement equals 1 mm of deflection.

Unilateral weakness (UW) can be said to be present when the intensity of the nystagmus provoked by irrigation of the right ear differs from that elicited by left ear irrigations. Unilateral weakness is expressed as a percentage and is calculated by using the formula:

$$UW = \frac{(RW + RC) - (LW + LC)}{(RW + RC + LW + LC)} \times 100$$

RW = peak slow-phase eye speed after 44° irrigation of the R ear; RC = peak slow-phase eye speed after 30° irrigation of the R ear; LW = peak slow-phase eye speed after 44° irrigation of the L ear; LC = peak slow-phase eye speed after 30° irrigation of the L ear.

Directional preponderance (DP) is the difference between the intensity of the right beating caloric nystagmus and the left beating caloric nystagmus. Using the same parameters as those used to determine unilateral weakness, the formula for directional preponderance is as follows:

$$DP = \frac{(RW + LC) - (LW + RC)}{(RW + LC + LW + RC)} \times 100$$

The fixation index (FI) indicates the ability of the patient to effectively suppress the caloric nystagmus with visual fixation. The following formula is used to determine the fixation index:

$$FI = \frac{SPEC\ (EO)}{SPEC\ (EC)}$$

SPEC = slow phase eye speed; EO = eyes open; EC = eyes closed.

Normal caloric responses range from 6° to 80° per second, but all four irrigation responses will be approximately the same intensity for any one individual. Normal variations for unilateral weakness is 25 percent; for directional preponderance, 30 percent. Alpert (1974) has reported the 95 percent limit for normal variation of the fixation index as 0.6 (Figure 15.12).

When determining directional preponderance, it is important to consider whether any spontaneous nystagmus or strong direction-fixed positional nystagmus may be affecting the caloric responses. If the caloric responses are being facilitated by a pre-existing nystagmus, the calorics should not be considered truly asymmetric. Even a significant directional preponderance is of little clinical import since it indicates only that something is probably wrong but does not correlate well with either peripheral or central pathology.

A decided unilateral weakness is an important finding and usually suggests a peripheral vestibular lesion on the weak side (Fig. 15.13). Bilateral weakness may be seen in patients treated with ototoxic drugs such as streptomycin or gentamicin. Other causes of bilateral weakness include various peripheral vestibular lesions, as well as CNS lesions. Among peripheral vestibular lesions that cause bilateral weakness of caloric responses are bilateral 8th nerve tumors, bilateral temporal bone fracture, bilateral Ménière's disease and Cogan's syndrome.

Simmons (1973) found 43 of 2,500 consecutively tested patients to have no vestibular responses bilaterally to stimulation with 5 cc ice water. Of these 43, 9

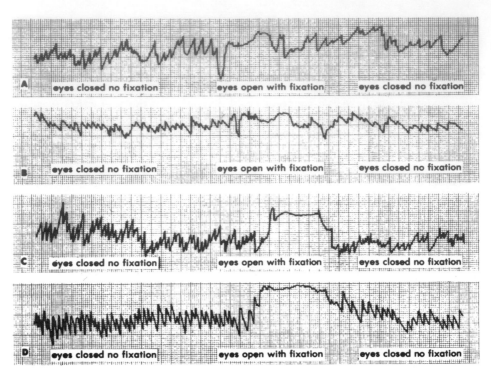

Fig. 15.12. *Normal caloric responses. A. Right cold; B. Left cold; C. Left hot; D. Right hot.*

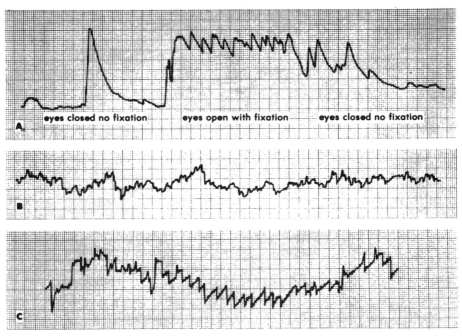

Fig. 15.13. *Abnormal caloric responses. A. Absence of fixation suppression; B. No labyrinthine responses to 5 cc ice water; C. No labyrinthine response; superimposed left beating spontaneous nystagmus seen with 5 cc ice water on the left.*

had CNS neoplasms (6 in the midline posterior fossa), 6 had autoimmune or collagen disease, 6 had infections (otitis, meningitis, syphilis), 5 had congenital abnormalities involving only the ear, 5 were drug-induced, and 4 had combined visual and 8th nerve hereditary disorders.

Hyperactive caloric responses (above 50° per second from cool stimulation and 80° per second for warm stimulation) are uncommon unless the patient has a tympanic membrane perforation or a mastoidectomy cavity. Very alert or nervous patients sometimes have hyperactive caloric responses which have not been correlated with any pathogenic state.

Failure of fixation suppression will only be seen in patients with CNS disease. The caloric nystagmus intensity with eyes open will be nearly equal to, equal to, or exceed that of nystagmus with eyes closed, in one nystagmus direction or both. Normal individuals and patients with peripheral vestibular disorders will suppress caloric nystagmus with visual fixation (Fig. 15.13). Some CNS pathology, such as Wernicke's metabolic encephalopathy or barbiturate intoxication, inhibits eyes closed caloric responses so that the nystagmus is seen only with eyes open. With this sort of extreme failure of fixation suppression, it is important to be certain that the patient is alert during testing since cases have been reported of non-alerted (often deaf) patients whose caloric nystagmus is suppressed except with visual fixation. Alerting such a patient when his eyes are closed will elicit the suppressed nystagmus.

Congenital nystagmus superimposed on caloric responses sometimes makes it impossible to interpret these responses. Congenital nystagmus that is abolished with eye closure will not, of course, affect caloric nystagmus interpretation except with regard to evaluating failure of fixation suppression, which may be difficult to discern.

Drug Effects

All patients referred for ENGs are asked to discontinue all but life-supporting medications for 48 hours before the test and to discontinue all vestibular medications for 72 hours before the test. Drug-induced abnormal eye movements are most often seen with antihistamines, tranquilizers, barbiturates, alcohol, and diphenylhydantoin (Dilantin) sodium. Antihistamines and tranquilizers have a mild sedative effect, presumable from action on the CNS. Overall reduction of caloric responses is common with patients taking diazepam (Valium) or other similar drugs. Alcohol will cause direction-changing positional nystagmus, abnormal tracking, and inadequate saccadic eye movements.

Barbiturates and Dilantin affect the CNS at times, causing bilateral gaze nystagmus and abnormal tracking. They may, in high doses, cause vertical (usually upbeating) nystagmus or oblique-upbeating nystagmus, and they can inhibit or obliterate the fast component of caloric nystagmus. If it is impossible to discontinue all medications before ENG testing, as happens with hospital inpatients, medications being taken should be noted on the patient's ENG record.

CONCLUDING COMMENT

ENG testing can provide useful information concerning disturbances of eye movements in patients with various neurologic disorders. It has a particularly useful role in the detection of nystagmus that may not otherwise be readily apparent, and it provides a permanent record of eye movement that can be used for comparative purposes and for making quantitative measurements. Moreover, it has a particularly important role in providing valuable diagnostic information to the clinician who is attempting to determine whether a patient who complains of dysequilibrium has central or peripheral pathology. Table 15.2 summarizes the distinguishing features that may be seen in either instance with the various testing procedures in current use. In some cases, however, the findings may be inconclusive, and in all cases they need to be incorporated with the clinical and other laboratory data. The importance of this is emphasized by our recent observation that the clinical and ENG findings in patients with small cerebellar infarcts, as recognized by CT scanning, may mimic those of patients with a peripheral vestibulopathy.

Table 15.2. RESPONSES IN PERIPHERAL AND CENTRAL VESTIBULOPATHIES

ENG Tests	Peripheral (End Organ) Vestibulopathy	Central Vestibulopathy
Calibration	Normal	Ocular dysmetria
Gaze	Symmetric	Asymmetric
Positional	Geotropic	Ageotropic
Tracking	Sinusoidal	Ataxic
Optokinetic	Symmetric	Asymmetric
Caloric	Fixation suppression	Failure of fixation suppression

REFERENCES

Alpert, J. N. (1974). Failure of fixation suppression: a pathologic effect of vision on caloric nystagmus. Neurology, *24:*891.

Barber, H. (1973). Positional vertigo and nystagmus. Otolaryngol. Clin. North Am., *6:*169.

Barber, H. O. and Wright, G. (1973). Positional nystagmus in normals. Adv. Otorhinoloaryngol., *19:*276.

Benitez, J. T. (1970). Eye-tracking and optokinetic tests. Diagnostic significance in peripheral and central vestibular disorders. Laryngoscope, *80:*834.

Capps, M. J., Preciado, M. C., Paparella, M. M., and Hoppe, W. E. (1973). Evaluation of the air caloric test as a routine examination procedure. Laryngoscope, *83:*1013.

Foti, T. M. and Foti, G. (1977). A closed-flow water caloric system. J.A.M.A., *69:*303.

Hood, J. D., Kayan, A., and Leech, J. (1973). Rebound nystagmus. Brain, *96:*507.

Money, K. E., Myles, W. S., and Hoffert, B. M. (1974). The mechanism of positional alcohol nystagmus. Can. J. Otolaryngol., *3:*302.

Morissette, Y., Abel, S. M., and Barber, H. O. (1974). Optokinetic nystagmus in otoneurological diagnosis. Can. J. Otolaryngol., *3:*348.

Simmons, F. B. (1973). Patients with bilateral loss of caloric response. Ann. Otol. Rhinol. Laryngol., *82:*175.

16

The Polysomnographic Evaluation of Sleep Disorders in Man

ELLIOT D. WEITZMAN, CHARLES P. POLLAK,
and PETER McGREGOR

INTRODUCTION

During the past 20 years, major advances in our knowledge of the normal physiology of sleep (Figs. 16.1, 16.2, 16.3, 16.4) and the development of improved recording technology have led several major sleep research centers to confront the clinical disorders of sleep. It rapidly became evident that the range of patient complaints and clinical syndromes, and the prevalence of sleep disorders in the population, are very large. To insure that this emerging new medical discipline would be based on the highest clinical and scientific standards, utilize the best and latest polygraphic technology, and be responsive to a wide range of patient needs, the Association of Sleep Disorder Centers (ASDC) has been formed. This association has formulated an explicit nosology of the Sleep Disorders and will soon publish minimal standards for polysomnography.

An outline of the diagnostic classification of sleep and arousal disorders, recently formulated by the Nosology Committee of the ASDC, is shown in Table 16.1. Although this nosology will almost certainly be revised during the next several years, it is an important first step. It will not be possible to review

TYPICAL
SLEEP PATTERN

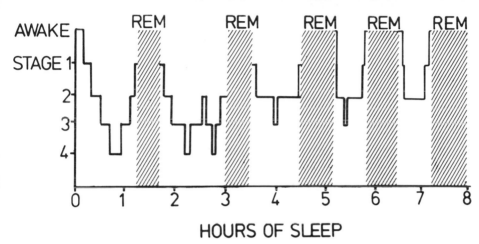

Fig. 16.1 Pattern of sequential sleep stages in a normal young adult (from McGregor, P. A., Weitzman, E. D., and Pollak, C. P.: Polysomnographic recording techniques used for the diagnosis of sleep disorders in a sleep disorders center. Am. J. EEG Technol. 18, 107, 1978. Raven Press, New York).

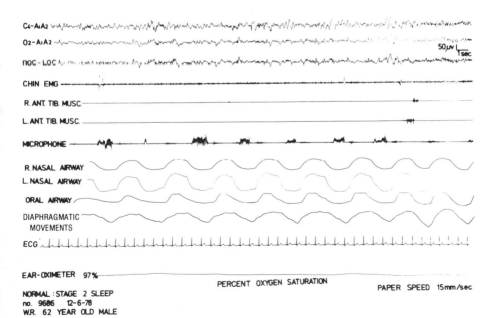

Fig. 16.2. Polysomnogram (PSG) of normal Stage 2 sleep in a 62-year-old man.

Table 16.1. ASSOCIATION OF SLEEP DISORDERS CENTERS
DIAGNOSTIC CLASSIFICATION OF SLEEP AND AROUSAL DISORDERS *

A. Disorders of Initiating and Maintaining Sleep: DIMS (The Insomnias)
  1. *Psychophysiologic*
     a. Transient and Situational
     b. Persistent
  2. *Psychiatric Disturbances*
     associated with
     a. Personality and Neurotic Character Disorders
     b. Affective Disorders
     c. Acute Schizophrenia and Other Psychoses
  3. *Use of Drugs and Alcohol*
     associated with
     a. Tolerance to or Withdrawal from CNS Depressants
     b. Sustained Use of CNS Stimulants
     c. Sustained Use of or Withdrawal from Other Drugs
     d. Habitual Use of or Withdrawal from Alcohol
  4. *Sleep Induced Ventilatory Impairment*
     a. Sleep Apnea
     b. Hypoventilation Syndromes
  5. *Nocturnal Myoclonus and "Restless Legs" Syndromes*
     associated with
     a. Nocturnal Myoclonus Syndrome
     b. "Restless Legs" Syndrome
  6. associated with *Other Medical, Toxic, and Environmental Conditions*
  7. *Childhood Onset*
  8. *Other DIMS Conditions*
     associated with
     a. Parasomnias
     b. Repeated REMS Interruptions
     c. Atypical Polysomnographic Features
  9. *No DIMS Abnormality*
     a. Short Sleeper ("Healthy Insomniac")
     b. Subjective DIMS Complaints without Objective Findings

B. Disorders of Excessive Somnolence: DOES
  1. *Psychophysiologic*
     a. Transient and Situational
     b. Persistent
  2. associated with *Psychiatric Disorders*
  3. *Use of Drugs and Alcohol*
     associated with
     a. Tolerance to or Withdrawal from CNS Stimulants
     b. Sustained Use of CNS Depressants
  4. *Sleep Induced Ventilatory Impairment*
     a. Sleep Apnea
     b. Hypoventilation Syndromes

5. *Nocturnal Myoclonus and "Restless Legs" Syndrome*
   associated with
   a. Nocturnal Myoclonus Syndrome
   b. "Restless Legs" Syndrome
6. *Narcolepsy*
7. *Idiopathic CNS Hypersomnolence*
   a. Familial
   b. Nonfamilial
8. associated with *Other Medical, Toxic, and Environmental Conditions*
9. *Other DOES Conditions*
   a. Intermittent DOES (Periodic Syndrome)
      i. Klein-Levin Syndrome
      ii. Menstrual Associated
      III. Other
   b. Insufficient Sleep
   c. Disorder of Initiating Wakefulness (Sleep Drunkenness)
   d. Not Otherwise Specified
10. *No DOES Abnormality*
    a. Long Sleeper
C. Dyssomnias Associated with Disruptions of 24-hour Sleep-Wake Cycle
   1. *Phase Shift*
      associated with
      a. Rapid Time Zone Change ("Jet Lag" Syndrome)
      b. Unconventional or Changing Sleep-Work Schedule (Shift Work)
      c. Delayed Sleep Phase
   2. *Non-24 Hour Sleep-Wake Syndrome*
   3. *Irregular Sleep-Wake Pattern*
D. Dysfunctions Associated With Sleep, Sleep Stages, or Partial Arousals (Parasomnias)
   1. *Sleepwalking (Somnambulism)*
   2. *Night Terrors (Pavor Nocturnus, Incubus)*
   3. *Nocturnus Enuresis*
   4. *Other Dysfunctions*
      a. Bruxism
      b. Jactatio Capitus Nocturnus
      c. Painful Erections
      d. Familial Sleep Paralysis
      e. Hyperactive Gag Reflex
      f. Dream Anxiety Attacks (Nightmares)
      g. Paroxysmal Nocturnal Hemoglobinuria
      h. Nocturnal Epileptic Seizures
      i. Cluster Headaches and Chronic Paroxysmal Hemicrania
      j. Nocturnal Cardiovascular Symptoms
      k. Nocturnal Asthma
      l. Nocturnal Gastroesophageal Reflux
      m. Not Otherwise Specified (N.O.S.)

---

* A full description of this classification will be available from the Secretary of the ASDC, Dr. Merril Mittler, State University of New York at Stony Brook, Department of Psychiatry, New York.

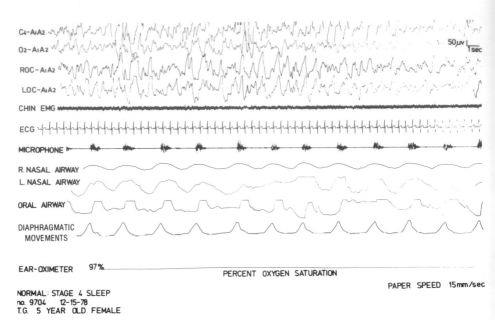

Fig. 16.3. PSG of normal Stage 4 sleep in a 5-year-old girl.

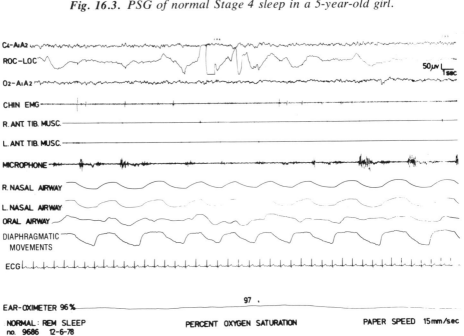

Fig. 16.4. PSG of normal REM sleep in a 62-year-old man.

all these clinical entities seen in a typical sleep disorders center and we will, therefore, emphasize those syndromes which are common, reasonably well-defined, and which require special expertise to obtain a proper polygraphic recording during sleep.

NORMAL SLEEP IN THE HUMAN YOUNG ADULT

For a complete description of the normal sleep polysomnogram, the reader is referred to the "Sleep Scoring Manual" edited by Rechtschaffen and Kales (1968), as only a brief summary can be given here.

There are two distinct phases of sleep, "nonrapid eye movement" sleep (nonREM sleep), and "rapid eye movement" sleep (REM sleep). NonREM sleep consists of four stages, designated 1, 2, 3, and 4.

Three major physiologic parameters are commonly used in the polygraphic measurement of sleep stages: (1) the electroencephalogram (EEG), (2) the electro-oculogram (EOG) and (3) the mentalis electromyogram (EMG). Electrodes are attached to the scalp at the C3 and C4 locations (international classification) and referred to the mastoids. The EOG electrodes are applied to the skin at the outer canthus of both eyes and also referred to the mastoids (to measure lateral eye movements). EMG electrodes are attached to the skin overlying the chin muscles (mentalis) and are referred to each other.

Sleep Stage Characteristics

The characteristics of the various sleep stages are shown in Figures 16.2, 16.3, and 16.4. Stage 1 sleep is characterized by low voltage mixed frequency EEG activity, associated with slow rolling eye movements recorded on the EOG channel. The chin EMG is typically of moderately high amplitude, but is decreased compared to the waking state. Stage 2 sleep is represented by a moderately low voltage background EEG interspersed with brief (0.2 to 0.75 sec) high voltage discharges (K-complexes) and 12 to 15 Hz low to moderate amplitude coherent discharges (spindles). Stage 3 sleep consists of high amplitude background activity of theta (5 to 7 Hz) and delta (1 to 3 Hz) waves, as well as K-complexes and spindle activity. This high voltage slow wave activity is present between 20 and 50 percent of the epoch (one page of polygraph recording). Stage 4 sleep consists of high voltage delta waves (75 μV or greater) with a frequency of 0.5 to 3.0 Hz. Spindles may or may not be present. This delta wave activity is present for 50 percent or more of the epoch. Tonic chin muscle potentials are usually present during these nonREM sleep stages. Electrical activity seen on the EOG channels represents the EEG transmitted from the frontal and anterior temporal regions of the brain.

REM sleep consists of low voltage, mixed frequency EEG activity which resembles that seen during Stage 1 sleep; however, saw-tooth waves are often seen. These are moderately high amplitude, 3 to 5 Hz, triangular shaped waveforms. The EOG shows rapid groupings of conjugate eye movements in all directions of gaze (rapid eye movements). Tonic EMG activity from the chin is either totally absent or markedly suppressed. Phasic muscle potential discharges, however, are prominent and irregularly present.

REM sleep alternates with nonREM sleep at approximately every 90 to 100 minutes (Fig. 16.1), the first REM period occurring about 90 to 100 minutes after sleep onset. The sequence of Stages 1, 2, 3 and 4 typically occurs at the time of going to sleep. The sequence is then reversed (Stages 4, 3, 2) and REM sleep then ensues. The normal sleep pattern of the night consists of 3 to 5 such "short term sleep cycles" with an increasing duration and percentage of the REM sleep period during the later half of the night. Stages 3 and 4 occur predominantly during the first one third of the night. Stage 1 sleep occupies approximately 5 to 10 percent, Stage 2 about 50 percent, Stage 3 some 15 percent, Stage 4 about 10 percent, and REM sleep approximately 20 percent of the average of 450 minutes of total sleep.

SELECTED SPECIFIC SLEEP DISORDERS

As can be seen from Table 16.1, the number of presenting problems and range of clinical entities seen in a sleep disorders center is very large. The reader is referred to several recent reports, reviews, and monographs, which together provide an extensive sleep disorders bibliography (Broughton, 1968; Kales et al, 1974a; Aschoff, 1976; Guilleminault, Dement, and Passouant, 1976a; Hauri, 1977, Guilleminault and Dement, 1978. We will here provide brief summaries, illustrations with case reports of a few common clinical entities, followed by a detailed description of polysomnographic (PSG) recording methods.

The Insomnias

This heterogenous group of disorders is organized around the symptoms of difficulty in initiating and/or maintaining sleep. It is important to emphasize that such complaints do not define a specific disease entity—"insomnia" is not a disease. The range of different polysomnographic patterns seen in patients complaining of insomnia is large. Often the normal organization of sustained sleep stages is disrupted by frequent transient arousals and many sleep stage changes throughout the night. The patient may be unable to sustain long periods of sleep and demonstrates intrusive periods of wakefulness, lasting for minutes to several hours. The electroencephalographic pattern may show a variety of intrusive events not normally present. These include spindles occurring during REM sleep, and rapid eye movements during what is otherwise predominantly Stage 2 with spindles and K-complexes (Fig. 16.5). Alpha activity, not normally present during nonREM sleep, may persist for long periods in some patients, producing the so-called "alpha-delta" sleep pattern (Fig. 16.6). Sedative drugs, when used in high doses on an habitual basis, will produce electroencephalographic changes such as sustained beta activity (20 to 24 Hz)

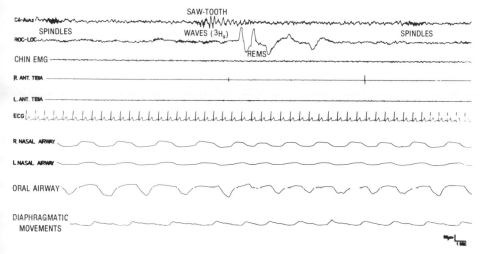

Fig. 16.5. REM-spindles in a 38-year-old man with a chief complaint of difficulty in falling asleep of 20 years' duration. He dated the onset of his difficulty in sleeping to childhood. He would often be unable to fall asleep until 2 A.M. and then had trouble awakening for school. There had been a long-standing tendency to delay the time of sleep onset relative to the usual social time. Polysomnography demonstrated a 37 minute latency from lights-out to sleep onset, absence of Stage 4 sleep, but adequate Stage 3 sleep. He demonstrated the REM-spindle abnormality often seen in patients with severe and prolonged sleep disturbance. There was no polygraphic evidence of nocturnal myoclonus or sleep apnea (from McGregor, P. A., Weitzman, E. D., and Pollak, C. P.: Polysomnographic recording techniques used for the diagnosis of sleep disorders in a sleep disorders center. Am. J. EEG Technol., 18, 107, 1978. Raven Press, New York).

(Figs. 16.7a, b, c). A specific syndrome of insomnia associated with chronic hypnotic drug use has been identified, in which partial drug withdrawal each night contributes to the complaint of disturbed sleep.

The association of the "Restless Legs Syndrome" with insomnia has been well-described. The presence of prolonged episodes of periodic leg movements alone, without the associated "restless legs" complaint, may also contribute to a disturbed and disrupted night's sleep. Unless identified by polysomnographic recording, it may go unrecognized. In a recent study by our Sleep Disorders Center group, we found that such periodic movements in sleep ("Nocturnal Myoclonus") occurred to a variable degree in 19 percent of patients complaining of insomnia. However, we also found that it was present during sleep in other patients, including those with narcolepsy and sleep apnea (Coleman, Pollak, and Weitzman, 1978). Although periodic movements in sleep may contribute to the disturbance of sleep in certain patients with chronic insomnia, they appear to be associated with, and perhaps caused by, chronic sleep-wake disturbances of many origins. The polysomnographic finding consists of highly periodic, unilateral or bilateral contractions of lower leg muscles every 20 to 40

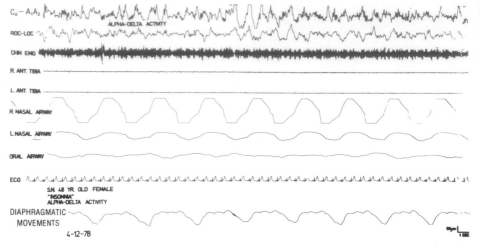

Fig. 16.6. *Alpha-delta sleep pattern in a 48-year-old woman with the complaint of insomnia for many years. She awakened too early in the morning and became sleepy too early in the evening. Throughout her life she had always been the first to go to bed and the first to be up in the morning. Her present schedule was to retire at 10:00 P.M., fall asleep at 11:00 P.M., awaken once or twice during the night, and awaken at 5:00 in the morning with inability to return to sleep after that hour. A polysomnogram was performed at a time when the patient was not taking any medication for this problem. The recording demonstrated a very short (1.7 minute) latency from lights-out to sleep onset; however, she slept only 77% of the time and had some decrease in REM sleep. The alpha-delta sleep EEG pattern was present for long periods of the night (from McGregor, P. A., Weitzman, E. D., and Pollak, C. P.: Polysomnographic recording techniques used for the diagnosis of sleep disorders in a sleep disorders center. Am. J. EEG Technol., 18, 107, 1978. Raven Press, New York).*

seconds during sleep (Fig. 16.8). Individual contractions last 1 to 2 seconds and are repetitive for many minutes or hours. Patients are typically unaware of these leg movements even though the EEG occasionally shows hundreds of brief (2 to 4 second) arousals.

An important differential diagnosis in patients who experience long standing difficulty falling asleep is the condition listed in the Nosology under Phase Shift Dyssomnia (see C), discussed later.

The Narcolepsy-Cataplexy Syndrome

In contradistinction to the heterogeneous nature of the "insomnias," narcolepsy-cataplexy is a distinct clinical syndrome with well-defined symptoms, age of onset, and natural history. In 1975, at the First International Symposium on Narcolepsy, the following definition was agreed to:

The word Narcolepsy refers to a syndrome of unknown origin that is characterized by abnormal sleep tendencies, including excessive daytime sleepiness, and often

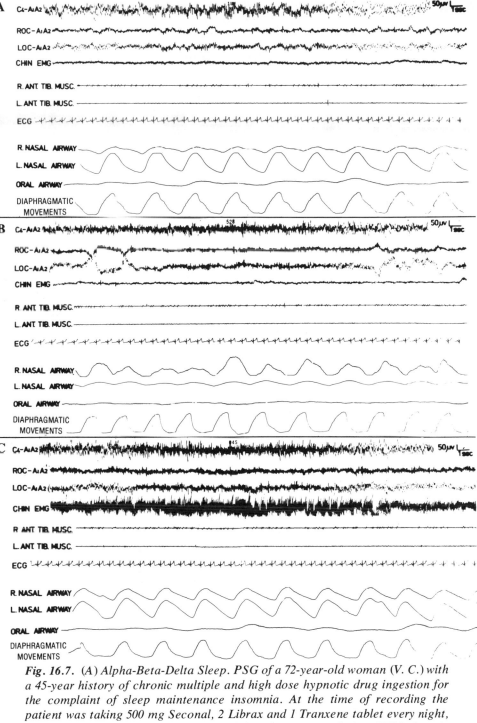

Fig. 16.7. (A) Alpha-Beta-Delta Sleep. PSG of a 72-year-old woman (V. C.) with a 45-year history of chronic multiple and high dose hypnotic drug ingestion for the complaint of sleep maintenance insomnia. At the time of recording the patient was taking 500 mg Seconal, 2 Librax and 1 Tranxene tablet every night, including the night of the PSG. (B) Alpha-Beta activity during REM sleep in patient V. C. Note the low amplitude chin EMG activity, irregular respiration, and rapid eye movements. (C) Alpha-Beta activity in patient V. C. while quietly awake. Note the high amplitude chin EMG activity. (Paper speed: 15 mm/sec.)

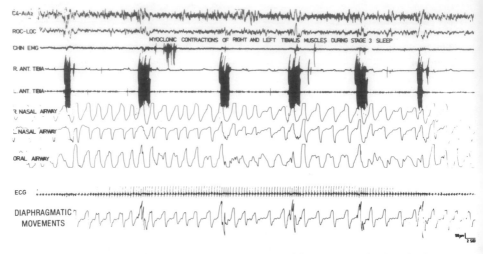

Fig. 16.8. *Nocturnal myoclonus in a 52-year-old woman with the chief complaint of insomnia for 20 years, that had increased during the past 3 years. She reported great difficulty in falling asleep upon retiring at 10:00 P.M., and would often lie awake for 3 or 4 hours. She would eventually sleep for 1 to 2 hours before awakening again, and then have trouble in returning to sleep for the rest of the night. She denied any history of restless leg syndrome, was not aware of any abnormal movements during sleep, and was unable to nap during the day. She had not taken medication for this problem for many years. Polysomnography during two consecutive nights demonstrated severe nocturnal myoclonus occurring in prolonged episodes, each lasting several hours. The myoclonus was synchronous in both legs (from McGregor, P. A., Weitzman, E. D., and Pollak, C. P.: Polysomnographic recording techniques used for the diagnosis of sleep disorders in a sleep disorders center. Am. J. EEG Technol., 18, 107, 1978. Raven Press, New York).*

disturbed nocturnal sleep, and pathological manifestations of REM sleep. The REM sleep abnormalities include sleep onset REM periods and the dissociated REM sleep inhibitory processes, cataplexy, and sleep paralysis. Excessive daytime sleepiness, cataplexy, and less often sleep paralysis and hypnagogic hallucinations are the major symptoms of the disease (Guilleminault et al, 1976a).

This condition typically begins during puberty or young adulthood. Once established, it remains a lifelong disease. There is an increased risk for narcolepsy to occur among the relatives of patients with proven narcolepsy as compared to the general population (Kessler, 1976). In addition, an animal (dog) model of the disease with genetic transmission to offspring has been found (Mitler, 1976). Narcolepsy is, therefore, clearly an organic neurologic disease with a well-defined and characteristic clinical picture.

The abnormal occurrence of a sleep onset REM period during an afternoon nap or at sleep onset at night is used as a polygraphic diagnostic test in sleep disorders centers, to aid in establishing the clinical diagnosis (Fig. 16.9a, b). If standard sleep conditions are met (recumbency in a comfortable bed), the probability of a sleep onset REM period (SOREMP) taking place during an afternoon nap and a night's sleep is certainly greater than 80 percent. Dement and his group found that each of 100 patients with cataplexy had at least one SOREMP when recorded during a standard nap or with a continuous 36-hour recording (Dement, 1976). The cessation of medication for 2 weeks will increase the probability of a SOREMP. SOREMP may also occur after prolonged sleep deprivation, circadian phase shifts of the sleep-wake cycle, and during "free-running" sleep-wake rhythms in conditions of temporal isolation in otherwise normal subjects. For normal subjects who sleep regularly at night, a SOREMP is an exceedingly infrequent event. A SOREMP is detected by a loss or marked reduction of tonic chin muscle tone, the presence of rapid conjugate eye movements, and a low-voltage, mixed frequency EEG pattern occurring within 15 minutes of sleep onset. Phasic chin muscle activity, irregular respira-

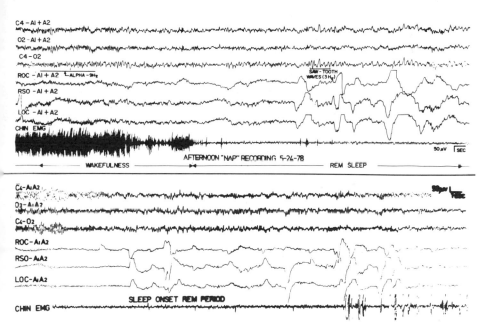

Fig. 16.9. (A) *Sleep onset REM period during an afternoon nap in a 28-year-old woman with a clear-cut history of narcolepsy. Polysomnographic recordings also demonstrated REM onset of the nocturnal sleep period (from McGregor, P. A., Weitzman, E. D., and Pollak, C. P.: Polysomnographic recording techniques used for the diagnosis of sleep disorders in a sleep disorders center. Am. J. EEG Technol., 18, 107, 1978. Raven Press, New York). (B) Sleep onset REM period during an afternoon nap in a 52-year-old woman with a clear history of the narcolepsy-cataplexy syndrome. Note the dramatic shift from high voltage alpha to mixed low voltage EEG activity, and the phasic chin EMG discharges in association with rapid eye movements. (Paper speed: 15 mm/sec.)*

tion, and "REM spindles" may also be found during it. The patient will often describe a hypnagogic hallucination (vivid dream) during this period and may also have an episode of sleep-paralysis. In addition to the frequent occurrence of a SOREMP, the nocturnal sleep of the narcoleptic is usually not normal. Although the disturbed nocturnal sleep pattern is not usually a prominent clinical complaint, most patients report having at least a few brief awakenings every night. Polysomnographic studies have shown that there is an increased amount of Stage 1 sleep, decreased Stages 3 and 4 sleep, more body movements and awakenings, and a normal amount and percent of REM sleep (Montplaisir, 1976).

The diagnosis of the narcolepsy-cataplexy syndrome is generally not difficult, provided a careful and thorough history is obtained. Since this is a lifelong disease that will significantly affect the patient's social, economic, and emotional life, and since pharmacologic therapy usually has a major beneficial impact, it is important to make as definitive a diagnosis as possible. We, therefore, strongly recommend that a daytime nap and an all-night PSG be obtained in all patients in whom the diagnosis is suspected.

Hypersomnia—Sleep Apnea Syndrome

The syndrome of excessive daytime sleepiness (hypersomnia) and recurring apnea during sleep (HSA) is an important clinical entity that is seen with increasing frequency in sleep disorders centers (Guilleminault and Dement, 1978). During the past 2 years we have diagnosed approximately 75 patients with this illness. During the past 6 months alone it has represented approximately 30 percent of all patients referred to our center. In addition to serious emotional, social, and economic disability produced by the daytime hypersomnia, the syndrome is associated with systemic hypertension, cardiac arrhythmias, erythremia, pulmonary hypertension, cardiac hypertrophy, and in some cases frank cerebral and myocardial infarcts. All patients with this syndrome seen by us have loud intermittent snoring during sleep and have had this prominent symptom for many years. It occurs predominantly in middle-aged men who are usually but not always obese, and who have typically gone undiagnosed for several years of increasing disability.

An analysis by our group of the upper airway, using multiview video fluoroscopy and fiber-optic endoscopic examination, has revealed that the specific site of functional airway obstruction during sleep is in the oral pharynx at the velo-pharyngeal sphincter. The mechanism involves recurrent apposition of the lateral pharyngeal walls and posterior movement of the base of the tongue (Weitzman et al, 1978a).

Following a complete medical history, general physical and neurologic examination, and laboratory tests, it is crucial that an all-night PSG be obtained with special emphasis on respiratory and cardiac monitoring. Airflow through the right and left nasal airways and the oral airway should be monitored using the thermistor technique. Thoraco-abdominal respiratory movements are recorded, as well as oxygen saturation using an ear oximeter, and a continuous one-channel electrocardiogram (Figs. 16.10, 16.11, 16.12, 16.13, 16.14). We typically record two EEG channels, one eye movement channel, one chin EMG channel, and right and left surface EMG anterior tibial muscle channels; and a miniature microphone is taped to the face to record snoring and breathing sounds. In special situations, we also record intrathoracic pressure using a midesophageal transducer (Fig. 16.12).

It is important to quantify the total number, duration, and types of apnea during sleep and to relate the apneas to changes in the EKG and decreases of oxygen saturation. This analysis provides the rational basis for subsequent therapeutic recommendations. It is generally agreed that a sleep apnea is defined as a cessation of airflow through the nose and mouth, lasting at least 10 seconds, and occurring during a polygraphically defined stage of sleep. Except for occasional apneas occurring at sleep onset and during REM sleep, sleep apneas rarely occur in normal young and middle-aged individuals. The normal older age group (over 65 years) has not been adequately studied. Most centers

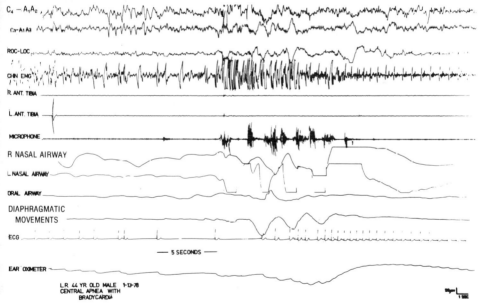

Fig. 16.10. *Central apneic episode associated with bradytachycardia and sinus arrest lasting up to 5 seconds in a 44-year-old man who complained of sleepiness during the day and had severe snoring and breathing abnormalities during sleep. He had recently gained 25 lb, bringing his weight when first seen to 245 lb. He had had several car accidents during the previous 6 months because he had fallen asleep at the wheel. He was a court stenographer and had fallen asleep so frequently during work that he had had to request sick leave from his job. Blood pressure was elevated. Other portions of his polysomnogram revealed obstructive sleep apnea. His symptoms were relieved by tracheostomy (from McGregor, P. A., Weitzman, E. D., and Pollak, C. P.: Polysomnographic recording techniques used for the diagnosis of sleep disorders in a sleep disorders center. Am. J. EEG Technol., 18, 107, 1978. Raven Press, New York).*

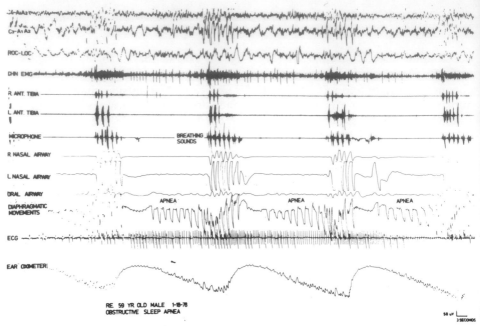

Fig. 16.11. *Obstructive apneic episodes in a 59-year-old company executive who had a 15-year history of increasingly severe daytime sleepiness, progressive systemic hypertension, coronary artery disease, and cardiac arrhythmias. Note the diaphragmatic movements during apnea, and also the irregular ECG, demonstrating multiple ventricular premature contractions with trigeminy and bigeminy (from McGregor, P. A., Weitzman, E. D., and Pollak, C. P.: Polysomnographic recording techniques used for the diagnosis of sleep disorders in a sleep disorders center. Am. J. EEG Technol., 18, 107, 1978. Raven Press, New York).*

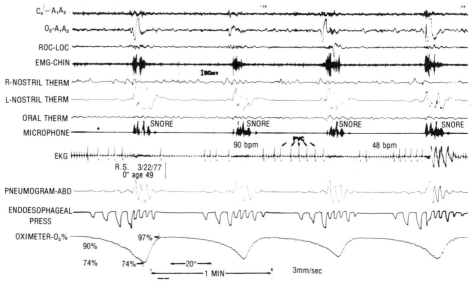

Fig. 16.12. *Mixed (obstructive and central) sleep apnea in a 49-year-old man (R.S.) with progressive sleepiness of 4 years' duration. Note the bradytachycardia pattern associated with multiple premature ventricular contractions. There were frequent falls in oxygen saturation below 75% (PO$_2$ approx. 40 mm Hg).*

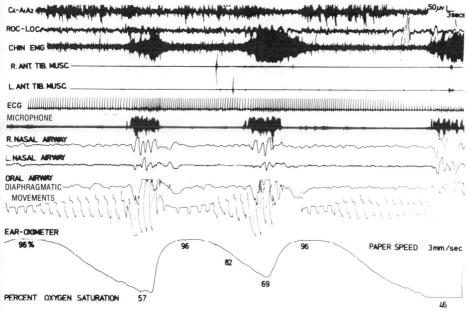

Fig. 16.13. *Pure obstructive sleep apnea in a 38-year-old man (V.P.) with a 5-year history of progressive daytime sleepiness, loud snoring, and systemic hypertension. Note marked recurrent drop in oxygen saturation to values below 50% (46% O_2 saturation $\cong PO_2$ 25 mm Hg) and bradytachycardia ECG pattern.*

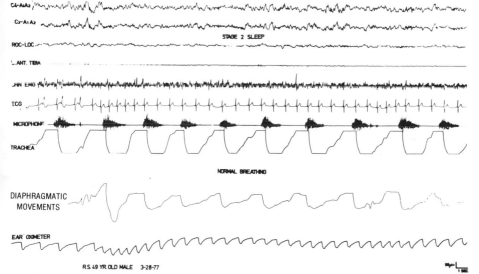

Fig. 16.14. *Improved polysomnogram 1 week following tracheostomy in a 49-year-old male with the chief complaint of excessive daytime sleepiness and severe snoring at night, progressive during the past 4 years. His wife described periods during sleep when he appeared to stop breathing for 30 seconds to 1 minute at a time. A thorough evaluation demonstrated severe obstructive sleep apnea. Tracheostomy was performed with dramatic and sustained improvement in his symptoms. Pretracheostomy PSG for this patient is shown in Fig. 16.12 (from McGregor, P. A., Weitzman, E. D., and Pollak, C. P.: Polysomnographic recording techniques used for the diagnosis of sleep disorders in a sleep disorders center. Am. J. EEG Technol., 18, 107, 1978. Raven Press, New York).*

diagnose a sleep apnea syndrome if there are more than 30 apneic episodes during 7 hours of nocturnal sleep. However, there is rarely a problem of arriving at a diagnosis in patients with the classical symptoms of HSA. In a series of 25 patients analyzed quantitatively by us, no patient had fewer than 200 separate apneic episodes during sleep in one 6-to-8-hour nocturnal recording.

Three types of apnea have been defined using the above recording technique. Diaphragmatic (central) apnea is characterized by a cessation of both airflow and respiratory movements (Fig. 16.10). Obstructive (upper-airway) apnea consists of no airflow through either the nasal passages or mouth, but with persistent respiratory movements of the thorax or diaphragm (Fig. 16.13). In mixed apnea, there is an initial cessation of all airflow and respiratory effort, followed by obstructive apnea with respiratory effort but no airflow (Figs. 16.11, 16.12). The predominant patterns seen during sleep in patients with HSA syndrome are the obstructive and mixed apnea types. Predominantly diaphragmatic apneas have been found to occur in patients with insomnia, narcolepsy, and several rare conditions (Guilleminault and Dement, 1978).

Cardiac arrhythmias are prominent during sleep in patients with HSA and are one of the major indications for prompt therapeutic intervention. The most common abnormality is recurrent bradycardia-tachycardia, in association with the cyclic apneic and oxygen saturation-desaturation pattern (Figs. 16.12, 16.13). Heart rates typically alter between 40 to 50 and 90 to 110 beats per minute. Multiple premature ventricular contractions are frequently found during sleep (Fig. 16.12). More serious arrhythmias can occur, including extreme sinus bradycardia (to less than 30 per minute), asystole for up to 10 seconds or longer (Fig. 16.10), ventricular tachycardia, bigeminy (Fig. 16.14), trigeminy, and second-degree AV block (Guilleminault, Tilkian, and Dement, 1976b; Burack et al, 1977).

The only proven effective treatment for the HSA syndrome is to perform a tracheostomy and thereby allow the patient an open tracheal airway during sleep. This procedure bypasses the upper airway obstruction and the patient sleeps with normal respiratory air exchange (Fig. 16.14). The improvement in symptoms is dramatic, rapid, and in most cases sustained. The hypersomnia and sleep disturbance disappear, cardiac arrhythmias either disappear or are markedly improved, the elevated blood pressure falls, and often the hematocrit drops (Kuhlo, Doll, and Franc, 1969; Tilkian et al, 1975; Guilleminault et al, 1976b; Pollak et al, 1978). The availability of a proven effective form of therapy for this serious, life-threatening medical illness emphasizes the importance of a thorough clinical evaluation and well-recorded polysomnogram.

The Parasomnias

These sleep disorders, listed in Table 16.1, are complex behaviors which either occur during sleep or interrupt sleep and are clinical problems in their own right. It has been suggested that these sleep disturbances are related to a partial arousal that often, but not always, occurs during sleep stages 3 or 4

(Broughton, 1968). Somnambulism, night terror attacks (Fig. 16.15) and enuresis have been shown to be rarely related to the REM-dreaming stages of sleep. The EEG pattern is typically a complex mixture of slow wave, alpha, and beta activities, accompanied by superimposed movement and muscle activity artifacts obscuring the polygraphic recording. These sleep-disturbing phenomena occur more often in children, are present early in the night's sleep (usually about 1 to 2 hours after falling asleep), may assume different forms in the same individual, produce a dissociated behavioral state, and are usually not remembered in detail by the patient in the morning (Kales and Kales, 1974b).

A sleep-related seizure disorder may go unrecognized for years and may be identified for the first time by polysomnography if an adequate (6 or more channel) montage is employed (Figs. 16.16, 16.17). Continuous video-taping and monitoring of the patient's behavior during sleep can be extremely useful and diagnostic of specific seizure patterns such as focal motor, generalized, and temporal lobe seizures. The use of nasopharyngeal and sphenoidal leads during sleep is useful if seizures originating in the temporal lobe are suspected, but this requires special expertise. It is most important that the polysomnographic technician be alerted beforehand to the possible occurrence of a parasomnia. He should be prepared to protect the patient from possible injury, describe clearly any abnormal behavior, and modify the recording program as often as necessary to document fully the events of the night.

The Phase Shift Dyssomnias (C.1 in Table 16.1) may be related to rapid time zone changes ("jet lag"), to shiftwork, or to a delayed sleep phase. Delayed Sleep Phase is a debilitating functional disorder that is being increasingly recognized in patients seen at sleep disorders centers. The history is characteris-

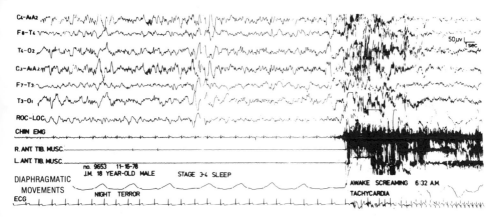

Fig. 16.15. PSG of an 18-year-old male with a 6-year history of nightly night terror and violent episodes of somnambulism. This PSG episode took place during Stage 3 sleep. Note the absence of any change in respiration, heart rate, or EEG just prior to the sudden onset of the event. A video tape recording dramatically showed that the patient abruptly sat up in bed, screamed incoherently, and appeared to be confused with nonpurposeful hand and arm movements. No clinical seizure activity could be identified.

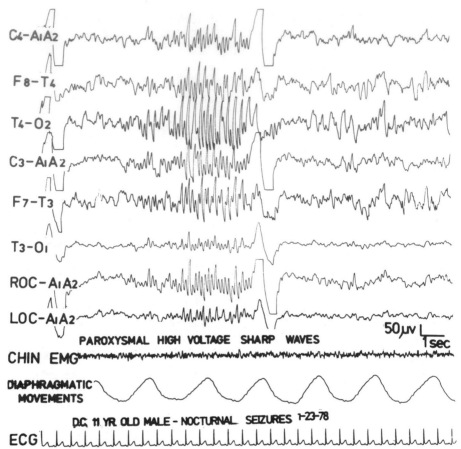

Fig. 16.16. *Paroxysmal, hypersynchronous, bilaterally symmetrical 6 to 7 Hz activity in an 11-year-old boy with the complaint of "having some kind of spell associated with nightmares." His parents noted that after falling asleep, he would sit up with a sudden start associated with rapid shallow breathing. At times he had fallen off the bed. There was no history of tonic or clonic activity, tongue biting, or incontinence during sleep; however, there were symptoms suggesting daytime seizures as well as daytime "sleepiness." He would suddenly fall off a chair and roll over on the floor until striking an obstacle. At such times he was very difficult to awaken. The daytime episodes lasted for several seconds to 1 minute. Although the illustrated discharges were not noted to be associated with any abnormal motor activity, their paroxysmal intrusive quality indicated the possibility of a seizure disorder. A clinical EEG was then performed which showed two episodes of bilaterally synchronous spike and wave activity. The final diagnosis was probable temporal lobe epilepsy with major behavioral component (from McGregor, P. A., Weitzman, E. D., and Pollak, C. P.: Polysomnographic recording techniques used for the diagnosis of sleep disorders in a sleep disorders center. Am. J. EEG Technol., 18, 107, 1978. Raven Press, New York).*

tic: the patient has experienced difficulty in falling asleep for years ("sleep onset insomnia") but then sleeps soundly. If allowed to sleep late in the morning, the patient spontaneously awakens after 7 or 8 hours, feeling well-rested. Individuals with this sleep-wake pattern experience difficulties whenever they are confronted with responsibilities (school, work) that begin relatively early in the morning. They make futile attempts to retire earlier and may resort to sleeping pills. They may become chronically sleep-deprived due to a late hour of sleep onset combined with a forced early awakening, and compensate partially on weekends by sleeping very late in the morning. A sleep-wake log kept by the patient for several weeks will often reveal this pattern, and a polysomnogram obtained at the patient's best hours of sleep, e.g. 0500 to 1300 h, often discloses a strikingly normal sleep pattern. Our Center is presently investigating a nonpharmacologic treatment of this disorder in which a 24+ hour sleep-wake schedule is temporarily imposed ("chronotherapy").

A less common, but even more debilitating, disorder of the 24-hour sleep-wake cycle is the non-24 hour day, or as we have termed it, the "Hyper-nychthermeral Syndrome" (Kokkoris et al, 1979). Affected individuals display

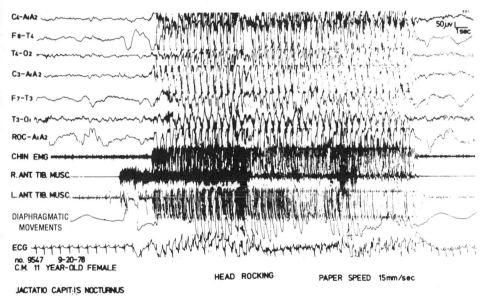

Fig. 16.17. PSG recording of an 11-year-old girl with a 9-year history of head rocking at the onset of, and recurrently during, sleep. A video tape recording revealed that while lying on her back with her head on a pillow, she would suddenly make rhythmic flexion-extension movements of her head lasting 20 to 40 seconds. These would be followed by several seconds of alpha EEG activity, but then she would rapidly resume sleeping. Note the similarity to electrographic seizure discharge. However, the patient never had any evidence of clinical seizures, nor any abnormality in standard clinical electroencephalograms.

a variable tendency to sleep and wake at intervals that are somewhat longer than 24 hours (24.5 to 27.0 hours). Sleep onset and termination, therefore, occur at progressively later solar hours. This pattern is particularly likely to emerge during vacations when occupational and other social temporal demands are reduced, but is also present at other times in the most severe cases. As a result, patients may be occupationally disabled by their inability to maintain the socially conventional work-rest schedule, and their social and family activities may be disrupted.

It has repeatedly been demonstrated that normal individuals, living in an environment isolated from time cues, will develop a sleep-wake rhythm which is longer than 24 hours (free-running rhythm) (Aschoff, 1976). Recent data obtained by polygraphic recording of sequential sleep periods of such normal subjects have shown that there are characteristic internal sleep stage changes. For example, we have shown that REM sleep shifts to an earlier time of the sleep period, producing a shortened REM latency and an increased amount of REM sleep during the first 3 hours (Weitzman et al, 1978b).

Chronic disturbances of the circadian sleep-wake cycle occur in patients who have intermittent or permanent occupational shift-work jobs. Frequent phase shifts and sleep deprivation have been shown to lead to very disturbed daily sleep stage pattern organization. Polysomnographic recordings obtained in such individuals can be quite abnormal.

The application of the concepts of biologic rhythm research to a wide variety of sleep disorders, including changes associated with aging, manic-depressive and endogenous depression, drug withdrawal syndromes, etc., is now only in its infancy, but those working in sleep disorders centers and polysomnographic laboratories will increasingly be aware of new developments in this area of clinical investigation.

POLYSOMNOGRAPHIC RECORDING ARRANGEMENTS

General Aspects

Clinical polysomnography is the term used to define a complex, multichannel continuous polygraphic recording of several physiologic functions during an extended period of sleep for diagnostic purposes. It typically includes the assessment of central nervous system measures (including autonomic, complex motor, and electroencephalographic activity), and of respiratory, cardiac, gastrointestinal, endocrine, and genitourinary functions, depending on the clinical indications. It is important to emphasize that, as in any diagnostic laboratory procedure, the indications for performing polysomnography depends on an adequate medical and psychiatric history and general physical and neurologic examination.

Since there are differences in techniques and clinical emphasis in different sleep disorders centers, we will describe the methods presently used at the Sleep-Wake Disorders Center at Montefiore Hospital and Medical Center

(Bronx, New York) (Fig. 16.18). The ASDC is presently compiling a set of guidelines for the technical aspects of clinical polysomnography, and the description here generally conforms to those guidelines, although our Center uses some additional techniques and equipment. Techniques are rapidly evolving in this area as new clinical findings, instrumentation, and data processing methods are applied.*

It is of the utmost importance that the examination be performed under pleasant, respectful conditions which provide those amenities that are found in most people's homes. A comfortable bed in an attractive, private bedroom should be provided. This bedroom should be quiet, able to be darkened, and separated from the polygraphic recording equipment and the sounds of technicians' conversations.

The polysomnographic technician must be present and vigilant throughout the entire 8 to 10 hours of recording. The technician is responsible for making observations and documenting the time and description of special events such as apneic periods, night terror attacks, somnambulism, and seizures, and he must be able to recognize and handle emergencies, including cardiopulmonary resuscitation.

Every competent technician knows that a good EEG recording will result only if the electrodes are well applied. This becomes especially important when recording an all-night polysomnogram (PSG). Electrodes and sensors are attached to a patient who will sleep in bed for periods of 8 to 10 hours. Poorly applied electrodes will produce artifacts and have to be reapplied, and this will inevitably lead to some disturbance of the patient. Special attention must, therefore, be paid to the technique of applying electrodes. Skin resistance should be reduced to less than 5,000 ohms. A few spare electrodes should be applied to especially troublesome areas such as the chin (EMG) and scalp (EEG).

Our Sleep-Wake Disorders Center uses a variety of electrodes and sensors. For EEG recording, gold-plated cup electrodes (Grass Instruments, Inc.) and the International 10–20 Placement System is followed. Beckman electrodes (Beckman Inc.) are small, lightweight, silver/silver chloride sensors which are nonpolarizable and are attached to the skin with small double-sided adhesive collars. These electrodes are usually used for facial and non-scalp areas, and also for surface EMG recordings from the legs to detect periodic movements.

To record respiratory airflow, small thermistors are placed at each nostril and in front of the mouth. These devices are sensitive to temperature change and produce an electrical potential with each breath which is recorded on the polygraph. A small 1.5 V battery is included in a wheatstone bridge circuit.

Thermocouples may also be used to measure airflow. A thermocouple consists of two dissimilar metal wires, such as constantin and copper, which

---

* Portions of the following material appeared in McGregor, P. A., Weitzman, E. D., and Pollak, C. P.: Polysomnographic recording techniques used for the diagnosis of sleep disorders in a sleep disorders center. Am. J. EEG Technol., *18:*107–132, 1978. Raven Press, New York.

SLEEP-WAKE DISORDERS UNIT
PHYSICIAN'S PSG REQUEST (VERSION: 10/76)
Department of Neurology - Montefiore Hospital and Medical Center, New York

1. Patient's Name _____ 2. Age _____ 3. Soc. Sec. # _____

4. Date of Request_____ 5. Working diagnosis_____

6. Patient's usual bedtime_____ am/pm 7. Usual arising_____ am/pm

8. Priority: ASAP _____Within 3 weeks_____Other_____

9. Select the recording array(s) to be used if "Standard". Enter individual sensors
   if a "Special" array is requested.

Chan	Standard					Special			
	A	B	C*	D	E	W	X	Y	Z
1	C4-A1+2	C4-A1+2	C4-A1+2	C4-A1+2	URO				
2	ROC-A1+2	F8-T4	O2-A1+2	ROC-A1+2	F8-T4				
3	RSO-A1+2	T4-O2	ROC-A1+2	LOC-A1+2	T4-O2				
4	LOC-A1+2	C3-A1+2	LOC-A1+2	CHIN	F7-T3				
5	CHIN	F7-T3	CHIN	RAT	T3-O1				
6	RAT	T3-O1	RAT	LAT	ROC-A1+2				
7	LAT	ROC-LOC	LAT	RQ	LOC-A1+2				
8	RNA	CHIN	RNA	LQ	CHIN				
9	LNA	RAT	LNA	RNA	RAT				
10	OA	LAT	OA	LNA	LAT				
11	TAM	TAM	TAM	OA	TAM				
12	ECG	ECG	ECG	ECG	ECG				

10.

Check one	Common indications	Night				ABBREVIATION KEY
		1	2			EEG: use std.internat.10-20 system
	General use	A				EOG: ROC,LOC - right, left outer canthus / RSO,LSO - right, left supraobital
	Noct. seiz.	B				EMG: CHIN - mentalis muscle / RAT,LAT - right,left anterior tibial / RQ,LQ - right,left quadriceps
	Sleep apnea	C				RESP: RNA,LNA- right,left nasal airflow (thermistor)
	Noct.myclon.	D				OA - oral airflow (thermistor) / TAM - thoracoabdominal movements (strain gauge or equivalent)
	Noct.eneur.	E				ECG: electrocardiogram / URO: urometer

11. VIDEOTAPE. Yes_____ No
    Describe possible behavior of interest below.
12. Special instructions:
    *On the C montage, add 13 - ear oximeter
                           14 - mini-microphone

Staff Physician

Fig. 16.18. Physician's request form, showing arrays used in polysomnography (from McGregor, P. A., Weitzman, E. D., and Pollak, C. P.: Polysomnographic recording techniques used for the diagnosis of sleep disorders in a sleep disorders center. Am. J. EEG Technol., 18, 107, 1978. Raven Press, New York).

change temperature at different rates. The difference in rate of temperature change establishes an electrical voltage which can be used as a measure of respiration. The thermocouple leads can be plugged directly into the electrode miniboard since no wheatstone bridge is required.

Diaphragmatic movements can be indicated by a mercury strain gauge strapped around the chest or abdomen. Long leads from the strain gauge are connected to a wheatstone bridge, the output of which is amplified by a DC amplifier. We prefer to use a pneumograph to record chest/abdomen movements. The pneumograph consists of a cylindrical rubber bellows strapped to the chest, and connected to a volumetric pressure transducer. The movements of the chest create a change in air pressure in the bellows, and the transducer converts these pressure changes into electrical potentials. These signals should also be recorded on a DC amplifier, using a long time constant of 0.1 sec or, preferably, a DC setting.

The Ear Oximeter

The ear oximeter is an instrument which provides a continuous measurement of the oxygen saturation of the arterial blood by means of a photoelectric pick-up placed on the ear. The color spectrum of the ear reflects the percentage of oxyphenoglobin. A photoelectric device attaches to the ear, and its output can be read directly on the control panel and simultaneously recorded with a DC amplifier on the polygraphic recording. The pen zero control should be used to set the pen almost at the upper position of its deflection range. This setting should represent normal oxygen levels (approximately 95 percent). As the saturation level of oxygen drops, the pen will show a downward deflection.

The Urometer

In order to determine the stage of sleep in which enuresis occurs, and whether it is associated with epileptiform EEG activity, a special electrode can be made and attached to the inside seat of the patient's pajamas. Details of the construction of this simple device are given elsewhere (McGregor, Weitzman, and Pollak, 1978). The device is connected to a 1.5 V battery-operated relay which closes when the electrode insulation is made wet by urine, causing plates in the device to short-circuit and pass the signal from a 60 Hz wave generator to a polygraph amplifier.

Miniature Microphone

A miniature microphone is used to record breathing sounds from patients with sleep apnea. The microphone, which measures ½″ x ⅜″, is taped on the face between the nose and mouth. The signal from the microphone amplifier goes to the soundtrack of a videotape recorder or other audio recorder. The signal is also monitored with a loudspeaker and recorded on the polygraph.

Polygraphic Recording Equipment

Details of the equipment used for recording purposes have been given elsewhere (McGregor et al, 1978), and the interested reader will also find addresses of commercial suppliers in that publication.

The Audiovisual System

All patients with sleep apnea, as well as those with suspected behavioral and movement disorders during sleep, are continuously viewed on TV monitors. These data can be simultaneously recorded on a time-lapse video tape recorder. A control panel on the instrument rack will enable the bedroom cameras to be controlled remotely. The camera direction is controlled by a pan-tilt switch, and a zoom lens control permits a close-up of special features or can provide a view of the entire bed.

A special effects generator will permit recording from two cameras simultaneously. Two patients may be recorded at the same time and each seen on one half of the screen, or one patient can be recorded on one half of the screen and the PSG recording simultaneously displayed and recorded on the other half. This technique is very valuable for monitoring seizure patients.

A speed selector switch on the video tape recorder permits the tape to run at normal speed (real time). However, operation at this speed would require the use of about eight tapes during a typical night. Time-lapse speeds are, therefore, used such that 1 to 12 hours of data can be recorded on one tape. This is accomplished by taking a reduced number of frames per second. An electronic date-time generator provides a digital display of the year, month, day, hour, minute, and second on the TV monitor. This information is also recorded on videotape and is very useful for matching original PSG graphed data with information played back from the video tapes.

RECORDING PROCEDURES

Calibration

The standard calibration used is such that a 50 μV signal produces a pen deflection of 7 mm. The ½ amplitude points of the low frequency filters are set at 0.3 Hz and the high frequency filters at 60 Hz. The DC amplifiers are set either on a long time-constant (0.1 sec), or on the DC mode. Sensitivity is set on both preamplifier and driver amplifiers such that 100 mV equals 2 cm on the driver, and 2 mV equals 2 cm on the preamplifier pen deflection. The driver amplifier can be set between 0.1 and 75 Hz, depending on the desired response. For DC recording, Grass oscillographs providing a 2-inch pen deflection are used instead of the 1-inch deflection galvanometers used for AC recordings. This permits DC signals to be recorded at high gain for quantification purposes. The paper speed normally used is 15 mm per second, but is increased to the standard clinical EEG speed of 30 mm per second at intervals during the PSG. At times, very slow paper speeds of 3 or 6 mm per second are used at intervals to better display certain rhythmic abnormalities, such as sleep apnea or periodic leg movements.

Recording the Afternoon Nap

This has become a standard procedure to confirm and document the diagnosis of narcolepsy. The test is positive when REM sleep begins within 15 minutes of sleep onset. The test should always be made in the afternoon (approximately 1300 h) to avoid "false positives" that may occur during morning naps. More commonly, the recording will be "false negative." A common and avoidable cause of a negative recording in a patient with many of the clinical features of narcolepsy is a nap taken shortly before the recording begins. Patients must, therefore, be instructed to remain awake for several hours before the test; when the patient arrives in the laboratory, the technician should be vigilant to prevent premature napping, especially while electrodes are being applied.

This procedure requires few electrode placements, since length of recording (less than 1 hour) is not adequate to evaluate other diagnostic possibilities. Two EEG electrodes are connected to the C4 and O2 positions. Beckman electrodes are connected as closely as possible to the eye placements: right outer canthus (ROC), left outer canthus (LOC), and right supra-orbital ridge (RSO). All of the above electrodes are referred to both mastoids connected together electrically. This is accomplished by referring the electrodes to A1 and A2. This method provides symmetry during monopolar recordings from the right and left eyes so that the antiphase signal seen during lateral eye movements will have equal amplitude. In addition, connecting both reference placements together usually produces lower electrode resistance. Two Beckman electrodes are attached to the chin (mentalis) muscles and are referred to each other ("bipolar"). The amplifier settings are as follows:

Channel 1, C4–A1,A2	Low filters 0.3, Hi filters 60 Hz
Channel 2, O2–A1,A2	Low filters 0.3, Hi filters 60 Hz
Channel 3, ROC–A1,A2	Low filters 0.1, Hi filters 60 Hz
Channel 4, RSO–A1,A2	Low filters 0.1, Hi filters 60 Hz
Channel 5, LOC–A1,A2	Low filters 0.1, Hi filters 90 Hz
Channel 6, Right chin–left chin	Low filters 3.0, Hi filters 90 Hz

Note that in EMG from the chin, emphasis is placed on the higher frequencies. Sensitivity is increased to maximal during EMG recording, and it is important that this setting remain at the highest gain.

The Nocturnal Sleep PSG

It is often observed that patients with complaints of insomnia, as well as narcoleptics, may show apneic episodes or periodic leg movements during the PSG. For this reason a "screening montage" with a minimum 12-channel recording is routine practice at our center. This montage consists of the following:

Channel 1, C4–A1,A2
Channel 2, ROC–A1,A2
Channel 3, RSO–A1,A2
Channel 4, LOC–A1,A2
Channel 5, Left chin–right chin
Channel 6, RAT (right anterior tibial muscle) bipolar
Channel 7, LAT (left anterior tibial muscle) bipolar
Channel 8, RNA (right nasal airflow)
Channel 9, LNA (left nasal airflow)
Channel 10, OA (oral airflow)
Channel 11, TAM (thoracoabdominal movements) pneumogram
Channel 12, ECG (electrocardiogram)

The techniques used to record the EEG, EOG, and chin EMG are the same as used in the nap recording. The other physiologic parameters may be recorded from electrodes and sensors applied in the following way: Beckman electrodes with long leads are attached to the skin overlying both anterior tibial muscles. The epidermis from this region is rather thick, and in order to reduce the electrical resistance, the skin may be rubbed slightly with fine sandpaper or a tiny scratch may be made with a sterile needle. The electrodes should be placed about 3 to 4 cm apart and fixed to the legs with adhesive collars, reinforced with pieces of adhesive tape. The long leads are passed under the pajamas, taped to the sides of the thighs, and then passed under the shirt to emerge at the shirt collar. Polygraph settings for right and left anterior tibial muscles (RAT and LAT) are the same as the chin EMG settings. Right nasal airflow (RNA), left nasal airflow (LNA), and oral airflow (OA) are recorded with thermistors or thermocouples. RNA and LNA sensors are placed just into the right and left nostrils, and the OA sensor is attached vertically to the chin just in front of the mouth. These sensors are held firmly in place with strips of thermotape. The leads are led up the sides of the face to converge at the top of the head along with the EOG, EMG, EEG, and reference electrodes. They are taped in a bunch close to the head. The combined leads are then taped together at intervals to form a cable. All leads should be labeled at the pin ends. If thermistors are used with a bridge circuit, the μV/mm-mV/cm switch should be set on the mV/cm range. Thermocouples are usually set on the μV/mm range. The time-constants for both should be set at "Low" ½ A frequency 0.1 Hz, "Hi" ½ A frequency 60 Hz. The individual gain control setting will depend upon the amplitude of the specific signal being recorded.

The ECG recording taken during sleep is derived from one channel. One electrode is placed under the center of the left breast, equivalent to the V4 exploring position. This electrode is referred to another placed just to the right of the sternum in the second intercostal space. Although this ECG arrangement is limited, most cardiac arrhythmias and other abnormalities can be demonstrated. These potentials are recorded with an AC amplifier. The μV/mm-mV/cm switch is set at mV/cm. The filters are set at "Low" 0.1 Hz, "Hi" 60 Hz. The amplitude of the QRS complex should be adjusted for a deflection of approximately 1 cm.

Other Recording Protocols

The recording arrays used for patients with nocturnal seizures, enuresis, and periodic movements are described in the specific illustrations.

REFERENCES

Aschoff, J. (1976). Circadian systems in man and their implications. Hosp. Pract., *11:*51.

Broughton, R. J. (1968). Sleep disorders: disorders of arousal. Science, *159:*1070.

Burack, B., Pollak, C., Borowiecki, B., and Weitzman, E. D. (1977). The hypersomnia-sleep apnea syndrome (HSA): A reversible major cardiovascular hazard. (Abstract). American Heart Association, Miami Beach, Florida.

Coleman, R. M., Pollak, C. P., and Weitzman, E. D. (1978). Periodic nocturnal myoclonus occurs in a wide variety of sleep-wake disorders. Trans. Am. Neurol. Assoc., *103:*23.

Dement, W. C. (1976). Daytime sleepiness and sleep "attacks." In: Narcolepsy, Guilleminault, C., Dement, W. C. and Passouant, P., Eds., p. 17, Spectrum, New York.

Guilleminault, C., and Dement, W. C., Eds. (1978). Sleep Apnea Syndromes, Alan R. Liss, New York.

Guilleminault, C., Dement, W. C., Passouant, P., Eds. (1976a). Narcolepsy, Spectrum, New York.

Guilleminault, C., Tilkian, A., and Dement, W. C. (1976b). The sleep apnea syndromes. Ann. Rev. Med., *27:*465.

Hauri, P. (1977). The Sleep Disorders. Current Concepts, Upjohn, Michigan.

Kales, A. and Kales, J. D. (1974b). Sleep disorders. Recent findings in the diagnosis and treatment of disturbed sleep. N. Engl. J. Med., *290:*487.

Kales, A., Bixler, E. O., Tan, T. L., Scharf, M. B., and Kales, J. D. (1974a). Chronic hypnotic-drug use. Ineffectiveness, drug-withdrawal insomnia, and dependence. J.A.M.A., *227:*513.

Kessler, S. (1976). Genetic Factors in Narcolepsy. In: Narcolepsy, Guilleminault, C., Dement, W. C., and Passouant, P., Eds., p. 285, Spectrum, New York.

Kokkoris, C. P., Weitzman, E. D., Pollak, C. P., Spielman, A. J., Czeisler, C. A., and Bradlow, H. (1979). Long term ambulatory temperature monitoring in a subject with a hypernychthemeral sleep-wake cycle disturbance. Sleep, *1:*177.

Kuhlo, W., Doll, E., and Franc, M. (1969). Exfolgreich behandlung eines Pickwick syndrome durch eine dauertracheal kanule. Dtsch. Med. Wochenschr., *94:*1286.

McGregor, P. A., Weitzman, E. D., and Pollak, C. P. (1978). Polysomnographic recording techniques used for the diagnosis of sleep disorders in a sleep disorders center. Am. J. EEG Technol., *18:*107.

Mitler, M. M. (1976). Toward an Animal Model of Narcolepsy-Cataplexy. In: Narcolepsy, Guilleminault, C., Dement, W. C., and Passouant, P., Eds., p. 387, Spectrum, New York.

Montplaisir, J. (1976). Disturbed Nocturnal Sleep. In: Narcolepsy, Guilleminault, C., Dement, W. C., and Passouant, P., Eds., p. 43, Spectrum, New York.

Pollak, C. P., Kahn, E., Borowiecki, B., and Weitzman, E. D. (1978). The effect of tracheostomy on sleep and apneas in patients with hypersomnia-sleep apnea syndrome. (Abstract). APSS, Eighteenth Annual Meeting, Palo Alto, Calif.

Rechtschaffen, A. and Kales, A. (1968). A Manual of Standardized Serminology, Techniques and Scoring System for Sleep Stages of Human Subjects, Government Printing Office, Washington, D. C.

Tilkian, A., Guilleminault, C., Schroeder, J., Lehrman, K., Simmons, F. B., and Dement, W. C. (1975). Sleep-induced apnea syndrome: reversal of serious arrhythmias after tracheostomy. Circulation, *52:* Suppl. 11, 131.

Weitzman, E. D., Czeisler, C. A., and Moore Ede, M. (1978b). Sleep-wake, neuroendocrine and body temperature circadian rhythms under entrained and non-entrained (free running) conditions in man. NAITO International Symposium on Biorhythm and its central mechanism, Tokyo, Japan, Elsevier North-Holland. In press.
Weitzman, E. D., Pollak, C. P., Borowiecki, B. Burack, B., Shprintzen, R., and Rakoff, S. (1978a). The hypersomnia-sleep apnea syndrome: site and mechanism of upper airway obstruction. In: Sleep Apnea Syndromes, Guilleminault, C. and Dement, W. C., Eds. Alan R. Liss, New York.

17

Electrophysiologic Evaluation of Brain Death: A Critical Appraisal

GIAN EMILIO CHATRIAN

INTRODUCTION

Traditionally, death has been defined in medicine as the permanent cessation of heart beat and respiration. Whenever the loss of these functions is not promptly reversed by appropriate resuscitative measures, profound and irreversible pathologic alterations occur in the brain within minutes under normothermic conditions. During the last quarter of a century, the increasing effectiveness of resuscitative techniques and life-support systems made it possible to restore and artificially maintain cardiovascular and respiratory functions in countless individuals. However, it soon became apparent that the extreme vulnerability of the brain to anoxia, which exceeded that of other systems of the body, was a major limiting factor in assuring the favorable outcome of resuscitation. In patients who had suffered sufficiently prolonged cardiorespiratory arrest, the restoration and maintenance of pulmonary, cardiac, and other functions was not accompanied by recovery of conscious adaptive behavior and of those higher faculties that represented the very essence of human life. Tragic cases of individuals who harbored dead brains in technically living bodies became common observation in intensive care units throughout the world.

In France, Mollaret and Goulon (1959) and Mollaret, Bertrand, and Mollaret, (1959) coined the term "coma dépassé" (a "state beyond coma") to describe a condition in which even autonomic control was lost and that was believed to be associated with destruction of the brain. In the United States, Adams and Jequier (1969) proposed the term "brain death syndrome" to designate these states.

The study of these conditions demonstrated that when brain functions were completely and permanently abolished, the preservation of other organs was inconsequential, that is, the death of the brain was equivalent to death of the person. Moreover, it was recognized that the futile use of extraordinary measures to support certain body functions in individuals with dead brains demanded unreasonable expenditure of human and financial resources, unnecessarily prolonged the sorrow and grief of relatives and friends, and was contrary to the individual's "right to die with dignity." Some religious authorities saw fit to speak on these issues. In an address to an International Congress of Anesthesiologists, Pope Pius XII (1958) stated that "human life continues for as long as its vital functions, distinguished from the simple life of the organs, manifest themselves without the help of artificial processes." He further indicated that "It is incumbent on the physician to take all reasonable, ordinary means of restoring the spontaneous vital functions and consciousness, and to employ such extraordinary means as are available to him to this end. It is not obligatory, however, to continue to use extraordinary means indefinitely in hopeless cases."

The advent of transplant surgery provided a major impetus to redefining death of the individual as death of the brain, since its success depended on the use of viable organs removed from patients with permanently abolished brain function before their circulation failed (Hamburger and Crosnier, 1968). The concept of brain death won the support of numerous medical organizations including the Twenty-Second World Medical Assembly ("Declaration of Sydney," Gilder, 1968), the American Neurological Association (Plum and Masland, 1973), the American Medical Association (1974), and the American Bar Association (1975). In the United States, this notion has won statutory recognition in many states (Saunders, 1975; Walker, 1977b; Black, 1978). The legal status of brain death in other countries has been summarized by Walker (1977b).

Acceptance of the notion of brain death made it necessary to formulate operational criteria for diagnosing this condition in individuals with artificially sustained cardiac and/or respiratory functions. The definition of these standards was intended to help physicians identify the circumstances under which continuation of extraordinary supportive measures was both unnecessary and inadvisable, as well as to protect patients against premature termination of these efforts. This task was undertaken by individual neurologists, electroencephalographers, neurosurgeons, and other medical and surgical specialists, as well as by medical organizations throughout the world. With rare exceptions (Mohandas and Chou, 1971; Conference of Royal Colleges and Faculties of the United Kingdom, 1976) most criteria for determining brain death consisted of combinations of clinical and laboratory findings, with the latter generally represented by results of EEG recordings and/or studies of cerebral circulation. Readers interested in the evolution of these standards may find it profitable to consult the bibliography on brain death by Smith and Penry (1972) and the comprehensive book by Walker (1977b).

GUIDELINES FOR ESTABLISHING BRAIN DEATH

One of the milestones in the development of guidelines for determining brain death in the United States was the definition by an Ad Hoc Committee of the "Harvard Criteria" of "irreversible coma," a term used synonymously with brain death (Beecher, 1968). These standards required that the following criteria be met:

1. Unreceptivity and unresponsivity. "There is total unawareness to externally applied stimuli and inner need and complete unresponsiveness. . ." "Even the most intensely painful stimuli evoke no vocal or other response. . ."
2. No movements or breathing. "Observation covering a period of at least one hour by physicians is adequate to satisfy the criteria of no spontaneous muscular movements or spontaneous respiration or response to stimuli . . ." ". . . the total absence of spontaneous breathing may be established by turning off the respirator for three minutes and observing whether there is any effort on the part of the subject to breathe spontaneously." This requires that the carbon dioxide tension be normal before the trial with the patient breathing room air for at least 10 minutes before the test.
3. No reflexes. "The pupil will be fixed and dilated and will not respond to a direct source of bright light." "Ocular movements (to head turning and to irrigation of the ears with ice water) and blinking are absent . . ." "There is no evidence of postural activity (decerebrate or other). Swallowing, yawning, vocalization are in abeyance. Corneal and pharyngeal reflexes are absent." "As a rule the stretch or tendon reflexes cannot be elicited . . ."
4. Flat electroencephalogram. "Of great confirmatory value is the flat or isoelectric EEG." (Technical guidelines include: the requirement that instrumental sensitivities of 10, 5 and 2.5 μV/mm be used during the recording, the suggestion that maximal sensitivities be employed for a brief period of 5-100 seconds, and the recommendation that the ECG and environmental noise be monitored, the latter by means of electrodes over the dorsum of one hand).

"At least ten full minutes of recording are desirable, but twice that would be better."

"All of the above tests shall be repeated at least 24 hours later with no change."

"The validity of such data as indications of irreversible cerebral damage depends on the exclusion of two conditions: hypothermia (temperature below 90°F. [32.2°C.]) or central nervous system depressants, such as barbiturates."

Practical clinical application of the Harvard criteria revealed the need for revisions and modifications. This prompted the National Institute of Neurological Diseases and Stroke (NINDS) to promote a prospective collaborative investigation of brain death which was jointly conducted by nine medical centers in the United States between 1971 and 1973. Criteria for admission of patients to the American Collaborative Study included: cerebral unresponsivity (deep coma) and apnea. The former was characterized as "a state in which the patient did not respond purposively to externally applied stimuli, obeyed no commands, and did not phonate spontaneously or in response to a painful stimulus." The latter was defined as "the absence of spontaneous respiration, manifested by the need for controlled ventilation . . . for at least 15 minutes" (Walker, 1977a). These admission criteria were sufficiently broad to include all individuals in danger of imminent death, yet restrictive enough to exclude as many patients with reversible brain damage as possible (Walker, 1977b). A final report on this study has not yet been released. However, a summary statement of this research (Walker, 1977a) indicated that:

> Based on the findings in a collaborative study of 503 comatose and apneic patients, the establishment of cerebral death requires (1) that all appropriate examinations and therapeutic procedures have been performed, (2) that cerebral unresponsivity, apnea, dilated pupils, absent cephalic reflexes and electrocerebral silence be present for 30 minutes at least six hours after the ictus, and (3) that if one of these standards is met imprecisely or cannot be tested, a confirmatory test be made to demonstrate the absence of cerebral blood flow. This would allow the diagnosis of a dead brain to be made in patients with small amounts of sedative drugs in the blood, in patients undergoing therapeutic procedures that make examination of one or more of the cranial nerves impossible, and in patients otherwise meeting the criteria whose pupils are small.

The application of these standards to the data base of the Collaborative Study "identified patients, all of whom died within a week with evidence of a dead brain."

Even before the publication of the summary statement of the Collaborative Study, awareness of the results of this investigation prompted the Inter-Agency Committee on Irreversible Coma and Brain Death and the American Neurological Association to promulgate guidelines designed to assist the physician in determining that the brain is dead.

The standards of the Inter-Agency Committee or IAC (Masland, 1975) state that:

> . . . for the patient who following appropriate diagnostic and therapeutic procedures remains apneic and unresponsive with circulation maintained, the following conditions provide assurance that the brain is dead:
>
> 1) Cerebral unresponsivity
> 2) Apnea
> 3) Absent cephalic reflexes, including:
>   a) pupillary
>   b) corneal
>   c) audio-ocular
>   d) oculocephalic

4) Dilated pupil (> 5.0 mm). In the event that the pupil is less than 5.0 mm, the possibility of a toxic factor is heightened, and blood drug levels and/or studies of the cerebral circulation may be required to eliminate this possibility.

5) Electrocerebral silence. The EEG criteria must be observed for a minimum recording period of 30 minutes at a time when the clinical criteria have persisted for at least 6 hours. These criteria should be reexamined and confirmed on a second occasion at least 6 hours later. (These criteria may be inapplicable for children under 5 years of age, since there are indications that the immature nervous system can survive significant periods of electrocerebral silence).

6) Arrest of cerebral circulation. In any instance where there is a possibility of drug effect, or any question regarding the true nature of the intracranial process, the condition of brain death may be verified by cerebral perfusion studies demonstrating complete cessation of intracranial circulation.

The guidelines of the American Neurological Association or ANA (1976) are said to:

. . . apply to the person who remains apneic and unresponsive in spite of appropriate diagnostic and therapeutic procedures, including those directed toward remediation of hypothermia and/or circulatory collapse.

Under these circumstances, the following conditions provide assurance that the brain is dead:

A. Cerebral unresponsivity
B. Apnea
C. Absent cephalic reflexes, including:
   1. Pupillary
   2. Corneal
   3. Audio-ocular
   4. Oculocephalic
D. Electrocerebral silence. The EEG criteria must be observed for a minimum recording period of 30 minutes, carried out in accordance with the techniques currently specified by the American EEG Society * and carried out at a time when the clinical criteria have persisted for at least 6 hours.

All these criteria should be reexamined and confirmed on a second occasion, at least 6 hours later. (These criteria may be inapplicable for children under 5 years of age, since there are indications that the immature nervous system can survive significant periods of electrocerebral silence.)

In any instance where there is a possibility of drug effect, or any question regarding the true nature of the intracranial process, the existence of brain death may be verified by persistence of the above described conditions for a period exceeding 48 hours.

The standards of the IAC and of the ANA differ from the earlier Harvard Criteria (Beecher, 1968) in several respects. First, they prescribe an interval of 6 hours after the onset of coma and apnea and the lack of evidence of car-

---

* cf. American Electroencephalographic Society (1976)

diovascular shock as prerequisites for the determination of brain death. This is intended to provide adequate time for all appropriate diagnostic and therapeutic measures to be completed and for the cardiovascular system to stabilize. Second, they exclude from the criteria of brain death the loss of spinal reflexes. The state of these responses in patients with suspected brain death depends upon the persistence or regression of spinal shock, a phenomenon not directly relevant to the determination of permanent loss of brain function (Ivan, 1973; Jørgensen, 1973; Walker, 1977a and b). Third, they require the indicators of brain death to be present for a period shorter than the 24 hours prescribed by the Harvard Criteria, except in certain specified instances. Fourth, the ANA mandates more stringent technical conditions for EEG recording than were originally prescribed by the Harvard Committee.

Disagreements exist among the criteria of brain death formulated by the American Collaborative Study, the IAC, and the ANA with regard to the following requirements:

1. the demonstration of dilated pupils which is included among the criteria of brain death by the Collaborative Study and the IAC but not the ANA

2. the confirmation of EEG or clinical and EEG criteria of brain death on a second occasion at least 6 hours later which is advocated by the IAC and the ANA, respectively, but not by the Collaborative Study

3. the verification of the diagnosis of brain death by cerebral perfusion studies in all questionable cases. This is suggested by the Collaborative Study and the IAC whereas the ANA recommends in the same circumstances verification of the specified clinical and EEG criteria for a period exceeding 48 hours.

Dilated pupils have been shown not to be essential to the diagnosis of brain death (Schwartz and Vendrely, 1969; Paillas, 1970; Sims and Bickford, 1973; Jørgensen, 1973; Walker, 1977a and b; Arfel, 1976). However, the finding of constricted pupils is of special diagnostic interest because it is common among individuals suffering from intoxications with CNS depressants, except those produced by glutethimide (Doriden) and scopolamine (Walker, 1977a and b).

Medical organizations and individual investigators throughout the world disagree on whether or not EEG or clinical and EEG criteria of brain death should be routinely confirmed on a separate occasion. The evidence reviewed in this chapter suggests that when these standards of brain death are unambiguously fulfilled at least 6 hours after onset of coma and apnea, and certain sources of error are ruled out beyond suspicion, their verification after an interval of at least 6 hours is likely to be redundant (cf. p. 540). In these circumstances, repetition of some or all examinations after an additional interval of at least 6 hours may prolong agonizing uncertainty for families and friends, further burden hospital staffs, and cause loss of potential organ donors succumbing to circulatory arrest (Walker, 1977b). It should be added that very few medical centers in the United States have a team of physicians and EEG and other technologists with expertise in brain death determination available on short notice around the clock. Hence, in practice, in most hospitals the time elapsed between the onset of apneic coma and the first application of clinical and EEG criteria of brain death probably is as long as 12 to 24 hours, if not longer. The duration of this interval offers additional margin for error.

Whenever ambiguity exists on the diagnosis of brain death, verification of clinical and EEG findings and additional investigations such as cerebral perfusion studies are indicated. Wertheimer, Jouvet, and Descotes (1959) first reported that "coma dépassé" was accompanied by arrest of cerebral circulation. This finding led them to postulate that total cerebral infarction was the pathologic substrate of brain death. Subsequent authors confirmed that a high correlation existed between clinical and EEG criteria of permanent failure of brain function and arrest of cerebral circulation by angiography (Vlahovitch et al, 1971, 1972; Greitz et al, 1973; Jørgensen, Jørgensen, and Rosenklint, 1973; Rosenklint and Jørgensen, 1974). Thus, especially in Europe, some guidelines have included the angiographic proof of arrest of cerebral circulation among the cardinal criteria of brain death (Ingvar and Widén, 1972). In the United States, contrast cerebral angiography has not encountered much favor for routine use in brain death suspects, chiefly because of fears that prolonged contact of high density contrast materials with cerebral blood vessels may have toxic effects on the brains of patients with slowed cerebral circulation and severe neurologic deficits (Walker, 1977b). However, in recent years, the advent of intravenous radioisotope angiography (Maynard, Prior, and Scott, 1969) has provided safe alternatives to contrast angiography in patients with suspected brain death (Goodman, Mishkin, and Dyken, 1969; Arfel et al, 1972; Ouaknine et al, 1973). Especially promising is the relatively simple and innocuous bedside radioisotopic "bolus" technique described by Braunstein et al (1972, 1973) and Korein et al (1975, 1977). This method studies the time/activity curves of the initial passage through the cerebral circulation of an intravenously injected radioisotopic bolus. The absence of a "bolus tracing" through the head (Fig. 17.1) is indicative of a cerebral circulatory deficit which correlates highly with clinical, EEG, and neuropathologic findings of cerebral death.

Recognition of the existence of a variety of methods for determining brain death prompted Walker (1977b) to formulate a more flexible approach to the diagnosis of this condition than was recommended by earlier guidelines. This was summarized in an "algorithm for cerebral death" (Table 17.1) which suggested various courses of action that might be taken for establishing this diagnosis depending on the facilities and skills available in each hospital and the nature of the primary condition.

Standards of brain death continuously evolve under the influence of new clinical observations and with the advent of new technologies. Thus, no guidelines should be looked upon as final, immutable rules such as are alien to the practice of medicine. In keeping with this concept, this review will not confine itself to an inquiry into the contribution of traditional scalp EEGs to the diagnosis of brain death, but also will attempt to evaluate the potential of other, including new, electrophysiologic methods for assessing brain viability in humans.

Table 17.1. ALGORITHM FOR CEREBRAL DEATH

The patient, normothermic and normotensive *, must be comatose, apneic, and without cephalic reflexes

and

The case must meet the conditions specified in A, B, or C.

A.

1. This state must be present for at least 3 days

or

B.

1. The primary condition must be known to be an irreparable lesion of the brain
2. The patient, by appropriate examinations, must be shown to have for at least 30 minutes:

   (a) electrocerebral silence in the EEG

   or

   (b) absence of cerebral blood flow **

   or

   (c) no cerebral metabolism ***

   or

C.

1. The primary condition, not a known irreparable lesion of the brain, has not responded to appropriate treatment
2. The patient's EEG must be isoelectric for 2 days

   or

   at least 6 hours after the ictus, the EEG must be isoelectric for 30 minutes and either there must be no evidence of cerebral blood flow, or no cerebral metabolism for 30 minutes.

* The rectal temperature should be above 90°F (32°C) and the systolic blood pressure should be above 80 mm Hg, for hypothermia and hypopiesia may so depress cerebral activity that areflexia and ECS result; if these vital functions cannot be restored to a normal level, cerebral death may be declared on the basis of the other criteria and the absence of cerebral blood flow for 30 minutes.

** This may be determined by quantitative measurements of CSF, four vessel angiography, isotopic angiography, bolus passage of isotopes intravenously injected, or demonstration of the absence of a midline echo.

*** A $CMRO_2$ level below 1 ml/gm/min, or an $AVDO_2$ of less than 2 vols percent, or a lactic acid level greater than 6 mEq/l.

From Walker, A. E., 1977. Cerebral Death. Professional Information Library, Dallas.

Abbreviations: ECS—electrocerebral silence; CSF—cerebrospinal fluid; $CMRO_2$—cerebral metabolic rate of O_2; $AVDO_2$—arteriovenous difference of O_2 content across the brain.

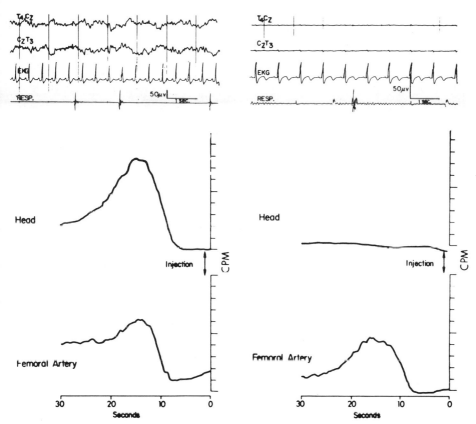

Fig. 17.1. *From top to bottom: EEGs, EKG, respiration monitor, and time/ activity curves of initial passage through the intracranial circulation and one femoral artery of an intravenously injected bolus of 99m TC 04 in two comatose, apneic individuals. In one patient (left) EEG activity is recorded, although abnormal, and a "head bolus" curve is present suggesting persistence of cerebral blood flow. In the other individual (right), the scalp record is electrocerebrally inactive and a "head bolus" is absent indicating abolition of cerebral blood flow. Normal control femoral curve is obtained in both individuals (from Korein, J., Braunstein, P., Kricheff, I., Lieberman, A., and Chase, N. 1975. Radioisotopic bolus technique as a test to detect circulatory deficit associated with cerebral death. Circulation, 51, 924, by permission of the American Heart Association, Inc.).*

EEG IN DETERMINATION OF BRAIN DEATH

Demonstration of Electrocerebral Inactivity

Brain death implies "total and permanent abolition of brain function" (Walker, 1977b). To the extent that the EEG is an indicator of brain and, more specifically, cerebral cortical function, it seemed natural that it be called upon to provide objective proof of failure of this function. Fischgold and Mathis (1959) were the first to report that scalp records of patients in coma grade IV ("coma dépassé") showed absence of demonstrable EEG potentials, a finding they termed "cerebral silence." Subsequent studies confirmed that brain death was characterized by an enduring state of electrocortical inactivity (Jouvet, 1959; Arfel and Fischgold, 1961; Hockaday et al, 1965; Muller, 1966; Scharfetter and Schmoigl, 1967; Spann, Kugler, and Liebhardt, 1967; Pampiglione and Harden, 1968; Rosoff and Schwab, 1968). Scalp records demonstrating this finding were variously referred to as "flat," a term employed earlier in a different context by Jasper, Fitzpatrick, and Solomon (1939); "nul" (Arfel et al, 1963); "isoelectric" (Scharfetter and Schmoigl, 1967); "equipotential" (Pampiglione and Harden, 1968); and tracings of "electrocerebral silence" (Silverman et al, 1969). Following earlier formulations of Silverman et al (1969), the American Electroencephalographic Society (1976) defined "electrocerebral silence" as "no electrocerebral activity over 2 μV when recording from scalp or referential electrode pairs 10 or more cm apart with interelectrode resistances under 10,000 ohms (or impedances under 6,000 ohms), but over 100 ohms." This somewhat awkward definition could be construed to imply that a scalp record which demonstrated electrocerebral activity having an amplitude of 2 μV or less indicated electrocerebral silence. Presumably, its authors intended to state that, because international regulations required that modern electroencephalographs have noise levels mostly no greater than 2 μV (Barlow et al, 1974), only cerebral activity exceeding 2 μV in amplitude was potentially discernible from instrumental noise. Because the demonstration of electrocerebral activity of any amplitude and in any amount is manifestly incompatible with the notion of "electrocerebral silence," the Terminology Committee of the International Federation of Societies for Electroencephalography and Clinical Neurophysiology (Chatrian et al, 1974) suggested that "electrocerebral inactivity" denoted "the absence over all regions of the head of identifiable electrical activity of cerebral origin, whether spontaneous or induced by physiological stimuli and pharmacological agents." The term "electrocerebral inactivity" (ECI) is preferred in this review to its equivalent "electrocerebral silence" (ECS).

Techniques for demonstrating ECI in brain death suspects have been refined through the years under the influence of improvements in EEG instrumentation, advances in EEG technology, and experience with the use of the EEG in assessing brain viability. The "Minimum Technical Standards for EEG Recording in Suspected Cerebral Death" of the American Electroencephalographic Society (1976) represents the current "state of the art" in this field, and the standards are widely accepted throughout the United States. These guidelines require that the following minimal conditions be fulfilled for determining ECI:

1. use of a minimum of eight scalp electrodes and two ear lobe reference electrodes
2. measurement of electrode impedances under 10,000 but over 100 ohms
3. performance of certain tests of integrity of the entire recording system
4. recording from electrode pairs having interelectrode distances of at least 10 cm

5. use of instrumental sensitivities of at least 2 μV per mm during most of the recording and inclusion of appropriate calibrations
6. use of time constants of 0.3 to 0.4 seconds during part of the procedure
7. monitoring of artifacts originating in the surroundings or produced by the patients, especially the electrocardiogram, and elimination of electromyographic (EMG) artifacts by administration of neuromuscular blocking agents
8. performance of tests of EEG reactivity to intense noxious, auditory and, whenever possible, photic stimuli
9. recording time of at least 30 minutes
10. performance of the record by a qualified technologist experienced in recording EEGs in intensive care units and working under the supervision of a qualified electroencephalographer
11. repetition of the whole test after an interval, such as 6 hours, whenever electrocerebral inactivity is doubtful
12. abstention from using telephone transmission of the EEG.

These guidelines of the American Electroencephalographic Society include detailed explanations for each individual recommendation and a warning that the significance of electrocerebral inactivity in infants and small children is not clearly established.

It is imperative that scalp records demonstrating complete absence of electrocerebral activity (Fig. 17.2) be distinguished from:

1. records displaying bursts of EEG potentials separated by periods of apparent inactivity lasting from a few seconds to as long as 10 to 15 minutes (Fig. 17.3). This pattern of "suppression bursts" or "periodic silences" is frequently observed in intoxications with CNS depressants (Wulff, 1950; Mellerio, 1964; Mantz et al, 1965, 1971; Kubicki, Rieger, and Bharckow, 1970; Haider, Matthew, and Oswald, 1971) as well as in other encephalopathies such as those due to anoxia (Pampiglione, 1962; Hockaday et al, 1965; Pampiglione and Harden, 1968; Prior and Volavka, 1968; Binnie et al, 1970; Lemmi, Hubbert, and Faris, 1973; Prior, 1973; Brenner, Schwartzman, and Richey, 1975). In some extreme cases, isolated waves with long intervening periods of low voltage activity are detected (Fig. 17.4A).

2. EEGs consisting primarily of delta waves of relatively low voltage, such as are seen in certain severe diffuse encephalopathies with widespread cortical damage

3. records showing no detectable electrocerebral activity over limited areas of the heads, and

4. "low voltage" EEGs displaying "activity of amplitude not greater than 20 μV over all head regions" (Chatrian et al, 1974), such as are found in a proportion of normal subjects (Chatrian, 1976).

Technical and Interpretive Aspects

To obtain records in the intensive care unit that satisfy or exceed the minimal requirement of the American Electroencephalographic Society (1976) is a

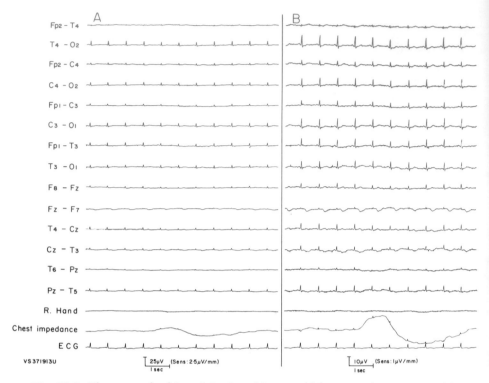

Fig. 17.2. *Electrocerebral inactivity in a 23-year-old hypertensive woman with intracerebral hemorrhage. Patient was deeply comatose and had absent spontaneous respiration, no cephalic reflexes, and dilated pupils.*

task which often seriously challenges the competence, experience, ingenuity, and determination of the EEG technologist. Major difficulties and conflicting pressures are generated by : (1) the existence of multiple and ever-changing electrically operated life supporting devices connected to the patient, (2) the periodic performance of therapeutic maneuvers by nurses and other paramedical personnel, (3) the need to identify beyond doubt and to eliminate or reduce and monitor all possible sources of artifact, and (4) the desire to conclude the procedure within a reasonable time. This last goal must be achieved to permit other examinations and expedite the final diagnosis anxiously awaited by relatives, physicians in charge, and transplant teams.

Artifacts, i.e., electrical potentials due to extracerebral sources, frequently contaminate EEG records taken in intensive care units (Mowrey, 1962; Montoya and Hill, 1968; Grass, 1969; Redding, Wandel, and Nasser, 1969; Trojaborg, 1970; Saunders, 1972; Sims et al, 1973; Westmoreland et al, 1975). These spurious potentials are especially troublesome in the particular recording conditions intended to establish brain death. Bennett et al (1976) reported that in the American Collaborative Study 22.3 percent of all records required special efforts to identify and eliminate artifacts, although only 5.2 percent were con-

sidered technically unsatisfactory because artifactual contamination significantly interfered with the interpretation. These artifacts, described in detail and
richly illustrated in these authors' atlas, included:

1. electrical potentials generated by instrumentations close to or connected
   to the patient such as ECG monitors, cardiac pacemakers, and dialysis
   units, and
2. biopotentials of extracerebral origin generated by the patient, including
   those of muscular, respiratory, and cardiovascular origin.

Electromyographic (EMG) potentials may make it difficult to rule out the
presence of electrocerebral activity in scalp records of brain death suspects.
However, it is possible to eliminate them in patients receiving respiratory support by administering neuromuscular blocking agents such as succinylcholine
(Mosier, 1968; Wood-Smith, Stewart, and Vickers, 1968; Vourc'h, 1973; Suter,
1974; Suter and Brush, 1978) or pancuronium bromide (Speight and Avery,
1972).

Delivery of a bolus of air to the patient through flexible tubes generates

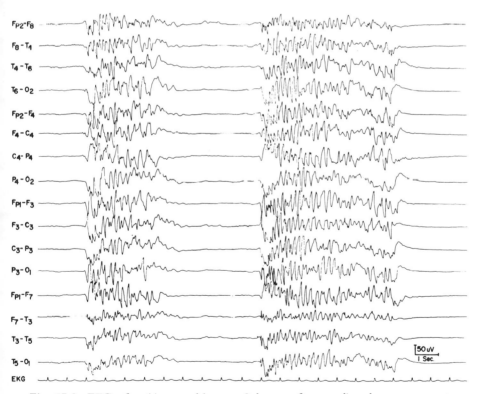

*Fig. 17.3. EEG of a 44-year-old man, 9 hours after cardiopulmonary arrest.
Patient was comatose, artificially ventilated, and was under the influence of
pancuronium bromide to suppress bilateral myoclonus.*

vibrations of these tubes and/or head movements that may cause the appearance in some or all scalp derivation of large potentials resembling periodic paroxysmal discharges or rhythmic activity at various frequencies. Monitoring these mechanical artifacts with appropriate transducers is often desirable to distinguish them from EEG potentials. On occasion, it may even be necessary to briefly stop the respirator to assess questionable activity (Bennett et al, 1976).

The most frequent and disturbing of all patient-generated artifacts appearing in scalp records of brain death suspects is the electrocardiogram (ECG or EKG) (Fig. 17.2). Its prominence in these conditions is said to be related to factors including: (1) the extremely high instrumental sensitivities employed, (2) the tendency for some montages used to assess brain viability to differentially enhance certain ECG components (Berger et al, 1974), (3) the disproportionately large amplitude of some ECG components due to myocardial infarction or ischemia (Walker, 1977b), and (4) the existence of active feedback in many intensive care unit ECG monitors operated simultaneously with the EEG apparatus (Berger et al, 1974). Moreover, because the electrical fields generated

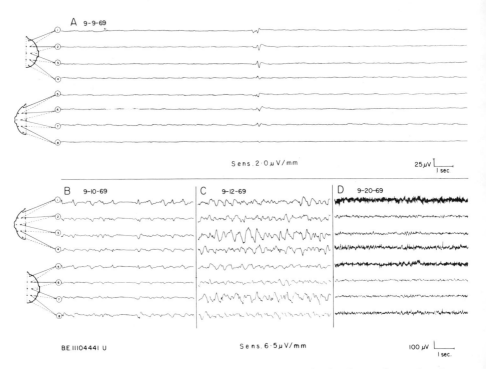

Fig. 17.4. *EEGs of a 30-year-old woman with secobarbital overdose. On the second day of hospitalization (A), she was deeply comatose and had absent spontaneous respiration, no cephalic reflexes, constricted pupils, and a blood barbiturate level of 36 mg/100 ml. On the following day (B), she was clinically unchanged. Four days after admission (C), she withdrew to noxious stimuli and her pupils reacted to light. Eight days later (D), she was alert and responded appropriately to commands.*

at the surface of the scalp are different for each component of the ECG (Walker, 1977b), the amount of ECG artifact varies considerably from one montage to the other, and within a given montage from one derivation to the next. Referential montages utilizing an ear reference frequently display an amount of ECG contamination incompatible with proper assessment of electrocerebral inactivity. By contrast, this artifact tends to be less forbidding in bipolar montages even when using long interelectrode distances (Fig. 17.2). Bennett et al (1976) pointed out that, in certain circumstances, the ECG potentials detected in scalp records of brain death suspects resemble sharp-and-slow wave complexes characterizing some epileptic disorders or "triphasic waves" associated with certain systemic metabolic derangements. In other instances, the ECG generates in scalp records quasi-sinusoidal rhythms at twice or three times the frequency of the cardiac rhythm. Irregularities of this rhythm such as premature ventricular contractions and more severe arrhythmias, such as ventricular tachycardia, may produce potentials which appear on the scalp as sharp transients and theta or delta rhythms, respectively. Moreover, rhythms of faster (mostly alpha) frequency occasionally are produced in scalp records by mechanical vibrations of the head associated with the cardiac cycle (ballistocardiogram).

Disconnecting existing ECG monitors, repositioning the patient's head, and selecting montages less prone to ECG pickup may reduce, but generally do not eliminate, the ECG artifact. Thus, having attempted these and other maneuvers, the technologist generally can do little but acknowledge the presence of this artifact and endeavor to provide a proof of its origin by monitoring on the electroencephalograph an ECG lead simultaneously with the scalp activity (Fig. 17.2). The subsequent interpretation of the record requires that the ECG and related potentials be visually subtracted from the activity displayed by each individual channel to determine whether or not any ECG-unrelated activity is present. This is not always an easy task. Bickford et al (1971) attempted to assess the extent to which electroencephalographers can recognize by visual estimates the last remnants of EEG activity in the presence of ECG artifact. By means of tape recording techniques, measured amounts of ECG were mixed with EEG activity recorded on comatose subjects prior to brain death. Visual analysis of these "synthetic" records were said to indicate that "fully trained electroencephalographers are unable to recognize reliably EEG slow wave activity that is less than 25 percent of the amplitude of the EKG (measured by the R-wave) appearing in the record." The authors felt that the difficulty of recognizing EEG in the presence of ECG was attributable mainly to 2 to 5 Hz activity generated by the S-T segment of the ECG, although the spike-like appearance of the R-wave contributed to "hide low voltage EEG components." These synthetic tracings may not have exactly reproduced the features of records obtained on brain death suspects. However, a survey of 40 "isoelectric" EEG records taken on patients with "irreversible coma" suggested that ECG contamination was "sufficient in approximately 30 percent of cases to mask significant EEG activity (above an assumed noise level of 2 microvolts)." It would seem logical to argue that records in which "significant EEG activity" could be identified, by definition were not "isoelectric." However, the authors deserve credit for emphasizing the importance of the problems posed by ECG contamination of scalp records of individuals whose brain viability is in question.

Because of difficulties in assessing the EEGs of brain death suspects, one may wonder about the degree of reliability of interpretation of these records rendered by different electroencephalographers. In the American Collaborative Study it was estimated that, had all records been reviewed by senior EEG consultants, the disagreement between them and the interpreters in the individual participating centers probably would have been limited to about 3 percent of cases (Walker, 1977b). However, it should be pointed out that only a small minority of technologists and physicians throughout the country are adequately trained in recording and interpreting EEGs, especially in the difficult environment of the intensive care unit and in the demanding circumstances of suspected brain death. Thus, to what extent the Collaborative Study can be regarded as representative of the standards of practice prevailing outside a few major, selected medical centers remains to be determined.

Limitations and Validity

To inquire into the validity of the concept that ECI indicates permanent failure of brain function, it appears essential to review the information available on: (1) the conditions that might produce temporary, reversible ECI, (2) the reports of recovery of EEG activity in individuals not suffering from these conditions, and (3) the relationships between ECI and clinical outcome.

Conditions Causing Temporary Electrocerebral Inactivity. Temporary, reversible ECI is said to occur in the following conditions:

1. overdoses with CNS depressants
2. hypothermia
3. cardiovascular shock

Patients rendered comatose by massive overdoses of CNS depressants frequently display in their EEGs a pattern of "suppression bursts" (cf. p. 535 and Fig. 17.4A). In rare instances, records said to demonstrate absence of electrocerebral activity for periods up to 24 hours or longer have been reported (Bird and Plum, 1968; Haider and Oswald, 1970; Jørgensen, 1970; Kirschbaum and Carollo, 1970; Mantz et al, 1971; Bennett et al, 1976). Because of the use of relatively low instrumental sensitivities, the records described in most of these studies probably were not electrocerebrally inactive by present standards. However, the occurrence of ECI in drug overdoses has been confirmed by the inquiry of the American EEG Society (Silverman et al, 1969) and by the American Collaborative Study (Bennett et al, 1976; Walker, 1977a and b) among others. Drugs most commonly producing loss of electrocerebral activity were said to include barbiturates, methaqualone, diazepam, mecloqualone, meprobamate, and trichloroethylene (Powner, 1976). Both ECI and the more common suppression burst pattern detected in these conditions generally are associated with clinical signs of profound depression of brain function with the possible exception of pupillary dilatation (Walker, 1977a and b). The possibility that clinical and EEG criteria of brain death may be met or may be closely approximated in these drug intoxications prompted Walker (1977b) to suggest that whenever the pupils of brain death suspects were small and/or blood assays for drugs were not available, the determination of brain death required not only the fulfillment of other clinical and EEG criteria of failure of brain function but also the demonstration of absent cerebral circulation or metabolism. In the American Collaborative Study, although drug assays were available in all centers, their usefulness was found to be unexpectedly limited by factors including: occasional omissions to obtain them, excessive time required for the reports to become available, variability between the barbiturate levels determined by local and central laboratories, and the frequent finding that these levels were no higher than those regarded as therapeutic for epilepsy. Potentiation of the effects of barbiturates by other drugs and local or systemic conditions that modify the blood-brain barrier were regarded as possibly responsible for the poor correlation between clinical states and barbiturate blood levels. Because of this, the presence of even small amounts of CNS depressants in the blood was felt to be a sign of possible drug toxicity requiring prompt treatment (Walker and Molinari, 1977; Walker, 1977b). By analogy, it seems appropriate to recommend that caution be exercised in interpreting as indicative of brain death the finding of ECI in comatose patients whose blood demonstrates even small amounts of CNS depressants.

Hypothermia has been shown to produce transient and reversible ECI (Arfel and Weiss, 1962). Thus, a rectal temperature above 32.2°C (90°F) has been regarded as a prerequisite for reliably determining brain death with the aid of the EEG. It should be noted that in the collaborative investigation reported by Walker (1977b), only 12 of 503 patients were hypothermic, and most of them could be warmed by external heat to temperatures within the normal range.

Of some interest is the report of a case of profound depression, without complete abolition, of EEG activity by hyperthermia (rectal temperature of 42.5°C or 104°F) in the course of a febrile episode. This finding led the authors to the conclusion, unwarranted by their data, that "in hyperthermia, as well as in hypothermia, an isoelectric EEG may not indicate irreversible brain damage" (Cabral et al, 1977).

EEG activity (and clinical signs of brain function) may be abolished by cardiovascular shock with consequent low cerebral perfusion pressure, and may be restored when blood pressure is raised above shock levels. Hence, Walker (1977b) included a systolic blood pressure above 80 mm Hg as a prerequisite to the application of criteria of brain death. However, the same author pointed out that the importance of cardiovascular shock should not be overestimated because in intensive care units patients are ordinarily treated with intravenous volume expanders and vasopressor drugs. Moreover, in the Collaborative Study, only about 25 percent of patients required the administration of vasopressor agents (Walker, 1977b). The prescribed interval of at least 6 hours between the onset of coma and apnea and the application of criteria of brain death (Masland, 1975; American Neurological Association, 1976; Walker, 1977a and b) is generally felt to be adequate to permit stabilization of the cardiovascular system.

The belief is sometimes expressed in the literature that various endogenous intoxications may contribute to the generation of ECI (Masland, 1975). The identification of such potentially treatable disorders, especially those due to dysfunction of the liver, kidney, and pancreas, is one of the goals of the diagnostic procedures that must be performed before the condition of brain death is established. However, to our knowledge, the exact role of these factors in determining ECI has not been investigated in detail.

It is frequently stated that ECI may not have the same ominous significance in children below the age of 5 years that it has in older individuals (Masland, 1975; American Electroencephalographic Society, 1976; American Neurological Association, 1976; Walker, 1977b). However, the information on the significance of ECI in comatose infants and children is scarce. Harden (1969) reported results on 60 infants, 1 day to 6 months of age, who were resuscitated after cardiocirculatory arrest. She found that the interpretation of the EEG findings in these patients was complicated by a variety of factors including the frequent existence of congenital anomalies, and the occurrence of severe systemic metabolic derangements and repeated cardiocirculatory disturbances. The combined effects of these conditions, and of transient cerebral ischemia and anoxia, generated a greater variety of EEG patterns than was seen after cardiocirculatory arrest in older individuals. However, the analysis of 2,180 EEGs recorded over a period of 20 years on 363 children resuscitated after an ischemic/anoxic episode recently enabled Pampiglione, Chaloner, and Harden (1978) to state that there was "little difficulty in predicting that cerebral functions were irreparably lost when electrocerebral silence persisted for 6–12 hours in repeated records."

Reported Recovery of EEG from Electrocerebral Inactivity of Other Causes. Reports have been published of recovery of EEG activity in individuals who did not suffer from conditions known to produce temporary, reversible ECI yet displayed at a given time "flat," "nul," "isoelectric," or other EEGs interpreted as electrocerebrally inactive. The patients described in these studies had suffered: cardiorespiratory arrest (Lundervold, 1954; Tentler et al, 1957; Kurtz et al, 1966; Levin and Kinnel, 1966; Riehl and McIntyre, 1968; Jørgensen, 1971; Green and Lauber, 1972; Bennett et al, 1976—cases V-9 and V-10; Hughes, Boshes, and Leestma, 1976); cerebral embolism (Fischgold and Mathis, 1959); encephalitis (Bental and Leibowitz, 1961; Houtteville et al, 1970); head injury (Bricolo et al, 1971) and severe hyperthermia (Cabral et al, 1977). On close scrutiny, none of these cases represents a fully acceptable example of ECI. In some instances, inspection of the illustrations reveals manifest or probable low voltage EEG activity. In other cases, the criteria for ECI were either unspecified or inadequate to determine that EEG activity was absent by present standards (American Electroencephalographic Society, 1976). This inadequacy generally was related to the use of low instrumental sensitivites and, occasion-ally, to insufficient recording time, topographically limited recordings or dis-turbing artifacts. In two instances, effects of CNS depressants (Levin and Kinnel, 1966), or a combination of these effects with those of hypothermia and hypotension (Tentler et al, 1957), may have played a role in the manifestation of extreme EEG depression. It should be added that in several of these cases, even clinical criteria of brain death were not or were inadequately specified, or were not or were incompletely fulfilled at the time EEG activity was said to be absent.

Because, in this reviewer's opinion, loss of electrocerebral potentials was not established beyond doubt in any of the cases reported so far, the sub-sequent demonstration of EEG activity in these individuals cannot be con-strued as credible evidence of recovery from electrocerebral inactivity. It would seem reasonable to conclude that whenever ECI is unambiguously dem-onstrated (American Electroencephalographic Society, 1976), subsequent re-covery of EEG activity is extremely unlikely, if at all possible, in individuals who are not under the effect of CNS depressants and are not suffering from hypothermia or extreme hypotension. However, it should be pointed out that this belief is primarily based on records taken several hours after the onset of coma and apnea as is the case in the vast majority of clinical situations. Adequate information is not available on the EEG changes immediately follow-ing catastrophic cerebral insults in unanesthetized humans. This is an addi-tional reason for acquiring that EEG (as other) criteria of brain death not be applied until at least 6 hours after the onset of coma and apnea (Masland, 1975; American Neurological Association, 1976; Walker, 1977a and b).

Electrocerebral Inactivity and Clinical Outcome. Several investigations have inquired into the relationships between ECI and clinical outcome. The largest survey was conducted by the American EEG Society's Ad Hoc Committee on EEG Criteria for the Determination of Cerebral Death (Silverman et al, 1969). Of 2,650 comatose patients with EEGs regarded as "isoelectric" by 279 elec-troencephalographers, 23 were believed to have survived. The Committee re-viewed 14 of these cases in which additional information could be obtained and determined that in 5 instances the report of survival was erroneous, and in 6 cases the EEGs were not truly isoelectric but only of low voltage. The remain-ing 3 patients who had recovered after displaying apparently true "isoelectric" EEGs had suffered intoxication with CNS depressants. These results suggested that "the EEG of electrocerebral silence, properly recorded, together with a neurological picture of totally unresponsive coma, usually absent reflexes and always absent spontaneous respiration, is strong presumptive evidence of total brain death, except in the situation of central nervous system depressant drugs and the theoretical one of hibernation." This concept received support from several other investigations including those of Kimura, Gerber, and McCor-mick (1968), Korein and Maccario (1971), Ingvar and Widén (1972), Prior (1973), Jørgensen (1974), and the American Collaborative Study. In this last research, only 2 of 187 individuals with ECI in their first records lived, and both suffered from drug overdoses (Walker, 1977b).

It should be emphasized that the notion that all nonintoxicated patients with ECI ultimately expired has little meaning unless the circumstances of death are specified. Because standards of clinical practice cannot be subverted for purposes of investigation, in most recent clinical series, brain death suspects with electrocerebral inactivity who ultimately succumbed included individuals who died of spontaneous "cardiac death" while receiving artificial ventilation as well as patients whose respiratory support was deliberately terminated once they met clinical and EEG criteria of permanent loss of brain function. The latter demises can hardly be adduced as proofs of the validity of those same criteria of brain death the application of which played a decisive role in their occurrence. Yet, the frequently quoted survey of Silverman et al (1969) did not clarify this crucial point.

In the American Collaborative Study, of 185 patients with ECI in their initial EEGs, 110 succumbed of cardiac and 75 of brain death (Walker, 1977b). However, no information was given on the deaths of those individuals who developed ECI in subsequent records.

In spite of some ambiguities, the findings analyzed so far in this review indicate that the unequivocal demonstration of electrocerebral inactivity in adults whose brain viability is in question several hours after the onset of coma and apnea, denotes cessation of cerebral cortical function. It should be emphasized that absent electrocerebral activity per se does not imply loss of function of the whole brain or even of the whole cerebrum. However, this finding is customarily associated with clinical signs of deep coma, apnea, and cephalic areflexia. The combination of these EEG and clinical deficits attests to a global failure of brain function. In the presence of CNS depressant drugs, deep hypothermia, or profound hypotension, this functional failure must be regarded as potentially reversible, whereas when these conditions can be excluded, it is highly likely to be permanent, and to indicate brain death. Although infrequently, total failure of cortical function, as indicated by electrocerebral inactivity, may be associated with some degree of preservation of brainstem function. In other instances, brainstem function may be lost while electrocortical activity is variously preserved. These eventualities are discussed on page 548 of this review in the section which deals with persistent vegetative and de-efferented states.

Neuropathology and EEG Changes

Early work by Bertrand et al (1959) and Mollaret et al (1959) suggested that marked edema, extensive softening, and necrosis, particularly in the gray matter, and severe neuronal alterations without inflammatory reaction or vascular thrombosis characterized the brains of individuals who had been in "coma dépassé." However, subsequent publications revealed a far greater diversity of findings in individuals with brain death. These were described in detail by several investigators including Walker, Diamond, and Moseley (1975), Walker (1977b), and Black (1978).

In the American Collaborative Study, complex relationships were found between neuropathologic and EEG alterations in individuals who expired after a period of apneic coma. Patients with electrocerebrally inactive records had a significantly higher incidence of swollen brains, cerebral herniations, and "respirator brains" (Kimura et al, 1968; Walker et al, 1975), than did individuals with preservation of EEG activity. Persons with records classified as equivocal displayed pathologic changes intermediate between these two groups (Walker et al, 1975; Walker, 1977b). Although ECI did not correlate well with the specific nature of the pathology, there appeared to be a trend for the EEG to be more commonly abolished in cases with hemorrhage, edema, and necrosis than with other types of lesions (Walker et al, 1975; Walker, 1977b). A poor correlation existed between ECI and distribution of primary pathology, in that the proportion of patients with brainstem lesions who had ECI (63 percent) was approximately the same as that of individuals with diffuse cerebral (60 percent) or focal cortical (62 percent) alterations.

Although in general the finding of ECI in the last scalp record correlated highly with the pathologic demonstration of a respirator brain, discrepancies between electrical and pathologic findings were observed in the Collaborative Study. For instance, some of the patients with ECI who died less than 24 hours after the onset of coma and apnea had brains displaying minimal or no pathologic alterations. This finding was in keeping with observations indicating that 12 to 36 hours, but usually 24 hours, must elapse after the onset of coma and apnea for the changes of the respirator brain to develop (Schneider, Masshoff, and Neuhaus, 1969; Lindenberg, 1972; Matakas, Cervos-Navarro, and Schneider, 1973; Nedey et al, 1974; Walker et al, 1975; Hughes et al, 1976). Contrariwise, a respirator brain was found at times in patients with some preservation of EEG activity in their last record. The significance of this last finding was difficult to assess. Especially when days or hours had elapsed between the last EEG recording and death, the possibility existed that, had an EEG been obtained closer to the patient's demise, ECI may have been demonstrated. Of additional interest was the persistence of at least some EEG activity in patients whose brains showed only patchy swelling, edema, infarction, and necrosis classified as "partial respirator brains" (Walker et al, 1975; Walker, 1977b).

The likelihood of occurrence of ECI appears to be related to certain postulated pathogenetic mechanisms. Thus, a group of cerebrally dead patients who had suffered cerebral trauma with consequent major increase in intracranial pressure, arrest of cerebral circulation, and rapid and severe ischemia, revealed a higher proportion of records of ECI than did a group of individuals who had suffered cardiac arrest with consequent inadequate perfusion of the intracranial contents (Walker et al, 1975; Walker, 1977b).

Prognostic Significance of EEG Activity in Comatose, Apneic Individuals

In a proportion of comatose, apneic patients, scalp records disclose unambiguous EEG activity. This finding was evident in the initial records of 241 of 503 patients admitted to the American Collaborative Study (Bennett et al, 1976; Walker, 1977b). The EEGs of these individuals displayed a variety of patterns,

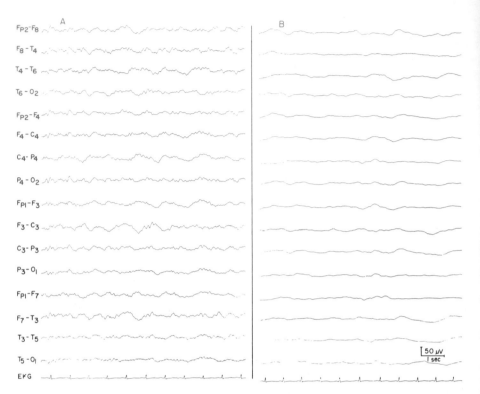

Fig. 17.5. *EEG of a 26-year-old individual following an episode of ventricular fibrillation sustained during strenuous exercise. On admission (A), patient was comatose but had spontaneous respiration and preserved corneal and oculocephalic reflexes. Ten days later (B), he required artificial ventilation and his corneal reflexes could no longer be elicited.*

including: slow waves of delta and theta frequency, bilateral, unilateral or focal, and continuous or intermittent (Fig. 17.5); beta potentials frequently intermixed with slow waves; triphasic waves; suppression bursts (Figs. 17.3 and 17.4A) and other periodic patterns (Fig. 17.6); epileptiform discharges (Fig. 17.6) and electrical seizures; low voltages over limited areas of the scalp; and even rhythms of alpha frequency (Fig. 17.7) and patterns of sleep. The demonstration of any type of EEG activity in comatose, apneic patients had a less ominous prognostic significance than did the finding of ECI. In fact, 42 of 241 patients (17.4 percent) with EEG activity in their initial records survived, whereas only 2 of 187 individuals with ECI (1.07 percent), both suffering from drug overdoses, lived. However, no individual pattern of activity observed in the initial EEG of brain death suspects proved predictive of the likelihood of occurrence of ECI in subsequent examinations or of the clinical outcome (Bennett et al, 1976; Hughes et al, 1976; Walker, 1977b; Suter and Brush, 1978). By contrast, other authors including Pampiglione (1962), Hockaday et al (1965), Pampiglione and Harden (1968), Binnie et al (1970), Kurtz et al (1970), Prior

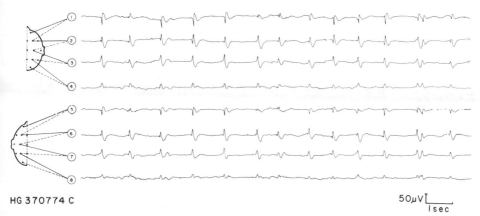

HG 370774 C   50μV└─────┘
                                                              I sec

Fig. 17.6. *EEG of a 37-year-old man, 2 days after cardiopulmonary arrest due to food aspiration. Patient was deeply comatose, artificially ventilated, and was under the influence of pancuronium bromide to control bilateral myoclonus. Pseudoperiodic epileptiform discharges were temporally unrelated to ECG (not shown here).*

(1973), Brenner et al (1975) and Pampiglione et al (1978) found the EEG helpful in establishing prognosis in patients resuscitated after cardiac or respiratory arrest. Of special interest is the admirable work of Prior (1973), which indicated that accurate prognostic information could be derived from the EEGs of comatose patients, provided that the abnormalities were carefully and consistently graded, and analyzed by sensitive statistical techniques. In Prior's experience, visual rating of EEGs using a 5-point scale enabled outcome to be predicted in approximately 80 percent of patients. Computer-aided discriminant function

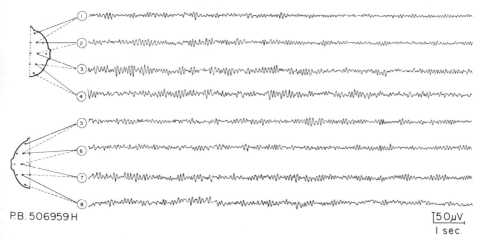

P.B. 506959 H   ⌈50μV
                                                           I sec.

Fig. 17.7. *EEG of a 29-year-old man, 3 days after cardiopulmonary arrest due to accidental strangulation. Patient was comatose, decerebrate, with small, reactive pupils and spontaneous hyperventilation. Note widespread EEG activity of alpha frequency. Patient survived 5 days (from Vignaendra, V., Wilkus, R. J., Copass, M. K., and Chatrian, G. E. 1974. Neurology, 24, 582).*

analyses of large numbers of visually assessed variables further increased the accuracy of prognostication. Only in patients with drug overdoses, brain damage sparing the cerebral cortex, or mild damage compatible with survival were discriminant scores erroneous or equivocal. To what extent these methods can be employed to predict the outcome of brain death suspects within hours of the precipitating event remains to be determined. However, until these elegant techniques have been applied on a sufficiently large series of cases, it seems premature to conclude that the EEG has no predictive value in the investigation of individuals whose brain viability is in doubt. It should be added that the demonstration of a normal or minimally altered EEG is of decisive importance in the rare instances in which the clinical signs of brain death may be simulated by pharmacologic effects such as succinylcholine sensitivity (Prior, 1973; Tyson, 1974).

Persistent Vegetative and De-efferented States

Among the conditions that deserve mention in this review are those described by Jennett and Plum (1972) as "persistent vegetative states," a term characterizing certain patients who survive devastating brain damage due to head injury, cardiopulmonary arrest, or other pathologic conditions. Most commonly, these individuals lie for variable periods of time with their eyes open, have roving eye movements, and blink spontaneously or to threat, whereas at other times their eyes are closed and they appear asleep. These patients generally display extensor and/or flexor postures (Fig. 17.8). Noxious and, occasionally, other stimuli may produce eye opening, grimacing, teeth grinding, and primitive postural or reflex responses. Although grunting or groaning occasionally occurs with stimulation, these individuals do not speak or otherwise communicate with the environment. Sucking, chewing, and swallowing movements are frequent. Control of respiration, heart rate, blood pressure, and body temperature is preserved and these functions are frequently modified by stimulation. The observation of these unfortunate individuals suggests that they are capable of "wakefulness without awareness" (Jennett and Plum, 1972) and are deprived of any form of mental functioning. During the last three decades, numerous terms have been employed in the literature to describe variations of these persistent vegetative states. These include the following: "apallic syndrome" (Kretschmer, 1940), "akinetic mutism" (Cairns et al, 1941), "anoetic symptom complex" (Duensing, 1949), "prolonged unconsciousness" (French, 1952), "coma vigil" or vigilant coma (Alajouanine, 1957), "severe post-traumatic dementia" (Strich, 1956), "post-comatose hypertonic stupor" (Fischgold and Mathis, 1959), "vegetative life" (Arnaud, Vigouroux, and Vigouroux, 1963), "prolonged post-traumatic coma" (Bricolo, 1976), "vegetative survival" (Vapalahti and Troupp, 1971), and "irreversible coma" (Walker, 1977a and b). It should be noted that the use of the term "irreversible coma" to designate these conditions differs from that of Beecher (1968) who employed it to describe brain death.

Pathologic alterations characterizing persistent vegetative states frequently consist of multiple lesions of the cerebral cortex, subcortical structures of the cerebral hemispheres, and brainstem. However, severe degenerative changes of the white matter of the cerebral hemispheres have been found to be most characteristic of cases secondary to head injury (Strich, 1956, 1969). Anoxic alterations predominating in the cerebral cortex have been reported in rare cases of "neocortical death" following cardiopulmonary arrest (Brierley et al, 1971) whereas in other infrequent instances the primary lesions selectively involved the mesencephalic and rostral pontine tegmentum (Ingvar et al, 1964; Ingvar and Sourander, 1970).

In a few cases, scalp records of individuals whose comatose conditions later evolved into persistent vegetative states or who were in such a state at the time of recording were said to be "flat," "isoelectric," or otherwise electrocerebrally inactive (Lundervold, 1954; Gerstenbrand, 1967; Brierley et al, 1971; Ingvar and Brun, 1972; Bricolo et al, 1969, 1971; Crow and Winter, 1969; Bennett et al, 1971, 1976—cases V-9 and V-10; Ingvar, 1971). It is possible that some if not all records so described actually demonstrated EEG activity of very low voltage (Bricolo, 1976) rather than ECI as currently defined (American Electroencephalographic Society, 1976). Moreover, subsequent tracings on the same individuals as well as records of other patients who were in a persistent vegetative state or were recovering from such a condition demonstrated a wide

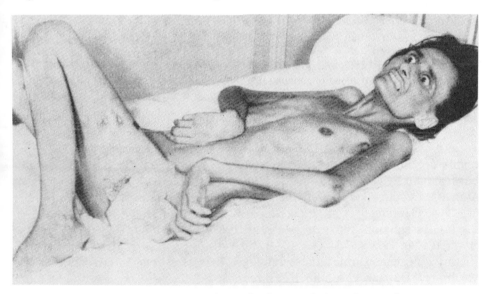

Fig. 17.8. *32-year-old woman with cerebral air embolism due to abortive maneuvers. Her comatose condition had evolved into a "hypertonic decerebrate stupor" during which she did not communicate with the environment and did not give any evidence of mental functioning. Patient died after 4 months (from Fischgold, H. and Mathis, P. 1959. Electroencephalogr. Clin. Neurophysiol., Supplement 11. Masson, Paris).*

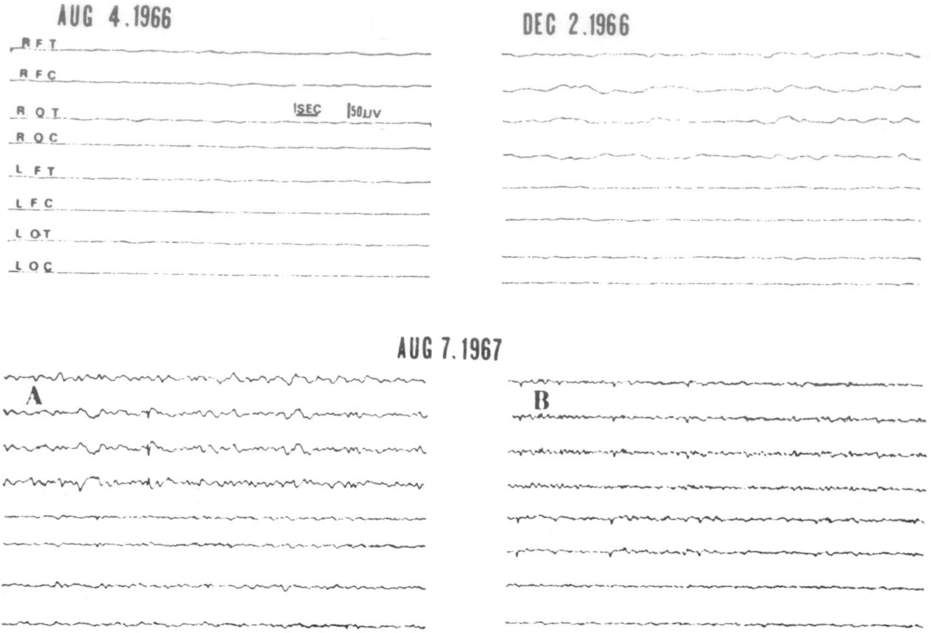

Fig. 17.9. *EEGs of a 17-year-old woman who developed "bulbar syndrome" following severe head injury. This evolved into complete, "apallic syndrome" with "severe postural disturbances and manifestations of primitive motor patterns." "Persistently 'flat' but not 'silent'" EEGs were initially obtained (top). Fully developed apallic syndrome was associated with more prominent EEG activity (bottom) and behavioral signs of sleep (A) and wakefulness (B). Patient survived 5 years without improvement (from Bricolo, A. 1976. In: Handbook of Clinical Neurology, Volume 24, Vinken, P. J. and Bruyn, G. W., Eds. American Elsevier, New York, p. 699).*

variety of EEG activities, ranging from barely discernible delta potentials to highly organized waking and sleep patterns (Lundervold, 1954; Cravioto, Silberman, and Feigin, 1960; Jouvet, Pellin, and Mounier, 1961; Ingvar et al, 1964; Mansuy, Lecuire, and Jouvet, 1965; Ingvar and Sourander, 1970; Vigouroux et al, 1964; Gentilomo et al, 1966; Lepetit et al, 1966; Dolce and Kaemmerer, 1967; Gerstenbrand, 1967; Bricolo et al, 1968a and b, 1969, 1971; Ingvar, 1971; Bennett et al, 1971, 1976—cases V-9 and V-10; Bricolo, 1976; Beresford, 1977). Figure 17.9 demonstrates these findings. It is of special interest that in the celebrated Quinlan case the EEG recorded "during wakefulness" demonstrated "only mild, diffuse slowing" (Beresford, 1977).

Studies of Gentilomo et al (1966), Dolce and Kaemmerer (1967), Rosadini and Gentilomo (1967), Bricolo et al (1968a and b), Bergamasco et al (1968a and b), and Bricolo (1976) have alluded to the finding that although most patients with persistent vegetative states succumb, often after periods of hospitalization lasting months or years, a few survive, generally with various neurologic sequelae. These authors have suggested that the progressive restoration of organized sleep EEG patterns and nocturnal sleep cycles in patients with post-traumatic "apallic syndrome" represents a favorable prognostic sign with respect to survival. However, these studies require around-the-clock polygraphic monitoring. Moreover, there is no definite evidence that the EEG is helpful in prognosticating the "quality" of survival in these individuals—that is, the likelihood of recovery of "cognition" "including speech, comprehension, thought, reasoning, sentience, and the capacity to respond in a purposeful way to external stimuli." In the Quinlan case, a state supreme court authorized withdrawal of artificial ventilation from an individual in a chronic vegetative state with a well-preserved EEG, provided that the attending physicians and an "ethics committee" agreed that there was no reasonable possibility of her regaining cognition and sapience (Beresford, 1977). Unfortunately, there are at present no adequate statistical data on the outcome of persistent vegetative states and no methods for reliably distinguishing between brain-damaged individuals who have totally and irreversibly lost cognition and those who may conceivably regain it. Hence, the possible emergence of the concept that persistently vegetating individuals who are capable of waking behavior, make primitive movements and sounds, grimace or withdraw when stimulated, and display various degrees of preservation of electrocerebral activity may be "legally dead" (Beresford, 1977) is likely to generate passionate controversy among physicians, judicial and religious authorities, and the public.

Persistent vegetative states with abolished mental faculties must be clearly distinguished from "de-efferented states" characterizing individuals whose higher mental functions are preserved but who are tetraplegic and mute, with variable preservation of vertical eye and eyelid movements by which they communicate with the examiner. The interactions of most patients in this condition are limited to opening or closing the eyes, moving the eyes upward or downward on written or, occasionally, spoken command, or blinking once or twice to answer "yes" or "no" (Halsey and Downie, 1966; Plum and Posner, 1966; Kemper and Romanul, 1967; Chase, Moretti, and Prensky, 1968; Shafey et al, 1968; Nordgren et al, 1971; Hawkes and Bryan-Smith, 1974; Markand, 1976). However, occasional patients are capable of more elaborate communication, for instance by blinking according to the Morse code as did the individual described by Feldman (1971).

Most patients suffering from this "locked-in syndrome" have lesions, usually infarcts or hemorrhages, destroying major portions of the basis pontis bilaterally without or with at most unilateral involvement of the pontine tegmentum (Halsey and Downie, 1966; Plum and Posner, 1966; Chase et al, 1968; Bottinelli et al, 1969; Nordgren et al, 1971; Hawkes and Bryan-Smith, 1974; Markand, 1976). The site of pathology in de-efferented states accounts for the use of the term "ventral pontine syndrome" by some to designate them (Shafey et al, 1968). However, bilateral midbrain lesions have been reported to produce a similar state (Karp and Hurtig, 1974). The waking EEGs of these de-efferented individuals generally are normal or minimally altered (Fig. 17.10)

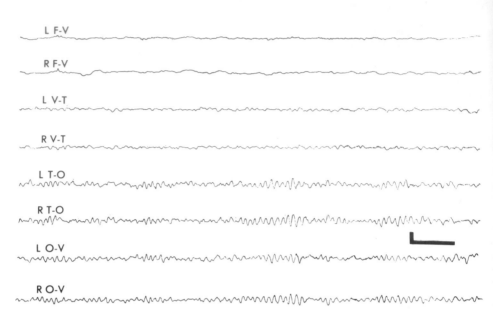

Fig. 17.10. *Waking EEG of a 36-year-old woman with locked-in syndrome due to traumatic occlusion of the basilar artery. Patient was tetraplegic and mute but alert and capable of communicating by eyeblinks and jaw movements. This condition persisted for 2 years. F, frontal; V, vertex; T, temporal; O, occipital; L, left; R, right. Calibrations: 50 μV; 1 second (modified from Feldman M. H. 1971. Neurology, 21, 459).*

and frequently are reactive to eye opening and stroboscopic and other stimuli. Non-REM sleep patterns are usually well-preserved (Fig. 17.11), whereas alterations of REM sleep are demonstrated by polygraphic records (Chase et al, 1968; Bottinelli et al, 1969; Feldman, 1971; Nordgren et al, 1971; Hawkes and Bryan-Smith, 1974; Markand, 1976). As opposed to the locked-in patients, individuals with more extensive lesions producing virtually complete transection of the pons up to its junction with midbrain (Fig. 17.12) generally are unable to communicate with the examiner by eyelid and eye movements. When spontaneous respiration also is abolished, only the demonstration of well-preserved EEG activity permits differentiating these individuals from persons with dead brains. Characteristically, their waking EEGs are normal or slightly abnormal (Fig. 17.13) and may be reactive to passive eye opening and stroboscopic stimulation. Moreover, their non-REM sleep patterns are well-developed as opposed to loss or marked alterations of REM sleep (Loeb and Poggio, 1953; Lundervold, Hauge, and Loken, 1956; Loeb, Rosadini, and Poggio, 1959; Kaada, Harkmark, and Stokke, 1961; Chatrian, White and Shaw, 1964; Chase et al, 1968; Wilkus et al, 1971; Hughes et al, 1972; Ferguson and Bennett, 1974; Freemon, Salinas-Garcia, and Ward, 1974; Obrador et al, 1975). Because failure of effectors mechanisms precludes all responses, it is difficult to determine with certainty whether awareness is preserved or lost in these unfortunate individuals.

SPECIAL METHODS FOR MONITORING AND ANALYZING THE EEGs OF BRAIN DEATH SUSPECTS

Visual analysis of adequate samples of EEG activity simultaneously recorded from multiple regions of the scalp is at present the method of choice for assessing electrophysiologically the viability of the brain. However, the use of special-purpose analog devices and digital computers has been proposed to expand the scope of these recordings, facilitate their analysis, and quantify their results. A special-purpose analog instrument designed with these intents was the "Cerebral Function Monitor" devised by Maynard et al (1969) for continuous single-channel EEG recordings in the intervals between complete EEG examinations. The activity detected by a pair of symmetric parietal electrodes was passed first through a filter designed to reject most waves below 2

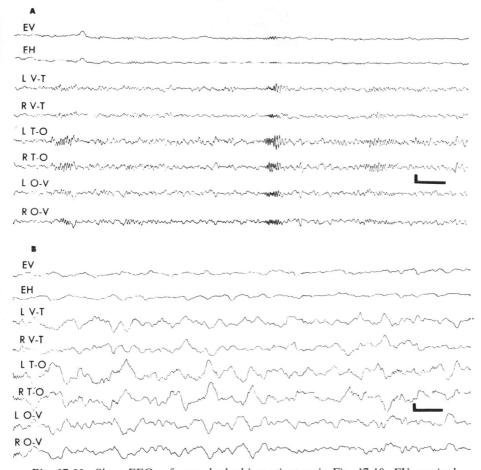

Fig. 17.11. *Sleep EEGs of same locked-in patient as in Fig. 17.10. EV, vertical eye movement leads; EH, horizontal eye movement leads; other symbols and calibration as in Fig. 17.10 (from Feldman, M. H. 1971. Neurology, 21, 459).*

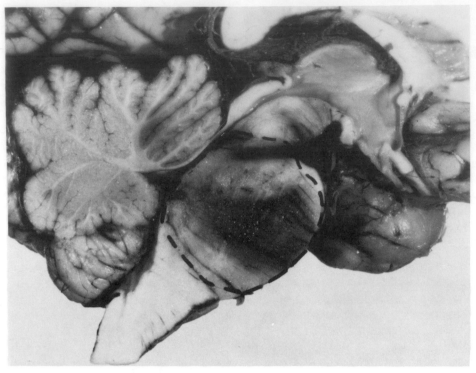

Fig. 17.12. *Sagittal midline section of the brain of a 59-year-old man who was unresponsive and decerebrate following infarct transecting the pons and lowermost portion of the midbrain. Dotted line indicates limits of infarct (from Chatrian, G. E., White, L. E., Jr., and Shaw, Ch-M. 1964. Electroencephalogr. Clin. Neurophysiol., 16, 285).*

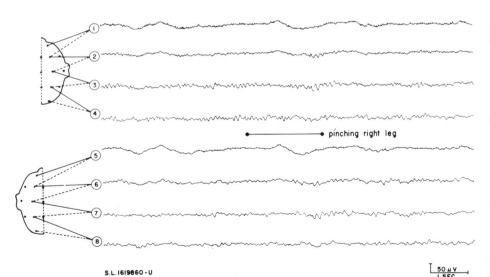

pinching right leg

S.L. 1619860-U

50 µV
1 SEC.

Fig. 17.13 *EEG of same patient as in Fig. 17.12 (modified from Chatrian, G. E., White, L. E., Jr., and Shaw, Ch-M. 1964. Electroencephalogr. Clin. Neurophysiol., 16, 285).*

and above 15 Hz, and then through a semi-logarithmic amplitude compression network. After peak-to-peak rectification, the output of this device was written out at very low speed (50 to 90 mm per hour). The compressed records so obtained gave a measure of the highest and lowest amplitudes of the filtered EEG. A separate network monitored electrode impedance to provide information on the state of conductivity of the electrodes and the occurrence of artifacts of short duration, as well as amplifier blocking or failure. This device proved useful in determining that the electrocerebral silence, once established, persisted for the duration of the study (Fig. 17.14) and for demonstrating increasing or decreasing levels of EEG activity over long periods of time (Fig. 17.15) in comatose patients (Prior et al, 1971; Prior, 1973, 1979).

Bickford et al (1971) described a "Bedside EEG Monitor" of simpler design to continuously monitor the electrical activity detected between the left frontal and the right occipital electrodes. The output of this device, expressed in "microvolts of integrated activity" included instrumental and biologic noises as did that of Maynard's monitor. However, the belief was expressed by the authors that the noise could be assayed at the time of recording, expressed as "microvolts of integrated noise activity" and subtracted from the total activity to yield a measure of actual integrated brain activity in the dimension of microvolts ("Brain Activity Number", BAN). Using this system, patients with dead brains would have a BAN of zero, whereas BANs between 15 and 40 would characterize comatose patients with preservation of cerebral electrical

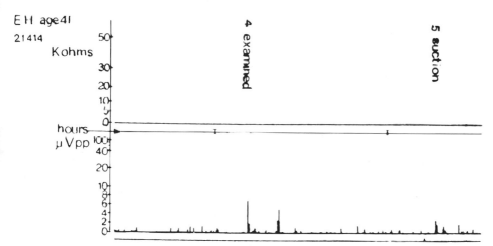

Fig. 17.14. *Impedance (top) and Cerebral Function Monitor (CFM) (bottom) records of a 41-year-old patient with "isoelectric" EEG for 6 days following drug overdose with respiratory arrest. CFM tracing shows "zero level" of cerebral activity (lower margin of tracing) with small peaks (upper margin) due to artifacts, particularly when the patient was manipulated by medical and nursing staff. Time marker indicates hourly intervals. Patient died and was found to have extensive brain damage (from Prior P. F. 1979. Monitoring Cerebral Function. J. B. Lippincott, Philadelphia, previously published in Prior, P. F. 1973. The EEG in Acute Cerebral Anoxia, Excerpta Medica, Amsterdam).*

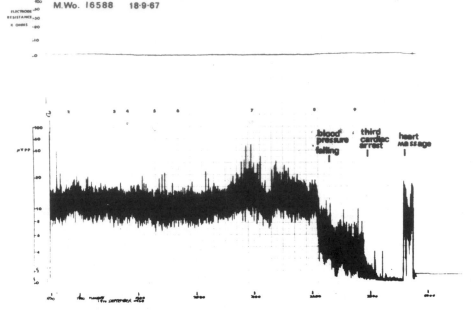

Fig. 17.15. *CFM record from a 73-year-old woman 3 days after successful resuscitation from two cardiac arrests occurring during esophagectomy. Initially, patient was conscious and CFM level was steady at 8 to 15 μV peak-to-peak, until steep fall in level occurred at about 22:00 hours. Blood pressure was found to be falling and cardiac arrest ensued. Resuscitation efforts proved ineffective (from Prior, P. F. 1973. The EEG in acute cerebral anoxia. Excerpta Medica, Amsterdam, and Prior, P. F. 1979. Monitoring Cerebral Function. J. B. Lippincott, Philadelphia. Originally from Maynard, D., Prior, P. F. and Scott, D. F. 1969. Br. Med. J. 4, 545).*

activity. Artifacts introduced by nursing and other procedures would be readily recognizable in the integrated trace and easily identified by appropriate notations. It was not clear how the noise detected in scalp records of brain death suspects was assayed and subtracted from the total activity. However, an analog method for subtracting the ECG artifact from scalp records of brain death suspects was subsequently described in Bickford's laboratory by Berger et al (1974). This technique consisted of obtaining from electrodes placed on various areas of the neck a record displaying an ECG artifact identical to the scalp ECG. This neck ECG was subtracted from the scalp record by mixing the two tracings by means of an operational amplifier. In this reviewer's opinion, searching for an ECG at the neck which closely matches the ECG artifact on the scalp is likely to be a laborious task of questionable practicality. Moreover, the ECG frequently is only one of the artifacts contributing to the total activity recorded from the scalp of brain death suspects.

More recently, Walsh (1974) reported testing successfully a small, portable, commercial device intended to screen patients for "possible or impending electrocerebral silence" by sounding an alarm whenever the amplitude of the electrical activity monitored between a pair of electrodes over each hemisphere fell below 12, 8, or 4 microvolts. The author emphasized that whenever this device indicated the possibility of electrocerebral inactivity, the recording of a complete EEG was mandatory. No information was provided on the design of this instrument. It should be pointed out that, should gross screening methods of this last type be uncritically accepted in intensive care units as substitutes for complete scalp records, their use could result in adverse medical and legal consequences.

The utilization of digital computer techniques in the determination of brain death by EEG recording was pioneered by Rivano et al (1969) and Ferrillo et al (1969). The latter continuously monitored 15 patients with "coma dépassé" from the time their scalp records no longer revealed electrocerebral activity detectable by visual inspection to the time of final cardiac arrest. Autocorrelation and power spectral analysis (Rosadini et al, 1968) of these apparently "silent" tracings demonstrated in 10 patients the presence of rhythmic activity of delta, theta and, in 3 cases, alpha, frequency as long as 48 hours after the cessation of cerebral activity had been first visually recognized (Fig. 17.16). In some instances, visual, auditory, and noxious stimuli produced alterations of

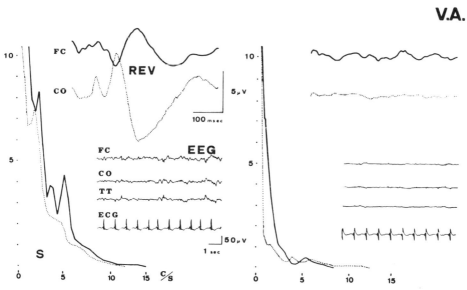

Fig. 17.16. Patient with deeply seated cerebral tumor studied while in deep coma (left-hand section) and in "coma dépassé" (right-hand section). Within each section, top two tracings (REV) depict averaged records from frontocentral (FC) and centro-occipital (CO) areas of scalp, time-locked to flash stimulation. Next three traces are records from frontocentral (FC), centro-occipital (CO), and temporotemporal (TT) regions of the scalp and last tracing is an ECG. Power spectra (S) of EEG records (0 to 15 Hz) are displayed on left-hand side of each section (from Ferrillo, F., Giunta, F., Rivano, C., Rodriquez, G., Rosadini, G., Rossi, G. F., Sannita, W., Siani, C., Turella, G., and Zattoni, J. 1969. Riv. Neurol., 39, 589).

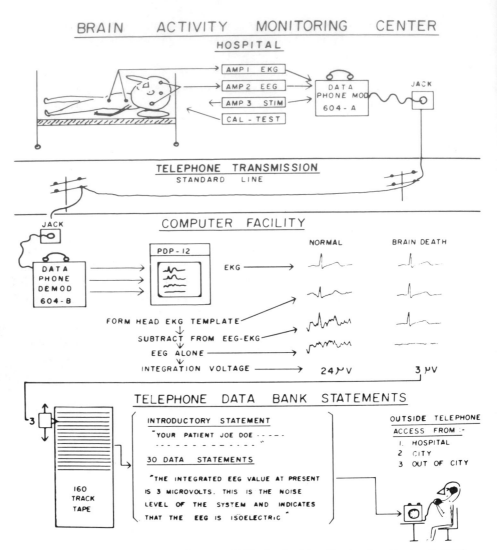

Fig. 17.17. Diagrammatic layout of "Brain Activity Monitoring Center." EKG (ECG) and EEG information are continuously transmitted through a data phone system over a standard telephone line. At the computer facility, a template of the scalp EKG is constructed by averaging the EKG-EEG mixture with the R-wave used as a trigger. This template is then subtracted from the EKG-EEG mixture yielding the EEG alone which is integrated and expressed in microvolts. This process and its results are shown for normal subject (left) and cerebrally dead individual (right). Depending on the results of these computations, the computer moves the tape head to an appropriate track to generate an interpretive verbal statement that can be obtained by accessing the system from an outside telephone (copyrighted by Matthew Bender Company, Inc. and reprinted with permission from Bickford, R. G., Sims, J. K., Billinger, T. W., and Aung, M. H. 1971. Problems in EEG estimation of brain death and use of computer techniques for their solution. Trauma, 12, 61.

the power spectra which displayed increased amplitude of peaks in the delta and theta bands. This evidence of "reactivity" was obtained as long as 30 hours after apparent extinction of EEG activity. These findings were felt to indicate that the apparent absence of electrocerebral activity in visually analyzed scalp records was compatible with some preservation of cerebral function and did not justify the diagnosis of brain death. Close inspection of the figures illustrating this work reveals that the instrumental sensitivities employed were inadequate by today's standards (American Electoencephalographic Society, 1976) to rule out the presence of EEG activity in scalp records. Moreover, it has become increasingly apparent in recent years that activities throughout the EEG band can be generated in recordings of brain death suspects by a variety of extracerebral sources, both instrumental and biologic (cf. p. 536). Hence, it is likely that adventitious potentials including ECG, pulse, and other artifacts were responsible for the activity demonstrated by the authors' computer analyses. Similar results were reported by Zattoni, Fritz, and Giasotto (1971).

An ambitious attempt to use computer techniques for the study of brain death suspects was the design by Bickford et al (1971) of a "Brain Activity Monitoring Center" (Fig. 17.17). This consisted of a central computer facility capable of processing EEG (and ECG) information transmitted to the center via a data phone system utilizing a standard telephone line. Samples of the ECG-contaminated scalp record were averaged using the R-wave of the scalp ECG as a trigger. Because the ECG, but not the EEG, potentials were time-locked to the R-wave, a relatively pure "template" of the ECG component of the scalp record was obtained. This template was subtracted from the primary ECG-contaminated record and the ECG-free remainder was integrated to estimate "brain output." The computer was interfaced with a special multiple-track tape recorder containing interpretive verbal statements for each microvolt interval of integrated brain output. These interpretations were available by telephone to anyone in the hospital, city, or country who had the proper access number. The system was said to have been satisfactorily tested on 10 patients (Bickford et al, 1971). This Brain Activity Monitoring Center represents an imaginative, bold attempt to create "a complete medical diagnostic system combined with a medical information system designed for easy use by the practitioner" in determining brain death (Bickford, 1974). However, its concept does not adequately consider present instrumental limitations and suffers from certain oversimplifications that should not be uncritically accepted. As recently as 1976, the American Electroencephalographic Society and the American Society of Electroencephalographic Technologists jointly inquired into the problems involved in telephone transmission of EEGs and concluded that "at the present time, telephone transmission of EEGs cannot be used for determination of electrocerebral silence in the diagnosis of brain death because of the inherent and unpredictable electrical noise present in telephone networks relative to the very low signal amplitudes in the EEG recording itself, in ECS." The reliability of the ECG subtraction method proposed by Bickford et al (1971) remains to be determined, especially in circumstances such as those of brain death in which the ECG may be severely altered and is subject to abrupt variations (Drory et al, 1975). Moreover, the assumption that the electrical activity remaining after ECG subtraction provides an estimate of "brain output" does not appear justified. In practice, instrumental and biologic artifacts other than those time-locked to the cardiac cycle may represent a significant proportion of the activity recorded from the head of certain brain death suspects. The possible intrusion of these intermittent and unpredictable artifacts mandates that any scalp-detected electrical activity remaining after ECG subtraction be as carefully scrutinized as are the ECG-contaminated primary records. Should this condition be met, it is conceivable that improved ECG subtraction methods could be useful in assessing brain viability in the future. By contrast, it is likely that major imprecision will cloud this assessment should any ECG-purged scalp activity exceeding the instrumental noise level be automatically quantified and unhesitatingly characterized as brain activity. One may further object to the concept of the Brain Activity Monitoring Center that the disadvantages of single-channel scalp records as substitutes for complete EEG examinations are likely to outweigh the advantages of continuous monitoring. The potential ability of computers to successively sample different scalp derivations does not entirely overcome this criticism. Awareness of these limitations accounts for the view prudently held by Prior et al (1971) and Prior (1973, 1979) that topographically limited continuous monitoring should supplement, rather than replace, more comprehensive EEG studies.

Monitoring and quantification of electrocerebral activity over long periods of time should be welcome as a useful, additional tool for the study of patients whose brain viability is in question. However, it is important to realize that indiscriminate quantification of electrical potentials recorded from the scalp of brain death suspects would do little to clarify and much to confound the problem of their cerebral or artifactual origin, which is the primary concern of those charged with the responsibility of assessing their clinical significance.

OTHER ELECTROPHYSIOLOGIC TECHNIQUES FOR DETERMINING BRAIN DEATH

This review has confirmed the notion that scalp recording of the spontaneous EEG is a valuable aid in assessing brain viability in humans. Other electrophysiologic techniques have been proposed to provide additional information when the survival of brain function is in question. These include:

1. cortical and depth recordings
2. measurements of the cortical DC potential and
3. recordings of sensory evoked potentials

Cortical and Depth Recordings

Electrodes applied over the cerebral cortex or implanted within the brain substance have been used in rare instances to record from, and occasionally electrically stimulate the brain of, individuals presumed cerebrally dead (Jouvet, 1959; Carbonell et al, 1963; Ferrillo et al, 1969; Jonkman, 1969; Visser, 1969; Findji et al, 1970; Gaches, 1970; Waltregny, Bonnal, and Le Jeune, 1970; Velasco et al, 1971). On close analysis of these reports, only the studies of Waltregny et al (1970) and Velasco et al (1971) appear to have been conducted with techniques satisfying current EEG criteria for brain death (Fig. 17.18). Both of these studies showed absence of electrical activity at all cortical and subcortical levels explored. The significance of the preservation of some EEG activity in the cerebral cortex and deep brain areas in the cases described by Ferrillo et al (1969), Jonkman (1969), Visser (1969), and Findji et al (1970), is unclear because the available information does not permit the determination of whether or not the scalp records of their patients demonstrated ECI acceptable by contemporary criteria (American Electroencephalographic Society, 1976). In the case reported by Carbonell et al (1963), whether or not electrocerebral activity was absent in scalp records by current standards, cerebral regions above the thalamus failed to display evidence of electrical activity, whereas EEG potentials were detected in and below this structure. However, it should be pointed out that this patient displayed some clinical evidence of preserved brainstem function at variance with current criteria of brain death (cf. p. 527).

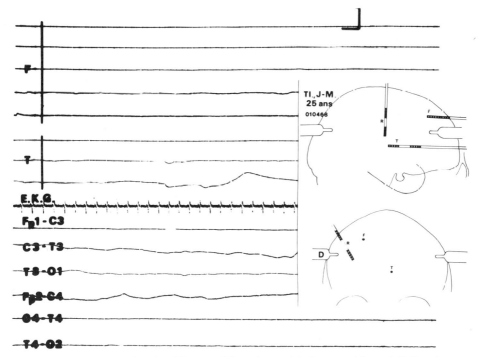

Fig. 17.18. Records of a 25-year-old patient with "coma dépassé." Tracings above the EKG were taken by means of multielectrode probes stereotactically implanted into the depths of the brain. Simultaneous scalp records are depicted below the EKG. Calibrations are 1 sec and 20 µV (from Waltregny, A., Bonnal, J., and LeJeune, G. 1970. Rev. Neurol., 122, 406)

Thus, it appears that studies utilizing cortical and depth electrodes so far have not provided conclusive evidence that patients with unequivocal brain death actually have preserved electrical activity either at cortical or at lower levels. By contrast, well-developed EEG activity was detected in the globus pallidus and the ventralis anterior nucleus of the thalamus of a patient with "apallic syndrome" (cf. p. 548), and EEG changes and behavioral arousal were produced by prolonged electrical stimulations of these same subcortical areas (Hassler et al, 1969). Less conclusive results were obtained by Bennett et al (1976) in another persistently vegetating patient with questionable electrocerebral inactivity in her scalp records.

It has been suggested that depth recording "might be used as confirmatory when a very early statement regarding death is required" (Walker, 1977b). However, we feel that the implantation of electrodes within the brain substance of individuals hovering between life and death carries risks of quantifiable magnitude. Moreover, how much recordings from restricted and often poorly defined areas of the depths of the brain conclusively contribute to the determination of brain death is open to debate. Hence, it seems reasonable to question whether or not, in the usual clinical circumstances, depth recordings are fully justifiable medically, legally, and ethically as a method for assessing brain viability.

Measurement of Cortical DC Potential

The existence of a DC ("steady" or "standing") potential of the cerebral cortex was first described by Caton (1875) in his brief, germinal report on "the electric currents of the brain." Working with rabbits and monkeys, he observed that when two electrodes were applied, one on the external surface of the brain and the other on the surface of a vertical section through it, a current flowed through the connecting galvanometer, the external surface generally being positive relative to the vertical section. Weaker currents of varying direction also were detected when both electrodes were applied on the external surface of the brain or one was placed on that surface and the other on the skull. These "electric currents of grey matter" were altered at the time of death and "fell to near zero after death" (Caton, 1877).

Modern experimental studies have confirmed Caton's findings. Asphyxiation by arrest of artificial ventilation or circulatory arrest was shown to produce a characteristic sequence of DC potential variations culminating in a large negativity that was referred to as "terminal negative shift" or "terminal depolarization." These changes were found to be related to alterations in pO_2, pCO_2, and/or pH, with the terminal negative shift primarily depending on the development of tissue anoxia (Caspers and Speckmann, 1971). Bushart and Rittmeyer (1968, 1969) and Bushart (1969) made similar observations in three patients with suspected brain death and no sign of cerebral activity in their EEGs. A large DC potential in the millivolt range was measured between electrodes placed on the scalp or cortical surface and a cheek reference. In one subject, transient hypoxia produced by arrest of artificial ventilation repeatedly caused a reduction of this potential by as much as 3.7 mV at the cortex, with return to the initial values upon reinstitution of respiration. Reductions of the DC potential greater than 7.2 mV at the cortex and 5.1 mV at the scalp followed the final discontinuation of ventilation. Similar phenomena were observed in the second individual, whereas the third patient demonstrated no changes with either cessation of ventilation or final circulatory collapse. Manaka and Sano (1972) measured the DC potential with two electrodes placed on the vertex and the tip of the nose, respectively, and found it to be 17.7 to 9.6 mV in normal humans. This potential generally fell to zero in patients with brain death, whereas in cases of brain damage due to anoxia, hypoglycemia, or other factors, it decreased by an amount roughly proportional to the degree of damage. These authors expressed the belief that DC measurement from the scalp could help determine brain death or the degree of cerebral damage.

DC recordings require the use of special nonpolarizable electrodes and low-drift DC amplifiers, and pose technical and interpretive difficulties (Gumnit, 1974). Moreover, the detection of a steady potential difference between a scalp and a reference electrode by no means implies that this potential is cerebral in origin. DC voltages obscuring the steady potential of the cerebral cortex can arise from nonbiologic sources, such as the electrodes themselves and the electrode-tissue interfaces. Biologic generators of these potentials may include not only neurons but also glial cells, the blood-brain barrier, and the meninges (O'Leary and Goldring, 1964; Caspers and Speckmann, 1969). The location of the reference electrode relative to extracerebral sources of DC potential is an additional complicating factor (Gumnit, 1974). This reviewer believes that, using available electrodes and techniques, it would be exceedingly difficult to obtain reliable measurements of DC potential from the scalp of brain death suspects in the intensive care unit. Should technically dependable determinations be achieved, it is doubtful that the potentials so measured could be interpreted with confidence as specifically reflecting the DC potential of the cerebral cortex. It should be added that careful experiments based on cortical DC recordings in animals (Caspers and Speckmann, 1971) have led to the conclusion that "the presumption that the so-called terminal depolarization might represent a suitable indicator for the revival of all cortical functions has been disproved" (Caspers and Speckmann, 1974).

Recording of Sensory Evoked Potentials

The determination of ECI in scalp EEGs requires special efforts visually to resolve minute electrical oscillations of cerebral origin from extraneous potentials, including instrumental and other noises and biologic activity of extracerebral origin. Because computer-averaging techniques are uniquely capable of extracting small neural signals time-locked to sensory stimuli from unrelated noise, it would seem natural to resort to these methods when attempting to assess brain viability. "Sensory evoked potentials" demonstrated by these techniques include electrical events elicited by sensory stimuli at successive levels along sensory pathways, i.e., in: (1) sensory organs ("sensory organ potentials''), (2) peripheral nerves and nuclei and fiber tracts of the spinal cord and/or brainstem, cerebrum, and cerebellum (''far-field evoked potentials''), and (3) the cerebral cortex (''cerebral evoked potentials'').

Cerebral Evoked Potentials. Scalp-recorded cerebral evoked potentials, i.e., electrical responses of the cerebral cortex to sensory stimuli, have long been employed to provide objective information on human brain function. The use of these measures in assessing brain viability was pioneered by Jouvet (1959), who reported that in four patients with evidence of abolished brain function, including absent spontaneous EEG activity on the scalp and at all levels from the cerebral cortex to the thalamus, no scalp responses were recorded (without averaging) in response to electrical stimulation of peripheral nerves or the thalamus. Absence of averaged cerebral flash-evoked potentials was similarly noted by Arfel (1967, 1970), and Walter and Arfel (1972) in patients in ''coma dépassé'' with ''tracé nul,'' and by Sament, Alderete, and Schwab (1969) in cerebrally dead individuals with ''flat isoelectric EEGs.''

More recently, Trojaborg and Jørgensen (1973) investigated 50 patients who, following severe cerebral anoxia, were comatose, artificially ventilated, and had an ''isoelectric'' EEG apparently satisfying present standards of ECI (American Electroencephalographic Society, 1976). The authors attempted to average visual and somatosensory evoked potentials and to correlate the results of these studies with the presence or absence of cephalic reflexes and intracranial circulation. In all but 1 of 31 patients with cephalic areflexia, flash-evoked potentials could not be demonstrated. Electrical stimulation of the median nerve evoked no detectable response in 16 of these individuals, whereas the remaining 15 patients displayed a small, short-latency (mean:12 msec) potential over the central areas of both sides but no later response components (Fig. 17.19). Evidence was adduced by the authors that this early potential presumably was extracranial in origin, i.e., due to pick-up by the ear reference of the ''nerve action potential travelling up to the level of the foramen magnum.'' Aortocervical angiography performed in 20 of these patients with cephalic areflexia revealed no intracranial circulation in 19. The one individual who had preserved visual, but absent somatosensory, evoked potentials also had preserved circulation in the carotid arteries with venous filling but no circulation in the basilar artery. None of the patients in this group survived.

In the same study of Trojaborg and Jørgensen, 19 of 50 persons with ''isoelectric'' EEGs who had preserved cephalic reflexes displayed visual and somatosensory evoked potentials, although these were simple in form, devoid of late components, and apparently delayed in latency (Fig. 17.20). These responses were demonstrated as late as 8 days after disappearance of spontaneous EEG activity. However, at this late stage, the somatosensory responses mainly consisted of a positive wave of small amplitude and relatively short latency (mean:22 msec). This was felt to represent the first surface-positive wave of the scalp-recorded human somatosensory evoked potential, and was believed to be related to the arrival at the cortex of the volley conducted by the thalamocortical fibers (cf. also Cracco 1972). Following resuscitation, nine of these patients with preserved cephalic reflexes recovered first the evoked and then the spontaneous EEG. The visual responses of these individuals were of larger amplitude than those of patients who did not regain spontaneous electrocerebral activity and their initially simple form increased in complexity as recovery took place. In two patients who initially had preserved cephalic reflexes and cerebral evoked potentials, the subsequent loss of cephalic reflexes was accompanied by disappearance of the cerebral responses. Aortocervical angiography performed in six persons with preserved cephalic reflexes showed the presence of intracranial circulation in all. Repetition of this procedure in the two individuals who subsequently lost these reflexes revealed absence of intracranial circulation. Three of the patients who displayed preservation of cephalic reflexes and certain cerebral evoked potential components "recovered consciousness" and one was "discharged from the hospital."

The above-mentioned observations of Trojaborg and Jørgensen indicate that in deeply comatose, apneic patients without spontaneous electrocerebral activity, the preservation or loss of both visual and somatosensory evoked potentials correlates closely with the presence or absence of cephalic reflexes and intracranial circulation. Moreover, the finding that cerebral evoked potentials persist in brain death suspects in circumstances in which spontaneous electrocerebral activity is absent suggests that these responses might represent more sensitive indices of cerebral function than the spontaneous EEG. The experimental literature lends support to this conjecture and the interested

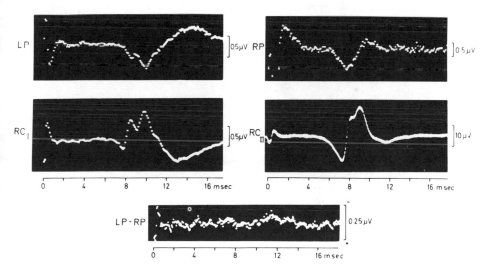

Fig. 17.19. Averaged evoked potentials to electrical stimulation of right median nerve of a 7-year-old girl who was unconscious after respiratory arrest and had no cephalic reflexes. Aortocervical angiography showed absent intracranial circulation. Top 4 records were taken between electrodes over the left and right somatosensory scalp areas (LP and RP) and the neck (RC$_I$ and RC$_{III}$), and ipsilateral earlobe reference leads. Bottom record was obtained bipolarly between the two somatosensory areas (LP-RP) (from Trojaborg W. and Jørgensen E. O. 1973. Electroencephalogr. Clin. Neurophysiol., 35, 301).

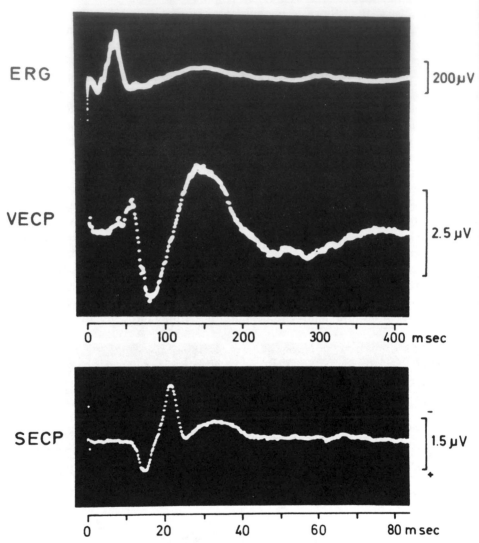

Fig. 17.20 *Averaged responses in a 75-year-old man after cardiac arrest. Patient was comatose, artificially ventilated, and had preserved cephalic reflexes. Top two traces depict flash-evoked electroretinogram (ERG) from right eye and cerebral evoked potential from left occipital region (VECP). Bottom record is response from left somatosensory scalp area (SECP) to electrical stimulation of right median nerve (from Trojaborg, W., and Jørgensen E. O. 1973. Electroencephalogr. Clin. Neurophysiol., 35, 301).*

reader is referred to the elegant work of Meldrum et al (1968), Brierley et al (1969), and Meldrum and Brierley (1969), and to that of Hossman and Kleihues (1973) and Stockard, Bickford, and Aung (1975).

Of additional interest are the observations made by Brierley et al (1971) on two patients who were unconscious for a period of 5 months after cardiac arrest but resumed spontaneous respiration and had preservation of some cephalic, including pupillary, reflexes. Both these persistently vegetating patients (cf. p. 548) had "isoelectric" EEGs except for the appearance in a single record of one subject of "low voltage 12 Hz rhythmical activity in both occipital lobes." Flashes, clicks, and, in one case, peripheral stimulation failed to elicit responses other than eyeblinks and electroretinograms in one individual and myogenic potentials in the other. The abolition of both spontaneous and evoked electrocerebral activity in the face of at least partial preservation of brainstem and spinal reflexes suggested the diagnosis of "neocortical death." Postmortem studies confirmed the primarily cortical distribution of the pathology.

It is important to recognize that computer averaging does not automatically provide simple answers to the question of whether or not cerebral responses are present or absent in cases of suspected brain death. Painstaking precautions and special maneuvers often are essential to assess the possible contamination of the averages by potentials which are time-locked to the stimulus but are generated by extracranial sources. These include: electroretinographic and eyeblink potentials that may complicate averaged flash-evoked scalp activity; early components of somatosensory evoked potentials presumably arising outside the cranial cavity (Trojaborg and Jørgensen, 1973); and myogenic contaminants (Cracco and Bickford, 1968). Even when cerebral evoked potentials are unambiguously present, the significance of the alterations of their form, latency, amplitude, and topography is incompletely known at present. Moreover, the possibility of differences in vulnerability of cerebral responses to stimuli of different sensory modality deserves consideration. Further investigations of brain death suspects correlating cerebral evoked potentials with the spontaneous EEG, clinical findings, and neuropathologic alterations, as well as studies of cerebral blood flow and metabolism, are needed. Until this information becomes available, cerebral evoked potentials should be prudently used as adjuncts to rather than substitutes for EEG recordings in brain death suspects. These responses may prove especially useful in circumstances in which ambiguity exists as to the presence or absence of spontaneous EEG activity in scalp records. In these instances, the preservation of cerebral evoked potentials should suggest special circumspection to the interpreter. By contrast, the lack of demonstrable cerebral responses may add substance to the suspicion that brain function has failed.

Far-field Evoked Potentials. Both brainstem auditory evoked potentials and short latency somatosensory evoked potentials have been studied in patients with suspected brain death, and will therefore receive brief consideration here.

Brainstem Auditory Evoked Potentials. The spontaneous EEG and cerebral evoked potentials primarily reflect cerebral cortical activity and give only indirect information on the functional integrity of the brainstem. Because current concepts of brain death imply permanent cessation of function of both the cerebrum and brainstem, the electrophysiologic assessment of brain viability ideally should include objective measures of functional brainstem capacities. Such information was not available until recently, when the method of recording "far-field" evoked potentials was introduced. The first of these responses to be reported were the "brainstem auditory evoked potentials" (BAEPs) which provided unique measures of functioning of the auditory pathway from the cochlea to the thalamus (Jewett, 1970; Jewett and Williston, 1971). These responses and their application to neurologic diagnosis are discussed in detail in Chapter 12. Starr (1976) studied with this technique 27 patients fulfilling contemporary clinical and EEG criteria of brain death. He found that all components of BAEPs were absent in 16 patients, whereas the remaining 11 patients showed preservation of wave I to stimulation of one or both ears. When present, this wave was prolonged in latency and often showed greater variability on repeated measurements than it did in normal subjects. Repeated BAEP recordings were obtained over a period of 2 to 13 days on four patients who had suffered acute anoxia while their clinical condition evolved from coma with evidence of preserved cerebral and brainstem functions to a state meeting the criteria of brain death. Initially, all BAEP components were present and of normal latency and amplitude. As clinical evidence of deteriorating brainstem function became apparent, first components IV and V decreased in amplitude and increased in latency while waves I-III were normal, then alteration of these earlier components also became manifest. Finally, when clinical criteria of brain death were fulfilled, the whole BAEP was abolished or was restricted to wave I which displayed prolonged latency and decreased amplitude (Fig. 17.21). These serial changes provided graphic evidence of "gradual dissolution of brainstem function in a rostrocaudal direction" reminiscent of that described clinically by Plum and Posner (1966) in comatose states due to supratentorial mass lesions. In one patient, the changes of BAEPs also paralleled the progressive deterioration of the spontaneous EEG. Neuropathologic findings in three of these individuals consisted of widespread necrotic changes of the brain with patchy vacuolization of the gray and white matter throughout the brainstem, including portions of the fiber tracts and nuclei of the auditory pathway. Stock-

Fig. 17.21. Brainstem auditory evoked potentials (BAEPs) to monaural clicks at 65 dB SL in patient following anoxic episode. Designations on left (D4, D7, etc.) refer to day of hospitalization. On days 7 and 8, top tracings were taken in the morning and bottom tracings in the afternoon, On day 4, patient was comatose but withdrew to noxious stimuli and had spontaneous respiration and preserved cephalic reflexes. One day earlier his EEG showed widespread delta activity. On the 7th day, cephalic reflexes were no longer present, there were decerebrate responses to noxious stimuli and low voltage delta activity was present in the EEG. Lack of spontaneous breathing and "isoelectric" EEG were noted on day 8 and on day 10 all responses to noxious stimuli were absent. Patient expired 14 days after admission (from Starr, A. 1976. Brain, 99, 543).

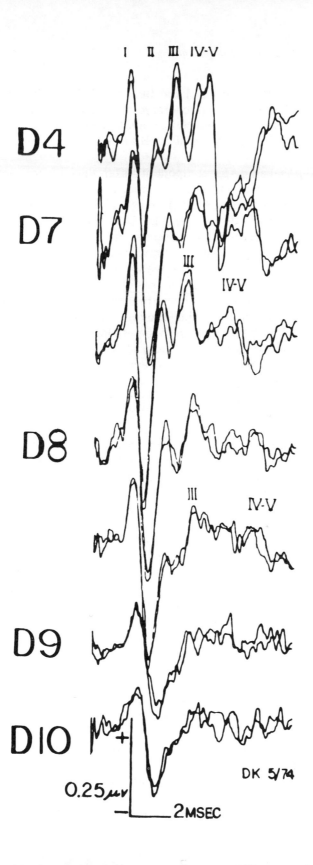

ard and Rossiter (1977) and Uziel and Benezech (1978) confirmed this sequential loss of BAEP components generated at progressively lower levels of the brainstem in patients displaying clinical evidence of rostrocaudal deterioration and the abolition in brain death of all BAEPs with the possible exclusion of wave I.

The finding that all BAEP components after wave I were abolished in brain death, but were little or not at all influenced by CNS depressants, suggested that these responses were of special assistance in evaluating the possibility of drug overdose in brain death suspects (Starr and Achor, 1975; Starr, 1977; Stockard, 1978). The expeditious assessment of this eventuality often is hampered by lack of adequate history, the virtual impossibility of obtaining accurate blood analyses of toxic agents within hours, and the ambiguous significance of the findings of minimal amounts of drugs in the blood (cf. p. 540). In the presence of clinical signs of severe brainstem dysfunction including absent spontaneous respiration and cephalic reflexes, the demonstration of normal or near-normal BAEPs suggests a metabolic etiology such as a massive overdose of CNS depressants rather than a structural brainstem lesion (Starr and Achor, 1975; Starr, 1977; Stockard, 1978). However, in the face of clinical signs of less than global brainstem dysfunction, the preservation of normal brainstem responses to auditory stimulation does not necessarily imply a metabolic or otherwise reversible cause (Stockard, 1978). Normal responses have been observed in patients rendered irreversibly comatose by structural lesions of the midbrain tegmentum sparing the auditory pathway (Stockard, 1978). Similarly, widespread cortical anoxic damage with relative preservation of the brainstem may produce decerebrate or decorticate states with intact BAEPs (Starr, 1977; Pollack and Kellaway, 1979).

The notion that brain death is consistently associated with abolition of all BAEP components after wave I (Starr, 1976) is undergoing critical reappraisal. Recently, Goldie, Chiappa, and Young (1979) reported their findings that 1 of 13 patients with clinical and EEG evidence of brain death displayed both wave I and wave II to stimulation of either ear. Persistence of wave II was also noted by Stockard et al in a case of brain death (Ch. 12). This finding may suggest that wave II of human BAEPs has extra-axial as well as intra-axial sources. Preservation of the former component may account for the persistence of this wave in rare cases of brain death (Stockard et al, Ch. 12).

The recording of BAEPs requires appropriate equipment, a suitable environment, and special technical expertise and interpretive skills. The instrumentation and methodology for reliably demonstrating these responses presently are unfamiliar not only to most clinicians but also to many EEG technologists and clinical electroencephalographers. This is not surprising because the time and voltage parameters of far-field evoked potentials represent entirely new dimensions in human electroencephalography which demand special training and thorough understanding.

These difficulties require careful consideration but are by no means unsurmountable. Hence, it appears reasonable to hope that brainstem auditory evoked potentials, if judiciously used, will significantly contribute to the assessment of brain viability in humans. It seems well-established at present that when certain sources of error are ruled out, abolition of all components of BAEPs except for, or including, the initial positive wave represents further evidence of lack of brain viability in individuals fulfilling clinical and EEG criteria of brain death.

Short latency somatosensory evoked potentials. Short latency components of somatosensory evoked potentials (SLSEPs), elicited by electrical stimulation of peripheral nerves such as the median nerve, have been described in laboratory animals and in man (Fig. 17.22), and their origin is considered in Chapters 13 and 14.

Alterations of SLSEPs have been reported in various neurologic disorders by Anziska et al (1978). Anziska and Cracco (1979) studied eight patients who fulfilled all clinical criteria for brain death, and found in all cases preservation of the first positive component which relates to activity in primary somatosensory fibers. In three patients, all subsequent potentials were abolished. However, the second positive potential was recorded in two pa-

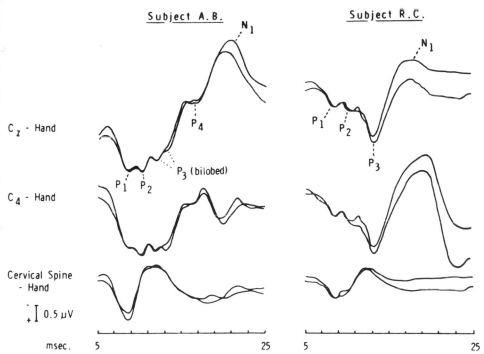

Fig. 17.22. Short latency somatosensory evoked potentials (SLSEPs) to electrical stimulation of left median nerve in two normal subjects. Two superimposed averages of 2,048 trials each, recorded from electrodes located over the vertex (Cz), the right central regions of the scalp (C4), and the cervical spine with reference lead on the dorsum of one hand (from Anziska, B., Cracco, R. O., Cook, A. W., and Feld, E. W. 1978. Electroencephalogr. Clin. Neurophysiol., 45, 602).

tients, the third positive potential in three individuals and the first negative potential in one. Subsequent, cortical potentials were not demonstrated in any of these patients. No information was given as to whether or not these individuals also fulfilled EEG criteria of brain death. In a patient in whom all, including EEG, criteria of brain death were met, Chiappa, Choi, and Young (1979) demonstrated persistence of a positive wave which was recorded over the brachial plexus (Erb's point) in close temporal relationship to the first positive potential detected on the scalp (vertex). Subsequent SLSEP components were absent. Normal potentials at Erb's point also were found by Goldie et al (1979) in 10 patients with brain death determined by similar criteria. Of these individuals, nine also displayed a normal or slightly decreased potential which culminated at 14 msec in recordings from the neck and probably corresponded to the third positive potential characterizing scalp (vertex) records.

Because, at the time of this writing, uncertainty exists as to the exact nature of the structures giving rise to the second and third positive components of human scalp-recorded SLSEPs (Cracco and Cracco, 1976; Chiappa et al, 1979), it is difficult to assess the significance of the preservation of these waves in some brain death suspects. Further investigation of these findings and detailed clinicopathologic correlations are likely to dispel these uncertainties in the future. To what extent SLSEPs will prove helpful in assessing brain viability is unclear at present.

Whatever the outcome of future investigations, the study of far-field in addition to near-field (cerebral) evoked potentials and to the scalp EEG promises to provide a more complete evaluation of brain function than is possible by using these last two techniques alone.

Sensory Organ Potentials. Sensory organ potentials recordable in individuals with brain death include the electroretinogram and the electrocochleogram.

The electroretinogram. The electroretinogram (ERG) is a mass response of the retina to flash stimulation. This response arises in the outer retinal layers where the photoreceptors (rods and cones) and the Müller cells are believed to be its main sources (Tomita, 1950, 1965; Armington, Johnson, and Riggs, 1952; Brown and Watanabe, 1962; Miller and Dowling, 1970). Although it is best recorded by corneal electrodes, the ERG also can be detected by electrodes placed over the face and head, especially when averaging methods are employed.

Arfel (1967) first reported that patients in "coma dépassé" with "nul" EEG displayed in averaged records from the anterior regions of the scalp a response to flashes which included an initial negative-positive component. This biphasic potential persisted from several hours to several days after the disappearance of the spontaneous EEG. When repeatedly studied over successive days, it showed increasing latency and decreasing amplitude of its component waves until it became extinguished. The distribution of this response with a maximum close to the eyes suggested that it was retinal in origin. Subsequent studies confirmed that ERGs could be recorded with or without averaging techniques from the scalp of patients with brain death (Figs. 17.23 and 17.24).

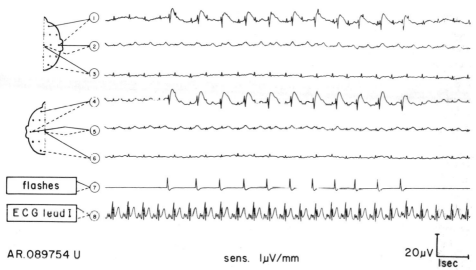

AR.089754 U   sens. 1μV/mm   20μV
                                              ⌐
                                              1sec

Fig. 17.23. Electroretinograms (ERGs) to light flashes recorded from anterior scalp leads (channels 1 and 4) in a patient who was deeply comatose, artificially ventilated, and had no cephalic reflexes (from Wilkus R. J., Chatrian, G. E., and Lettich, E. 1971. Electroencephalogr. Clin. Neurophysiol., 31, 537).

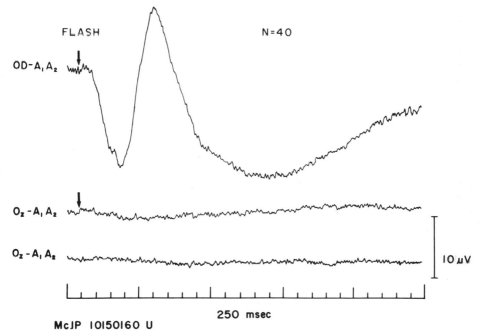

McJP 10150160 U

Fig. 17.24. Top two traces are simultanenous averaged records from right infraorbital (OD) and midline occipital (Oz) electrodes using interconnected ear reference (A1-A2). Bottom trace is averaged control record with no stimulus. Same patient as in Fig. 17.23. Note presence of ERG as opposed to absence of cerebral evoked response (from Wilkus, R. J., Chatrian, G. E., and Lettich, E. 1971. Electroencephalogr. Clin. Neurophysiol., 31, 537).

Some authors attempted to assess certain quantitative aspects of the ERG detected in brain death suspects with the intent of determining whether or not they deviated from the normal. Lobstein, Mantz, and Mack (1968) and Mantz et al (1971) described attenuation of the a-wave of the ERG in patients with "coma dépassé." Sament et al (1969) reported that the ERGs of patients with "irreversible coma" and "isoelectric" EEG had features observed in individuals with circulatory disturbances of the retina and resembled the ERGs of the "cone" type of retinas. Sament (1969) further characterized the ERGs of 8 of 18 patients satisfying the same clinical and EEG criteria as demonstrating an a-wave or a ratio between the a- and the b-wave which was larger than normal. Walter and Arfel (1972) also commented on the lower amplitude of the ERG displayed by patients with "coma dépassé" as compared to those of normal individuals. Reliable quantitative assessment of ERG parameters such as the amplitude of the a-wave, the voltage of the total ERG, the a/b amplitude ratio, and the latency of individual ERG components requires stringent control of the conditions of stimulation including position of light source, flash intensity, and intensity of background illumination (Gouras, 1970; Berson, 1975). This can hardly be achieved in intensive care units without the use of specially designed instrumentation. Moreover, adequate normative data on periorbitally averaged ERGs were not available prior to the study of Noonan et al (1973). Hence, the significance of ERG abnormalities described so far in patients with brain death is unclear at best. It is significant that ERGs apparently indistinguishable from those of alert volunteers were obtained on patients with brain death by Sims et al (1972) who achieved better control of stimulus parameters by using special goggles incorporating light-emitting diodes. Normal ERGs were similarly reported in less controlled circumstances in 10 of 18 patients studied by Sament (1969), 2 individuals with "coma dépassé" and electrocerebral "silence" investigated by Ferrillo et al (1969), and 1 patient with "neocortical death" following cardiac arrest described by Brierley et al (1971).

Some investigators inquired into the possible usefulness of the ERG in the study of brain death suspects. Recognizing that the ERG can be present in circumstances suggesting brain death, Ferrillo et al (1969), Arfel (1970), Wilkus, Chatrian, and Lettich (1971), Sims et al (1972) and Walker (1977b) suggested that the preservation of ERG responses had neither diagnostic nor prognostic value in brain death suspects. Ferrillo et al (1969) reported that in two individuals with normal ERGs but absent electrocerebral activity, carotid angiography demonstrated arrest of contrast at the level of the carotid siphon, distal to the origin of the ophthalmic artery which was normally visualized. In 3 percent of cases the external carotid artery is the main source of blood to the ophthalmic artery. Moreover, the facial artery provides collateral circulation to the ophthalmic artery. These anatomic factors probably account for the preservation of retinal perfusion in the face of abolished cerebral circulation in cases of brain death (Sims et al, 1972; Walker, 1977b). Somewhat different beliefs were expressed by Sament (1969) who felt that the persistence of an ERG was not in itself a favorable prognostic factor. However, he postulated that, because of the remarkable resistance of the ERG to anoxia, those patients who displayed abnormal ERGs were likely to have suffered very severe anoxia with consequent gross brain damage. He further predicted that in patients with acute barbiturate intoxication and "reversible flat" EEG, an abnormal ERG would indicate severe anoxia and represent a poor prognostic sign whereas a normal ERG would predict a favorable course. There appears to be little basis for this belief. Because high doses of barbiturates sharply alter the ERG (Berson, 1975), recordings of this response in patients with massive overdoses are unlikely to provide reliable information on the severity of anoxia possibly suffered and the likelihood of recovery.

Although the ERG appears to be of little diagnostic and prognostic value in the study of brain viability in humans, awareness that it may be preserved in patients with brain death is important. When this response is evident in scalp records, its ocular rather than cerebral origin can be demonstrated by successively covering one eye, the other eye, and both eyes during stroboscopic stimulation. This maneuver abolishes the response detected by electrode(s) close to the occluded eye(s). Moreover, when attempting to computer-average cerebral responses to flashes in brain death suspects, the possibility that the ERG may contaminate, if not stimulate, these responses must be carefully assessed (Arfel, 1967; Jørgensen and Trojaborg, 1971; Trojaborg and Jørgensen, 1973; Stockard et al, 1975; Starr, 1976, 1977). In these circumstances, the anterior distribution of the ERG and its asymmetry on the two sides of the head when it is monocularly elicited, help differentiate it from cerebral responses. Trojaborg and Jørgensen also have suggested that subtracting from an averaged occipital record contaminated by ERG potentials a certain number of ERG responses detected by a corneal electrode further contributes to ascertain the absence of cerebral responses in brain death suspects.

The electrocochleogram. AC recordings of the electrical potentials generated in the human cochlea by auditory stimuli or "electrocochleogram" demonstrate two concurrent responses: the "cochlear microphonics" (CM) and the "eighth nerve compound action potential" (cf. Eggermont, 1976). The cochlear microphonics are piezo-electric potentials which arise in the cochlear haircells, whereas the compound action potential reflects the discharge of afferent fibers of the auditory nerve. Some authors have recorded both responses by means of electrodes inserted through the tympanic membrane into the cochlear promontory (Aran and Le Bert, 1968; Yoshie, 1971; Eggermont, 1976). However, techniques which do not require penetration of the middle ear also have been developed. These utilize electrodes which are applied on the tympanic membrane (Cullen et al, 1972), inserted under or applied on the skin of the external auditory canal (Yoshie et al, 1967; Coats and Dickey, 1970; Coats, 1974) or of the earlobe (Sohmer and Feinmesser, 1967). Figure 17.25 illustrates this finding. Clicks of opposite phase producing "condensation" and "rarefaction," respectively, elicit microphonic potentials of opposite polarity, whereas the polarity of the eighth nerve compound action potential is not influenced by stimulus phase. Thus, when responses to clicks of alternating polarity are summated, cancellation of cochlear microphonic potentials occurs and only the

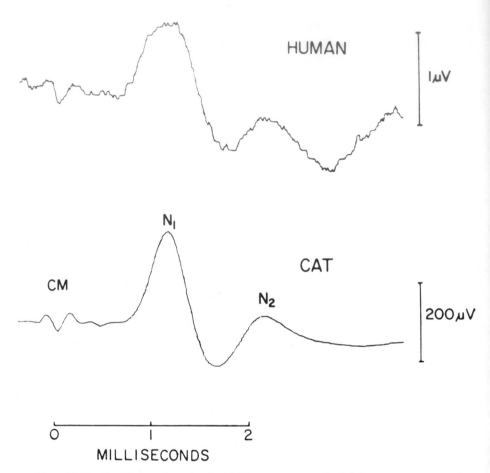

Fig. 17.25. *Cochlear microphonic (CM) response and eighth nerve compound action potential (N1, N2) recorded from human (by needle electrode in external auditory canal) and cat (by silver ball electrode on round window). Click intensity was 55 dB. Records from human and cat are averages of 1,024 and 20 trials, respectively (from Coats, A. C. and Dickey, J. R. 1970. Ann. Otol. Rhinol. Laryngol., 79, 844).*

eighth nerve action potential can be appreciated. Because most clinical studies of brainstem auditory evoked potentials in cerebrally dead individuals (BAEPs, cf. p. 567) published so far have been conducted in these conditions and have not attempted to record from the external auditory canal, wave I, a component of the eighth nerve action potential, has been the earliest indicator of activity in the auditory pathway. An exception is the report of Uziel and Benezech (1978), who investigated a patient with brain death displaying loss of all BAEP components after a wave I of increased latency and decreased amplitude. Transtympanic promontory recordings demonstrated persistence of cochlear microphonics, a finding which was felt to indicate "the absence of cochlear disturbance." Cochlear microphonics also have been described by Stockard, Stockard, and Sharbrough (1978) in an individual with "brainstem death" and well-preserved EEG. Additional studies are needed to determine whether or not noninvasive recordings of the electrocochleogram are helpful and practical adjuncts to the technique of eliciting BAEPs in brain death suspects.

SUMMARY AND CONCLUSIONS

This chapter has reviewed the concept of brain death defined as total and permanent abolition of brain function and the criteria on which the diagnosis of this condition is currently based in the United States. An attempt has been made to evaluate the usefulness of electrophysiologic methods to confirm the diagnosis of brain death suggested by clinical observation. Available data indicate that, in the appropriate clinical circumstances, the absence of any spontaneous EEG activity in scalp records, obtained and interpreted according to stringent standards, provides reliable evidence of failure of cerebral cortical function. Thus, the use of the EEG is desirable to confirm brain death whenever the necessary instrumentation and skills are available. Other methods, including cortical and depth recordings and measurements of the cortical DC potential, have contributed to a degree to the understanding of the electrophysiologic events underlying failure of brain function, but are of questionable practical value. By contrast, recordings of sensory evoked potentials promise to develop into useful tools for assessing brain viability. Brainstem auditory evoked potentials are especially likely to provide measures of brainstem function that will effectively complement the information derived from the spontaneous EEG. These relatively new techniques must be used prudently, and the utility of other methods for confirming brain death, including studies of cerebral perfusion and metabolism, must be borne in mind.

REFERENCES

Adams, R. D. and Jequier, M. (1969). The brain death syndrome: hypoxemic panencephalopathy. Schweiz. Med. Wochenschr., 99:65.

Alajouanine, J. (1957). Les altérations des états de conscience causées par les désordres neurologiques. Acta Med. Belg., 2:19.

American Bar Association. (1975). Insurance, negligence and compensation law section. Euthanasia—symposium issue. 27 Baylor Law Rev., 1:1 (cited by Walker, 1977b).

American Electroencephalographic Society. (1976). Minimum technical standards for EEG recording in suspected cerebral death. In: Guidelines in EEG, p. 21.

American Electroencephalographic Society and American Society of Electroencephalographic Technologists. (1976). Provisional Recommendations for Telephone Transmission of EEGs. In: Guidelines in EEG, p. 28.

American Medical Association. (1974). House of Delegates Substitute Resolution 18 (cited by Walker, 1977b).

American Neurological Association. (1976). Statement regarding method for determining that the brain is dead. Trans. Am. Neurol. Assoc., 101:322.

Anziska, B. and Cracco, R. Q. (1979). Somatosensory evoked short latency potentials in brain dead patients. Electroencephalogr. Clin. Neurophysiol. (in press).

Anziska, B., Cracco, R. Q., Cook, A. W., and Feld, E. W. (1978). Somatosensory far field potentials: studies in normal subjects and patients with multiple sclerosis. Electroencephalogr. Clin. Neurophysiol., *45:*602.

Aran, J. M. and Le Bert, G. (1968). Les réponses nerveuses cochléaires chez l'homme image du fonctionnement de l'oreille et nouveau test d'audiométrie objective. Rev. Laryngol. Otol. Rhinol. (Bord), *89:*361.

Arfel, G. (1967). Stimulations visuelles et silence cérébral. Electroencephalogr. Clin. Neurophysiol., *23:*172.

Arfel, G. (1970). Problèmes électroencéphalographiques de la mort. Masson, Paris.

Arfel, G. (1976). Brain death. In: Handbook of Clinical Neurology, Vol. 24, Vinken, P. J. and Bruyn, G. W., Eds., p. 757, American Elsevier, New York.

Arfel, G. and Fischgold, H. (1961). Significance of electrical silence of the brain. Electroencephalogr. Clin. Neurophysiol., *13:*653.

Arfel, G. and Weiss, J. (1962). Électroencéphalogramme et hypothermie profonde. Ann. Chir. Thorac. Cardiovasc., *16:*666.

Arfel, G., Fischgold, H., and Weiss, J. (1963). Le silence cérébral. In: Problèmes de Base en Électroencéphalographie, Fischgold, H., Dreyfus-Brisac, C., and Pruvot, P., Eds., p. 118. Masson, Paris.

Arfel, G., Akerman, M., Hertzog, E., and Bamberger-Bozo, C. (1972). Données radiologiques, électro-encéphalographiques et isotopiques dans les comas dépassés. Acta Radiol. (Stockh.), *13:*295.

Armington, J. C., Johnson, E. P., and Riggs, L. A. (1952). The scotopic A-wave in the electrical response of the human retina. J. Physiol. (Lond.), *118:*289.

Arnaud, M., Vigouroux, R., and Vigouroux, M. (1963). États frontière entre la vie et la mort en neuro-traumatologie. Neurochirurgia (Stuttg.), *6:*1.

Barlow, J. S., Kamp, A., Morton, H. B., Ripoche, A., and Shipton, H. (1974). EEG Instrumentation Standards: Report of the Committee on EEG Instrumentation Standards of the International Federation of Societies for Electroencephalography and Clinical Neurophysiology. Electroencephalogr. Clin. Neurophysiol., *37:*549.

Beecher, H. K. (1968). A definition of irreversible coma. Report of the Ad Hoc Committee of the Harvard Medical School to examine the definition of brain death. J.A.M.A., *205:*337.

Bennett, D. R., Hughes, J. R., Korein, J., Merlis, J. K., and Suter, C. (1976). Atlas of electroencephalography in coma and cerebral death. EEG at the bedside or in the intensive care unit. Raven Press, New York.

Bennett, D. R., Nord, N. M., Roberts, T. S., and Mavor, H. (1971). Prolonged "survival" with flat EEG following cardiac arrest. Electroencephalogr. Clin. Neurophysiol., *30:*94.

Bental, E. and Leibowitz, U. (1961). Flat electroencephalograms during 28 days in a case of "encephalitis." Electroencephalogr. Clin. Neurophysiol., *13:*457.

Beresford, H. R. (1977). The Quinlan decision: problems and legislative alternatives. Ann. Neurol., *2:*74.

Bergamasco, B., Bergamini, L., and Doriguzzi, T. (1968a). Clinical value of the sleep electroencephalographic patterns in post-traumatic coma. Acta Neurol. Scand., *44:*495.

Bergamasco, B., Bergamini, L., Doriguzzi, T., and Fabiani, D. (1968b). EEG sleep patterns as a prognostic criterion in post-traumatic coma. Electroencephalogr. Clin. Neurophysiol., *24:*347.

Berger, E. L., Stockard, J. J., Aung, M. H., and Bickford, R. G. (1974). Removal of EKG artifact from EEG in brain death and other recordings. Electroencephalogr. Clin. Neurophysiol., *37:*202.

Berson, E. L. (1975). Electrical phenomena in the retina. In: Adler's physiology of the eye. Clinical application, Moses, R. A., Ed., p. 453. C. V. Mosby Co., St. Louis.

Bertrand, I., Lhermitte, F., Antoine, B., and Ducrot, H. (1959). Nécroses massives du système nerveux central dans une survie artificielle. Rev. Neurol., *101:*101.

Bickford, R. G. (1974). Quantitative techniques in EEG. In: Medical Engineering, Ray, C. D., Ed., p. 385. Year Book Medical Publishers, Chicago.

Bickford, R. G., Sims, J. K., Billinger, T. W., and Aung, M. H. (1971). Problems in EEG estimation of brain death and use of computer techniques for their solution. Trauma, *12:*61.

Binnie, C. D., Prior, P. F., Lloyd, D. S. L., Scott, D. F., and Margerison, J. H. (1970). Electroencephalographic prediction of fatal anoxic brain damage after resuscitation from cardiac arrest. Br. Med. J., *4:*265.

Bird, T. D. and Plum, F. (1968). Recovery from barbiturate overdose coma with a prolonged isoelectric electroencephalogram. Neurology, *18:*456.

Black, P. McL. (1978). Brain death (Second of Two Parts). N. Engl. J. Med., *299:*393.

Bottinelli, M. D., Maslenikov, V., Medoc, J., and Purriel, J. A. (1969). The ventral pontine syndrome: a clinical, pathological, and 24 hour EEG study. Fourth Internat. Congr. Neurol. Surg., Ninth Internat. Congr. Neurol., Excerpta. Med. Internat. Congr. Series No. 193, p. 192.

Braunstein, P., Korein, J.,and Kricheff, I. (1972). Bedside assessment of cerebral circulation. Lancet, *1:*1291.

Braunstein, P., Korein, J., Kricheff, I., Corey, K., and Chase, N. (1973). A simple bedside evaluation for cerebral blood flow in the study of cerebral death: A prospective study on 34 deeply comatose patients. Am. J. Roentgenol., *118:*757.

Brenner, R. P., Schwartzman, R. J., and Richey, E. T. (1975). Prognostic significance of episodic low amplitude or relatively isoelectric EEG patterns. Dis. Nerv. Syst., *36:*582.

Bricolo, A. (1976). Prolonged post traumatic coma In: Handbook of Clinical Neurology, Vol. 24, Vinken, P. J. and Bruyn, G. W., Eds., p. 699. American Elsevier, New York.

Bricolo, A., Benati, A., Mazza, C., and Bricolo, A. P. (1969). Studio longitudinale di un coma postraumatico esordito con 130 giorni di silenzio elettrico. Riv. Neurol., *29:*598.

Bricolo, A., Benati, A., Mazza, C., and Bricolo, A. P. (1971). Prolonged isoelectric EEG in a case of post-traumatic coma. Electroencephalogr. Clin. Neurophysiol., *31:*174.

Bricolo, A., Gentilomo, A., Rosadini, G., and Rossi, G. F. (1968a). Akinetic mutism following cranio-cerebral trauma. Physiopathological considerations based on sleep studies. Acta Neurochir. (Wien), *18:*67.

Bricolo, A., Gentilomo, A., Rosadini, G., and Rossi, G. F. (1968b). Long lasting post-traumatic unconsciousness. Acta Neurol. Scand., *44:*512.

Brierley, J. B., Adams, J. H., Graham, D. I., and Simpson, J. A. (1971). Neocortical death after cardiac arrest. A clinical, neurophysiological, and neuropathological report of two cases. Lancet, *2:*560.

Brierley, J. B., Brown, A. W., Excell, B. J., and Meldrum, B. S. (1969). Brain damage in the rhesus monkey resulting from profound arterial hypotension. I. Its nature, distribution and general physiological correlates. Brain Res., *13:*68.

Brown, K. T. and Watanabe, K. (1962). Isolation and identification of a receptor potential from the pure fovea of the monkey retina. Nature, *193:*958.

Bushart, W. (1969). Significance of DC recording in man. Electroencephalogr. Clin. Neurophysiol., *26:*433.

Bushart, W. and Rittmeyer, P. (1968). Elektroencephalographische Verlaufsüberwachung und Kriterien der irreversiblen Hirnschädigung in der Intensivpflege. Verh. Dtsch. Ges. Inn. Med., *74:*865.

Bushart, W. and Rittmeyer, P. (1969). Kriterien der irreversiblen Hirnschädigung bei Intensivbehandlung: Elektroenzephalographische und klinische Verlaufsüberwachung. Med. Klin., *64:*184.

Cabral, R., Prior, P. F., Scott, D. F., and Brierley, J. B. (1977). Reversible profound depression of cerebral electrical activity in hyperthermia. Electroencephalogr. Clin. Neurophysiol., *42:*697.

Cairns, H., Olfield, R. C., Pennybacker, J. B., and Whitteridge, D. (1941). Akinetic mutism with an epidermoid cyst of the 3rd ventricle. Brain, *64:*273.

Carbonell, J., Carrascosa, R., Dierssen, G., Obrador, S., Oliveros, J. C., and Sevillano, M. (1963). Some electrophysiological observations in a case of deep coma secondary to cardiac arrest. Electroencephalogr. Clin. Neurophysiol., *15:*520.

Caspers, H. and Speckmann, E.-J. (1969). DC potential shifts in paroxysmal states. In: Basic Mechanisms of the Epilepsies, Jasper, H. H., Ward, H. H. Jr., and Pope, A., Eds., p. 375. Little, Brown and Co., Boston.

Caspers, H. and Speckmann, E.-J. (1971). Gleichspannungsverschiebungen an der Hirnringe bei Asphyxie. Arzneim Forsch., *25:*241.

Caspers, H. and Speckmann, E.-J. (1974). Cortical DC Shifts associated with changes of gas tension in blood and tissue. In: DC potentials recorded directly from the cortex. Handbook of Electroencephalography and Clinical Neurophysiology, Vol. 10A, Caspers, H., Ed., p. 41. Elsevier, Amsterdam.

Caton, R. (1875). The electrical currents of the brain. Br. Med. J., *2:*278.

Caton, R. (1877). Interim report on investigation of the electric current of the brain. Br. Med. J., Supplement Vol *1:*62.

Chase, T. N., Moretti, L., and Prensky, A. L. (1968). Clinical and electroencephalographic manifestations of vascular lesions of the pons. Neurology, *18:*357.

Chatrian, G. E. (1976). The low voltage EEG. In: The EEG of the waking adult. Handbook of Electroencephalography and Clinical Neurophysiology, Vol. 6A, Chatrian, G. E. and Lairy, G. C., Eds., p. 77. Elsevier, Amsterdam.

Chatrian, G. E., White, L. E., Jr., and Shaw, Ch.-M. (1964). EEG pattern resembling wakefulness in unresponsive decerebrate state following traumatic brain-stem infarct. Electroencephalogr. Clin. Neurophysiol., *16:*285.

Chatrian, G. E., Bergamini, L., Dondey, M., Klass, W. D., Lennox-Buchthal, M., and Petersen, I. (1974). A glossary of terms most commonly used by clinical encephalographers. Electroencephalogr. Clin. Neurophysiol., *37:*538.

Chiappa, K. H., Choi, S. K., and Young, R. R. (1979). Short latency somatosensory evoked potentials following median nerve stimulation in patients with neurological lesions. In: Progress in Clinical Neurophysiology, Vol. 7, Desmedt, J. E., Ed., S. Karger, Basel (in press).

Coats, A. C. (1974). On electrocochleographic electrode design. J. Acoust. Soc. Am., *56:*708.

Coats, A. C. and Dickey, J. R. (1970). Nonsurgical recording of human auditory nerve action potentials and cochlear microphonics. Ann. Otol. Rhinol. Laryngol., *79:*844.

Conference of Royal Colleges and Faculties of the United Kingdom. (1976). Diagnosis of brain death. Lancet, *2:*1069.

Cracco, R. Q. (1972). The initial positive potential of the scalp recorded somatosensory evoked response. Electroencephalogr. Clin. Neurophysiol., *32:*623.

Cracco, R. Q. and Bickford, R. G. (1968). Somatomotor and somatosensory evoked responses—median nerve stimulation in man. Arch. Neurol., *18:*52.

Cracco, R. Q. and Cracco, J. B. (1976). Somatosensory evoked potentials in man: far-field potentials. Electroencephalogr. Clin. Neurophysiol., *41:*460.

Cravioto, H., Silberman, J., and Feigin, I. (1960). A clinical and pathologic study of akinetic mutism. Neurology, *10:*10.

Crow, H. J. and Winter, A. (1969). Serial electrophysiological studies (EEG, EMG, ERG, evoked responses) in a case of 3 months survival with flat EEG following cardiac arrest. Electroencephalogr. Clin. Neurophysiol., *27:*332.

Cullen, J. K., Ellis, M. S., Berlin, C. I., and Lousteau, R. J. (1972). Human acoustic nerve action potential recordings from the tympanic membrane without anesthesia. Acta Otolaryngol., *74:*15.

Dolce, G. E. and Kaemmerer, E. (1967). Contributo anatomico ed elettroencefalografico alla conoscenza della sindrome apallica. Studio dell'evoluzione dell'EEG da sonno in 5 casi. Sist. Nerv., *29:*12.

Drory, Y., Ouaknine, G., Kosary, I. Z., and Kellerman, J. J. (1975). Electrocardiographic findings in brain death; description and presumed mechanism. Chest, *67:*425.

Duensing, F. (1949). Das Elektroenzephalogramm bei Störungen der Bewubstseinslage, Arch Psychiatr. Nervenkr., *183:*71.

Eggermont, J. J. (1976). Electrocochleography. In: Handbook of Sensory Physiology, Vol. V/3. Auditory system. Clinical and special topics, Keidel, W. S. and Neff, W. D. Eds., p. 625. Springer-Verlag, Heidelberg.

Feldman, M. H. (1971). Physiological observations in a chronic case of "locked-in" syndrome. Neurology, *21:*459.

Ferguson, J. M. and Bennett, D. R. (1974). Sleep in a patient with a pontine infarction. Electroencephalogr. Clin. Neurophysiol., *36:*210.

Ferrillo, F., Giunta, F., Rivano, C., Rodriquez, G., Rosadini, G., Rossi, G. F., Sannita, W., Siani, C., Turella, G., and Zattoni, J. (1969). Analisi dell'attivitá elettrica cerebrale spontanea ed evocata nel coma profondo e nella "morte del cervello." Riv. Neurol., *39:*589.

Findji, E., Gaches, J., Houtteville, J. P., Creissard, P., and Caliskan, A. (1970). Enregistrements électroencéphalographiques corticaux, transcorticaux et souscorticaux dans dix cas de coma profound ou dépassé (note préliminaire). Neurochirurgia (Stuttg.), *13:*211.

Fischgold, H. and Mathis, P. (1959). Obnubilations, comas et stupeurs. Electroencephalogr. Clin. Neurophysiol., Suppl. 11, Masson, Paris.

Freemon, F. R., Salinas-Garcia, R. F., and Ward, J. W. (1974). Sleep patterns in a patient with a brainstem infarction involving the raphe nucleus. Electroencephalogr. Clin. Neurophysiol., *36:*657.

French, J. D. (1952). Brain lesions associated with prolonged unconsciousness. Arch. Neurol. Psychiatr, *68:*727.

Gaches, J., Galiskan, A., Findji, F., and LeBeau, J. (1970). Contribution à l'étude du coma dépassé et de la mort cérébrale. Etude de 71 cas. Sem. Hop. Paris, *46:*1487.

Gentilomo, A., Rivano, C., Rosadini, G. E., and Rossi, G. F. (1966). Studio elettroclinico longitudinale del coma cerebrale evolvente verso la sindrome apallica. Rass. Arch. Chir., *4:*816.

Gerstenbrand, F. (1967). Das traumatische apallische Syndrom. Springer, Wien, p. 344 (cited by Bricolo 1976).

Gilder, S. S. B. (1968). Twenty-Second World Medical Assembly. Br. Med. J., *3:*493.

Goldie, W. D., Chiappa, K. H., and Young, R. R. (1979). Brainstem auditory evoked responses and short latency somatosensory evoked responses in the evaluation of deeply comatose patients. Neurology (in press).

Goodman, J. M., Mishkin, F. S., and Dyken, M. (1969). Determination of brain death by isotope angiography. J.A.M.A., *209:*1869.

Gouras, P. (1970). Electroretinography. Some basic principles. Invest. Ophthalmol. Vis. Sci., *9:*557.

Grass, E. R. (1969). Technological aspects of electroencephalography in the determination of death. Am. J. EEG Technol., *9:*77.

Green, J. B. and Lauber, A. (1972). Return of EEG activity after electrocerebral silence: two case reports. J. Neurol. Neurosurg. Psychiatry, *35:*103.

Greitz, T., Gordon, E., Kolmodin, G., and Widén, L. (1973). Aortocranial and carotid angiography in determination of brain death. Neuroradiology, *5:*13.

Gumnit, R. J. (1974). Recording techniques. In: DC potentials recorded directly from the cortex. Handbook of Electroencephalography and Clinical Neurophysiology. Vol 10A, Caspers, H., Ed., p. 7. Elsevier, Amsterdam.

Haider, I. and Oswald, I. (1970). Electroencephalographic investigation in acute drug poisoning. Electroencephalogr. Clin. Neurophysiol., *29:*105.

Haider, I., Matthew, H., and Oswald, I. (1971). Electroencephalographic changes in acute drug poisoning. Electroencephalogr. Clin. Neurophysiol., *30:*23.

Halsey, J. H., Jr. and Downie, A. W. (1966). Decerebrate rigidity with preservation of consciousness. J. Neurol. Neurosurg. Psychiatry, *29:*350.

Hamburger, J. and Crosnier, J. (1968). Moral and ethical problems in transplantation. In: Human Transplantation, Rapaport, F. T. and Dausset, F. T., Eds., p. 37. Grune and Stratton, New York.

Harden, A. (1969). EEG studies following resuscitation after cardiac arrest in 60 babies. Electroencephalogr. Clin. Neurophysiol., *27:*333.

Hassler, R., Dalle Ore, G., Dieckman, G., Bricolo, A., and Dolce, G. (1969). Behavioral and EEG arousal induced by stimulation of unspecific projection systems in a patient with post-traumatic apallic syndrom. Electroencephalogr. Clin. Neurophysiol., *27:*306.

Hawkes, C. H. and Bryan-Smyth, L. (1974). The electroencephalogram in the "locked-in" syndrome. Neurology, *24:*1015.

Hockaday, J. M., Potts, F., Epstein, E., Bonazzi, A. and Schwab, R. S. (1965). Electroencephalographic changes in acute cerebral anoxia from cardiac or respiratory arrest. Electroencephalogr. Clin. Neurophysiol., *18:*575.

Hossman, K. A. and Kleihues, P. (1973). Reversibility of ischemic brain damage. Arch. Neurol., *29:*375.

Houtteville, J. P., Gaches, J., Garreau, J., and Teman, G. (1970). Méningoencéphalite gravissime avec silence EEG total au cours d'une mononucléose infectieuse. Guérison. Ann. Med. Interne (Paris), *121:*347.

Hughes, J. R., Boshes, B., and Leestma, J. (1976). Electro-clinical and pathological correlations in comatose patients. Clin. Electroencephalogr., *7:*13.

Hughes, J. R., Cayaffa, J. J., Leestma, J., and Mizuno, Y. (1972). Alternating "waking" and "sleep" EEG patterns in a deeply comatose patient. Clin. Electroencephalogr., *3:*86.

Ingvar, D. H. (1971). EEG and cerebral circulation in the apallic syndrome and akinetic mutism. Electroencephalogr. Clin. Neurophysiol., *30:*272.

Ingvar, D. H. and Brun, A. (1972). Das komplette apallische Syndrom. Arch. Psychiatr. Nervenkr., *215:*219.

Ingvar, D. H. and Sourander, P. (1970). Destruction of the reticular core of the brainstem. Arch. Neurol., *23:*1.

Ingvar, D. H., and Widén, L. (1972). Brain death—Summary of a symposium. Lakartidningen, *34:*3804.

Ingvar, D. H., Häggendal, E., Nilsson, H. J., Sourander, P., Wickbom, I., and Lassen, N. A. (1964). Cerebral circulation and metabolism in a comatose patient. Arch. Neurol., *11:*13.

Ivan, L. P. (1973). Spinal reflexes in cerebral death. Neurology, *23:*650.

Jasper, H. H., Fitzpatrick, C. A., and Solomon, P. (1939). Analogies and opposites in schizophrenia and epilepsy. Am. J. Psychiatry, *95:*835.

Jennett, B. and Plum, F. (1972). Persistent vegetative state after brain damage—A syndrome in search of a name. Lancet, *1:*734.

Jewett, D. L. (1970). Volume conducted potentials in response to auditory stimuli as detected by averaging in the cat. Electroencephalogr. Clin. Neurophysiol., *28:*609.

Jewett, D. L. and Williston, J. S. (1971). Auditory-evoked far fields averaged from the scalp of humans. Brain, *94:*681.

Jonkman, E. J. (1969). Cerebral death and the isoelectric EEG (Review of the literature). Electroencephalogr. Clin. Neurophysiol., *27:*215.

Jørgensen, E. O. (1970). The EEG during severe barbiturate intoxication. Acta. Neurol. Scand., Suppl. *43:*281.

Jørgensen, E. O. (1971). The EEG following circulatory and respiratory arrest. Electroencephalogr. Clin. Neurophysiol., *30:*273.

Jørgensen, E. O. (1973). Spinal man after brain death. The unilateral extension-pronation reflex of the upper limb as an indication of brain death. Acta Neurochir., *28:*259.

Jørgensen, E. O. (1974). EEG without detectable cortical activity and cranial nerve areflexia as paramenters of brain death. Electroencephalogr. Clin. Neurophysiol., *36:*70.

Jørgensen, E. O. and Trojaborg, W. (1971). Visual evoked potentials and the diagnosis of cortical death, a comment. Nord. Med., *86:*1054.

Jørgensen, P. B., Jørgensen, E. O., and Rosenklint, A. (1973). Brain death pathogenesis and diagnosis. Acta Neurol. Scand., *49:*355.

Jouvet, M. (1959). Diagnostic électro-sous-cortico-graphique de la mort du système nerveux central au cours de certains comas. Electroencephalogr. Clin. Neurophysiol., *11:*805.

Jouvet, M., Pellin, B., and Mounier, D. (1961). Étude polygraphique des différentes phases du sommeil au cours des troubles de conscience chroniques (comas prolongés). Rev. Neurol. *105:*181.

Kaada, B. R., Harkmark, M. D. W., and Stokke, O. (1961). Deep coma associated with desynchronization in EEG. Electroencephalogr. Clin. Neurophysiol., *13:*785.

Karp, J. S. and Hurtig, H. I. (1974). "Locked-in" state with bilateral midbrain infarcts. Arch. Neurol., *30:*176.

Kemper, T. L. and Romanul, F. C. A. (1967). State resembling akinetic mutism in basilar artery occlusion. Neurology, *17:*74.

Kimura, J., Gerber, H. W. and McCormick, F. (1968). The isoelectric electroencephalogram. Significance in establishing death in patients maintained on mechanical respirators. Arch. Intern. Med., *121:*511.

Kirschbaum, R. J. and Carollo, V. J. (1970). Reversible isoelectric EEG in barbiturate coma. J.A.M.A., *212:*1215.

Korein, J. and Maccario, M. (1971). On the diagnosis of cerebral death: a prospective study on 55 patients to define irreversible coma. Clin. Electroencephalogr., *2:*178.

Korein, J., Braunstein, P., Kricheff, I., Lieberman, A., and Chase, N. (1975). Radioisotopic bolus technique as a test to detect circulatory deficit associated with cerebral death. Circulation, *51:*924.

Korein, J., Braunstein, P., George, A., Wichter, M., Kricheff, I., Lieberman, A., and Pearson, J. (1977). Brain death: I. Angiographic correlation with the radioisotopic bolus technique for evaluation of critical deficit of cerebral blood flow. Ann. Neurol., *2:*195.

Kretschmer, E. (1940). Das apallische Syndrom. Zentralbl. Neurol. Psychiatr., *169:*576.

Kubicki, S., Rieger, H., and Bharckow, D. (1970). EEG in fatal and near fatal poisoning with soporific drugs. II—Clinical significance. Clin. Electroencephalogr., *1:*14.

Kurtz, D., Cornette, M., Tempe, J. D., and Mantz, J. M. (1970). Prognostic value of the EEG following reversible cardiac arrest. From 90 cases. Electroencephalogr. Clin. Neurophysiol., *29:*530.

Kurtz, D., Mantz, J. M., Tempe, J. D., and Feuerstein, J. (1966). Silence électrique cérébral prolongé et réversible: à propos de trois observations. Rev. Neurol., *115:*423.

Lemmi, H., Hubbert, C. H., and Faris, A. A. (1973). The electroencephalogram after resuscitation of cardiocirculatory arrest. J. Neurol. Neurosurg. Psychiatry, *36:* 997.

Lepetit, J. M., Vallat, J. N., Mathieu, S., Radvanyi, M. F., Eliet-Flescher, J. and Fischgold, H. (1966). Étude du nycthémère dans un état comateux prolongé. Étude électro-clinique. Rev. Neurol., *115:*526.

Levin, P. and Kinnel, J. (1966). Successful cardiac resuscitation despite prolonged silence of EEG. Arch. Intern. Med., *117:*557.

Lindenberg, R. (1972). Systemic oxygen deficiencies: the respirator brain. In: Pathology of the Nervous System, Vol. 2, Minckler, J., Ed., p. 1583. McGraw-Hill, New York, (cited by Walker, 1977).

Lobstein, A., Mantz, J-M., and Mack, G. (1968). Circulation rétinienne, électrorétino-gramme et coma dépassé. Bibl. Ophthalmol., *76*:237.

Loeb, C. and Poggio, G. F. (1953). Electroencephalograms in a case with pon-tomesencephalic hemorrhage. Electroencephalogr. Clin. Neurophysiol., *5*:295.

Loeb, C., Rosadini, G. and Poggio, G. F. (1959). Electroencephalograms during coma. Normal and borderline records in 5 patients. Neurology, *9*:219.

Lundervold, A. (1954). Electroencephalographic changes in a case of acute cerebral anoxia unconscious for about three years. Electroencephalogr. Clin. Neurophysiol., *6*:311.

Lundervold, A., Hauge, T., and Loken, A. (1956). Unusual EEG in unconscious pa-tient with brainstem atrophy. Electroencephalogr. Clin. Neurophysiol., *8*:665.

Manaka, S. and Sano, K. (1972). Study of stationary potential (SP) II. Its value in various animals and its use for the estimation of cerebral death. Brain Nerve, *24*:1573.

Mansuy, L., Lecuire, J., and Jouvet, M. (1965). A clinical study of traumatic lesions of the brainstem. Proc. Third Int. Congr. Neurol. Surg. Excerpta Med., Internat. Congr. Ser. No. 110. p. 411.

Mantz, J. M., Kurtz, D., Otteni, J. C., and Rohmer, F. (1965). EEG aspects of six cases of severe barbiturate coma. Electroencephalogr. Clin. Neurophysiol., *18*:426.

Mantz, J. M., Tempe, M. D., Jaeger, A., Kurtz, D., Lobstein, A., and Mack, G. 1971 Silence électrique cérébral de vingt-quatre heures au cours d'une intoxication mas-sive par 10 g de pentobarbital. Hémodialise, Guérison. Presse Med., *79*:1242.

Markand, O. N. (1976). Electroencephalogram in "locked-in" syndrome. Electroen-cephalogr. Clin. Neurophysiol., *40*:529.

Masland, R. L. (1975). Report of the Inter-Agency Committee on Irreversible Coma and Brain Death. Trans. Am. Neurol. Assoc., *100*:280.

Matakas, F., Cervos-Navarro, J., and Schneider, H. (1973). Experimental brain death. 1. Morphology and fine structure of the brain. J. Neurol. Neurosurg. Psychiatry, *36*:497.

Maynard, D., Prior, P. F., and Scott, D. F. (1969). Device for continuous monitoring of cerebral activity in resuscitated patients. Br. Med. J., *4*:545.

Meldrum, B. S. and Brierley, J. B. (1969). Brain damage in the rhesus monkey resulting from profound arterial hypotension. II. Changes in the spontaneous and evoked electrical activity of the neocortex. Brain Res., *13*:101.

Meldrum, B. S., Excell, B. J., Brierley, J. B., Brown, A. W., and McSheehy, M. A. (1968). The production of brain damage in the rhesus monkey by arterial hypoten-sion and its correlation with changes in the spontaneous and evoked electrocortical activity. Electroencephalogr. Clin. Neurophysiol., *24*:594.

Mellerio, F. (1964). L'électroencéphalographie dans les intoxications aigües. Masson, Paris.

Miller, R. F. and Dowling, J. E. (1970). Intracellular responses of the Müller (glial) cells of the mudpuppy retina: their relation to b-waves of the electroretinogram. J. Neurophysiol., *33*:323.

Mohandas, A. and Chou, S. N. (1971). Brain death. A clinical and pathological study. J. Neurosurg., *35*:211.

Mollaret, P. and Goulon, M. (1959). Le coma dépassé (mémoire préliminaire). Rev. Neurol., *101*:3.

Mollaret, P., Bertrand, I., and Mollaret, H. (1959). Coma dépassé et nécroses nerveuses centrales massives. Rev. Neurol., *101*:116.

Montoya, M. L. and Hill, G. (1968). EEG recording in intensive care units. Am. J. EEG Technol., *8*:85.

Mosier, J. M. (1968). The use of succinylcholine in EEG. Electroencephalogr. Clin. Neurophysiol., *24*:394.

Mowery, G. L. (1962). Artifacts. Am. J. EEG Technol., *2*:41.

Muller, H. R. (1966). Zur Problematik der flaschen Hirnstromkurve und der Diagnose "Hirntod" nach akuter zerebraler Anoxie. Med. Klin., *61*:1955.

Nedey, R., Brian, S., Jedynak, P., and Arfel, G. (1974). Neuropathologie du coma dépassé. Ann. Anesthesiol. Fr., *15:*3.

Noonan, B. D., Wilkus, R. J., Chatrian, G. E., and Lettich, E. (1973). The influence of direction of gaze on the human electro-retinogram recorded from periorbital electrodes: a study utilizing a summating technique. Electroencephalogr. Clin. Neurophysiol., *35:*495.

Nordgren, R. E., Markesbery, W. R., Fukuda, K., and Reeves, A. G. (1971). Seven cases of cerebromedullospinal disconnection: the "locked-in" syndrome. Neurology, *21:*1140.

Obrador, S., Reinoso-Suarez, F., Carbonell, J., Cordoba, A., Martinez-Moreno, E., Navarro, V., Oliva, H., and Oliveros, J. C. (1975). Comatose state maintained during eight years following a vascular ponto-mesencephalic lesion. Electroencephalogr. Clin. Neurophysiol., *38:*21.

O'Leary, J. L. and Goldring, S. (1964). D-C potentials of the brain. Physiol. Rev., *44:*91.

Ouaknine, G., Kosary, I. Z., Braham, J., Czerniak, P., and Nathan, H. (1973). Laboratory criteria of brain death. J. Neurosurg., *39:*429.

Paillas, J. E. (1970). Les critères de la mort du donneur dans les transplantations d'organes. Marseille Méd., *5:*369.

Pampiglione, G. (1962). EEG studies after cardiac arrest. Proc. R. Soc. Med., *55:*653.

Pampiglione, G. and Harden, A. (1968). Resuscitation after cardiocirculatory arrest: prognostic evaluation of early electroencephalographic findings. Lancet, *1:*1261.

Pampiglione, G., Chaloner, J., and Harden, A. (1978). Early prediction of quality of survival after resuscitation. Programme of the Scientific Meeting of the EEG Society to be held in London, October 8, 1978.

Plum, F. and Masland, R. L. (1973). Resolution on brain death. Trans. Am. Neurol. Assoc., *98:*350.

Plum, F. and Posner, J. B. (1966). The diagnosis of stupor and coma. F. A. Davis, Philadelphia.

Pollack, M. A. and Kellaway, P. (1979). Cerebrocortical death vs. brain death: correlations of clinical, EEG, and evoked potential studies. Electroencephalogr. Clin. Neurophysiol. (in press).

Pope Pius XII. (1958). The prolongation of life. An address of Pope Pius XII to an International Congress of Anesthesiologists. The Pope speaks, *4:*393. Original French text in Acta Apostolicae Sedis, 1957, *49:*1033.

Powner, D. J. (1976). Drug-associated isoelectric EEGs—A hazard in brain-death certification. J.A.M.A., *236:*1123.

Prior, P. F. (1973). The EEG in acute cerebral anoxia. Excerpta Med., Amsterdam.

Prior, P. F. (1979). Monitoring cerebral function, J. B. Lippincott, Philadelphia.

Prior, P. F. and Volavka, J. (1968). An attempt to assess the prognostic value of the EEG after cardiac arrest. Electroencephalogr. Clin. Neurophysiol., *24:*593.

Prior, P. F., Maynard, D. E., Sheaff, P. C., Simpson, B. R., Strunin, L., Weaver, E. J. M., and Scott, D. F. (1971). Monitoring cerebral function: clinical experience with new device for continuous recording of electrical activity of brain. Br. Med. J., *2:*736.

Redding, F. L., Wandel, V., and Nasser, C. (1969). Intravenous infusion drop artifacts. Electroencephalogr. Clin. Neurophysiol., *26:*318.

Riehl, J. L. and McIntyre, H. B. (1968). Reliability of the EEG in the determination of cerebral death: Report of a case with recovery of an isoelectric tracing. Bull. Los Angeles Neurol. Soc., *33:*86.

Rivano, C., Rosadini, G., Rossi, G. F., and Turella, G. (1969). Correlografia e spettro di potenza nell'elettroencefalogramma nello stadio più profondo del coma (coma "dépassé"). Boll. Soc. Ital. Biol. Sper., *45:*307.

Rosadini, G. and Gentilomo, A. (1967). Quadri EEG di sonno nella sindrome apallica. Riv. Neurol., *37:*469.

Rosadini, G., Ferrillo, F., Puca, F. M., and Rivano, C. (1968). Spettro di potenza dell'elettroencefalogramma umano. 1) Tecnica. Boll. Soc. Ital. Biol. Sper., *44:*699.

Rosenklint, A. and Jørgensen, P. B. (1974). Evaluation of angiographic methods in the diagnosis of brain death. Correlation with local and systemic arterial pressure and intracranial pressure. Neuroradiology, *7:*215.

Rosoff, S. D. and Schwab, R. S. (1968). The EEG in establishing brain death. A 10-year report with criteria and legal safeguards in the 50 states. Electroencephalogr. Clin. Neurophysiol., *24:*283.

Sament, S., Alderete, J. F., and Schwab, R. S. (1969). The persistence of the electroretinogram in patients with flat isoelectric EEGs. Electroencephalogr. Clin. Neurophysiol., *26:*121.

Saunders, M. G. (1972). Physiological artifacts. Proc. Electrophysiol. Technol. Assoc., *19:*133.

Saunders, M. G. (1975). Medico-legal aspects of brain death. In: Handbook of Electroencephalography and Clinical Neurophysiology, Vol. 12, Harner, R. and Naquet, R., Eds., p. 129. Elsevier, Amsterdam.

Scharfetter, C. and Schmoigl, S. (1967). Zum isolektrischen Enzephalogram (Aussagewert nach Aussetzen der Spontanatmung). Dtsch. Med. Wochenschr., *92:*472.

Schneider, H., Masshoff, W., and Neuhaus, G. A. (1969). Klinische und morphologische Aspekte des Hirntodes. Klin. Wschr., *47:*844.

Schwartz, B. A. and Vendrely, E. (1969). Un des problèmes posés par le diagnostic du coma dépassé: EEG nul et diamètre pupillaire. Rev. Neurol., *121:*319.

Shafey, S., Scheinblum, A., Scheinberg, P., and Reinmuth, O. M. (1968). The ventral pontine syndrome. Trans. Am. Neurol. Assoc., *93:*21.

Silverman, D., Saunders, M. G., Schwab, R. S., and Masland, R. L. (1969). Cerebral death and the electroencephalogram. Report of the Ad Hoc Committee of the American Electroencephalographic Society on EEG Criteria for Determination of Cerebral Death. J.A.M.A., *209:*1505.

Sims, J. K. and Bickford, R. G. (1973). Non-mydriatic pupils occurring in human brain death. Bull. Los Angeles Neurol. Soc., *381:*24.

Sims, J. K., Aung, M. H., Bickford, R. G., Billinger, T. W., and Shattuck. C. M. (1973). Respirator artifact mimicking burst-suppression during electrocerebral silence. Am. J. EEG Technol., *13:*81.

Sims, J. K., Casler, J. A., Billinger, T. W., Aung, M. H., Shattuck, C. M., Fleming, N. I., and Bickford, R. G. (1972). The human electroretinogram in alert volunteers and in brain death patients: new recording techniques. Proc. San Diego Biomed. Symp., *11:*87.

Smith, A. J. K. and Penry, J. K., Eds. (1972). Brain death. NINDS Bibliography Series No. 1, DHEW Publication No. (NIH) 73–347.

Sohmer, H. and Feinmesser, M. (1967). Cochlear action potentials recorded from the external ear in man. Ann. Otol. Rhinol. Laryngol., *76:*427.

Spann, W., Kugler, J., and Liebhardt, E. (1967). Tod und elektrische Stille im EEG. Munch. Med. Wschr., *109:*2161.

Speight, T. M. and Avery, G. S. (1972). Pancuronium bromide: a review of its pharmacological properties and clinical application. Drugs, *4:*163.

Starr, A. (1976). Auditory brain-stem responses in brain death. Brain, *99:*543.

Starr, A. (1977). Clinical relevance of brainstem auditory evoked potentials in brainstem disorders in man. In: Progress in Clinical Neurophysiology, Vol. 2. Desmedt, J. E., Ed., p. l. Karger, Basel.

Starr, A. and Achor, J. (1975). Auditory brainstem responses in neurological disease. Arch. Neurol., *32:*761.

Stockard, J. J. (1978). Basics of brainstem auditory evoked response interpretation in neurologic disorders (Outline). Course in clinical electroencephalography, American Electroencephalographic Society, San Francisco, California, September 4–6, 1978.

Stockard, J. J. and Rossiter, V. S. (1977). Clinical and pathologic correlates of brainstem auditory response abnormalities. Neurology, *27:*316.

Stockard, J. J., Bickford, R. G., and Aung, M. H. (1975). The electroencephalogram in traumatic brain injury. In: Handbook of Clinical Neurology, Vol. 23, Vinken, P. J. and Bruyn, G. W., Eds., p. 317. American Elsevier, New York.

Stockard, J. J., Stockard, J. E., and Sharbrough, F. W. (1978). Non-pathologic factors influencing brainstem auditory evoked potentials. Am. J. EEG Technol., *18:*177.

Strich, S. J. (1956). Diffuse degeneration of cerebral white matter in severe dementia following head injury. J. Neurol. Neurosurg. Psychiatry, *19:*163.

Strich, S. J. (1969). The pathology of brain damage due to blunt head injuries. In: The Late Effects of Head Injury, Walker, A. E., Caveness, W. F., and Critchley, M., Eds., p. 501. C. C. Thomas, Springfield, Ill.

Suter, C. (1974). Clinical advances in the evaluation of deep coma. Med. Coll. Virginia Q., *10:*152.

Suter, C. and Brush, J. (1978). Clinical problems of brain death and coma in intensive care units. Ann. N.Y. Acad. Sci., *315:*398.

Tentler, R. L., Sadove, M., Becka, D. R., and Taylor, R. C. (1957). Electroencephalographic evidence of cortical "death" followed by full recovery: protective action of hypothermia. J.A.M.A., *164:*1667.

Tomita, T. (1950). Studies on the intraretinal action potential. I. Relation between the localization of micro-pipette in the retina and the shape of the intraretinal action potential. Jpn. J. Physiol., *1:*110.

Tomita, T. (1965). Electrophysiological study of the mechanisms subserving color coding in the fish retina. Cold Spring Harb. Symp. Quant. Biol., *30:*559.

Trojaborg, W. (1970). Artifacts in the "silent" EEG. Electroencephalogr. Clin. Neurophysiol., *29:*217.

Trojaborg, W. and Jørgensen, E. O. (1973). Evoked cortical potentials in patients with "isoelectric" EEGs. Electroencephalogr. Clin. Neurophysiol., *35:*301.

Tyson, R. N. (1974). Simulation of cerebral death by succinylcholine sensitivity. Arch. Neurol., *30:*409.

Uziel, A. and Benezech, J. (1978). Auditory brainstem responses in comatose patients: relationship with brain stem reflexes and levels of coma. Electroencephalogr. Clin. Neurophysiol., *45:*515.

Vapalahti, M. and Troupp, H. (1971). Prognosis for patients with severe brain injuries. Br. Med. J., *3:*404.

Velasco, M., Lopez-Portillo, M., Olvera-Rabiela, J. E., and Velasco, F. (1971). EEG y registros profundos en casos de coma post traumatico irreversible. Arch. Invest. Med., *2:*1.

Velupillay, V., Wilkus, R. J., Copass, M. K., and Chatrian, G. E. (1974). Electroencephalographic rhythms of alpha frequency in comatose patients after cardiopulmonary arrest. Neurology, *24:*582.

Vigouroux, R., Naquet, R., Baurand, C., Choux, M., Salamon, G. and Khalil, R. (1964). Évolution électro-radio-clinique de comas graves prolongés post-traumatiques. Rev. Neurol., *110:*72.

Visser, S. L. (1969). Two cases of isoelectric EEG. ("Apparent exceptions proving the rule"). Electroencephalogr. Clin. Neurophysiol., *27:*215.

Vlahovitch, B., Frèrebeau, P., Kuhner, A., Billet, M., and Gros, C. (1971). Les angiographies sous pression dans la mort du cerveau avec arrêt circulatoire encéphalique. Neurochirurgie, *17:*81.

Vlahovitch, B., Frèrebeau, P., Kuhner, A., Stopak, B., Allris, B. and Gros, C. (1972). Arrêt circulatoire intracrânien dans la mort du cerveau. Angiographie avec injection sous pression. Acta Radiol., *13:*334.

Vourc'h, P. (1973). Utilization de la succinylcholine dans le diagnostic des comas. Anesth. Analg., *30:*988.

Walker, A. E. (1977a). An appraisal of the criteria of cerebral death. A summary statement. A collaboration study. J.A.M.A., *237:*982.

Walker, A. E. (1977b). Cerebral death. Professional Information Library, Dallas.

Walker, A. E. and Molinari, G. F. (1977). Sedative drug surveys in coma. How reliable are they? Postgrad. Med., *61:*105.

Walker, A. E., Diamond, E. L., and Moseley, J. (1975). The neuropathological findings in irreversible coma. A critique of the "respirator brain." J. Neuropathol. Exp. Neurol., *34:*295.

Walsh, G. O. (1974). Small apparatus to monitor for possible impending electrocerebral silence. Bull. Los Angeles Neurol. Soc., *39:*154.

Walter, S. T. and Arfel, G. (1972). Réponses aux stimulations visuelles dans les états de coma aïgu et de coma chronique. Electroencephalogr. Clin. Neurophysiol., *32:*27.

Waltregny, A., Bonnal, J., and LeJeune, G. (1970). Mort cérébrale et homotransplant. Critères utilisés pour établir rapidement le diagnostic de coma dépassé. Rev. Neurol., *122:*406.

Wertheimer, P., Jouvet, M., and Descotes, J. (1959). À propos du diagnostic de la mort du système nerveux—dans les comas avec arrêt respiratoire traités par respiration artificielle. Presse Med., *67:*87.

Westmoreland, B. F., Klass, D. W., Sharbrough, F. W., and Reagan, T. J. (1975). Alpha coma: EEG, clinical, pathologic and etiologic correlations. Arch. Neurol., *32:*713

Wilkus, R. J., Chatrian, G. E., and Lettich, E. (1971a). The electroretinogram during terminal anoxia in humans. Electroencephalogr. Clin. Neurophysiol., *31:*537.

Wilkus, R. J., Harvey, F., Moretti-Ojemann, L., and Lettich, E. (1971b). Electroencephalogram and sensory evoked potentials. Findings in an unresponsive patient with pontine infarct. Arch. Neurol., *24:*538.

Wood-Smith, F. G., Stewart, H. C., and Vickers, M. D. (1968). Drugs in anesthetic practice. Third Ed., Appleton-Century-Crofts, New York.

Wulff, M. H. (1950). Electroencephalographic investigations in acute barbiturate poisoning. Electroencephalogr. Clin. Neurophysiol., *2:*111.

Yoshie, N. (1971). Clinical cochlear response audiometry by means of an average response computer: non-surgical technique and clinical use. Rev. Laryngol. Otol. Rhinol. (Bord), *92:*646.

Yoshie, N., Ohashi, T., and Suzuki, T. (1967). Non-surgical recording of auditory nerve action potentials in man. Laryngoscope, *77:*76.

Zattoni, J., Fritz, D., and Giasotto, G. (1971). Correlazione fra indici liquorali del metabolismo cerebrale e spettro di potenza dell'EEG nel coma profondo verso la morte cerebrale. Boll. Soc. Ital. Biol. Sper., *47:*798.

Index